D1348732

Comprehensive Handbook of Psychotherapy Integration

Comprehensive Handbook of Psychotherapy Integration

Edited by
George Stricker

Derner Institute of Advanced Psychological Studies
Adelphi University
Garden City, New York

and

Jerold R. Gold

Doctoral Program in Clinical Psychology
Long Island University
Brooklyn, New York

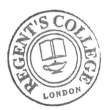

Plenum Press ● New York and London

Library of Congress Cataloging-in-Publication Data

Comprehensive handbook of psychotherapy integration / edited by George
  Stricker and Jerold R. Gold.
      p.   cm.
  Includes bibliographical references and index.
  ISBN 0-306-44280-9
  1. Psychotherapy--Handbooks, manuals, etc.   I. Stricker, George.
  II. Gold, Jerold R.
    [DNLM: 1. Psychotherapy--methods--handbooks.   WM 34 C737]
  RC480.5.C5774   1993
  616.89'14--dc20
  DNLM/DLC
  for Library of Congress   92-48871
                                                               CIP

ISBN 0-306-44280-9

©1993 Plenum Press, New York
A Division of Plenum Publishing Corporation
233 Spring Street, New York, N.Y. 10013

Printed in the United States of America

Contributors

David M. Allen
Department of Psychiatry
University of Tennessee
Memphis, Tennessee 38105

John D. W. Andrews
Psychological and Counseling Services
University of California, San Diego
La Jolla, California 92093

Diane B. Arnkoff
Department of Psychology
Catholic University of America
Washington, DC 20064

Mitchel Becker
The National Institute for the Rehabilitation of
  the Brain Injured
Tel Aviv, Israel

Larry E. Beutler
Counseling/Clinical/School Psychology
  Program
Department of Education
University of California
Santa Barbara, California 93106

James F. T. Bugental
Saybrook Institute and California School of
  Professional Psychology
Berkeley, California 94949

Robert T. Carter
Doctoral Program in Counseling Psychology
Teachers College
Columbia University
New York, New York 10031

Louis Georges Castonguay
Department of Psychology
State University of New York at Stony Brook
Stony Brook, New York 11794-2500

Sheila Coonerty
Doctoral Program in Clinical Psychology
Long Island University
Brooklyn, New York 11201

Nicholas A. Cummings
American Biodyne and the Foundation for
  Behavioral Health
South San Francisco, California 94080

Rebecca Curtis
Derner Institute of Advanced Psychological
  Studies
Adelphi University
Garden City, New York 11530

Mireille Cyr
Department of Psychology
University of Montreal
Montreal, Quebec
Canada H3C 3J7

Robert H. Dworkin
Departments of Anesthesiology and Psychiatry
College of Physicians and Surgeons
Columbia University
New York, New York 10032

Herbert Fensterheim
Department of Psychiatry
The New York Hospital–Cornell Medical
    Center
New York, New York 10021

Mary FitzPatrick
Department of Psychiatry
The New York Hospital–Cornell Medical
    Center
New York, New York 10021

Iris G. Fodor
Department of Applied Psychology
New York University
New York, New York 10003

Anderson J. Franklin
Doctoral Program in Clinical Psychology
City College of the City University of New
    York
New York, New York 10031

Carol R. Glass
Department of Psychology
Catholic University of America
Washington, DC 20064

Jerold R. Gold
Doctoral Program in Clinical Psychology
Long Island University
Brooklyn, New York 11201

Cynthia Grace
Department of Psychology
City College of the City University of New
    York
New York, New York 10031

Roy C. Grzesiak
Departments of Anesthesiology and Psychiatry
New Jersey Medical School
Newark, New Jersey 07103

Richard P. Halgin
Department of Psychology
University of Massachusetts
Amherst, Massachusetts 01003

Adele M. Hayes
Affective Disorders Program
Duke University Medical Center
Durham, North Carolina 27710

Bede J. Healey
The Menninger Clinic
Topeka, Kansas 66601-0829

David T. Hellkamp
Department of Psychology
Xavier University
Cincinnati, Ohio 45207

Amy B. Hodgson
Department of Education
University of California
Santa Barbara, California 93106

Thomas A. Inck
Derner Institute of Advanced Psychological
    Studies
Adelphi University
Garden City, New York 11530

Diana Adile Kirschner
Private Practice
Gwynedd Valley, Pennsylvania 19437

Sam Kirschner
Private Practice
Gwynedd Valley, Pennsylvania 19437

Richard I. Kleiner
Bay Counseling and Consulting
201 San Antonio Circle
Mountain View, California 94040

Conrad Lecomte
Department of Psychology
University of Montreal
Montreal, Quebec
Canada H3C 3J7

James Low
Psychotherapy Section, Division of Psychiatry
United Medical and Dental Schools
Guy's Hospital
London, SE1 9RT England

Leigh McCullough
Department of Psychology in Psychiatry
University of Pennsylvania
Philadelphia, Pennsylvania 19104

Derek J. McEntee
Department of Psychology
University of Massachusetts
Amherst, Massachusetts 01003

Cory F. Newman
Center for Cognitive Therapy
University of Pennsylvania
Philadelphia, Pennsylvania 19104-3246

Vicki Passman
Doctoral Program in Clinical Psychology
Long Island University
Brooklyn, New York 11201

Nicholas Papouchis
Doctoral Program in Clinical Psychology
Long Island University
Brooklyn, New York 11201

Jay Reeve
Derner Institute of Advanced Psychological
  Studies
Adelphi University
Garden City, New York 11530

Jeffrey B. Rubin
Private Practice
New York, New York and Westchester, New
  York

Anthony Ryle
Psychotherapy Section, Division of Psychiatry
United Medical and Dental Schools
Guy's Hospital
London, SE1 9RT England

Stéphane Sabourin
Department of Psychology
University of Montreal
Montreal, Quebec
Canada H3C 3J7

Jeremy Safran
Derner Institute of Advanced Psychological
  Studies
Adelphi University
Garden City, New York 11530

Robert N. Sollod
Department of Psychology
Cleveland State University
Cleveland, Ohio 44115

George Stricker
Derner Institute of Advanced Psychological
  Studies
Adelphi University
Garden City, New York 11530

Brian J. Victor
Department of Psychology
Catholic University of America
Washington, DC 20064

Paul L. Wachtel
Department of Psychology
City College of the City University of New
  York
New York, New York 10031

Eugene H. Walder
Institute for Integrated Training in
  Psychotherapy
New York, New York 10019

Joel Weinberger
Derner Institute of Advanced Psychological
  Studies
Adelphi University
Garden City, New York 11530

Richard L. Wessler
Department of Psychology
Pace University
Pleasantville, New York 10570

Michael A. Westerman
Clinical Psychology Doctoral Program
New York University
New York, New York 10003.

Preface

This *Handbook* is the culmination of an interest in psychotherapy integration that led to our first professional collaboration in 1978. At that time we undertook (in research conducted for a doctoral dissertation by the second editor and supervised by the senior editor) to understand, from and within a psychodynamic perspective, the experiences of patients who had completed behavioral therapies. At that time, psychotherapy integration was a topic considered viable and interesting by only a few clinicians and scholars, with little communication among them and less awareness, concern, and appreciation on the part of psychotherapists in general.

The situation today has changed. The appearance of this *Handbook* may be taken as a significant sign of maturation and legitimacy of work in psychotherapy integration. It is our hope and expectation that this volume will serve as an up-to-date and exhaustive overview of the status of ongoing scholarly and clinical work in the integration of the major schools of psychotherapy.

The *Handbook* opens with a section that will provide the reader with an overview of the history, sociocultural context, and empirical status of the broad field of psychotherapy integration.

The *Handbook* continues with six main substantive parts. The first of these is entitled Individual Approaches. Chapters herein have been contributed by authors who have developed and tested their own unique and professionally acknowledged methods of and for integrating discrete models of the processes and techniques of psychotherapeutic interventions drawn from competing schools of thought. These chapters include a description of the authors' conceptual approach to psychopathology and to the necessary ingredients of behavior change, as well as clinical examples of psychotherapeutic work carried out within those writers' specific methodologies.

The next part of the *Handbook*, The Integration of Traditional and Nontraditional Approaches, presents chapters concerned with the integration of spiritual, religious, philosophical, and folk medicine approaches to psychotherapy with standard and conventional treatment methods. The nontraditional approaches will include Oriental and Western viewpoints. Each chapter features a conceptual and theoretical integration, followed by clinical illustrations of the application of these ideas.

The next two parts of the *Handbook* are entitled, respectively, Psychotherapy Integration with Specific Disorders and Psychotherapy Integration with Specific Populations. In each part, the particular theoretical and clinical issues and dilemmas raised by integrative work with a specific type of psychopathology (depression, personality

ix

disorder, or organic disorders, among others), or by certain patient populations (children, families, minorities, the aged), are discussed and illustrated.

The penultimate part of the handbook is called Teaching Psychotherapy Integration, and contains chapters written by therapists who are involved in the instruction and supervision of work in this area, as well as by one therapist who is attempting to learn this way of thinking about and practicing psychotherapy. These chapters present discussions of the conceptual, professional, and personal issues and concerns involved in these endeavors.

The *Handbook* concludes with the chapter, The Current Status of Psychotherapy Integration, in which we attempt to pull together the varied contributions to the *Handbook* in order to come to some conclusions about current points of consensus, divergence, and controversy among workers in psychotherapy integration.

We would like to thank a number of people for their professional and personal contributions to this considerable project. Eliot Werner at Plenum deserves immediate mention for his attention to this *Handbook* and his efforts at all of the stages of planning, writing, and editing. Morton Bortner, Ph.D., was a model of interest and validation while some of the ideas that led to interest in the publication of this type of work were germinating and were being tested, and provided one of the first venues for the study and teaching of psychotherapy integration in an academic setting. Joseph Newirth, Ph.D., generously offered his ideas and personal support at all times and made this work seem tolerable and valuable when doubts and questions arose. He also modeled a sincere respect for, and appreciation of, scholarly activity even when the intellectual content deviated from his own ways of thinking. Jeffrey Rubin, Ph.D., is a much valued friend and colleague whose intellect, enthusiasm, and concern have been highly appreciated in this effort and in a much wider sense as well.

Most important, Roseann Ungaro, Ph.D., made all the work worthwhile by being who she is and by offering her strength, love, and confidence throughout. Daniel Nathan Gold was an equally important source of inspiration and delight. Joan Stricker, as always, was a constant and caring resource. Jocelyn and Geoffrey Stricker, and their spouses, Steven Mendelson and Laura Sweeney, continue to be what makes it all worthwhile.

Contents

PART III   THE INTEGRATION OF TRADITIONAL
           AND NONTRADITIONAL APPROACHES

PART IV PSYCHOTHERAPY INTEGRATION WITH SPECIFIC DISORDERS

PART V PSYCHOTHERAPY INTEGRATION WITH SPECIFIC POPULATIONS

PART VI   TEACHING PSYCHOTHERAPY INTEGRATION

PART VII   CONCLUSION

PART I

Introduction

CHAPTER 1

The Sociohistorical Context of Psychotherapy Integration

Jerold R. Gold

This handbook collects in one place a significant sampling of the most current and important work in psychotherapy integration. Psychotherapy integration is a subspeciality of the ongoing clinical, theoretical, and empirical scholarship in the general areas of psychotherapeutic process, technique, and outcome. It is a specialization and a field of inquiry with a relatively short but highly controversial history. Psychotherapy integration is both a set of ideas and theories and a group of technical procedures and innovations which arise from such academic and scholastic pursuits. In the last decade, the investigation of such constructs and methods of practice has moved from the fringes of respectability and clinical awareness to assume a more legitimate and prominent place in the broader fields of psychotherapeutic research and practice. The publication of this *Comprehensive Handbook of Psychotherapy Integration* is but one sign of the new respect and relative

prominence of these types of efforts. Other signs of this new status are found in the existence of two professional journals devoted exclusively to research concerned with integration. Each journal is published by a professional society whose memberships conduct integrated forms of psychotherapy and study it clinically, theoretically, or empirically. Studies of psychotherapy integration have appeared in increasing frequency in other older and more mainstream journals as well, and the topic of integration has been either the exclusive focus of, or a major agenda item within, many professional meetings and conferences. The number of books concerned with psychotherapy integration (many of them authored by contributors to this handbook) has multiplied enormously as well. In total, it seems that, as Arkowitz (1991) has announced, psychotherapy integration has come of age.

Such hard earned and newly found maturity and legitimacy as a field of inquiry and practice does not mean that all questions have been solved and all problems resolved. As will be apparent in the chapters that follow, psychotherapy integration is an open ended and ever evolving set of constructs and methods which cannot help but be influenced by new ideas and information.

In the remainder of this chapter, I will present a brief history of psychotherapy integration,

This chapter is dedicated to the memory of my mother and to my father, Gloria and Harry Gold, for teaching me about integration, as a personal, political, and intellectual ideal.

Jerold R. Gold • Doctoral Program in Clinical Psychology, Long Island University, Brooklyn, New York 11201.

Comprehensive Handbook of Psychotherapy Integration, edited by George Stricker and Jerold R. Gold. Plenum Press, New York, 1993.

and will follow it with discussions of some of the significant issues within the field of psychotherapy that encouraged work in integration. I will conclude with a look at some of the more important social, cultural, and historical developments which surrounded these more microscopic changes in our understanding of psychotherapy, and which perhaps were influential in promoting the growth of interest in psychotherapy integration.

A BRIEF HISTORY OF PSYCHOTHERAPY INTEGRATION

The first studies of psychotherapy which today we may recognize as integrative in nature or intent were concerned with the translation of concepts and methods from psychological or psychotherapeutic systems into the language and procedures of another. In the 1930s and 1940s several papers appeared which took as their task the conversion of Freudian psychoanalytic concepts into the terms of learning theories. Originally, these writers were concerned with the relationship between psychoanalysis and Pavlovian classical conditioning. As noted by Arkowitz (1984), whose fine history of psychotherapy integration has influenced extensively this more concise attempt, perhaps the first paper of this type was written by Ischlondy (1930), and his work was expanded upon by French (1933), and by Kubie (1934). French was concerned with the correspondences between the Pavlovian constructs of inhibition, differentiation, and conditioning; and the analytic concepts of repression, object choice, and insight. Kubie's expansion of these ideas moved him to consider the possibility of such phenomena as conditioning and disinhibition playing an important role in the relationship between the analyst and the analysand.

In certain subtle but important ways these early pioneers in integration were following a trend introduced into psychoanalysis by Freud (1909). He had noted the importance of compelling the phobic patient to actively face the phobic object—a preview of *in vivo* desensitization—and also experimented with setting times limits on the treatment in order to promote conflict and to gain access to deeper unconscious material.

As learning theorists began to include operant conditioning principles and organismic and complex psychological variables in their systems,

such ideas were applied to the dominant psychotherapeutic approaches of the era. In the 1940s and 1950s such writers as Sears (1944), Shoben (1949), and Dollard and Miller (1950) recast psychodynamic and client-centered therapies in the language and concepts of reinforcement and of the complicated internally mediated forms of learning which had been studied by neobehaviorists such as Hull (1952). These studies emphasized the reinforcement value of the therapist in terms of shaping or inhibiting changes in inner states or in behavior, and led, particularly in the case of Dollard and Miller (1950), to modifications in psychoanalytic technique which emphasized activity and instruction on the part of the therapist. Procedures which today are commonplace in cognitive-behavioral therapy and in many forms of integrative therapy were introduced by Dollard and Miller, and included the use of homework, role playing, and modelling, and active and graded confrontation of fearful situations and internal states. Wachtel (1977) and Arkowitz (1984) have noted that the work of Dollard and Miller was much more influential in general psychology and in learning theory than in psychotherapy studies, and that their direct impact on psychotherapy integration was not felt until much later.

Alexander (1963; Alexander & French, 1946) modified his psychoanalytically oriented approach to therapy by experimenting with active approaches to the induction of change which were informed by the then contemporary learning theories. A point crucial to later developments in psychotherapy integration was his introduction of the idea that insight into unconscious processes often *followed* behavioral change, rather than exclusively being the antecedent to change. This move away from a unidirectional view of change was highly influential in the thinking of many later students of integration.

A highly important trend in the study of psychotherapy which was occurring throughout the same period as the work just discussed was the search for generic change factors which were common to all psychotherapies. Although not aimed at integration or theoretical translations in themselves, these studies were crucial in breaking down barriers between adherents of specific theories and methods. Among the more important works of this type were the comparative therapeutic studies carried out by Fiedler (1950), who demonstrated that observers were unable to differentiate between psychoanalytic, Adlerian, and client-centered therapies or to identify the therapeutic ideology of different practitioners. Such research, as well as the investigations of Frank (1959), and London (1964), point to the commonalities between the variety of contemporary therapies, and collectively became, with the works of other authors, a voice arguing for a nonsectarian and generalist approach to psychotherapy. These arguments proved to be extremely generative of the more specifically integrative work that followed.

The 1950s, 1960s, and 1970s were marked by the flowering of modern behavior therapy, with its base in learning theory and its powerful technology. The study of behavior theory and of behavioral techniques by the minority of humanistic and dynamic therapists who immediately did not repudiate behavior therapy led to important integrations at the theoretical and technical levels. In a parallel development, as behavior therapy became more sophisticated and oriented toward complex clinical problems, certain of its theorists and practitioners came to look upon psychoanalysis, humanistic therapies, and systems approaches for guidance, ideas, and methods. Some pertinent examples of these truly integrative studies include the works of Marks and Gelder (1966), Weitzman (1967), Bergin (1968), Sloane (1969), Marmor (1971), and Birk and Brinkley-Birk (1974) among many others. These students shared a concern for searching out the underlying theoretical links and similarities between behavioral, humanistic, and dynamic methods. Workers such as Brady (1968), Birk (1970), and Feather and Rhoades (1972a,b) experimented with the technical integration of dynamic, systems, and behavioral methods within single cases. Increasing attention to the complex interpersonal transactions within the behavior therapy framework led certain behavioral workers toward the dynamic, humanistic, and interpersonal camps, as did the increasing emphasis within behavior therapy on covert cognitive and affective processes. A significant measure of integration from a behavioral vantage point was announced by the 1976 publication of *Clinical Behavior Therapy* by Goldfried and Davison, who acknowledged the utility of, and the need for, concepts and methods drawn from other systems of therapy.

If the history of developments in psychotherapy integration has a single watershed mo-

ment, it perhaps would be the publication of Wachtel's (1977) *Psychoanalysis and Behavior Therapy*. This volume remains the most frequently cited work in psychotherapy integration, and has served as a model of integration at both a theoretical and a technical level. Wachtel offered a theory of personality and psychopathology which fully integrated critical aspects of dynamic and behavioral theory into a unique and synergistic model. Just as important, this new and integrative theory also allowed interventions from a broad range of positions to be utilized clinically and in a way that was predictable and comprehensible.

The late 1970s, 1980s, and early 1990s have been marked by an explosion of integrative works, and by impassioned debate about the possibility and advisability of integrative efforts. Of particular note during this period was the collection of dialogues between supporters and opponents of psychotherapy integration which was compiled by Arkowitz and Messer (1984). Although the presence of this *Handbook* must be taken as an argument for integration, in fairness it must be noted that among the critics and opponents of psychotherapy have been some leading authorities on psychotherapy, including Wolpe (1984), Franks (1984), Messer (1984), and Lazarus (1989).

Much of the significant work done in psychotherapy integration in the last decade is considered in the chapters which follow in this volume, and therefore will not be discussed here. Readers who desire a more extensive discussion of the history of psychotherapy integration are referred to the excellent works by Arkowitz (1984) and Goldfried and Newman (1986).

FACTORS WITHIN PSYCHOTHERAPY WHICH HAVE PROMOTED INTEGRATION

The major schools of psychotherapy were developed in situations and at points in the history of mental health services which originally contributed to their isolation from each other. This segregation and the sectarian attitudes associated with it was responsible in large part for the unwillingness of psychotherapists of one orientation or another to learn from each others' theories, techniques, successes, and failures. As I have pointed out elsewhere, (Gold, 1990) developments in psychotherapy almost always are integrative in the broadest sense of the term. Psychotherapists have been willing and eager to incorporate ideas and methods from the social and natural sciences, from medicine, philosophy, theology, and literature, into the ideologies and procedures of psychotherapy. However, as a group, we have historically been most unwilling to learn from each other.

The consumption and practice of psychotherapy grew exponentially in the decades after World War II, and with this expansion came a breakdown in the geographic and professional boundaries which originally separated practitioners of different orientations. Departments of psychiatry, social work, and psychology in hospitals and in medical schools grew in size and in interaction within themselves and with each other. Clinical psychology programs in universities expanded and gradually were forced or chose to include faculty with alternative clinical and theoretical leanings. Psychoanalysis moved out of its traditional settings in free-standing institutes and entered academe, but its findings and techniques were challenged and tested by behaviorists, systems theorists, and humanists with more skeptical and empirically formed ideas. Similarly, as behavior therapists confronted more complex pathology which was far removed from the learning laboratory, some turned to the older insights and modalities of their dynamic and client-centered colleagues.

The degree of communication between, and integration of, therapeutic systems which this professional integration promoted was encouraged further by two challenges to the status and security of psychotherapy which arose during the 1970s and 1980s. I refer here first to the need for psychotherapists to respond to the shrinking economic resources that were available socially for mental health services by demonstrating the effectiveness of our efforts. The second pressure was that of the powerful trend within psychiatry and medicine, which spread into areas of psychology and into government- and private-funding sources, to conceptualize and treat psychopathology from a biomedical perspective. Both pressures were critical in changing the view of many therapists from looking for the "best" therapy to a more pragmatic search for the best of many therapies in order to survive economically and professionally. Accountability to insurance companies, governmental agencies, and to a better informed, more impatient, and more selective public became the key. The inability of psychotherapy outcome research to identify any psychotherapy as most effective across the board was a strong impetus in the search for the specific active ingredients in different therapies, and in the quest for theories and methodologies which could combine those ingredients in the most expedient and powerful ways. As practical eclecticism became more the norm among clinical practitioners, the seeds of a more sophisticated integration were sown. The possibility of such an integration became more attractive, and perhaps more vital to many therapists, and the existence of such "consumers" inevitably was stimulating and reinforcing to theorists and students of integration.

Another factor in the development of the larger field of psychotherapy which contributed to the flowering of integration is one of assimilation into the larger sociocultural environment. As in many families who are new to a society, there exists a dialectic tension between generations of psychotherapists with regard to remaining loyal to older traditions as opposed to assimilation and intermingling with others of new and different persuasions and beliefs. By the 1980s, the major schools of psychotherapy had each produced several generations of practitioners, many of whom had traveled the path from orthodox sectarianism to heterodox integration. In some of the systems, for example psychoanalysis or client-centered therapy, the founding generations had died, retired, or moved on to other interests. In behavior therapy, cognitive therapy, and systems approaches, key originators, such as Beck, Ellis, Minuchin, Wolpe, and others, remained vital and active, but did not or could not command the exclusive loyalty of a Freud, Rogers, or Skinner. As a result, many new therapists took what they had learned in their "families of origin" out into the larger sociocultural field where they struggled to mesh their traditions with new information and ways of working clinically.

SOCIAL AND HISTORICAL INFLUENCES ON PSYCHOTHERAPY INTEGRATION

The conduct of psychotherapy does not occur in a sociocultural or historical vacuum. Changes in the world around the therapist and around psychotherapy inevitably will affect the way psychotherapy is construed and practiced. The decades of the 1960s and 1970s were marked by a number of critical developments which surely encouraged the movement in psychotherapy integration.

Since the 1960s, traditional roles, boundaries, and reliance on governmental and social authority have come under assault in the United States and in much of western society. The civil rights movement and the women's liberation movement called for an end to social, political, and economic segregation. The rise of the "counterculture" with its sexual revolution, drug use, and rejection of the mores of the preceding generation shook the fabric of American life. The Vietnam war, the rise of crime, drug addiction, AIDS, and homelessness severely challenged smug and entrenched ideas about the stability, safety, and validity of the American way of life. Western European, scientific, and rational approaches to medical and social problems and to daily life were contradicted by a return by many people to a fundamentalist religious belief or by a choice of an "alternative" philosophy drawn from Asian, South American, or African societies and cultures. Developments in the philosophy of science and the history of ideas (Kuhn, 1962) have taught us that truth is rarely an issue in scientific discovery, and that theories are political, value laden, and are accepted or discarded for many reasons other than what we might think. Ethnic and minority groups challenged the exclusive hold on schools and universities with regard to the use of English as an instructional language, and with the reliance on curricula which promoted a single, Anglo-Saxon take on history, literature, and culture. As this chapter is being written, for example, the 500th anniversary of the "discovery" of the Americas by Columbus has prompted extensive, often venomous, and bitter revisionist debate about his place in history and the ways in which the European settling (or conquest, or decimation) of the Western hemisphere should be taught and understood.

Is it any wonder then that in the last 30 years many in the business of psychotherapy have been unable or unwilling to hold to a "one truth" ideology? The milieu in which we have lived, learned, and worked has not been conducive to an easy or ready acceptance of narrow and orthodox ideologies and methods. Instead, we have witnessed the breakdown of larger and more pat truths and belief systems, to be replaced by more relativistic theories or sometimes simply by blind uncertainty or ambiguity. The effects of these social changes on psychotherapy might be summed up by the questions raised by Klein (1971), a prominent and committed psychoanalyst. After observing the social unrest, generational turmoil, and emergence of alternative values and lifestyles in the Greenwich Village (New York City) setting of his university, he was moved to question whether the theory and methods to which he had devoted his professional life were of any relevance at that point in history.

Anyone who has lived, been educated, and worked in an academic or professional setting in the last three decades could not have avoided being touched by these and other social and historical changes. Regardless of each individuals' opinions and beliefs about such matters, these forces and changes have removed many of the contextual underpinnings of easy belief and faith for a large part of the population, while paradoxically stimulating a retreat or a return to fundamentalism for others. This schism is reflected in our theories about psychotherapy, as in most other segments of academic and intellectual life. Those students of psychotherapy who have embraced a pluralist approach to their subject are perhaps those who are the heirs of the social change and unrest of recent history.

In sum, the works contained in this handbook and throughout the field of psychotherapy integration are reflective of study, thought, and experimentation within this specific specialization. They are intrinsically intertwined with developments in the broader field of psychotherapy and with social, historical, and political forces which are the context for our lives.

REFERENCES

Alexander, F. (1963). The dynamics of psychotherapy in the light of learning theory. *American Journal of Psychiatry*, *120*, 440–448.

Alexander, F., & French, T. (1946). *Psychoanalytic therapy*. New York: Ronald Press.

Arkowitz, H. (1984). Historical perspective on the integration of psychoanalytic therapy and behavioral therapy. In H. Arkowitz & S. Messer (Eds.), *Psychoanalytic therapy and behavioral therapy: Is integration possible?* (pp. 1–30). New York: Plenum Press.

Arkowitz, H. (1991). Introductory statement: Psychotherapy integration comes of age. *Journal of Psychotherapy Integration, 1*, 1–4.

Arkowitz, H., & Messer, S. (Eds.). (1984). *Psychoanalytic therapy and behavioral therapy: Is integration possible?* New York: Plenum Press.

Bergin, A. E. (1968). Technique for improving desensitization via warmth, empathy, and emotional reexperiencing of hierarchy events. In R. Rubin & C. M. Franks (Eds.), *Advances in behavior therapy* (pp. 20–33). New York: Academic Press.

Birk, L. (1970). Behavior therapy: Integration with dynamic therapy. *Behavior Therapy, 1*, 522–526.

Birk, L., & Brinkley-Birk, A. (1974). Psychoanalysis and behavior therapy. *American Journal of Psychiatry, 131*, 499–510.

Brady, J. P. (1968). Psychotherapy by combined behavioral and dynamic approaches. *Comprehensive Psychiatry, 9*, 536–543.

Dollard, J., & Miller, N. E. (1950). *Personality and psychotherapy*. New York: McGraw-Hill.

Feather, B. W., & Rhoades, J. M. (1972a). Psychodynamic behavior therapy: I. Theory and practice. *Archives of General Psychiatry, 26*, 496–502.

Feather, B. W., & Rhoades, J. M. (1972b). Psychodynamic behavior therapy: II. Clinical aspects. *Archives of General Psychiatry, 26*, 503–511.

Fiedler, F. E. (1950). The concept of an ideal therapeutic relationship. *Journal of Consulting Psychology, 14*, 239–245.

Frank, J. D. (1959). *Persuasion and healing*. Baltimore: Johns Hopkins University Press.

Franks, C. M. (1984). On conceptual and technical integrity in psychoanalysis and behavior therapy: Two incompatible systems. In H. Arkowitz & S. Messer (Eds.), *Psychoanalytic therapy and behavior therapy: Is integration possible?* (pp. 223–248). New York: Plenum Press.

French, T. M. (1933). Interrelations between psychoanalysis and the experimental work of Pavlov. *American Journal of Psychiatry, 89*, 1165–1203.

Freud, S. (1909). Notes upon a case of obsessional neurosis. In J. Strachey (Ed. and Trans.), *The Standard edition of the complete psychological works of Sigmund Freud* (Vol. 10, pp. 153–318). London: Hogarth Press.

Gold, J. (1990). Culture, history, and psychotherapy integration. *Journal of Integrative and Eclectic Psychotherapy, 9*, 41–48.

Goldfried, M., & Davison, G. (1976). *Clinical behavior therapy*. New York: Holt, Rinehart, & Winston.

Goldfried, M., & Newman, C. (1986). Psychotherapy integration: An historical perspective. In J. C. Norcross (Ed.), *Handbook of eclectic psychotherapy* (pp.). New York: Brunner/Mazel.

Hull, C. E. (1952). *A behavior system*. New Haven: Yale University Press.

Ischlondy, N. E. (1930). *Neuropsyche und Hirnride: Bank II. Physiologische Grundlagen der Tiefenpsychologie unter besonder Berucksichting der Psychoanalyse*. Berlin: Urban and Schwarzenberg. Cited in Arkowitz, 1984.

Klein, G. S. (1971). *Psychoanalytic therapy: An exploration of essentials*. New York: International Universities Press.

Kubie, L. S. (1934). Relation of the conditioned reflex to psychoanalytic technique. *Archives of Neurology and Psychiatry, 32*, 1137–1142.

Kuhn, T. S. (1962). *The structure of scientific revolutions*. Chicago: University of Chicago Press.

Lazarus, A. (1989). *The practice of multimodal therapy*. Baltimore: Johns Hopkins University Press.

London, P. (1964). *The modes and morals of psychotherapy*. New York: Holt, Rinehart, & Winston.

Marks, I. M., & Gelder, M. G. (1966). Common ground between behavior therapy and psychodynamic methods. *British Journal of Medical Psychology, 39*, 11–23.

Marmor, J. (1971). Dynamic psychotherapy and behavior therapy: Are they reconcilable? *Archives of General Psychiatry, 24*, 22–28.

Messer, S. B. (1984). The integration of psychoanalytic therapy and behavior therapy: Summing up. In H. Arkowitz & S. Messer (Eds.), *Psychoanalytic therapy and behavior therapy: Is integration possible?* New York: Plenum Press.

Sears, R. R. (1944). Experimental analysis of psychoanalytic phenomena. In J. McV. Hunt (Ed.), *Personality and the behavior disorders* (pp. 191–206). New York: Ronald Press.

Shoben, E. J. (1949). Psychotherapy as a problem in learning theory. *Psychological Bulletin, 46*, 366–392.

Sloane, R. B. (1969). The converging paths of behavior therapy and psychotherapy. *American Journal of Psychiatry, 125*, 877–885.

Wachtel, P. L. (1977). *Psychoanalysis and behavior therapy: Towards an integration*. New York: Basic Books.

Weitzman, B. (1967). Behavior therapy and psychotherapy. *Psychological Review, 74*, 300–317.

Wolpe, J. (1984). Behavior therapy according to Lazarus. *American Psychologist, 39*, 1326–1327.

CHAPTER 2

Empirical Research on Integrative and Eclectic Psychotherapies

Carol R. Glass, Brian J. Victor, and Diane B. Arnkoff

In his recent chapter on the history of psychotherapy integration, Arkowitz (1992b) reviews a large number of articles and books on integration that have made significant theoretical and clinical contributions. In contrast, empirical evaluations of these ideas have lagged behind. He argues that until research on the effectiveness of integrative treatments and tests of hypotheses derived from integrative theories are carried out, the promise of these new approaches will remain unfulfilled.

The present chapter represents a review of the research to date on the nature and effectiveness of integrative and eclectic psychotherapy. Our goals are to encourage researchers to devote their energies to addressing the questions raised in the evergrowing theoretical and clinical publications in this field, and to encourage clinicians to become aware of the significant contributions made by research.

We have excluded several topics from our review. Although cognitive therapy has sometimes been described as an integration of behavioral and cognitive methods, we have chosen to consider cognitive-behavior therapy as a pure-form approach, and thus outside the scope of this chapter. Studies comparing different forms of psychodynamic therapy were also not included, nor were those comparing the outcome of different pure-form therapies. Because of our focus on psychosocial treatments, research on combinations of psychotherapy and pharmacotherapy was not addressed. Finally, a number of case studies on integrative or eclectic treatments without quantitative assessment of change were omitted.

Our review of empirical research on integrative and eclectic psychotherapies is organized into five major areas: (1) questionnaire surveys with therapists as subjects, (2) outcome research on combinations of techniques from psychodynamic and cognitive-behavioral approaches, (3) outcome research on interventions derived from integrative theories of disorders, (4) approaches to eclectic psychotherapy and prescriptive matching, and (5) tests of integrative models of therapy change.

Carol R. Glass, Brian J. Victor, and Diane B. Arnkoff • Department of Psychology, Catholic University of America, Washington, DC 20064.

Comprehensive Handbook of Psychotherapy Integration, edited by George Stricker and Jerold R. Gold. Plenum Press, New York, 1993.

QUESTIONNAIRE STUDIES: VIEWS OF ECLECTIC AND OTHER THERAPISTS

Surveys of clinical psychologists in the United States showed an increase in the mid-1970s in the percentage who called themselves "eclectic." Garfield and Kurtz (1976), in a landmark study, found that 55% of clinical psychologists who were surveyed called themselves eclectic. This increase in the eclectic percentage from previous surveys was largely at the expense of those holding psychodynamic points of view (Arnkoff & Glass, 1992).

Later surveys of psychologists have continued to find a high figure endorsing eclectic therapy (e.g., Norcross & Prochaska, 1982; Norcross, Prochaska, & Gallagher, 1989). In most surveys, between one-third and one-half call themselves eclectic (Arnkoff & Glass, 1992). Surveys that have included psychiatrists, social workers, and marital and family therapists also find a large proportion of eclectics (e.g., Jensen, Bergin, & Greaves, 1990). This phenomenon is not necessarily as widespread in other countries, however. Vasco and Garcia-Marques (1991), for example, found that eclecticism was the third most frequent orientation for Portuguese psychotherapists, after cognitive and psychodynamic, but accounted for only 13% of the respondents.

Since eclectic or integrative therapy is not an organized "school" of therapy, it is impossible to discern what the respondents actually *do* in therapy from these figures alone. Garfield and Kurtz (1977) did a follow-up survey of those who called themselves eclectic in their 1976 survey. Nearly half of these individuals reported that they previously had adhered to one school of therapy, primarily psychoanalytic. When they were asked to select the two orientations that were most characteristic of their current views, psychoanalytic plus learning theory was selected most often (21% of respondents), followed by neo-Freudian plus learning (16%). Subjects' most frequent definition of eclecticism was to select whatever approach seemed best for the client (called the "pragmatic" approach by Garfield and Kurtz), followed by integration of various orientations, and finally by the adherence to two or three orientations. Garfield and Kurtz (1977) concluded that "the designation eclectic covers a wide range of views, some of which are apparently quite the opposite of others" (p. 79).

In a short span of time, the interest of psychologists in eclecticism and integration shifted somewhat from the pragmatic approach found in Garfield and Kurtz (1977) toward an interest in integrating theories. For example, Norcross and Prochaska (1982) asked subjects who called themselves eclectic to choose a type of eclecticism that characterized their approach. By far the most frequent answer was *synthetic eclecticism* (integrating theories), followed by *technical eclecticism* (selecting procedures from different schools), and then *atheoretical eclecticism* (no preferred theory). Thus, Norcross and Prochaska (1988) concluded that the trend toward eclecticism has moved from a dissatisfaction with schools of therapy to a positive attempt at integration—from eclecticism "by default" to integration "by design" (p. 173).

As in the Garfield and Kurtz 1977 study, the Norcross and Prochaska (1988) survey of eclectic clinical psychologists found that the most frequent previous orientation among those psychologists who expressed a prior orientation was psychodynamic or psychoanalytic. When asked which orientations they combined, the three most frequent responses involved cognitive therapy: cognitive-behavioral, humanistic-cognitive, and psychoanalytic-cognitive. Overall, half of the clinicians chose a combination that included cognitive and/or behavior therapy. However, the survey by Jensen *et al.* (1990) found that eclectic psychiatrists most often chose psychodynamic as one of the schools they used in therapy (88% of respondents).

Several recent questionnaire studies grounded in an integrative perspective further examined the views and practices of psychotherapists. For example, Prochaska and Norcross (1983) asked psychologists to complete a questionnaire on the processes of change they employed with clients and in self-interventions. Eclectic therapists used counterconditioning/contingency control significantly more often with clients than did psychoanalytic or psychodynamic therapists, made more use of self-liberation than either humanistic or psychoanalytic therapists, and emphasized the helping relationship more than their cognitive-behavioral colleagues. Eclectic therapists had either the highest or the second highest means for each of the seven change processes, suggesting that they in fact do employ a wide range of interventions. Therapists' orientation did not, however, relate significantly to their reported use of change processes to deal with their own problems.

Heide and Rosenbaum (1988) asked psychotherapists to describe their experiences when conducting therapy using one orientation and when conducting therapy combining two or more orientations. Therapists described themselves as significantly more spontaneous, adventurous, and imaginative when combining orientations. The authors argued that the vitality that therapists report may be part of the current appeal of integrative and eclectic therapy, but that this advantage may be threatened if integrative approaches become solidified into new schools of therapy.

Finally, Giunta, Saltzman, and Norcross (1991) asked 30 prominent psychotherapists from various orientations to review the clinical formulations and treatment plans of nine cases published in the Clinical Exchange of the *Journal of Integrative and Eclectic Psychotherapy*. The therapists were asked to specify and justify their agreements and disagreements regarding the formulations and recommended techniques offered by their colleagues. The results indicated that there was more agreement than disagreement, especially for the therapeutic relationship and clinical strategies, whereas more frequent divergence was found regarding global theory, specific techniques, and client characteristics. A small minority of the respondents gave specific justification for their answers or cited research, and even fewer consistently referred to the empirical literature. The authors suggested that these results provide moderate support for the use of the therapeutic relationship and middle level clinical strategies in searching for consensus and integration among the various therapy schools.

These questionnaire surveys provide interesting information on what psychotherapists *say* they do in therapy and how they define their orientation or approach. However, a comprehensive picture of integrative therapy must rely more on research examining the actual practice of psychotherapy. The following section focuses on outcome research.

COMBINING TECHNIQUES FROM EXISTING APPROACHES

The possibility of integrating clinical techniques from different therapeutic schools and orientations has been a topic of great interest since the early 1970s, focusing primarily on the integration of methods from behavioral and psychodynamic therapies (Arkowitz & Messer, 1984; Marmor & Woods, 1980; Wachtel, 1977). Several theoretical and clinical strategies have been suggested, exemplified by the case studies of Feather and Rhoads (1972; Rhoads, 1984), which demonstrate different ways in which behavioral and psychodynamic therapies can complement each other. However, with only a few exceptions, very little empirical research has examined this issue.

The Sheffield Psychotherapy Project

Although the primary goal of the Sheffield Psychotherapy Project (Shapiro & Firth, 1987) was to compare a "prescriptive" cognitive and multimodal behavioral therapy with a more "exploratory" psychodynamic intervention, a crossover research design was selected that also allowed for a comparison of order effects within eclectic therapy. Clients completed 8 sessions of each therapy, receiving either prescriptive followed by exploratory (PE) methods or vice versa (EP). Results showed basically no differences in symptoms at the end of treatment that were due to the order in which the two treatments were offered, although there was a trend for greater symptom improvement at a 3-month follow-up for those who received the exploratory therapy first (Shapiro & Firth, 1987). A 2-year follow-up study showed that the significant gains made by the end of treatment were maintained (Shapiro & Firth-Cozens, 1990).

A report of results using the Personal Questionnaire, which was given 3 times a week to monitor patients' progress (e.g., symptoms, relationships, mood), found significant differences in subjects' experience of the order of therapy, with those in the EP sequence experiencing the process of therapy as smoother than most PE clients (Barkham, Shapiro, & Firth-Cozens, 1989). Specifically, improvement in the first period followed by deterioration in the second occurred for only

5% of EP patients compared to 29% of those in the PE order, suggesting that emphasizing aspects of relationships prior to developing coping strategies may be advantageous.

The Bergen Project

The Bergen Project on Brief Dynamic Psychotherapy (Nielsen *et al.*, 1987) had as a main objective the study of change in short-term dynamic therapy (e.g., Sifneos's Short Term Anxiety-Provoking Therapy (STAPP) and Malan's Intensive Brief Psychotherapy (BP)). In addition, a third, more integrative and pragmatic approach called the "FIAT" model (*F*lexibility, *I*nterpersonal orientation, *A*ctivity, and *T*eleologic understanding) was developed for use with patients who were not candidates for the other therapies because of insufficient ego resources and motivation for change. This intervention combined supportive, behavioral, and cognitive interventions as adjuncts to traditional psychodynamic (neo-Freudian and ego-analytic) techniques (Nielsen & Havik, 1989).

Seven clients with physical symptoms who received the integrative treatment showed statistically significant symptom change by the end of therapy, maintained such change at follow-up, and 86% were judged "much" or "very much" improved by independent raters (Nielsen *et al.*, 1988). Barth *et al.* (1988) compared 10 patients who completed the FIAT treatment with 22 patients assigned to either STAPP or BP. No outcome differences were found between the groups, although there was some indication that patients in the FIAT treatment may have reached their "peak of change" later in the process of therapy. More recently, Nielsen *et al.* (1991) reported that most of the 10 patients who were receiving integrative treatment showed significant symptom change, especially by the time of follow-up, and to a lesser extent judges also saw changes in adaptive functioning and underlying psychodynamics.

THERAPY DERIVED FROM INTEGRATIVE THEORIES OF DISORDERS

Both the Sheffield and the Bergen Projects provide evidence for the effectiveness of combined cognitive-behavioral and psychodynamic treatments for adult outpatients who show a range of clinical problems. Several integrative treatments have been developed that are targeted for *specific* types of disorders, where the interventions grew out of an integrative theory of the disorder itself.

Anxiety Disorders

Chambless, Goldstein, Gallagher, and Bright (1986) described agoraphobics as presenting with a broad range of problems, including susceptibility to panic attacks, sensitivity to separation stemming from childhood experience, current stress or conflict, catastrophizing over the consequences of anxiety, and avoidant behavior patterns. Consequently, Chambless *et al.* (1986) designed an intensive integrative treatment program, combining a large number of methods and therapy formats, and with active involvement of the patient's significant other.

The 35 clients in their study received group therapy as well as couples and family therapy. The group therapy included *in vivo* exposure followed by gestalt techniques to intensify and express feelings, paradoxical strategies, thought stopping, cognitive restructuring, yogic breathing, and self-reinforcement. In addition, clients explored contributing factors for anxiety, suppressed conflicts, and unresolved issues, such as grief, childhood trauma, and present interpersonal problems. By the end of treatment, clients showed significant changes in avoidance and on self-reports of social phobia, depression, assertiveness, and the cognitions and body sensations associated with agoraphobia. A very low dropout rate was found compared to previous exposure or drug treatments, and 58% were considered to be markedly or greatly improved/normal.

Hoffart and Martinsen (1990) have also tested the effectiveness of an integrated behavioral-psychodynamic treatment for 36 inpatient agoraphobics, and compared this program to 19 patients on two other wards, who completed a program of psychodynamic therapy alone. Integrated therapy included *in vivo* exposure, cognitive restructuring, anxiety coping strategies, and work on dynamic conflicts, such as autonomy and responsibility, unresolved grief, repressed anger, and marital difficulties. Both groups improved significantly on almost all measures by posttreatment, with no group differences. At a 1-year follow-up, however, only the integrative group was significantly improved on measures of anxiety and depression, and it had a significantly higher proportion of responders on measures of separation avoidance and fear of fear.

In his consideration of phobias and panic disorder, Wolfe (1989) has argued that the four major perspectives on etiology and treatment—psychoanalytic, behavioral, cognitive, and biological—each offer only partial explanations and partially effective treatments. His model postulates that phobias and panic disorders stem from childhood experiences that lead to the tacit processing of interpersonally related emotional conflicts or traumas. After a working therapeutic alliance is established, Wolfe's integrated therapy employs imaginal and *in vivo* procedures to elicit and explore these phobic and panic-related tacit catastrophic conflicts. Anxiety management strategies are then taught, and a major focus concerns the resolution of the core conflicts using cognitive-behavioral, psychoanalytic, and gestalt techniques. His integrative model, which has not yet been subjected to empirical test, represents an important future direction in the integrated treatment of anxiety.

Personality Disorders

A recent article by Westen (1991) described integrations of cognitive-behavioral and psychoanalytic psychotherapy in the treatment of borderline patients. Linehan's work on the development of an integrative, behavioral treatment for parasuicidal borderline patients is also based on a clear theory of the disorder (Linehan, 1987). She suggests that the behavior patterns of these individuals can be organized along three dialectical poles, emphasizing emotional vulnerability versus invalidation of affect, active passivity versus appearing competent, and unrelenting crises versus inhibited grieving. The borderline patient thus vacillates between each pole, between overreaction and underreaction. Linehan's Dialectical Behavior Therapy (DBT) contains both a behavioral focus on skill training and collaborative problem-solving, as well as an emphasis on dialectical processes to resolve the tendency to vacillate between the extremes of the dialectical poles. As she states, "the overriding dialectic is the neces-

sity of accepting patients . . . as they are within a context of trying to teach them to change" (Linehan, 1987, p. 272).

A recent report compared the effectiveness of a 1-year outpatient program of DBT to treatment as usual in the community (Linehan, Armstrong, Suarez, Allmon, & Heard, 1989). Although there was generally a high rate of parasuicide behavior, DBT patients showed a significant reduction in the frequency and medical severity of parasuicidal behavior, in the likelihood of attempting suicide, and in days of inpatient psychiatric hospitalization compared to controls. Linehan's DBT was also very effective in keeping patients in therapy. Although significant pre-post changes were found on questionnaire measures of depression, hopelessness, suicidal ideation, and reasons for living, no group differences on these measures were obtained.

ECLECTIC PSYCHOTHERAPY AND PRESCRIPTIVE MATCHING

Perhaps because of its logical, intuitive appeal, prescriptive matching of treatments to clients, what Stiles, Shapiro, and Elliott (1986) have called the "matrix paradigm" (p. 168), has a long history in psychotherapy research. An early entry in the field, which generated a flurry of empirical research, was the A-B therapist variable (see Berzins, 1977, and Razin, 1977, for a comprehensive review). In the mid-1970s, when the problem of equivalent therapeutic outcomes began to become apparent, the matrix paradigm provided a potential solution by redirecting research toward uncovering differential treatment outcomes for specific diagnoses (Stiles *et al.*, 1986). Unfortunately, much of the research with regard to aptitude-treatment interaction (ATI) for specific client diagnostic categories or behavior disorders (i.e., anxiety, depression, pain, smoking cessation, and weight loss) has yielded disappointing results (see Dance & Neufeld, 1988, for a comprehensive review). Along these lines, Rude and Rehm (1991) reviewed the literature on client factors that predicted outcome in the cognitive and behavioral treatment of depression. Interestingly, they found that, while matching client deficits to treatment focus did not predict outcome, several studies indicated that clients *without* the targeted deficits responded better to treatment. Recently, there has been a renewed interest in ATI research, as evidenced by the special series on client-therapy interaction in the *Journal of Consulting and Clinical Psychology* (1991).

Several systems of eclectic psychotherapy are based on a strategy of client-treatment matching to improve therapy outcome. After assessing specific client characteristics, interventions are then tailored to each client regardless of the theoretical framework in which the techniques originated. There are several excellent examples of this approach.

Multimodal Therapy

Perhaps the best-known system of eclectic psychotherapy is *multimodal therapy* (Lazarus, 1981), in which therapy is tailored to clients' problem areas and favored modalities based on a thorough assessment and analysis of seven factors: *B*ehavior, *A*ffect, *S*ensation, *I*magery, *C*ognition, *I*nterpersonal relationships, and (*D*rug) biological functioning (the BASIC I.D.). Although the interventions used are primarily cognitive and behavioral because of their demonstrated effectiveness, Lazarus employs a total of perhaps four dozen actual techniques, including medication, imagery and fantasy, Rogerian reflection, and gestalt empty chair exercises (Lazarus, 1986b).

Given the popularity of and the amount written about Lazarus' approach, it is surprising that so little empirical research has been conducted to evaluate its effectiveness. The utility of modality and structural profiles, and of tracking modality firing orders to select techniques, is also untested. Lazarus (1989) reviews a number of studies, but many have been dissertations dealing with the reliability and validity of related assessment techniques. In his own practice, he says that more than 75% of clients have achieved their major treatment goals, and that data from other multimodal clinicians are consistent with these findings (Lazarus, 1986a, 1987). A survey of 100 clients (Lazarus, 1989), all of whom had failed to respond to at least three other therapists before beginning multimodal therapy and were considered "intractable," found 61 who achieved "unequivocal, measurable, and objective benefits" (p. 221). Those for whom multimodal therapy appeared least effective were populations of substance abusers, severe personality disorders, some bipolar depressives and those with florid psychoses, as well as clients receiving secondary gains for maladaptive behavior (Lazarus, 1987). Although Lazarus (1989) makes the claim that "multimodal assessment and therapy often succeed where less comprehensive and/or systematic approaches fail" (p. 221), more empirical tests are needed.

A few uncontrolled group studies have demonstrated the effectiveness of a multimodal approach. Kertesz (personal communication, January, 1991) wrote us from Argentina that his 1982 dissertation showed that 80% of a group of 20 outpatients treated for a period from 2 months to 3 years experienced moderate or excellent rates of improvement. Kwee, Duivenvoorden, Trijsburg, and Thiel (1986) found that multimodal therapy with 84 adult neurotic inpatients helped 78% of obsessive-compulsives and 52% of phobics to improve by time of discharge, with 64% and 55%, respectively, judged improved at a 9-month follow-up. Finally, a study by Olson (1979) compared a weight-loss program tapping four of the BASIC I.D. modalities to one employing all seven. Both groups were equally effective, and the more comprehensive treatment did not increase effectiveness.

Several applications of the multimodal approach have been undertaken in the area of school counseling. Gerler, Kinney, and Anderson (1985) randomly assigned 41 underachieving elementary school children to either multimodal individual and group counseling or to a control group. The treatment group improved significantly on self-rated classroom behavior, math, and language grades, while the control group did not. More recently, Gerler, Drew, and Mohr (1990) developed a 10-week multimodal counseling program for potential middle-school dropouts. They found that attitudes of girls (but not boys) in the treatment group became significantly more positive while the control group did not change, yet no significant change was observed on a teacher behavior-rating scale or on academic performance.

Systematic Treatment Selection

A second important model of eclectic psychotherapy was developed by Beutler (1983), Frances, Clarkin, and Perry (1984), and Beutler and Clarkin (1990). This model has led to an impressive series of empirical studies. Since this approach is described in detail in Beutler and Hodgson's chapter in this volume (Chapter 12), we will only briefly describe this work.

Systematic eclectic psychotherapy (Beutler, 1983) is a method of prescribing discrete treatment procedures, independent of their theoretical foundations, and based on an array of decision criteria that are closely related to empirical literature. Some of the dimensions of systematic eclectic psychotherapy have gained empirical support; for example, several studies have identified the type of treatments best matched with various client-coping, reactance, and personality styles (Beutler, 1979; Beutler & Mitchell, 1981; Calvert, Beutler, & Crago, 1988). *Differential therapeutics* (Frances *et al.*, 1984) is a less specific model of technical eclecticism that outlines the enabling factors and indicators necessary for success across a wide range of therapeutic treatments.

Both of these models are based on anticipated client responses, with the intent to assign clients selectively to treatments, therapists, and settings. However, as Beutler and Clarkin (1990) have noted, differential therapeutics is less specific regarding the actual selection of treatment procedures, and systematic eclectic psychotherapy fails to specify treatment parameters, such as treatment setting or format. As a result, Beutler and Clarkin (1990) have proposed a new model of differential treatment selection, which integrates the two prior models and relationship variables and, to a lesser extent, the role of stages and phases of change (e.g., Beitman, 1987; Prochaska & DiClemente, 1984) and core conflictual relationship themes (e.g., Luborsky & Crits-Christoph, 1989).

The new systematic treatment selection model (Beutler & Clarkin, 1990) incorporates a constellation of fine-grained, interactive decisions organized around four progressive, temporally related classes of variables. The first class, *patient predisposing variables*, includes the client's diagnosis; personality; coping, and conflictual style; and environmental and social system resources. The second class, *treatment contexts*, includes such variables as the treatment setting, mode, format, duration, and frequency. The third class, *relationship variables*, includes client and therapist compatibility regarding backgrounds, beliefs, rela-

tionship styles, and treatment formats, as well as efforts to enhance the therapeutic alliance through role induction and the accommodation of client expectations. The fourth class, *tailoring strategies and techniques*, includes selecting focal change targets; selecting the appropriate level of experience (e.g., behavioral, affective, cognitive, or unconscious); specifying mediating subgoals with respect to the stages or phases of change; and selecting specific strategies based on directiveness, level of arousal, reactance, etc. (cf. Beutler, 1989; Beutler, 1991).

Several extensive empirical studies based on Beutler and Clarkin's (1990) model have emerged recently. Beutler and his colleagues at the University of Arizona (Beutler, Engle, *et al.*, 1991) undertook a large-scale psychotherapy project of clients with major depression who were randomly assigned to one of three manualized treatment conditions (group cognitive therapy, group experiential therapy, and self-directed therapy). These treatments were selected and developed to encompass ranges of both internal/external focus (insight vs. cognitive-behavior change objectives) and therapist directiveness (self-directed vs. authority-directed). The project was designed to investigate the interaction effects of two client variables (coping style and reactance) with treatment types.

Beutler, Engle, *et al.* (1991) found that behavioral and cognitive procedures were best indicated for clients with an externalizing coping style. Clients who were less externalizing did somewhat better in insight-oriented or self-directed therapy. The results also revealed that directive treatments yielded poor results among reactant clients, and that among such clients improvement may be bolstered by assuming a non-authoritative and nondirective treatment stance. This finding confirms the conclusions of other research on paradoxical interventions for reactance (Shoham-Salomon, Avner, & Neeman, 1989; Shoham-Salomon & Rosenthal, 1987; Westerman, Frankel, Tanaka, & Kahn, 1987).

In a more recent article, Beutler, Mohr, Grawe, Engle, and MacDonald (1991) reported a cross-cultural validation of these findings with the Bernese Psychotherapy Project (Grawe, 1991). The Bernese project compared individual treatment in broad-band behavior therapy and client-centered therapy, which were representative of the dimensions of internal/external focus and therapist directiveness/nondirectiveness. This study replicated Beutler, Engle, *et al.* (1991) with regard to coping style and reactance. The correlations between externalization and improvement were largely positive in behavior therapy and largely negative in client-centered therapy. In addition, high reactance was negatively associated with improvement in directive (behavior) therapy, and positively associated with improvement in nondirective (client-centered) therapy.

Conclusions from research by Beutler and his colleagues are based upon correlations between certain personality variables and treatment outcome. Although such analyses are a useful and necessary first step, stronger support for this or any treatment selection model could be obtained by initially assessing clients on relevant dimensions and then randomly assigning subjects to different treatment approaches (H. Arkowitz, personal communication, November 23, 1991).

Other Models of Eclectic Psychotherapy

Garfield's (1980, 1986, 1989) writings on eclectic brief psychotherapy have had an important influence on the field. He highlights the role of common therapeutic variables (e.g., the therapeutic relationship), mechanisms that facilitate patient change (e.g., emotional release, desensitization), and therapist activities, such as reflection, interpretation, confrontation, and modeling. Although Garfield (1986) asserts that "no systematic research has been conducted on this approach" p. 157), research on common factors provides indirect support.

Adaptive Counseling and Therapy (ACT) (Howard, Nance, & Myers, 1987) is an integrative, metatheoretical model based on concepts from organizational psychology. In ACT, therapeutic styles are matched with the level of the client's task-relevant readiness or "developmental maturity" on three dimensions (ability, self-confidence, and motivation), in order to optimize progress. To date, this interesting model has not been tested.

There are several additional approaches to eclectic psychotherapy that have also, unfortunately, not been empirically tested. Norcross (1986, 1987) presents excellent conceptual and clinical descriptions of these interventions. We will instead focus on six larger models of therapy change that suggest more integrative forms of treatment, some of which are accompanied by empirical studies attesting to their validity and to the effectiveness of integrative therapy.

INTEGRATIVE MODELS OF THERAPY CHANGE

The Transtheoretical Model

The most thoroughly tested model is that of Prochaska and DiClemente (1984), whose transtheoretical integrative model of change (both within and outside of psychotherapy) is based on three dimensions. One or more of 10 *processes* of change (e.g., helping relationship, stimulus control) are used to modify problem behaviors. These curative factors can be matched to one of 4 client *stages* of change, reflecting readiness to take action. Finally, they suggest that there are 5 *levels* of change, representing aspects that need changing (e.g., maladaptive cognitions, interpersonal and intrapersonal conflicts). Prochaska and DiClemente recognize that specific theoretical orientations typically employ only a few of these change processes, but advocate that therapists need to be able to use all of them, and to be cognizant of which change processes work best in which stages of change (Prochaska & DiClemente, 1986). In the present chapter, we will review a few of the studies that have stemmed from this model.

An early study on the *processes of change* asked members of the American Psychological Association's Division 29 (Psychotherapy) to complete a questionnaire pertaining either to how they treat clients or to their self-interventions (Prochaska & Norcross, 1983). As described in the earlier section on therapist surveys, eclectic therapists employed a wide range of interventions, and differed from their psychoanalytic, psychodynamic, cognitive-behavioral, and humanistic colleagues in the use of several change processes.

McConnaughy, DiClemente, Prochaska, and Velicer (1989) used a 32-item scale to assess which of four *stages of change* adult outpatient clients were in at the start of treatment. The highest correlations were obtained between adjacent stages, suggesting that clients move from one stage to the next in order, but can be engaged in more than one stage at a time.

A major study of the process of smoking cessation recruited a large number of smokers at each of the stages of change (DiClemente et al., 1991). Those at the "prepared for action" stage had the same smoking history, but were smoking fewer cigarettes per day, had more prior quit attempts, and had higher levels of confidence to stop smoking compared to those in earlier stages of change. These stages were also predictive of subjects' participation in a minimal smoking cessation intervention, such that those in stages more prepared for action made more attempts to quit and had greater success than individuals in the preceding contemplation or precontemplation stages.

Prepared smokers also were the most active (and precontemplaters the least) on almost all of the 10 processes of change, suggesting that processes of change do vary in use across the stages of change model (DiClemente et al., 1991). This same treatment study, which compared four types of interventions, found that the "interactive" treatment (employing transtheoretical manuals with procedures individualized to each participant's stage of change plus individualized written feedback based on questionnaires) was more than twice as effective as the standardized American Lung Association manual for subjects in the prepared for action stage (Prochaska & DiClemente, 1992). This latter paper also provides an excellent review of their entire program of research.

In a study on psychotherapy, three clients were asked to complete two different Processes of Change Questionnaires, one prior to each session to reflect processes between session, and one immediately after each session to assess processes within sessions (Prochaska, Rossi, & Wilcox, 1991). One client who remained in the contemplation stage, and who did not improve, used few action-related processes. In contrast, a second client who did improve progressed from the contemplation to the action stage, had almost all change processes used in sessions (compared to a sample of outpatient adults), and used increasingly more action-related processes between sessions. These studies provide support for the transtheoretical model, suggesting that people move from one stage to the next by changing their reliance from one group of change processes to

another more effective for the next stage (Prochaska et al., 1991).

Brief SASB-Directed Reconstructive Learning Therapy

Benjamin (1991) asserts that successful therapy, regardless of therapy orientation, helps clients learn about the nature and roots of patterns that are interpersonal and intrapsychic in nature, as well as to develop new and better alternatives. The Structural Analysis of Social Behavior (SASB) (Benjamin, 1974) can be used as a model for deriving information about these historical patterns, as well as a means to analyze the ongoing process of therapy. These SASB Intrex questionnaires can quantify clients' perceptions of key people in their present and past, stimulate memories, and provide computer-generated "maps" of specific relationships to help change client perceptions (Benjamin, 1987a).

Benjamin's brief SASB-directed reconstructive learning therapy (SASB-RCL) starts from a baseline of empathy, and combines views from psychoanalytic, learning, and developmental perspectives with situation and person variables (Benjamin, in press). Both situational and interpersonal/personality factors are important, and affect each other in important ways. Any method or technique can be used, as long as the interventions consist of one of five classes: those that enhance collaboration, facilitate learning about patterns, block maladaptive patterns, mobilize the will, or teach new patterns (Benjamin, 1991).

Although there is not yet a great deal of research evidence on this approach, Benjamin (1991) asserts that clients in three year-long intensively studied cases all showed major improvement. These clients each met the criteria of difficulties of at least 10 years' duration and two failed previous therapy attempts. Details of the treatment and measurable changes in symptomatology and personalty traits can be found in the references cited above. Benjamin (1987b) also provides an interesting illustration of the clinical use of client-centered, rational-emotive, cognitive, and psychoanalytic interventions with a female client, where the SASB was used to compare the approaches and to describe the therapy process as well as the content of the patient's speech.

Martin's Cognitive-Mediational Model of Change

A cognitive-mediational model of generic therapeutic change has been proposed by Martin (1989, 1992). The model is based on a theory of cyclic therapeutic interaction that centers on the schemata, plans, intentions, behaviors, perceptions, and cognitive operations of both the client and the therapist. Although Martin's cognitive-mediational approach does not lead to a specific model of conducting therapy, the theory attempts to understand the interaction between cognitive and social information processing and construction that leads to client change across different therapies. Martin notes that the primary task of treatment is to help clients achieve a level of cognitive functioning that will expedite attaining personal goals. He proposes that three types of cognitive structural change result from the therapeutic interaction: (1) elaborating clients' problem-representation schemata, (2) building and/or refining problem-solving structures relevant to the problem, and (3) empowering clients' self-schemata through elaboration and integration of these structures with information from the first two types of change.

Research on Martin's cognitive-mediational model has yielded three general results (summarized in Martin, 1992). First, recognizable, relatively stable patterns of therapist behaviors and client cognitive operations are associated with specific therapist intentions. Second, despite considerable individual variation, there are gradual increases during therapy in the complexity, orderliness, comprehensiveness, and integration of clients' problem-related and self-related knowledge structures. Finally, clients have long-term maintenance of insight, understanding, and awareness achieved in therapy, particularly when the therapeutic dialogue was deep, elaborative, and conclusion-oriented.

Generic Model of Psychotherapy

After an extensive review of research on psychodynamic, experiential, cognitive, and interpersonal therapies, Orlinsky and Howard (1987) developed a generic model of psychotherapy, attempting to define elements that are common to various schools and to describe therapy in terms of its "active ingredients." They argued that every form of therapy can be characterized in terms of one of five components: therapeutic contract, therapeutic interventions, therapeutic bond, personal self-relatedness, and therapeutic realizations. In addition to this description of process variables, Orlinsky and Howard related process to input variables (society, treatment setting, significant others, personal characteristics of patient and therapist), as well as to output or outcome factors (taking into account the length of time change takes to unfold). Orlinsky (1989) has described several initial studies based on the generic model.

A dissertation by Kolden (1988, 1991) examined the relationship between three components of the model (client perceptions of therapeutic bond, self-relatedness, and therapeutic realizations) and both immediate postsession and ultimate outcome. The first two components contributed significantly to the amount of variance accounted for in the prediction of both therapeutic realizations and session outcome with psychotherapy outpatients; session outcome was significantly associated with termination outcome. In addition to providing support for the empirical validity of the generic model, Kolden's research illustrates a methodology for studying process-outcome relationships in psychotherapy.

Cognitive-Analytic Therapy

Ryle also presents an approach to psychotherapy that is not confined by the "language, concepts, values, or methods of any existing school" (Ryle, 1982, p. 1). His time-limited cognitive-analytic therapy (CAT) (Ryle, 1990) draws upon a range of theories and methods, especially object relations and cognitive-behavioral (Beard, Marlowe, & Ryle, 1990). Beard *et al.* also present details on three cases, and illustrate the use of sequential diagrammatic reformulation. Since this approach is discussed in Ryle and Low's chapter in this volume (Chapter 7), we have summarized it only briefly and will describe some clinical and research findings.

Brockman, Poynton, Ryle, and Watson (1987) assigned outpatient adult clients to either CAT or a 12-session psychoanalytically based "interpretive" therapy. Although both interventions led to significant improvement on self-report questionnaires of depression and general health, the CAT group exhibited significant additional improvement in positive self-attitudes. When subjects were matched on pretreatment depression and obsessionality scores, the groups did not differ at posttest on ratings of target problems and target problem procedures.

In an earlier series of single case studies, Ryle (1980) reported the outcome for 15 patients who had received from 5 to 30 sessions of integrated psychotherapy. Most patients reported having made gains by the end of therapy in the areas of target problems and target problem procedures. Self-ratings of change were also typically related to changes in cognitive structures.

Active Self in Psychotherapy

A final integrative framework with empirical support is Andrews' (1991) model of the active self in psychotherapy. Since this approach is described in Andrews' chapter in this volume (Chapter 13), we will offer only a brief summary here. Using terms and constructs derived from self-confirmational theory, Andrews (1991) described three levels of interventions (supportive therapeutic relationship, complementary or anticomplementary interactions between client and therapist, and target-specific methods), coupled with nine intervention styles or stages of the confirmation cycle.

Therapy is seen as a way to help clients interrupt or rechannel their self-confirming feedback cycles, and Andrews (1988) delineated 18 distinctive interventions (corresponding to the 9 stages, with interventions focusing either on gaining awareness of patterns or developing change experiments). Andrews postulated that, unlike existing schools of psychotherapy that primarily focus on a subset of these interventions, an integrated approach dealing with all aspects of this feedback cycle would be maximally effective.

Transcripts were analyzed from different pure-form therapists (e.g., Rogers, Ellis, Wolpe, and Wolberg), using a content analysis system to describe how therapists interact with clients and using the confirmation cycle model to delineate their core style, parallels, and dissimilarities (An-

drews, 1988, 1991). His Intervention Style Inventory may allow us to examine the question of whether "differences in style also influence therapy outcome" (Andrews, 1991, p. 171).

A recent study examined the role of therapists in providing complementary or anticomplementary responses to clients, using Leary's interpersonal system (Andrews, 1990). A rank profile of the importance of each of 8 interpersonal styles was developed for each of 45 clients and 6 therapists in a university counseling center. Although many results were not significant, moderate-to-high levels of interpersonal challenge were associated with greatest client progress. Andrews (1990) concluded that there may be two types of clients, with different therapy goals that have implications for client-treatment-therapist matching: those who are looking for support and validation and those who are looking for push and challenge.

Other Integrative Models

A number of additional integrative models have been proposed that are still in need of empirical support. Feixas (1990a,b) described personal construct theory (PCT) as a constructivist framework for integrating individual and family-systems therapy. He suggested that PCT is an approach to psychotherapy "capable of integrating technical procedures coming from different psychotherapeutic traditions under [a] constructivist framework" (Feixas, 1990a, p. 31).

Mahoney's (1991) recent book on human change processes highlights what he terms "developmental psychotherapy," based on general principles of human development and human helping. This approach seeks to integrate a number of different streams of thought: contributions from cognitive and developmental psychology; psychoanalytic, existential, behavioral, and humanistic perspectives; and findings from psychotherapy outcome and process research. His approach is derived from lifespan development and evolutionary epistemology, with the role of the therapist to encourage and facilitate client exploration (Mahoney, 1990). With this goal in mind, Mahoney (1991) described the use of creative clinical techniques, such as writing unsent letters, personal journals, streaming, and mirror time.

Caspar and Grawe (1989) argued for a heuristic model of therapy, which is based on perspectives from cognitive and developmental psychology and is related to current constructivist cognitive models. After identifying maladaptive "plans" (cognitive or emotional structures), appropriate schemata are activated and changed. Caspar and Grawe called on therapists to shed specific methods tied to theoretical orientations. Instead, they suggested using specific methods as prototypes or "heuristic strategies" of common therapeutic functions, in order to construct a more flexible adaptation of treatment to the particular client and problem.

Integrating cognitive and interpersonal perspectives, Safran (1990a,b) suggested that dysfunctional interpersonal schemas (representations of self–other relationships) interact with interpersonal behavior, and that the therapeutic relationship can be used to assess and challenge these core cognitive structures and cognitive-interpersonal cycles. In their recent book, Safran and Segal (1990) extended this integration to include affective processes, arguing that emotional engagement facilitates therapeutic exploration, and they highlighted the importance of interpersonal "markers" in therapy that signal a potential place for cognitive/affective exploration. Thus, their approach draws from cognitive, interpersonal, gestalt, and client-centered therapies.

FUTURE DIRECTIONS

The research reviewed in this chapter is a solid beginning, but it is clear that there are nearly unlimited avenues for future study. To begin with, as noted above, survey studies of psychologists in the United States indicate that from one-third to one-half consider themselves eclectic. Yet we have very little information on what these therapists do in therapy, and how (if at all) they differ from noneclectic therapists. Observational studies of eclectic therapists in comparison with those with single orientations would inform us about the decision-making process in eclectic therapy (Wolfe & Goldfried, 1988). Therapists could be peer-nominated so that good examples of such therapy could be represented. It is likely that several types of eclectic models are used in practice, so that group means would obscure

findings. Thus, as in Hill (1989), aggregated case studies could be used, with quantitative combined with qualitative data.

Goldfried (1991) has emphasized that the "ultimate goal for research in psychotherapy integration is to develop empirically based procedures that can enhance our effectiveness in dealing with different types of clinical problems" (p. 21). The bottom line, therefore, is to demonstrate that integrative or eclectic approaches to therapy are at least as effective as pure-form approaches. Or, as Arkowitz (1992a) suggests, integrative and pure-form therapies that claim unique or specific effects could be compared to a "common factors" therapy in which the therapist provides whatever factors are common across all treatments for a given disorder. Regardless of what comparison groups are deemed appropriate, well-controlled outcome studies are crucial before we can conclude that integrating or adding interventions to those already in existence leads to positive therapy outcome. This is no easy task, requiring very large numbers of clients and a careful consideration of the measures selected to assess therapy change and the maintenance of change. The information obtained from these studies can be greatly enhanced if change process research is incorporated into the research plan (Garfield, 1990; Marmar, 1990), as it was in the Sheffield study (e.g., Llewelyn, Elliott, Shapiro, Hardy, & Firth-Cozens, 1988).

It is also important to note that "integrative therapy" is not a fixed approach that can easily be contrasted with other fixed types of therapy. Rather, integrative psychotherapies are more likely to share an underlying rationale that encourages a *strategy* of treatment, in which different techniques are selected, combined, and integrated at different stages of therapy (H. Arkowitz, personal communication, November 23, 1991). The development of such innovative treatments represents an important direction for both clinical and research efforts. At a 1991 National Institute of Mental Health (NIMH) workshop, for example, integrative psychotherapy was considered to be a fruitful area for treatment development research (B. Wolfe, personal communication, January 6, 1992).

Goldfried and Padawer (1982) encouraged researchers to collaborate with clinicians and develop research methodologies for applied settings, where "our knowledge about what works in therapy must be rooted in clinical observations, but it must also have empirical verification" (p. 33). Wolfe and Goldfried (1988) and Goldfried (1991) further suggested that archives of audiotapes, videotapes, and transcripts of therapy sessions from varying orientations be made available for future research.

In this chapter, we have highlighted a number of eclectic and integrative therapies that should receive this kind of attention. Lazarus' (1989) multimodal therapy, with its specific clinical procedures and assessment techniques, needs to be evaluated against approaches that are more restricted in their interventions. Wolfe's (1989) model of phobias and panic also is in need of empirical confirmation. Based on his theory of the etiology of these disorders, it would be predicted that the addition of psychodynamic and experiential techniques to cognitive-behavioral methods should enhance treatment effectiveness, since this would allow for exploration of tacit catastrophic conflicts in addition to teaching anxiety management strategies. This example illustrates that integrative theories of specific disorders, which suggest specific integrative interventions, may be useful in guiding future outcome research.

Outcome research is also needed in order to evaluate the effectiveness of traditional cognitive therapy compared to Safran and Segal's (1990) interpersonal-cognitive approach, Mahoney's (1991) integrative therapy based on his theory of human change processes, Ryle's (1990) cognitive-analytic therapy, the constructivist approaches described by Neimeyer and Feixas (1990), and the ACT theory of Howard et al. (1987).

Not all patients will benefit from a specific therapy, and there may be types of clients who benefit most from integrative therapies. The Bergen project (Nielsen et al., 1987), for example, administered the integrative treatment only to clients who did not meet the criteria for one of two brief dynamic therapies. Unfortunately, since subjects were not randomly assigned to treatments, we do not know whether those individuals who were judged to have high levels of ego resources and motivation for change would have fared even better if given access to the integrative treatment.

To investigate specific effects and optimal matches of clients to treatments, Frances, Sweeney, and Clarkin (1985) proposed that future research should have sufficient sample size for division of the treatment cells to search for specific effects, sufficient subject specificity to locate optimal matches, well-defined treatments that are sufficiently different from each other to find specific effects, measures that are specific to the disorders and treatments studied, and process-outcome measurement throughout treatment. It would be important, for example, to test the Beutler and Clarkin (1990) matching prescription against random assignment to therapists and treatments to see if the matching resulted in benefits. Even if no difference in ultimate outcome were found, the matching might result in earlier success or in fewer dropouts. Orlinsky and Howard (1987) argued that research on matching patient and therapist characteristics to make for good therapeutic bonds should be a priority, since outcome is less associated with interventions than with the quality of the therapeutic relationship.

More empirical studies of client aptitude by treatment interactions, like those on client coping style and reactance in the Arizona and Bernese psychotherapy projects, are needed to support theoretical treatment matching models. Regarding Beutler and Clarkin's (1990) model, such studies will need to extend to different client presenting problems, client predisposing interpersonal styles, and treatment contexts. It would also be important to investigate the relationship variables, which might mediate any of the interaction effects.

In addition, it would be useful to analyze both treatment successes and failures across the different approaches. This is consistent with the consensus recommendations of the NIMH workshop on psychotherapy integration held in 1986, where it was proposed that systematic analyses of treatment failures and partial successes from pure-form therapies be conducted in order to learn what was "missing" that could have enhanced treatment effectiveness (Wolfe & Goldfried, 1988).

Another recommendation from the NIMH workshop concerns the need for research comparing the effects of different decision rules for selecting and sequencing therapy procedures (Wolfe & Goldfried, 1988). When different interventions are used with the same client, how should we decide whether to use them sequentially or simultaneously, with different approaches targeting different aspects of the client's presenting problems? Several years ago, Rhoads (1984) presented at least four ways in which behavioral and psychodynamic therapies could complement each other (e.g., to use behavior therapy initially for immediate symptom relief followed by psychodynamic therapy to address more characterological problems, or to move back and forth from one to another depending on the methods most useful for the problems addressed at the time). The Sheffield Psychotherapy Project (Shapiro & Firth, 1987) compared the use of these approaches one at a time, in two different orders. An interesting program of research could investigate each of Rhoads's suggestions for sequencing, as well as those of Wachtel (1977), to discover which manner of integration of behavioral and psychodynamic approaches works best for which clients.

In the investigation of new integrative models of psychotherapy, the question arises as to what standard we should hold these treatments. Should we require that such therapies be *more* successful than standard treatments in order to recommend that they be adopted? In addressing this question, it seems important to take into account the issue of how difficult it is to train therapists to do the integrated treatment. There does not seem to be any reason to hold new treatments to a higher standard *unless* they are more difficult to learn than current treatments. For example, it is likely to be more difficult to learn to be an expert in both psychodynamic and behavior therapy separately and in combination than in one of these treatments alone. If an integrated treatment required the expanded expertise, then an advantage over existing treatments would need to be demonstrated.

In conclusion, future research on integrative and eclectic psychotherapies is likely to be a complex and expensive endeavor. As Elkin (1991) pointed out, pilot studies would first need to be conducted to test the feasibility of larger scale clinical trials. This, we would suggest, should also involve the validation of measures and constructs. Focusing on integrative interventions for specific presenting problems would allow the treatment to follow from an integrative theory of the disorder in question. We hope that researchers

will not be discouraged by the difficulty of this task, but will instead see it as an opportunity to seek out creative and collaborative ways of exploring psychotherapy integration empirically.

REFERENCES

Andrews, J. (1988). Self-confirmation theory: A paradigm for psychotherapy integration. Part I. Content analysis of therapeutic styles. *Journal of Integrative and Eclectic Psychotherapy, 7,* 359–384.

Andrews, J. (1990). Interpersonal self-confirmation and challenge in psychotherapy. *Psychotherapy, 27,* 485–504.

Andrews, J. (1991). *The active self in psychotherapy: An integration of therapeutic styles.* Boston: Allyn & Bacon.

Arkowitz, H. (1992a). A common factors therapy for depression. In J. C. Norcross & M. R. Goldfried (Eds.), *Handbook of psychotherapy integration* (pp. 394–424). New York: Basic Books.

Arkowitz, H. (1992b). Integrative theories of therapy. In D. K. Freedheim (Ed.), *History of psychotherapy: A century of change* (pp. 261–303). Washington, DC: American Psychological Association.

Arkowitz, H., & Messer, S. B. (Eds.). (1984). *Psychoanalytic therapy and behavior therapy: Is integration possible?* New York: Plenum Press.

Arnkoff, D. B., & Glass, C. R. (1992). Cognitive therapy and psychotherapy integration. In D. K. Freedheim (Ed.), *History of psychotherapy: A century of change* (pp. 657–694). Washington, DC: American Psychological Association.

Barkham, M., Shapiro, D. A., & Firth-Cozens, J. (1989). Personal questionnaire changes in prescriptive vs. exploratory psychotherapy. *British Journal of Clinical Psychology, 28,* 97–107.

Barth, K., Nielsen, G., Havik, O. E., Haver, B., Mølstad, E., Rogge, H., Skåtun, M., Heiberg, A. N., & Ursin, H. (1988). Assessment for three different forms of short-term dynamic psychotherapy: Findings from the Bergen project. *Psychotherapy and Psychosomatics, 49,* 153–159.

Beard, H., Marlowe, M., & Ryle, A. (1990). The management and treatment of personality disordered patients: The use of sequential diagrammatic reformulation. *British Journal of Psychiatry, 156,* 541–545

Beitman, B. D. (1987). *The structure of individual psychotherapy.* New York: Guilford.

Benjamin, L. S. (1974). Structural analysis of social behavior. *Psychological Review, 81,* 392–425.

Benjamin, L. S. (1987a). Combined use of the MCMI and the SASB Intrex questionnaires to document and facilitate personality change during long-term psychotherapy. In C. Green (Ed.), *Conference on the Millon Clinical Inventories* (pp. 305–323). Minneapolis: National Computer Systems.

Benjamin, L. S. (1987b). Use of structural analysis of social behavior (SASB) to define and measure confrontation in psychotherapy. In W. Huber (Ed.), *Progress in psychotherapy research* (pp. 469–495). Louvain la Neuve, Belgium: Presses Universitaires de Louvain.

Benjamin, L. S. (1991). Brief SASB-directed reconstructive learning therapy. In P. Crits-Christoph & J. Barber (Eds.), *Handbook of short-term dynamic psychotherapy* (pp. 248–286). New York: Basic Books.

Benjamin, L. S. (in press). *Interpersonal diagnosis and treatment of DSM personality disorders*. New York: Guilford.

Berzins, J. I. (1977). Therapist-patient matching. In A. S. Gurman & A. M. Razin (Eds.), *Effective psychotherapy: A handbook of research* (pp. 222–251). New York: Pergamon Press.

Beutler, L. E. (1979). Toward specific psychological therapies for specific conditions. *Journal of Consulting and Clinical Psychology*, 47, 882–897.

Beutler, L. E. (1983). *Eclectic psychotherapy: A systematic approach*. New York: Pergamon Press.

Beutler, L. E. (1989). Differential treatment selection: The role of diagnosis in psychotherapy. *Psychotherapy*, 26, 271–281.

Beutler, L. E. (1991). Selective treatment matching: Systematic eclectic psychotherapy. *Psychotherapy*, 28, 457–462.

Beutler, L. E., & Clarkin, J. F. (1990). *Systematic treatment selection: Toward targeted therapeutic interventions*. New York: Brunner/Mazel.

Beutler, L. E., & Mitchell, R. (1981). Differential psychotherapy outcome in depressed and impulsive patients as a function of analytic and experiential treatment procedures. *Psychiatry*, 44, 297–306.

Beutler, L. E., Engle, D., Mohr, D., Daldrup, R., Bergan, J., Meredith, K., & Merry, W. (1991). Predictors of differential response to cognitive, experiential, and self-directed psychotherapeutic procedures. *Journal of Consulting and Clinical Psychology*, 59, 333–340.

Beutler, L. E., Mohr, D. C., Grawe, K., Engle, D., & MacDonald, R. (1991). Looking for differential treatment effects: Cross-cultural predictors of differential psychotherapy efficacy. *Journal of Psychotherapy Integration*, 1, 121–141.

Brockman, B., Poynton, A., Ryle, A., & Watson, J. P. (1987). Effectiveness of time-limited therapy carried out by trainees. *British Journal of Psychiatry*, 151, 602–610.

Calvert, S. C., Beutler, L. E., & Crago, M. (1988). Psychotherapy outcome as a function of therapist-patient matching on selected variables. *Journal of Social and Clinical Psychology*, 6, 104–117.

Caspar, F., & Grawe, K. (1989). Away from the method orientation in psychotherapy. *Bulletin der Schweizer Psychologen*, 3, 6–19.

Chambless, D. L., Goldstein, A. J., Gallagher, R., & Bright, P. (1986). Integrating behavior therapy and psychotherapy in the treatment of agoraphobia. *Psychotherapy*, 23, 150–159.

Dance, K. A., & Neufeld, W. J. (1988). Aptitude-treatment interaction in the clinical setting: A review of attempts to dispel the "patient uniformity" myth. *Psychological Bulletin*, 104, 192–213.

DiClemente, C. C., Prochaska, J. O., Fairhurst, S. K., Velicer, W. F., Velasquez, M. M., & Rossi, J. S. (1991). The process of smoking cessation: An analysis of precontemplation, contemplation, and preparation stages of change. *Journal of Consulting and Clinical Psychology*, 59, 295–304.

Elkin, I. (1991). Varieties of psychotherapy integration research. *Journal of Psychotherapy Integration*, 1, 27–33.

Feather, B. W., & Rhoads, J. M. (1972). Psychodynamic behavior therapy: II. Clinical aspects. *Archives of General Psychiatry*, 26, 503–511.

Feixas, G. (1990a). Approaching the individual, approaching the system: A constructivist model for integrative psychotherapy. *Journal of Family Psychology*, 4, 4–35.

Feixas, G. (1990b). Personal construct theory and systemic therapies: Parallel or convergent trends? *Journal of Marital and Family Therapy*, 16, 1–20.

Frances, A., Clarkin, J., & Perry, S. (1984). *Differential therapeutics in psychiatry: The art and science of treatment selection*. New York: Brunner/Mazel.

Frances, A., Sweeney, J., & Clarkin, J. (1985). Do psychotherapies have specific effects? *American Journal of Psychotherapy*, 39, 159–174.

Garfield, S. L. (1980). *Psychotherapy: An eclectic approach*. New York: Wiley.

Garfield, S. L. (1986). An eclectic psychotherapy. In J. C. Norcross (Ed.), *Handbook of eclectic psychotherapy* (pp. 132–162). New York: Brunner/Mazel.

Garfield, S. L. (1989). *The practice of brief psychotherapy*. New York: Pergamon Press.

Garfield, S. L. (1990). Issues and methods in psychotherapy process research. *Journal of Consulting and Clinical Psychology*, 58, 273–280.

Garfield, S. L., & Kurtz, R. (1976). Clinical psychologists in the 1970s. *American Psychologist*, 31, 1–9.

Garfield, S. L., & Kurtz, R. (1977). A study of eclectic views. *Journal of Consulting and Clinical Psychology*, 45, 78–83.

Gerler, E. R., Drew, N. S., & Mohr, P. (1990). Succeeding in middle school: A multimodal approach. *Elementary School Guidance & Counseling*, 24, 263–271.

Gerler, E. R., Kinney, J., & Anderson, R. F. (1985). The effects of counseling on classroom performance. *Journal of Humanistic Education and Development*, 23, 155–165.

Giunta, L. C., Saltzman, N., & Norcross, J. C. (1991). Whither integration? An exploratory study of contention and convergence in the Clinical Exchange. *Journal of Integrative and Eclectic Psychotherapy*, 10, 117–129.

Goldfried, M. R. (1991). Research issues in psychotherapy integration. *Journal of Psychotherapy Integration*, 1, 5–25.

Goldfried, M. R., & Padawer, W. (1982). Current status and future directions in psychotherapy. In M. R. Goldfried (Ed.), *Converging themes in psychotherapy* (pp. 3–49). New York: Springer.

Goldfried, M. R., Greenberg, L. S., & Marmar, C. (1990). Individual psychotherapy: Process and outcome. In M. Rosenzweig & L. Porter (Eds.), *Annual Review of Psychology*, 41, 659–688.

Grawe, K. (1991). The Bernese Psychotherapy Research Program. In L. E. Beutler and M. Crago (Eds.), *Psychotherapy research: An international review of programmatic studies* (pp. 202–211). Washington, DC: American Psychological Association.

Heide, F. J., & Rosenbaum, R. (1988). Therapists' experiences of using single versus combined theoretical models in psychotherapy. *Journal of Integrative and Eclectic Psychotherapy*, 7, 41–46.

Hill, C. E. (1989). *Therapist techniques and client outcomes: Eight cases of brief psychotherapy*. New York: Sage.

Hoffart, A., & Martinsen, E. W. (1990). Exposure-based integrated vs. pure psychodynamic treatment of agoraphobic inpatients. *Psychotherapy*, 27, 210–218.

Howard, G. S., Nance, D. W., & Myers, P. (1987). *Adaptive counseling and therapy*. San Francisco, CA: Jossey-Bass.

Jensen, J. P., Bergin, A. E., & Greaves, D. W. (1990). The meaning of eclecticism: New survey and analysis of components. *Professional Psychology: Research and Practice*, 21, 124–130.

Kolden, G. (1988). Process and outcome in psychotherapy:

An empirical examination of Orlinsky and Howard's generic model of psychotherapy. *Dissertation Abstracts International, 49*(05), 1945B. (University Microfilms No. AAC8811484)

Kolden, G. (1991). The generic model of psychotherapy: An empirical investigation of patterns of process and outcome relationships. *Psychotherapy Research, 1,* 62–73.

Kwee, M. G. T., Duivenvoorden, H. J., Trijsburg, R. W., & Thiel, J. H. (1986–1987). Multimodal therapy in an inpatient setting. *Current Psychological Research & Reviews, 5,* 344–357.

Lazarus, A. A. (1981). *The practice of multimodal therapy.* New York: McGraw-Hill.

Lazarus, A. A. (1986a). Multimodal psychotherapy: Overview and update. *International Journal of Eclectic Psychotherapy, 5,* 95–103.

Lazarus, A. A. (1986b). Multimodal therapy. In J. Norcross (Ed.), *Handbook of eclectic psychotherapy* (pp. 65–93). New York: Brunner/Mazel.

Lazarus, A. A. (1987). The multimodal approach with adult outpatients. In N. S. Jacobson (Ed.), *Psychotherapists in clinical practice* (pp. 286–326). New York: Guilford.

Lazarus, A. A. (1989). *The practice of multimodal therapy* (rev. ed.). Baltimore: Johns Hopkins University Press.

Linehan, M. M. (1987). Dialectical behavior therapy for borderline personality disorder. *Bulletin of the Menninger Clinic, 51,* 261–276.

Linehan, M. M., Armstrong, H., Suarez, A., Allmon, D., & Heard, H. L. (1989, November). *Comprehensive treatment for parasuicidal women with borderline personality disorder: Dialectical behavior therapy.* Washington, DC: Association for Advancement of Behavior Therapy.

Llewelyn, S. P., Elliott, R., Shapiro, D. A., Hardy, G., & Firth-Cozens, J. (1988). Client perceptions of significant events in prescriptive and exploratory periods of individual therapy. *British Journal of Clinical Psychology, 27,* 105–114.

Luborsky, L., & Crits-Christoph, P. (1989). A relationship pattern measure: The core conflictual relationship theme. *Psychiatry, 52,* 250–259.

Mahoney, M. J. (1990). Developmental cognitive therapy. In J. K. Zeig & W. M. Munion (Eds.), *What is psychotherapy? Contemporary perspectives* (pp. 164–168). San Francisco: Jossey-Bass.

Mahoney, M. J. (1991). *Human change processes.* New York: Basic Books.

Marmar, C. R. (1990). Psychotherapy process research: Progress, dilemmas, and future directions. *Journal of Consulting and Clinical Psychology, 58,* 265–272.

Marmor, J., & Woods, S. M. (Eds.). (1980). *The interface between the psychodynamic and behavioral therapies.* New York: Plenum Press.

Martin, J. (1989, June). *The social-cognitive construction of therapeutic experiences and memories.* Paper presented at the Society for Psychotherapy Research, Toronto.

Martin, J. (1992). Cognitive-mediational research on counseling and psychotherapy. In S. G. Toukmanian & D. L. Rennie (Eds.), *Psychotherapy process research: Paradigmatic and narrative approaches* (pp. 108–133). Newbury Park, CA: Sage.

McConnaughy, E. A., DiClemente, C. C., Prochaska, J. O., & Velicer, W. F. (1989). Stages of change in psychotherapy: A follow-up report. *Psychotherapy, 26,* 494–503.

Neimeyer, R. A., & Feixas, G. (1990). Constructivist contributions to psychotherapy integration. *Journal of Integrative and Eclectic Psychotherapy, 9,* 4–20.

Nielsen, G., & Havik, O. E. (1989). Korttids dynamisk psykoterapi Del II: Prinsipper for en pragmatisk integrativ arbeidsmodell [Brief psychodynamic psychotherapy. Part II: Principles for a pragmatic integrative model]. *Tidsskrift for Norsk Psykologforening, 26,* 451–466.

Nielsen, G., Havik, O. E., Barth, K., Haver, B., Mølstad, E., Rogge, H., & Skåtun, M. (1987). The Bergen Project on Brief Dynamic Psychotherapy: An outline. In W. Huber (Ed.), *Progress in psychotherapy research* (pp. 325–333). Louvain la Neuve, Belgium: Presses Universitaires de Louvain.

Nielsen, G., Barth, K., Haver, B., Havik, O. E., Mølstad, E., Rogge, H., & Skåtun, M. (1988). Brief dynamic psychotherapy for patients presenting physical symptoms. *Psychotherapy and Psychosomatics, 50,* 35–41.

Nielsen, G., Barth, K., Havik, O. E., Haver, B., Mølstad, E., Rogge, H., & Skåtun, M. (1991). ‹Uegnede› pasienter, eller egnet terapi? Erfaringer med korttids dynamisk psykoterapi for pasienter som ikke oppfyller ordinaere inklusjonskriterier. ["Unsuitable" patients, or suitable therapy?]. *Tidsskrift for Norsk Psykologforening, 27,* 91–98.

Norcross, J. C. (Ed.). (1986). *Handbook of eclectic psychotherapy.* New York: Brunner/Mazel.

Norcross, J. C. (Ed.). (1987). *Casebook of eclectic psychotherapy.* New York: Brunner/Mazel.

Norcross, J. C., & Prochaska, J. O. (1982). A national survey of clinical psychologists: Affiliations and orientations. *Clinical Psychologist, 35*(3), 1–2, 4–6.

Norcross, J. C., & Prochaska, J. O. (1988). A study of eclectic (and integrative) views revisited. *Professional Psychology: Research and Practice, 19,* 170–174.

Norcross, J. C., Prochaska, J. O., & Gallagher, K. M. (1989). Clinical psychologists in the 1980s: II. Theory, research, and practice. *The Clinical Psychologist, 42*(3), 45–53.

Olson, S. C. (1979). A multimodal treatment of obesity using Lazarus' BASIC ID model. *Dissertation Abstracts International, 40*(3), 1378B. (University Microfilms No. AAC7919028)

Orlinsky, D. E. (1989). Researchers' images of psychotherapy: Their origins and influence on research. *Clinical Psychology Review, 9,* 413–441.

Orlinsky, D. E., & Howard, K. I. (1987). A generic model of psychotherapy. *Journal of Integrative and Eclectic Psychotherapy, 6,* 6–27.

Prochaska, J. O., & DiClemente, C. C. (1984). *The transtheoretical approach: Crossing traditional boundaries of therapy.* Homewood, IL: Dow Jones-Irwin.

Prochaska, J. O., & DiClemente, C. C. (1986). The transtheoretical approach. In J. C. Norcross (Ed.), *Handbook of eclectic psychotherapy* (pp. 163–200). New York: Brunner/Mazel.

Prochaska, J. O., & DiClemente, C. C. (1992). Stages of change in the modification of problem behaviors. In M. Hersen, R. M. Eisler, & P. M. Miller (Eds.), *Progress in behavior modification* (Vol. 28, pp. 184–206). Sycamore, IL: Sycamore Publishing Co.

Prochaska, J. O., & Norcross, J. C. (1983). Psychotherapists' perspectives on treating themselves and their clients for psychic distress. *Professional Psychology, 14,* 642–655.

Prochaska, J. O., Rossi, J. S., & Wilcox, N. S. (1991). Change processes and psychotherapy outcome in integrative case research. *Journal of Psychotherapy Integration, 1,* 103–120.

Razin, A. M. (1977). The A-B variable: Still promising after twenty years? In A. S. Gurman & A. M. Razin (Eds.), *Effective psychotherapy: A handbook of research* (pp. 291–323). New York: Pergamon Press.

Rhoads, J. M. (1984). Relationships between psychodynamic and behavior therapies. In H. Arkowitz & S. B. Messer (Eds.), *Psychoanalytic therapy and behavior therapy: Is integration possible?* (pp. 195–211). New York: Plenum Press.

Rude, S. S., & Rehm, L. P. (1991). Response to treatments for depression: The role of initial status on targeted cognitive and behavioral skills. *Clinical Psychology Review, 11,* 493–514.

Ryle, A. (1980). Some measures of goal attainment in focussed integrated active psychotherapy: A study of fifteen cases. *British Journal of Psychiatry, 137,* 475–486.

Ryle, A. (1982). *Psychotherapy: A cognitive integration of theory and practice.* London: Academic Press.

Ryle, A. (1990). *Active participation in change: The theory and practice of brief cognitive-analytic therapy.* New York: Wiley.

Safran, J. D. (1990a). Towards a refinement of cognitive therapy in light of interpersonal theory: I. Theory. *Clinical Psychology Review, 10,* 87–105.

Safran, J. D. (1990b). Towards a refinement of cognitive therapy in light of interpersonal theory: II. Practice. *Clinical Psychology Review, 10,* 107–121.

Safran, J. D., & Segal, Z. V. (1990). *Interpersonal process in cognitive therapy.* New York: Basic Books.

Shapiro, D. A., & Firth, J. (1987). Prescriptive *v.* exploratory psychotherapy: Outcomes of the Sheffield Psychotherapy Project. *British Journal of Psychiatry, 151,* 790–799.

Shapiro, D. A., & Firth-Cozens, J. (1990). Two-year follow-up of the Sheffield Psychotherapy Project. *British Journal of Psychiatry, 157,* 389–391.

Shoham-Salomon, V., & Rosenthal, R. (1987). Paradoxical interventions: A meta-analysis. *Journal of Consulting and Clinical Psychology, 55,* 22–27.

Shoham-Salomon, V., Avner, R., & Neeman, K. (1989). "You are changed if you do and changed if you don't": Mechanisms underlying paradoxical interventions. *Journal of Consulting and Clinical Psychology, 57,* 590–598.

Stiles, W. B., Shapiro, D. A., & Elliott, R. (1986). "Are all psychotherapies equivalent?" *American Psychologist, 41,* 165–180.

Vasco, A. B., & Garcia-Marques, L. (1991, July). *Eclectic trends among Portuguese therapists.* Paper presented at the meeting of the Society for the Exploration of Psychotherapy Integration, London.

Wachtel, P. L. (1977). *Psychoanalysis and behavior therapy: Toward an integration.* New York: Basic Books.

Westen, D. (1991). Cognitive-behavioral interventions in the psychoanalytic psychotherapy of borderline personality disorders. *Clinical Psychology Review, 11,* 211–230.

Westerman, M. A., Frankel, A. S., Tanaka, J. S., & Kahn, J. (1987). Client cooperative interview behavior and outcome in paradoxical and behavioral brief treatment approaches. *Journal of Counseling Psychology, 34,* 99–102.

Wolfe, B. E. (1989). Phobias, panic and psychotherapy integration. *Journal of Integrative and Eclectic Psychotherapy, 8,* 264–276.

Wolfe, B. E., & Goldfried, M. R. (1988). Research on psychotherapy integration: Recommendations and conclusions from an NIMH workshop. *Journal of Consulting and Clinical Psychology, 56,* 448–451.

CHAPTER 3

Empirical Research on Factors in Psychotherapeutic Change

Diane B. Arnkoff, Brian J. Victor, and Carol R. Glass

INTRODUCTION

One of the prime reasons that psychotherapists have come to have a strong interest in psychotherapy integration is that the competition among schools of therapy has, on the whole, generated more heat than light (Arnkoff & Glass, 1992). Recently, therapists have become interested in the ways in which orientations are similar in spite of surface distinctions, as well as the ways in which they are truly different. This focus on common and specific factors has been accompanied by renewed curiosity about how psychotherapy accomplishes its goals, that is, the process of psychotherapy and how processes relate to outcome. In this chapter, we will first discuss empirical research on common and specific factors across schools of therapy. Then we will address new research programs and methodologies for studying the process of change, methods that we believe can be used by those interested in integration to increase our knowledge about what is effective in psychotherapy.

AN OVERVIEW OF COMMON AND SPECIFIC FACTORS

Wolfe and Goldfried (1988), in reporting on a National Institute of Mental Health (NIMH) workshop on psychotherapy integration held in 1986, argued that we need evidence about the common and specific factors across psychotherapies. Specifically, they noted that identification of common factors would show what has *already* been integrated, whereas the empirical delineation of specific factors would suggest what potentially *could* be integrated. Weinberger's chapter in this volume (Chapter 4) deals with a variety of perspectives on common and specific factors. Here we will provide merely an overview of the issues, to lead into a focus on empirical research.

Early History of Common Factors

Garfield (1980) explained the search for factors common across psychotherapies in this way:

To the extent that all approaches claim to be successful in alleviating the problems of the patients seeking their help, it seems plausible to assume that there may be variables or

Diane B. Arnkoff, Brian J. Victor, and Carol R. Glass • Department of Psychology, Catholic University of America, Washington, DC 20064.

Comprehensive Handbook of Psychotherapy Integration, edited by George Stricker and Jerold R. Gold. Plenum Press, New York, 1993.

processes common to most approaches which are the operative ones instead of the more specific ones advanced by
the separate approaches. (p. 133)

Common factors were discussed as early as 1936
by Rosenzweig, who argued that the effectiveness of therapies is due to similarity in their processes, such as providing an alternative view of
the client's problems.

Empirical research in the 1950s contributed
to the idea that psychotherapies were not as different as their theorists claimed. Fiedler (1950)
found that the nature of the therapeutic relationship established by experienced therapists was
more similar to that of experts from different
schools than to that of inexperienced therapists
from their own schools of therapy. Heine (1953)
found that clients treated by therapists with different orientations showed similar patterns of
changes, and attributed their changes to similar
factors.

Frank is probably the writer most associated
with the common-factors view. In his well-known
book *Persuasion and Healing*, Frank (1973) argued
that all healing endeavors, not just psychotherapy, operate through common factors. He later
hypothesized a common client factor of demoral-
ization, which is ameliorated through the four common therapy factors: (1) an emotionally charged,
confiding relationship with a helping person; (2) a
healing setting; (3) a rationale, conceptual scheme,
or myth; and (4) a ritual or therapeutic method
(Frank, 1982). Frank and his colleagues undertook research on the common factors and found
that a pill placebo group showed initial change
as great as that of psychotherapy groups (Frank,
1978).

In spite of these arguments and findings, the
common-factors idea had little impact on the
mainstream of psychotherapy until the late 1970s
(Arkowitz, 1992b). In fact, until recently it was
widely held to be necessary to demonstrate that a
form of psychotherapy was *more* successful than a
nonspecific or placebo group in order to claim its
effectiveness (see review by P. Horvath, 1988).
More recently, however, influential researchers
have argued that the placebo metaphor (e.g., Parloff, 1986), and, in fact, the entire pharmacology
metaphor (e.g., Butler & Strupp, 1986; Stiles &
Shapiro, 1989) is inappropriate for psychotherapy
research. The "active ingredients" of psychotherapy, in this view, are not synonymous simply

with those therapeutic interventions that differentiate schools of therapy, but rather encompass
the entire client–therapist interaction.

Recent Interest in Common Factors

Since the late 1970s, there has been an upsurge of interest in common factors. Omer and
London (1988) argued that the so-called nonspecific factors were formerly thought of as the
"noise" of psychotherapy research, whereas now
they are more often thought of as the "signal"
(though we would argue that they may be only
part of the signal). A number of reviewers have
concluded that techniques play a lesser role in
determining outcome than do client or common
factors (e.g., Frances, Sweeney, & Clarkin, 1985;
Lambert, Shapiro, & Bergin, 1986).

There is more agreement on the importance
of common factors than on what these common
factors are. Frank's list of the factors common
across all types of healing was described above.
Many others have been hypothesized (e.g., Garfield, 1980, 1989; Goldfried & Padawer, 1982; Karasu, 1986; Lambert, 1986; Nawas, Pluk, & Wojciechowski, 1985; Prochaska, 1984). In fact, so many
lists of common factors have been proposed that
categorization of the lists has been necessary.
Grencavage and Norcross (1990) examined 50 publications discussing common factors, and investigated which factors were most frequently proposed. They divided the commonalities into five
categories: (1) *client characteristics* (e.g., positive
expectation), (2) *therapist qualities* (e.g., ability to
cultivate hope, empathic understanding), (3) *change
processes* (e.g., opportunity for catharsis, acquisition and practice of new behaviors), (4) *treatment
structure* (e.g., use of techniques/rituals, focus on
"inner world"), and (5) *relationship elements* (e.g.,
development of alliance). Change processes were
listed most frequently by authors (41% of all commonalities listed, and at least one listed by 80% of
all authors); further, more change processes were
listed in more recent publications. Across categories, the most frequent common features listed
were the development of a therapeutic alliance
(listed by 56% of the authors), the opportunity for
catharsis (38%), the acquisition and practice of
new behaviors (32%), clients' positive expectancies (26%), beneficial therapist qualities (24%),
and the provision of a rationale (24%).

Not only is there disagreement on what is meant by common factors, but disagreement also exists on the level of abstraction at which to examine therapy (e.g., Goldfried, 1980). The goals of the search also differ, with some interested in using the commonalities as a basis for integration, some in simply exploring therapy, and some wishing to enrich their preferred therapy (Mahrer, 1989). Within psychotherapy integration, the goal of the investigation of common factors is generally said to be to identify the effective aspects of psychotherapy in order to combine the aspects into a new, powerful psychotherapy (e.g., Arkowitz, 1992b; Grencavage & Norcross, 1990), although some doubt that this is possible or useful (e.g., Haaga, 1986; Mahrer, 1989; Messer & Winokur, 1984). In a unique application of common factors, Arkowitz (1992a) presented a common-factors model of the treatment of depression, based on the provision of social support through the therapist–client relationship. He proposed that this common-factors therapy could be the standard against which more specific treatments for depression would be tested.

EVIDENCE FOR COMMON FACTORS

Lack of Differences in Outcome

A common conclusion from reviews of comparative outcome literature is that consistent differences in outcome between types of therapy are rarely demonstrated (e.g., Lambert et al., 1986; Smith, Glass, & Miller, 1980). Many writers on common factors cite this lack of differential effectiveness of treatments as evidence that is at least consistent with the common-factors view (e.g., Garfield, 1980; Goldfried, 1991). In fact, this lack of differential effectiveness is one of the reasons why eclectic and integrative therapies have become important recently (Arnkoff & Glass, 1992). However, the finding of no significant differences could come about for a myriad of other reasons besides factors common across therapies.

Stiles, Shapiro, and Elliott (1986) discussed various explanations for the lack of differential outcome findings, including the need to analyze change events more specifically. The "matrix paradigm," or the need to match treatments to clients, is also consistent with a global finding of no difference between treatments; such matching proposals are reviewed in Glass, Victor, and Arnkoff's chapter (Chapter 2) in this volume. Kazdin and Bass (1989) have shown that most comparative outcome studies have had too few subjects to find the small-to-moderate effect sizes that could differentiate treatments. An additional possibility is that treatments could cause change in different aspects of the client's functioning (e.g., interpersonal functioning versus cognitive schemata), but then these changes would generalize broadly by the time of therapy termination and posttest assessment, with the result that the therapies would appear to have acted similarly (Beckham, 1990; Hollon, DeRubeis, & Evans, 1987; Norcross, 1988).

Shoham-Salomon (1991) has also argued that from a clinical perspective, the lack of differential outcomes does not logically lead to the conclusion that all therapies operate in the same way. If therapies were the same, there would be no reason why practitioners would be interested in what other orientations could contribute to their own. Indeed, another reason for the interest in integration is that clinicians find that no one therapy seems sufficient for all clients (Garfield, 1989; Goldfried, 1991).

The rush to endorse common factors has now slowed to a more deliberate walk. Recent discussions of common factors have argued, for example, that proposed common factors, such as the therapeutic relationship, have sometimes been described in such vague terms as to be nearly meaningless (Arkowitz, 1992b; Haaga, 1986; Mahrer, 1989). We need greater specification of the hypothesized common factors (Mahrer, 1989), better theorizing about their role (Arkowitz, 1992b), as well as research on the components of the hypothesized constructs like the therapeutic alliance (Marmar, 1990). Further, there is no reason to think that the same factor, like the therapeutic relationship, operates identically in all types of therapy (Arkowitz, 1992b), so we need to guard against a uniformity myth about common factors.

The Therapeutic Alliance

The hypothesized common factor that has received the most empirical attention is the *therapeutic alliance*. Building on early work like that of Fiedler (1950), Rogers (1957), and Zetzel (1956), the therapeutic relationship has been a central theoretical and empirical focus in psychotherapy research over the past four decades. The concept of the alliance has become the primary construct for examining the therapeutic relationship. Much of the early theoretical and empirical work on the alliance centered on the psychodynamic and client-centered traditions, which produced a fair amount of empirical literature in support of predicting outcome from the nature of the therapeutic alliance (Gaston, 1990; A. O. Horvath & Symonds, 1991; Marmar, Gaston, Gallagher, & Thompson, 1989). However, over the past 15 years, theoretical support for the role of the alliance in eclectic, cognitive, behavioral, and pharmacological therapy has emerged (e.g., Bordin, 1979; Docherty & Fiester, 1985; Gelso & Carter, 1985; Rush, 1985; Wilson & Evans, 1977), providing more evidence for its place as a central change agent across a variety of treatment modalities.

As theoretical interest in the alliance spread beyond the psychodynamic and client-centered traditions, much confusion and controversy about divergent views of the alliance emerged. Clear illustrations of the controversy can be found in both the variety of definitions (working vs. helping vs. therapeutic alliance) and instruments developed and refined to measure the construct. A review of these definitions and instruments is beyond the scope of this chapter, but excellent theoretical and empirical overviews attempting to clarify the alliance concept have recently emerged (e.g., Frieswyk et al., 1986; Gaston, 1990; Gelso & Carter, 1985), as well as reports of alliance instrument validation (e.g., Gaston, 1991; A. O. Horvath & Greenberg, 1986, 1989). Despite the controversy, empirical research on the alliance has gained increasing momentum over the past 10 years.

Wolfe and Goldfried's (1988) report on the recommendations and conclusions of the NIMH workshop on psychotherapy integration noted that the therapeutic alliance is a focal variable for empirical research on integration, because it cuts across the various schools of therapy. Wolfe and Goldfried outlined three recommendations for alliance research: (1) clarifying whether different kinds of alliances are associated with various therapy orientations, (2) determining if different kinds of alliances are required for different kinds of therapy tasks or techniques, and (3) determining if client characteristics affect the alliance's role as a change vehicle in therapy.

A report of the results of empirical investigations of the alliance concept could fill several chapters. In order to focus more directly on alliance research that addresses psychotherapy integration, only results that bear directly on Wolfe and Goldfried's (1988) three recommended research directions will be briefly reviewed here. Loosely following Wolfe and Goldfried's first and third recommendations, a number of studies have investigated the role of the alliance within and across different theoretical orientations or in relation to client characteristics.

Alliance in Various Therapy Orientations. Raue, Castonguay, and Goldfried (1992) assessed observer ratings of the therapeutic alliance in single sessions from expert cognitive-behavioral and psychodynamic therapists. They found that the alliance was strong in both types of therapy, but significantly stronger for cognitive-behavioral, with more variability in the alliance in psychodynamic therapy. Further, client symptom scores were not significantly correlated with the alliance in cognitive-behavioral therapy, but in psychodynamic therapy, the more symptomatic the client, the poorer the therapeutic alliance.

In contrast to these findings, Salvio, Beutler, Wood, and Engle (1992) conducted a study of depressed outpatients who were randomly assigned to group cognitive therapy (CT), group gestalt-based therapy (Focused Expressive Therapy: FEP), or minimal contact treatment (Supportive/Self-Directed Therapy: S/SD). The levels of alliance, measured early and late in treatment, were not significantly different across the three treatment conditions. Similarly, Marmar et al. (1989) did not find differences in the strength of the alliance in behavior therapy, cognitive therapy, or brief dynamic therapy.

Several empirical studies have demonstrated that the alliance is related to outcome within various therapeutic orientations. A number of studies reviewed by A. O. Horvath and Symonds (1991) and Gaston (1990) lend support for the alliance-outcome association in brief dynamic therapy. In behavior therapy, relationship factors have been linked to outcome (e.g., Cross, Sheehan, & Khan, 1982; Marmar et al., 1989; Sloane, Staples, Cristol, Yorkston, & Whipple, 1975). Four studies have shown strong alliance to outcome links in cognitive therapy (Gaston, 1991; Luborsky, McLellan, Woody, O'Brien, & Auerbach,

1985; Marmar *et al.*, 1989; Safran & Wallner, 1991), whereas three reported no significant association (Crits-Christoph & Beebe, 1988; DeRubeis, Feeley, & Barber, 1988; Krupnick, 1988, cited in Safran & Wallner, 1991). Finally, one study involving gestalt therapy (Greenberg & Webster, 1982) reported a strong association between alliance and outcome.

There are also several studies that have simultaneously assessed alliance-outcome links across various treatment modalities. Marmar *et al.* (1989) conducted a study of depressed elderly outpatients who were randomly assigned to behavioral therapy (BT), cognitive therapy (CT), or brief dynamic therapy (BDT). As noted above, the levels of alliance, measured early in the treatment, were not significantly different across the three therapy conditions. The strongest relationships with outcome were found in the CT condition, with strong positive trends occurring in both CT and BDT and an opposite trend in BT. Marmar *et al.* also found that the alliance uniquely contributed to outcome variance (albeit modestly) over and above both initial level of symptomatology and symptom change at the middle of treatment.

Using the same client population and therapy modalities, Gaston, Marmar, Gallagher, and Thompson (1991) measured the alliance during the early, middle, and late phases of treatment. They found that there was no significant variation of alliance levels over time in any of the treatment conditions. Perhaps most importantly, Gaston *et al.* found that substantial amounts of the outcome variance were uniquely accounted for by the alliance in each of the three treatment conditions, with the strongest associations in the BT and CT conditions. Partial correlations of the various alliance dimensions were quite disparate when separated by treatment conditions, which is in accordance with Wolfe and Goldfried's (1988) suggestion that qualitatively different kinds of alliances may be active in diverse forms of therapy.

Gaston (1991) measured the four alliance dimensions of the patient version of the California Psychotherapy Alliance Scales (CALPAS-P) (Marmar *et al.*, 1989) in relation to outcome. The study included therapists representing psychodynamic, eclectic (dynamic and humanistic), and cognitive-behavioral orientations. Across treatment modalities, the alliance was significantly positively correlated with outcome. Only one alliance subscale showed a trend for differential association to outcome when the sample was divided by treatment modality. Although nonsignificant, the results showed a trend for a greater role for the alliance dimension labeled "client working capacity" in dynamic therapy.

There appears to be little strong empirical evidence for the differential effectiveness of the alliance across various forms of treatment. The equivocal findings across treatments are reflected in a recent meta-analysis by A. O. Horvath and Symonds (1991) on the relationship between alliance and long-term outcome in individual psychotherapy. They analyzed 24 studies, which were based on 20 distinct data sets employing a variety of alliance measures and evaluation perspectives. Seven of the data sets involved a psychodynamic treatment, 10 were based on eclectic or mixed treatments, 2 involved cognitive treatments, and 1 was based on gestalt therapy. The relationship between alliance and outcome was significant for each of the groups. Although there were no statistically significant differences between the groups, the effect sizes in the 24 individual studies were quite varied.

Client Characteristics and Alliance. In line with Wolfe and Goldfried's (1988) third recommendation, several studies have investigated client characteristics in relation to the alliance. In 1988, Gaston, Marmar, Thompson, and Gallagher studied the impact on the alliance of several client pretreatment characteristics in the same depressed, elderly population discussed above. Overall, the pretreatment characteristics in BT and CT showed similar patterns of relation to the alliance, whereas both BT and CT relationship patterns were different from the BDT condition. Gaston *et al.* (1988) found that client pretreatment quality of *interpersonal functioning* was not related to client contribution to the alliance in either form of therapy. Along similar lines, Marmar, Horowitz, Weiss, and Marziali (1986) found no relation between pretreatment level of ego functioning and alliance in clients with pathological grief. The results of several other studies, however, run counter to the findings of no association. Gaston (1991) found that clients with greater intimacy difficulties reported poorer alliances. Kokotovic and Tracey (1990) found that clients who were viewed by their therapists as expressing hostility and who had poor current and past interpersonal relationships tended to form worse alliances. Similar negative relationships were reported by Gomes-Schwartz (1978), Moras and Strupp (1982), Piper, DeCarufel, and Szkrumelack (1985), and Strupp (1980a,b,c).

Replicating the results of Marmar *et al.* (1986), Gaston *et al.* (1988) found no association between the pretreatment degree of *symptomatology* and the quality of the clients' contribution to the alliance. Similarly, Moras and Strupp (1982) found no relation between therapist ratings of overall client psychological health and the alliance. However, Eaton, Abeles, and Gutfreund (1988) and Gaston (1991) reported that alliance was adversely affected by higher levels of client symptomatology. Kokotovic and Tracey (1990) found that the therapist-rated level of client overall adjustment was related to the alliance, but the client's rating of overall adjustment was not.

Across all treatment conditions, Gaston *et al.* (1988) found that the clients' pretreatment degree of *defensiveness* was negatively related to therapists' ratings of their clients' ability to engage in the tasks of therapy. Also across treatments, Gaston *et al.* (1988) found that the degree of *family environmental support* was not significantly related to the client contributions to the alliance; however, positive trends emerged.

Although the results of these investigations are far from conclusive, they do suggest that clients' poor interpersonal functioning and higher degrees of defensiveness and hostility are negatively related to their ability to form an alliance, whereas clients' levels of symptomatology and environmental support yielded equivocal results in relation to the alliance. Overall, the results of the empirical literature suggest that the alliance is an important construct that is positively correlated with outcome in a wide variety of treatment modalities, and it is deserving of further examination.

INTEREST IN SPECIFIC FACTORS

In addition to common factors, psychotherapy integration is concerned with the possibility that there are also specific factors, or ways in which different forms of therapy have procedures, processes, or outcomes that are different. Of course, the competition among schools of therapy that has been the norm until recently focused almost exclusively on hypothesized specific factors. Research from this vantage point led to the seeming paradox that even though procedures in different types of therapy could be differentiated (e.g., DeRubeis, Hollon, Evans, & Bemis, 1982), their outcomes could not (e.g., Elkin *et al.*, 1989). Studies have also addressed whether differential change could be found on variables hypothesized to be more related to one form of therapy than to another; for example, interpersonal functioning in interpersonal therapy (IPT), and cognitive schemata in cognitive therapy. Findings in this area have been mixed; in one important study, Imber *et al.* (1990) found that most variables hypothesized to be more affected by IPT or cognitive therapy did not, in fact, result in differential outcomes, at least at termination.

Nevertheless, within psychotherapy integration, interest still runs high on the search for specific effects of therapy (e.g., Arkowitz, 1992b; Arnkoff, 1983; Wolfe & Goldfried, 1988). Just as Grencavage and Norcross (1990) sorted common factors into categories, so the same needs to be done for specific factors. Discussion and research would be more productive if it is clear whether the hypothesized specific factors are, for example, change processes or client characteristics. Further, rather than adopting the comparative outcome methodology, integrative researchers are calling for research on in-session behavior and proximal outcomes (as well as ultimate outcomes) in order to isolate common and specific effects (Goldfried, 1991).

RECENT RESEARCH PROGRAMS ON THE PROCESS OF CHANGE

Many research programs in psychotherapy are relevant to the factors in psychotherapeutic change, such as investigations of client expectations, client and therapist contributions to outcome, and the like. Because a review of all relevant studies is beyond the scope of this chapter, selected research programs will be highlighted that seem especially relevant to integration, specifically, current research on in-session behavior and psychotherapy process. As Elkin (1991) has noted, the resources for large-scale outcome studies are out of reach for many researchers.

Even though studies of change processes are also difficult and time-consuming, they may still be a realistic direction for psychotherapy integration researchers.

Orlinsky and Howard (1986) reviewed a large number of studies relating process to outcome. One facet of therapy that they reviewed was therapeutic interventions, including interpretation or giving insight, confrontation or giving feedback, exploration and questioning, giving support and encouragement, giving advice, reflection, self-disclosure, and therapist skillfulness. Only confrontation and therapist skillfulness were consistently found to be related to outcome. Stiles and Shapiro (1989), however, have criticized several aspects of Orlinsky and Howard's (1986) review, arguing that causal links have not been demonstrated, and that a nonsignificant correlation between intervention and outcome could actually reflect therapists' adaptation of procedures to individual client needs.

Stiles and Shapiro's (1989) conclusion is that more sophisticated research designs to understand therapy process are needed. In fact, some researchers have rejected the common and specific factors construct altogether (e.g., Butler & Strupp, 1986; Caspar & Grawe, 1991). Butler and Strupp (1986), for example, argued that "psychotherapy cannot be meaningfully reduced to 'factors' independent of a particular interpersonal context" (p. 31). The most important influence on therapy would seem to be "the interaction of the patient's interpersonal style with the therapist's skill in managing the interpersonal climate" (p. 36). They argued for a shift in research approach to the intensive study of process within dyads.

In keeping with Butler and Strupp's (1986) point of view, there appears to be a growing consensus on the importance of studying therapeutic activities *in context* (e.g., Greenberg, 1991; Marmar, 1990; Shoham-Salomon, 1990; Stiles *et al.*, 1986). Marmar (1990) identified some of the aspects important to study as "individual patient differences, phase of therapy, patient state, patient capacity for absorption of process, or related contextual problems" (p. 267). Stiles *et al.* (1986) posed a complementary question to the famous litany by Paul (1967): "Which specific therapist interventions, introduced in which momentary therapeutic contexts, will lead to which immedi-

ate and subsequent impacts (outcomes) for the client?" (Stiles *et al.*, p. 174). They noted that this type of research may be more useful for clinicians, in that it focuses on the moment-to-moment decisions that need to be made.

In addition to context, there is an agreement among current researchers that greater *specificity* of variables is needed than has commonly been the case (e.g., Jones, Cumming, & Horowitz, 1988; Mahrer, 1989; Stiles *et al.*, 1986). Finally, current researchers seem to agree that it is necessary to study *patterns* of variables (e.g., Greenberg, 1986; Marmar, 1990; Shoham-Salomon, 1990). Shoham-Salomon (1990) quoted Scarr (1985, p. 502) as proposing "a cloud of correlated events" as best representing the phenomena of interest; thus, patterns within interrelated variables may have greater meaning than any of the variables alone. Greenberg (1991, p. 7) has summarized the goal of contemporary change process research: "*in highly specified in-therapy contexts*, behavior and experience are lawfully explainable, and valid, specific models or micro-theory can be developed to help explain therapeutic change processes."

The observation-based research that will be described here can be contrasted with theory-driven research (Beutler, 1990; Luborsky, Barber, & Crits-Christoph, 1990). However, theory is not irrelevant to this research. Initial choices of questions and methods are influenced by theory, and the creation of new theory is the goal (Hill, 1990). Further, Shoham-Salomon (1990) has argued that theory-driven and observation-driven research can be integrated into a single program of alternating activities, with each type of research informing the other. Thus, integrative theory can be incorporated, tested, and improved in such research programs.

Hill (1990) has reviewed exploratory in-session process research programs in individual therapy. Most of these programs do not begin from a single theoretical orientation, so they may be particularly useful in research on psychotherapy integration. In addition to the Hill (1990) article, useful reviews are found in Russell (1989), Greenberg and Pinsof (1986), and Rice and Greenberg (1984). In the present chapter, we have chosen to focus on five areas of process research. The review here is not complete by any means; the illustrations were chosen because of their importance and relevance to psychotherapy integration.

Therapist Verbal Behavior

Research on therapist verbal behavior tries to categorize types of therapist interventions, and to observe their effects on immediate and more distal client behavior. For example, Mahrer and his colleagues have investigated "microstrategies," or patterns of sequences of interventions by therapists. In a study by Mahrer, Nifakis, Abhukara, and Sterner (1984), several sessions from well-known behavioral, client-centered, and gestalt therapists were examined. The three therapists tended to use distinctive microstrategies, and their microstrategies tended to be consistent across sessions and across clients.

Mahrer, Sterner, Lawson, and Dessaulles (1986), continuing the microstrategy research, examined a single session from six therapists with different orientations. Four of the therapists, but not the behavioral or client-centered therapist, commonly adopted the microstrategy of combining interpretation and explanation–description of the external world. With this exception, the microstrategies of the six therapists were consistent within each therapist but different from each other.

Elliott *et al.* (1987) compared six response mode systems in their ratings of therapy sessions from seven therapists who had different therapeutic orientations. Convergence was found for the six modes rated in all systems: question, advisement, information, reflection, interpretation, and self-disclosure. These six modes differentiated the seven therapists. Response modes, however, have not been found to account for a great deal of the variance in outcome, even immediate outcome (Hill, 1990).

Hill (1989) presented an analysis of eight case studies, assessing techniques (response modes) as well as context factors, such as therapist and client variables that moderate the influence of techniques. The therapists were peer-nominated experts, and the clients were anxious and depressed individuals who were given short-term therapy. Both therapists and clients completed measures immediately following each session, and judges used these measures to make ratings of the helpfulness of each of the therapist verbal response modes.

Therapist techniques were found to be influential in all eight cases. Interpretation and approval were helpful in all cases; direct guidance, open questions, and confrontation were helpful in some cases but not in others. Client factors influenced which techniques were most helpful; for example, passive/dependent clients preferred direct guidance and the provision of information. There was some influence of therapeutic orientation on choice of techniques. This study is notable for its combination of rigorous quantitative methodology with detailed client and therapy descriptions, as well as its emphasis on the context of the therapist's behavior.

Goldfried (1991) described a program of research currently being carried out to describe change processes using language that is neutral with regard to theory. He has chosen to study therapeutic feedback, or the effort on the part of the therapist to help the client become more aware of behavior, cognition, and affect, because it is described as an important principle in all schools of therapy (Goldfried & Padawer, 1982). It was anticipated that the study of feedback would allow both common and unique aspects of different schools of therapy to be identified.

The coding system of therapist responses devised by Goldfried and colleagues (Goldfried, 1991) consists of five sections: (1) *components* focused on in the therapist's response (e.g., situation, intention, action); (2) *general interventions* (a focus on broad aspects of the client's functioning, e.g., relationship of current material to a focal theme); (3) *links* (the type of connection the therapist is making, e.g., intrapersonal, between aspects of the client's functioning, or interpersonal between the client and another person); (4) *time frame*; and (5) *persons involved*.

One study carried out with this coding system (Kerr, Goldfried, Hayes, & Goldsamt, 1989) used data from the first Sheffield psychotherapy study (Hardy & Shapiro, 1985), which included eight sessions each of cognitive-behavior therapy and psychodynamic-interpersonal therapy. It was expected from theory that cognitive-behavior therapy would have feedback focused more in intrapersonal matters than interpersonal, and vice versa for psychodynamic-interpersonal therapy. The findings were that therapists in both treatments made more interpersonal than intrapersonal links (significantly so for psychodynamic-interpersonal therapy and approaching statistical significance for cognitive-behavior therapy). A study addressing outcome data (Castonguay *et al.*, 1990), however, found that the correlation between a focus on interpersonal links and improvement in social functioning was significant only for the psychodynamic-interpersonal therapy.

Castonguay *et al.* (1990) also addressed the relationship between outcome and an emphasis on what is real and unreal, that is, helping the client become aware of the way things really are versus the client's interpretation of events. The real–unreal focus was nearly significantly correlated with outcome, in a positive direction, for cognitive-behavior therapy, but there was a nearly significant *negative* correlation with outcome in psychodynamic-interpersonal therapy. Further investigation suggested that in cognitive-behavior therapy, the therapist was conveying the message "Things are not as *bad* as you think," whereas therapists in the psychodynamic-interpersonal treatment, when they focused on reality–unreality, were conveying the message "Things are not as *good* as you think."

Covert Therapist and Client Processes

In addition to overt behavior, such as therapist interventions, researchers have focused on covert processes, such as therapist intentions (e.g., Gaston & Ring, 1992; Hill & O'Grady, 1985) and client reactions to therapist interventions (e.g., Fuller & Hill, 1985; Martin, Martin, & Slemon, 1987). For example, Hill *et al.* (1988) found that therapist intentions accounted for more of the variance in immediate outcome than did therapist response modes.

It does not seem necessary, however, for clients to be aware of therapist intentions. Such awareness may even have a negative effect on therapy (Martin *et al.*, 1987), perhaps because clients need to be concentrating on their own work and not on that of the therapist (Hill, 1990). The research on client awareness of intentions is interesting in light of the emphasis on client–therapist collaboration in cognitive and behavior therapy. This collaboration may serve more to facilitate the therapeutic alliance than to inform the client of the therapist's intentions.

Client Experiencing and Behavior

Clients' experiences in psychotherapy (see review by Elliott & James, 1989) may be particularly applicable to psychotherapy integration. For example, Mahrer (1988) defined "good moments" as those "in-session events indicating a significant measure of client movement, improvement, progress, process, or change" (p. 81). Mahrer and his colleagues have developed a list of such good moments that was designed to cover all types of individual psychotherapy. The categories include provision of significant material about self and/or interpersonal relationships, expression of insight/understanding, and expression or report of change in target behaviors.

Mahrer, Nadler, Stalikas, Schachter, and Sterner (1988) asked judges to rate 12 categories of good moments in sessions from client-centered therapy, rational-emotive therapy (RET), and experiential therapy. "Providing meaningful material" was the most frequent category in client-centered and RET, and occurred with significantly greater frequency than in experiential therapy. "Expressive communication" occurred with significantly greater frequency in experiential therapy than in the other two therapies, though it was common in all therapies.

Mahrer, Nadler, Sterner, and White (1989) examined strings (common occurrences of one category) and clusters (combinations of at least two categories) of good moments from the same sessions described above. Client-centered and RET had characteristic clusters or strings, and all three therapies had both common and specific strings of good moments. The therapies also had distinctive sequences of strings and clusters.

Martin *et al.* (1987) also examined "good moments" in therapy. They found that the good moments in person-centered therapy tended to focus on client affective exploration and expression, whereas the good moments in RET tended to deal with client insight and understanding of new ways of behaving.

Stiles and his colleagues have studied client as well as therapist verbal response modes. They have found evidence that clients respond similarly regardless of the type of therapy they receive (e.g., Stiles, Shapiro, & Firth-Cozens, 1988). It would be interesting to study client responses in eclectic and integrative therapy to discover if there are unique patterns of client response as compared to pure-form therapies.

Finally, Glass and Arnkoff (1988) studied common and specific factors in clients' descriptions of changes made and explanations for these changes in four group treatment programs for shyness (cognitive restructuring, social skills training, problem solving, and unstructured interpersonal therapy as described by Yalom, 1985). As hypothesized, clients' reports focused both on components specific to the treatments they had received (e.g., learning to change negative thoughts in cognitive restructuring), and on factors common to all group therapies (e.g., taking part in a group). In fact, although the intended content was reported most often in subjects' explanations for change, the common factor of group process was the second most predominant code in the three structured group therapies. It is noteworthy as well that the primary changes subjects reported were consistent with the type of treatment they had received, but they also reported changes that had not been explicitly focused on in therapy (e.g., the cognitive restructuring subjects reported behavioral changes, and vice versa). Our research group is currently applying the same type of common and specific coding to client perceptions of change with data from the NIMH Treatment of Depression Collaborative Research Program (Elkin *et al.*, 1989).

Interpersonal Process in the Therapy Dyad

The study of interpersonal process in therapy is in keeping with the emphasis noted above on context and patterning. The client–therapist relationship is inherently reciprocal, and so there has been a dramatic increase in the study of interpersonal interactions. In fact, Henry, Schacht, and Strupp (1986) and Kiesler (1982) have argued that interpersonal transactions between the client and therapist should become the fundamental unit of psychotherapy process research.

Several researchers have developed complex process measures to capture the interrelated nature of interpersonal process. Three of the most extensively used measures are the Interpersonal Circle (Kiesler, 1982, 1983), the Structural Analysis of Social Behavior (SASB) (Benjamin, 1974; Ben-

jamin, Foster, Roberto, & Estroff, 1986), and the Core Conflictual Relationship Theme method (Luborsky, 1976; Luborsky & Crits-Christoph, 1989; Luborsky, Crits-Christoph, & Mellon, 1986). These measures have been used to investigate a wide range of interactions, for example, transference and the formation of symptoms from intrapsychic conflicts.

In 1986, Henry *et al.* reanalyzed the third-session interpersonal transactions of the four pairs of Strupp's (1980a,b,c,d) single-case studies from the Vanderbilt I psychotherapy project (Strupp & Hadley, 1979). Their purpose was to investigate client and therapist evoking and responding styles. Using a form of the SASB, they found that successful outcome cases were related to greater levels of client and therapist affiliative interactions, and poor outcome cases were related to more hostile interactions between the client and therapist. They also reported that therapists using multiple communication (i.e., containing both positive and negative messages in one thought) showed a greater trend toward poor outcome cases. Interestingly, despite wide differences in techniques, the interpersonal processes differentiating successful from poor outcome cases were similar across therapists.

A later finding in a similar study by Henry, Schacht, and Strupp (1990) confirmed the importance of the therapist's impact on interpersonal process in the relationship. In their study, poor outcome cases were differentiated early in therapy by therapist behaviors that were subtly hostile and controlling and confirmed clients' personality structures of hostility directed toward themselves. They also found that therapists who had a greater level of hostility toward themselves tended to treat their clients in a more hostile manner.

Kiesler and Watkins (1989), in a study relating interpersonal process to the alliance, found that interactions concerning hostile interpersonal behaviors were more important early in therapy. They reported that the closer clients and therapists complemented each other's interpersonal self-presentations in the third session, particularly for hostile behaviors, the better the alliance.

Clearly, the significance of the interpersonal process approach is that it examines the interaction in the therapy dyad or system as a process unit, rather than measuring each individual's unique contribution to process.

The Events Paradigm

In this final area of research with potential importance for integrative therapy, events of particular significance are chosen from theory or clinical observation and analyzed. This paradigm seeks to isolate those segments of therapy that are especially meaningful, with the notion that these are the events most likely to inform us about therapy process.

The recollection of important therapeutic events is one example of the events paradigm. Llewelyn, Elliott, Shapiro, Hardy, and Firth-Cozens (1988), in the first Sheffield psychotherapy project, asked clients who received eight sessions each of both psychodynamic-interpersonal and cognitive-behavior therapy to identify helpful and hindering events following each session and at the end of each treatment. The categories of problem solution and reassurance were more often reported in cognitive-behavior therapy, whereas awareness and personal insight were reported more in psychodynamic-interpersonal therapy. Events categorized as involvement, understanding, and awareness were reported more often in the first treatment, regardless of which type the client had received first. The prevalence of the events, however, was not correlated with outcome.

Martin and Stelmaczonek (1988) asked both counselors and clients to identify important events. They found that counselors and clients identified the same events as important in about one-third of the events reported. Llewelyn (1988) found that therapists and clients asked to identify helpful events following each session showed some similarities in their reports, but also some important differences. Therapists reported insight and awareness as helpful significantly more often then did their clients, whereas clients reported reassurance/relief and understanding as helpful significantly more often than did their therapists. Differences between clients and therapists in their report of events were most pronounced in a subgroup of clients with poor outcomes.

Rice and Greenberg (1984) proposed using a task analysis to study important change events (see also Safran, Greenberg, & Rice, 1988). Task analysis emphasizes the "discovery phase" of research far more than has been typical in research on psychotherapy. The task analysis begins with the intuitive description by an expert clinician of an important event in therapy. A rationally constructed model, with carefully developed measurement, is subject to empirical test in individual cases. A specific, refined model results that can then be tested in a verification phase (Greenberg, 1991). Greenberg (1984) has applied task analysis to intrapersonal conflict resolution in the gestalt two-chair technique. The ultimate outcome of the task analysis was a model in which the two sides of the individual, labeled the "experiencer" and the "harsh critic," start in an opposition phase, move to a merging phase, and finally unite in an integration phase. In this process, the harsh critic becomes softer and the experiencer more affiliative. The task analysis procedure holds promise for the investigation of common and specific factors in therapy, as well as the unique aspects (if any) of the new integrative treatment models. As Greenberg (1991) has argued, this type of research allows the cause of psychotherapeutic change to be discovered with more confidence than in standard correlational research.

FUTURE DIRECTIONS

In order to improve our investigations of common and specific factors across forms of therapy, several researchers have recommended strategies that look promising. Mahrer (1989) proposed a methodology to search for such factors: specify which therapies are proposed to share a factor in common, define the commonality in specific ways, and investigate whether the therapies "use the commonality under similar therapeutic conditions and to effect similar consequences" (p. 139). Because the correlational research designs currently in use cannot determine causality in the relationship between in-session behavior and more distal outcomes, both Arkowitz (1992b) and Hollon et al. (1987) advocate the use of structural modeling strategies.

In the investigation of common and specific factors, it seems especially important to investigate clients' perceptions of the factors involved in their changes (Glass & Arnkoff, 1988). Client behavior may form the common core of therapies; as noted earlier, clients have been shown to engage in similar behaviors regardless of the orientation of their therapists (Stiles et al., 1988). Interestingly, clients tend to see their therapists' interventions

(Fuller & Hill, 1985) and the helpful events of therapy (Llewelyn, 1988) differently from their therapists. Although the client's perception is not the only important vantage point, the client's views do have a significant influence on therapy. For example, clients make the decision to either drop out of or continue therapy. Thus clients' understanding of how therapy is benefitting or harming them is crucial, regardless of whether an observer or the therapist would call the client's understanding accurate, mistaken, incomplete, or a rationalization.

As discussed above, the therapeutic alliance is the one common factor that has already received considerable research attention. Although empirical literature on the therapeutic alliance suggests that there is little evidence for *quantitative* differences in the alliance-outcome relationship in various treatment modalities, more research is needed to determine if there are *qualitative* differences in the alliance across orientations. Future research might follow the lead of Gaston *et al.* (1991) in examining variations in the dimensions of the alliance across treatments. More microanalytic strategies for investigating changes and patterns in the alliance associated with various orientations, both within and between sessions, might also prove beneficial in teasing out if there are any differences. Following the recommendation of the NIMH workshop on psychotherapy integration (Wolfe & Goldfried, 1988), research should be conducted on specific therapeutic tasks and techniques, within and across orientations, to assess the impact of the alliance and variations in its dimensions.

Additionally, more research is needed regarding the impact of client characteristics on the alliance. Since a number of the results regarding client characteristics reported in this chapter were based on studies of depressed individuals, it will be important to assess these characteristics among different diagnostic populations.

Another interesting direction for study involves ruptures and repairs of the alliance (Safran, Crocker, McMain, & Murray, 1990; Safran & Segal, 1990). Safran *et al.* (1990) have suggested a model of the change process involved in resolving disruptions of the alliance, which is based on seven alliance rupture markers and five principles for their resolution. Their model is ripe for empirical validation, and it would be interesting to investigate the occurrence and/or variation of rup-

tures and repairs in the alliance across orientations.

Since the alliance is one particular type of interpersonal relationship, models and findings from other branches of psychology that deal with interpersonal influence could be profitably applied to the study of the therapeutic alliance (H. Arkowitz, personal communication, November 23, 1991; see also Arkowitz, 1991). Findings in such areas as attachment, social support, and self-disclosure may be useful and may help lead to an integrated model of the therapeutic relationship.

New directions in psychotherapy change research hold promise for studying integrated therapies and models. For example, a variety of therapist actions or intentions associated with different schools of therapy may actually lead to the same client behavior or experience (Goldfried & Safran, 1986). Studies that provide information on which therapist actions lead to which client experiences and behavior, and under which conditions, will allow us to recommend empirically sound integrated treatments. The research directions described above on interpersonal process, such as studies using the SASB, seem especially promising.

The events paradigm suggests many future directions relevant to integration. First, various pure-form therapies can be compared to each other, with the goal of identifying consistent similarities and differences in change events. For example, client markers (Rice & Greenberg, 1984) are those events that signal to the therapist that the client is ready for a certain type of intervention. Therapists may identify some similar markers, such as expression of dissatisfaction with an interpersonal relationship, and some different markers, such as negative thoughts in cognitive therapy and avoidance of expressing negative feelings toward the therapist in psychoanalytic therapy (Goldfried & Safran, 1986). Research focused on "process diagnoses" (Greenberg, 1991), that is, client states that call for intervention, could compare such diagnoses and what therapists do when they encounter them, across different types of therapy.

Second, the change events in integrated treatments can be compared to those in pure-form therapies. For example, as Elkin (1991) has suggested, a particular event, such as interpersonal conflict, could be compared in an insight-oriented treatment and in a treatment that attempted to combine insight with changes in interpersonal behavior.

Finally, it would be especially interesting to study the choices that pure-form and integrative therapists make when faced with *difficult* situations, as described by Strupp (1989, p. 719):

enactments that often put the therapist on the defensive, evoke boredom, irritation, anger, and hostility and in other respects "put pressure" on the therapist to behave in ways that are incompatible with his or her stance as an empathic listener and clarifier.

Strupp (1989) noted that even well-trained therapists often perform nontherapeutically when faced with such enactments, which can jeopardize all progress with the client. Thus, such situations are extremely important for us to investigate, both within pure-form and within eclectic and integrative therapy. The behavior of therapists who are therapeutic in the face of such client behavior is of special interest for therapy training and for building new models. Peer-nominated expert therapists could be studied for their decisions at such choice points.

In the research programs we envision, it becomes imperative to have a well-developed model of the treatments and processes to be studied (Goldfried & Safran, 1986). As Greenberg (1991) has argued, for research to lead to solid knowledge about the process of change, we need to engage extensively in discovery, which involves, as he says,

thought experiments, observations, prestudies, and unsuccessful initial experiments by which the scientist discovers the fuller meaning of the initial insight and the contexts in which the hypothesized relationship does and does not hold. (p. 6)

Therefore our major recommendations are twofold: first, that theoretical and clinical writers on psychotherapy integration develop their ideas specifically enough to encourage empirical observations, and second, that those who engage in empirical work develop their concepts, models, and measures sufficiently in a discovery phase before moving into costly experimentation and verification.

REFERENCES

Arkowitz, H. (1991, August). *Psychotherapy integration: Bringing psychotherapy back to psychology.* Paper presented at the meeting of the American Psychological Association, San Francisco.

Arkowitz, H. (1992a). A common factors therapy for depression. In J. C. Norcross & M. R. Goldfried (Eds.), *Handbook of psychotherapy integration* (pp. 394–424). New York: Basic Books.

Arkowitz, H. (1992b). Integrative theories of therapy. In D. K. Freedheim (Ed.), *History of psychotherapy: A century of change* (pp. 261–303). Washington, DC: American Psychological Association.

Arnkoff, D. B. (1983). Common and specific factors in cognitive therapy. In M. J. Lambert (Ed.), *Psychotherapy and patient relationships* (pp. 85–125). Homewood, IL: Dorsey.

Arnkoff, D. B., & Glass, C. R. (1992). Cognitive therapy and psychotherapy integration. In D. K. Freedheim (Ed.), *History of psychotherapy: A century of change* (pp. 657–694). Washington, DC: American Psychological Association.

Beckham, E. E. (1990). Psychotherapy of depression research at a crossroads: Directions for the 1990s. *Clinical Psychology Review, 10,* 207–228.

Benjamin, L. S. (1974). Structural analysis of social behavior. *Psychological Review, 81,* 392–425.

Benjamin, L. S., Foster, S. W., Roberto, L. G., & Estroff, S. E. (1986). Breaking the family code: Analysis of videotapes of family interactions by structural analysis of social behavior (SASB). In L. S. Greenberg & W. M. Pinsof (Eds.), *The psychotherapeutic process: A research handbook* (pp. 391–438). New York: Guilford.

Beutler, L. E. (1990). Introduction to the special series on advances in psychotherapy process research. *Journal of Consulting and Clinical Psychology, 58,* 263–264.

Bordin, E. S. (1979). The generalizability of the psychoanalytic concept of the working alliance. *Psychotherapy: Theory, Research, and Practice, 16,* 252–260.

Butler, S. F., & Strupp, H. H. (1986). Specific and nonspecific factors in psychotherapy: A problematic paradigm for psychotherapy research. *Psychotherapy, 23,* 30–40.

Caspar, F., & Grawe, K., (1991, July). *Therapy: An application of tools or a heuristic, integrating production process?* Paper presented at the meeting of the Society for the Exploration of Psychotherapy Integration, London.

Castonguay, L. G., Goldfried, M. R., Hayes, A. M., Raue, P. J., Wiser, S. L., & Shapiro, D. A. (1990, June). *Quantitative and qualitative analyses of process-outcome data for different therapeutic approaches.* Paper presented at the meeting of the Society for Psychotherapy Research, Wintergreen, VA.

Crits-Christoph, P., & Beebe, K. (1988, June). *Quality of cognitive therapy, alliance and the outcome of cognitive therapy with opiate addicts.* Paper presented at the meeting of the Society for Psychotherapy Research, Santa Fe.

Cross, D., Sheehan, P., & Khan, J. (1982). Short- and long-term follow-up of clients receiving insight-oriented and behavior therapy. *Journal of Consulting and Clinical Psychology, 50,* 103–112.

DeRubeis, R. J., Hollon, S. D., Evans, M. D., & Bemis, K. M. (1982). Can psychotherapies for depression be discriminated? A systematic investigation of cognitive therapy and interpersonal therapy. *Journal of Consulting and Clinical Psychology, 50,* 744–756.

DeRubeis, R. J., Feeley, M., & Barber, J. P. (1988, June). *Facilitative conditions, adherence, client cooperation and helping alliance in cognitive therapy for depression.* Paper presented at the meeting of the Society for Psychotherapy Research, Santa Fe.

Docherty, J. P., & Fiester, S. J. (1985). The therapeutic alliance and compliance with psychopharmacology. In

American Psychiatric Association (Ed.), *Psychiatry update* (Vol. 4, pp. 607–632). Washington, DC: American Psychiatric Association Press.

Eaton, T. T., Abeles, N., & Gutfreund, M. J. (1988). Therapeutic alliance and outcome: Impact of treatment length and pretreatment symptomatology. *Psychotherapy, 25,* 536–542.

Elkin, I. (1991). Varieties of psychotherapy integration research. *Journal of Psychotherapy Integration, 1,* 27–33.

Elkin, I., Shea, M. T., Watkins, J. T., Imber, S. D., Sotsky, S. M., Collins, J. F., Glass, D. R., Pilkonis, P. A., Leber, W. R., Docherty, J. P., Fiester, S. J., & Parloff, M. B. (1989). National Institute of Mental Health Treatment of Depression Collaborative Research Program. *Archives of General Psychiatry, 46,* 971–982.

Elliott, R., & James, E. (1989). Varieties of client experience in psychotherapy: An analysis of the literature. *Clinical Psychology Review, 9,* 443–467.

Elliott, R., Hill, C. E., Stiles, W. B., Friedlander, M. L., Mahrer, A. R., & Margison, F. R. (1987). Primary therapist response modes: Comparison of six rating systems. *Journal of Consulting and Clinical Psychology, 55,* 218–223.

Fiedler, F. E. (1950). A comparison of therapeutic relationships in psychoanalytic, nondirective and Adlerian therapy. *Journal of Consulting Psychology, 14,* 436–445.

Frances, A., Sweeney, J., & Clarkin, J. (1985). Do psychotherapies have specific effects? *American Journal of Psychotherapy, 39,* 159–174.

Frank, J. D. (1973). *Persuasion and healing* (rev. ed.). New York: Schocken Books.

Frank, J. D. (1978). Expectation and therapeutic outcome—The placebo effect and the role induction interview. In J. D. Frank, R. Hoehn-Saric, S. D. Imber, B. L. Liberman, & A. R. Stone, *Effective ingredients of successful psychotherapy* (pp. 1–34). New York: Brunner/Mazel.

Frank, J. D. (1982). Therapeutic components shared by all psychotherapies. In J. H. Harvey & M. M. Parks (Eds.), *The master lecture series. Vol. 1. Psychotherapy research and behavior change* (pp. 9–37). Washington, DC: American Psychological Association.

Frieswyk, S. H., Allen, J. G., Colson, D. B., Coyne, L., Gabbard, G. O., Horwitz, L., & Newsom, G. (1986). Therapeutic alliance: Its place as a process and outcome variable in dynamic psychotherapy research. *Journal of Consulting and Clinical Psychology, 54,* 32–38.

Fuller, F., & Hill, C. E. (1985). Counselor and helpee perceptions of counselor intentions in relation to outcome in a single counseling session. *Journal of Counseling Psychology, 32,* 329–338.

Garfield, S. L. (1980). *Psychotherapy: An eclectic approach.* New York: Wiley.

Garfield, S. L. (1989). *The practice of brief psychotherapy.* New York: Pergamon Press.

Gaston, L. (1990). The concept of the alliance and its role in psychotherapy: Theoretical and empirical considerations. *Psychotherapy, 27,* 143–153.

Gaston, L. (1991). Reliability and criterion-related validity of the California Psychotherapy Alliance Scales—Patient Version. *Psychological Assessment, 3,* 68–74.

Gaston, L., & Ring, J. M. (1992). Preliminary results on the Inventory of Therapeutic Strategies. *Journal of Psychotherapy Practice and Research, 1,* 135–146.

Gaston, L., Marmar, C. R., Thompson, L. W., & Gallagher, D. (1988). Relation of patient pretreatment characteristics to the therapeutic alliance in diverse psychotherapies. *Journal of Consulting and Clinical Psychology, 56,* 483–489.

Gaston, L., Marmar, C. R., Gallagher, D., & Thompson, L. W. (1991). Alliance prediction of outcome beyond in-treatment symptomatic change as psychotherapy processes. *Psychotherapy Research, 1,* 104–113.

Gelso, C. J., & Carter, J. A. (1985). The relationship in counseling and psychotherapy: Components, consequences, and theoretical antecedents. *The Counseling Psychologist, 13,* 155–243.

Glass, C. R., & Arnkoff, D. B. (1988). Common and specific factors in client descriptions of and explanations for change. *Journal of Integrative and Eclectic Psychotherapy, 7,* 427–440.

Goldfried, M. R. (1980). Toward the delineation of therapeutic change principles. *American Psychologist, 35,* 991–999.

Goldfried, M. R. (1991). Research issues in psychotherapy integration. *Journal of Psychotherapy Integration, 1,* 5–25.

Goldfried, M. R., & Padawer, W. (1982). Current status and future directions in psychotherapy. In M. R. Goldfried (Ed.), *Converging themes in psychotherapy* (pp. 3–49). New York: Springer.

Goldfried, M. R., & Safran, J. D. (1986). Future directions in psychotherapy integration. In J. C. Norcross (Ed.), *Handbook of eclectic psychotherapy* (pp. 463–483). New York: Brunner/Mazel.

Gomes-Schwartz, B. (1978). Effective ingredients in psychotherapy: Prediction of outcome from process variables. *Journal of Consulting and Clinical Psychology, 46,* 1023–1035.

Greenberg, L. S. (1984). Task analysis: The general approach. In L. N. Rice & L. S. Greenberg (Eds.), *Patterns of change: Intensive analysis of psychotherapy process* (pp. 124–148). New York: Guilford.

Greenberg, L. S. (1986). Research strategies. In L. S. Greenberg & W. M. Pinsof (Eds.), *The psychotherapeutic process: A research handbook* (pp. 707–734). New York: Guilford.

Greenberg, L. S. (1991). Research on the process of change. *Psychotherapy Research, 1,* 3–16.

Greenberg, L. S., & Pinsof, W. M. (Eds.). (1986). *The psychotherapeutic process: A research handbook.* New York: Guilford.

Greenberg, L. S., & Webster, M. C. (1982). Resolving decisional conflict by Gestalt two-chair dialogue: Relating process to outcome. *Journal of Counseling Psychology, 29,* 468–477.

Grencavage, L. M., & Norcross, J. C. (1990). Where are the commonalities among the therapeutic common factors? *Professional Psychology: Research and Practice, 21,* 372–378.

Haaga, D. A. (1986). A review of the common principles approach to integration of psychotherapies. *Cognitive Therapy and Research, 10,* 527–538.

Hardy, G., & Shapiro, D. A. (1985). Therapist response modes in prescriptive vs. exploratory psychotherapy. *British Journal of Clinical Psychology, 24,* 235–246.

Heine, R. W. (1953). A comparison of patients' reports on psychotherapeutic experience with psychoanalytic, nondirective and Adlerian therapists. *American Journal of Psychotherapy, 7,* 16–23.

Henry, W. P., Schacht, T. E., & Strupp, H. H. (1986). Structural Analysis of Social Behavior: Application to a study of interpersonal process in differential psychotherapeutic outcome. *Journal of Consulting and Clinical Psychology, 54,* 27–31.

Henry, W. P., Schacht, T. E., & Strupp, H. H. (1990). Patient and therapist introject, interpersonal process, and differential psychotherapy outcome. *Journal of Consulting and Clinical Psychology, 58,* 768–774.

Hill, C. E. (1989). *Therapist techniques and client outcomes: Eight cases of brief psychotherapy.* New York: Sage.

Hill, C. E. (1990). Exploratory in-session process research in individual psychotherapy: A review. *Journal of Consulting and Clinical Psychology, 58,* 288–294.

Hill, C. E., & O'Grady, K. E. (1985). A list of therapist intentions: Illustrated in a single case and with therapists of varying theoretical orientations. *Journal of Counseling Psychology, 32,* 3–22.

Hill, C. E., Helms, J. E., Tichenor, V., Spiegel, S. B., O'Grady, K. E., & Perry, E. S. (1988). Effects of therapist response modes in brief psychotherapy. *Journal of Counseling Psychology, 35,* 222–233.

Hollon, S. D., DeRubeis, R. J., & Evans, M. D. (1987). Causal mediation of change in treatment for depression: Discriminating between nonspecificity and noncausality. *Psychological Bulletin, 102,* 139–149.

Horvath, A. O., & Greenberg, L. S. (1986). The development of the Working Alliance Inventory. In L. S. Greenberg & W. M. Pinsof (Eds.), *The psychotherapeutic process: A research handbook* (pp. 529–556). New York: Guilford.

Horvath, A. O., & Greenberg, L. S. (1989). Development and validation of the Working Alliance Inventory. *Journal of Counseling Psychology, 36,* 223–233.

Horvath, A. O., & Symonds, B. D. (1991). Relation between working alliance and outcome in psychotherapy: A meta-analysis. *Journal of Counseling Psychology, 38,* 139–149.

Horvath, P. (1988). Placebos and common factors in two decades of psychotherapy research. *Psychological Bulletin, 104,* 214–225.

Imber, S. D., Pilkonis, P. A., Sotsky, S. M., Elkin, I., Watkins, J. T., Collins, J. F., Shea, M. T., Lever, W. R., & Glass, D. R. (1990). Mode-specific effects among three treatments for depression. *Journal of Consulting and Clinical Psychology, 58,* 352–359.

Jones, E. E., Cumming, J. D., & Horowitz, M. J. (1988). Another look at the nonspecific hypothesis of therapeutic effectiveness. *Journal of Consulting and Clinical Psychology, 56,* 48–55.

Karasu, T. B. (1986). The specificity versus nonspecificity dilemma: Toward identifying therapeutic change agents. *American Journal of Psychiatry, 143,* 687–695.

Kazdin, A. E., & Bass, D. (1989). Power to detect differences between alternative treatments in comparative psychotherapy outcome research. *Journal of Consulting and Clinical Psychology, 57,* 138–147.

Kerr, S., Goldfried, M. R., Hayes, A. M., & Goldsamt, L. A. (1989, June). *Differences in therapeutic focus in an interpersonal-psychodynamic and cognitive-behavioral therapy.* Paper presented at the meeting of the Society for Psychotherapy Research, Toronto.

Kiesler, D. J. (1982). Interpersonal theory for personality and psychotherapy. In J. C. Anchin & D. J. Kiesler (Eds.), *Handbook of interpersonal psychotherapy* (pp. 3–24). New York: Pergamon Press.

Kiesler, D. J. (1983). The 1982 interpersonal circle: A taxonomy for complementarity in human transactions. *Psychological Review, 90,* 185–214.

Kiesler, D. J., & Watkins, L. M. (1989). Interpersonal complementarity and the therapeutic alliance: A study of relationship in psychotherapy. *Psychotherapy, 26,* 183–194.

Kokotovic, A. M., & Tracey, T. J. (1990). Working alliance in the early phase of counseling. *Journal of Counseling Psychology, 37,* 16–21.

Lambert, M. J. (1986). Implications of psychotherapy outcome research for eclectic psychotherapy. In J. C. Norcross (Ed.), *Handbook of eclectic psychotherapy* (pp. 436–462). New York: Brunner/Mazel.

Lambert, M. J., Shapiro, D. A., & Bergin, A. E. (1986). The effectiveness of psychotherapy. In S. L. Garfield & A. E. Bergin (Eds.), *Handbook of psychotherapy and behavior change* (3rd ed., pp. 157–212). New York: Wiley.

Llewelyn, S. P. (1988). Psychological therapy as viewed by clients and therapists. *British Journal of Clinical Psychology, 27,* 223–237.

Llewelyn, S. P., Elliott, R., Shapiro, D. A., Hardy, G., & Firth-Cozens, J. (1988). Client perceptions of significant events in prescriptive and exploratory periods of individual therapy. *British Journal of Clinical Psychology, 27,* 105–114.

Luborsky, L. (1976). Helping alliance in psychotherapy: The groundwork for a study of their relationship to its outcome. In J. L. Claghorn (Ed.), *Successful psychotherapy* (pp. 92–116). New York: Brunner/Mazel.

Luborsky, L., & Crits-Christoph, P. (1989). A relationship pattern measure: The Core Conflictual Relationship Theme. *Psychiatry, 52,* 250–259.

Luborsky, L., McLellan, A. T., Woody, G. E., O'Brien, C. P., & Auerbach, A. (1985). Therapist success and its determinants. *Archives of General Psychiatry, 42,* 602–611.

Luborsky, L., Crits-Christoph, P., & Mellon, J. (1986). Advent of objective measures of the transference concept. *Journal of Consulting and Clinical Psychology, 54,* 39–47.

Luborsky, L., Barber, J. P., & Crits-Christoph, P. (1990). Theory-based research for understanding the process of dynamic psychotherapy. *Journal of Consulting and Clinical Psychology, 58,* 281–287.

Mahrer, A. R. (1988). Research and clinical applications of "good moments" in psychotherapy. *Journal of Integrative and Eclectic Psychotherapy, 7,* 81–93.

Mahrer, A. R. (1989). *The integration of psychotherapies: A guide for practicing therapists.* New York: Human Sciences Press.

Mahrer, A. R., Nifakis, D. J., Abhukara, L., & Sterner, I. (1984). Microstrategies in psychotherapy: The patterning of sequential therapist statements. *Psychotherapy, 21,* 465–472.

Mahrer, A. R., Sterner, I., Lawson, K. C., & Dessaulles, A. (1986). Microstrategies: Distinctively patterned sequences of therapist statements. *Psychotherapy, 23,* 50–56.

Mahrer, A. R., Nadler, W. P., Stalikas, A., Schachter, H. M., & Sterner, I. (1988). Common and distinctive therapeutic change processes in client-centered, rational-emotive, and experiential psychotherapies. *Psychological Reports, 62,* 972–974.

Mahrer, A. R., Nadler, W. P., Sterner, I., & White, M. V. (1989). Patterns of organization and sequencing of "good moments" in psychotherapy sessions. *Journal of Integrative and Eclectic Psychotherapy, 8,* 125–139.

Marmar, C. R. (1990). Psychotherapy process research: Progress, dilemmas, and future directions. *Journal of Consulting and Clinical Psychology, 58,* 265–272.

Marmar, C. R., Horowitz, M. J., Weiss, D. S., & Marziali, E. (1986). The development of the therapeutic alliance rating system. In L. S. Greenberg & W. M. Pinsof (Eds.), *The psychotherapeutic process: A research handbook* (pp. 367–390). New York: Guilford.

Marmar, C. R., Gaston, L., Gallagher, D., & Thompson, L. W. (1989). Alliance and outcome in late-life depression. *Journal of Nervous and Mental Disease, 177,* 464–472.

Martin, J., & Stelmaczonek, K. (1988). Participants' identification and recall of important events in counseling. *Journal of Counseling Psychology, 35,* 385–390.

Martin, J., Martin, W., & Slemon, A. G. (1987). Cognitive mediation in person-centered and rational-emotive therapy. *Journal of Counseling Psychology, 34,* 251–260.

Messer, S. B., & Winokur, M. (1984). Ways of knowing and visions of reality in psychoanalytic therapy and behavior therapy. In H. Arkowitz & S. B. Messer (Eds.), *Psychoanalytic therapy and behavior therapy: Is integration possible?* (pp. 63–100). New York: Plenum Press.

Moras, K., & Strupp, H. H. (1982). Pretherapy interpersonal relations, patient's alliance, and outcome in brief therapy. *Archives of General Psychiatry, 39,* 405–409.

Nawas, M. M., Pluk, P. W. M., & Wojciechowski, F. L. (1985). In search of the nonspecific factors in psychotherapy: A speculative essay. In M. A. van Kalmthout, C. Schaap, & F. L. Wojciechowski (Eds.), *Common factors in psychotherapy: Essays in honor of Emeritus Professor Dr. M. M. Nawas* (pp. 1–42). Lisse, The Netherlands: Swets & Zeitlinger.

Norcross, J. C. (1988). The exclusivity myth and the equifinality principle in psychotherapy. *Journal of Integrative and Eclectic Psychotherapy, 7,* 415–421.

Omer, H., & London, P. (1988). Metamorphosis in psychotherapy: End of the systems era. *Psychotherapy, 25,* 171–184.

Orlinsky, D. E., & Howard, K. I. (1986). Process and outcome in psychotherapy. In S. L. Garfield & A. E. Bergin (Eds.), *Handbook of psychotherapy and behavior change* (3rd ed., pp. 311–381). New York: Wiley.

Parloff, M. B. (1986). Placebo controls in psychotherapy research: A sine qua non or a placebo for research problems? *Journal of Consulting and Clinical Psychology, 54,* 79–87.

Paul, G. L. (1967). Strategy of outcome research in psychotherapy. *Journal of Consulting Psychology, 31,* 109–118.

Piper, W. E., DeCarufel, F. L., & Szkrumelack, N. (1985). Patient predictors of process and outcome in short-term individual psychotherapy. *Journal of Nervous and Mental Disease, 173,* 726–731.

Prochaska, J. O. (1984). *Systems of psychotherapy: A transtheoretical analysis.* Homewood, IL: Dorsey.

Raue, P. J., Castonguay, L. G., & Goldfried, M. R. (1992). *The working alliance: A comparison of two therapies.* Manuscript submitted for publication, State University of New York at Stony Brook.

Rice, L. N., & Greenberg, L. S. (1984). *Patterns of change: Intensive analysis of psychotherapy process.* New York: Guilford.

Rogers, C. R. (1957). The necessary and sufficient conditions of therapeutic personality change. *Journal of Consulting Psychology, 21,* 95–103.

Rosenzweig, S. (1936). Some implicit common factors in diverse methods in psychotherapy. *American Journal of Orthopsychiatry, 6,* 412–415.

Rush, A. J. (1985). The therapeutic alliance in short-term directive therapies. In American Psychiatric Association (Ed.), *Psychiatry update* (Vol. 4, pp. 562–572). Washington, DC: American Psychiatric Association Press.

Russell, R. L. (Ed.). (1989). Psychotherapy process research [Special issue]. *Clinical Psychology Review, 9*(4).

Safran, J. D., & Segal, Z. V. (1990). *Interpersonal process in cognitive therapy.* New York: Basic Books.

Safran, J. D., & Wallner, L. K. (1991). The relative predictive validity of two therapeutic alliance measures in cognitive therapy. *Psychological Assessment, 3,* 188–195.

Safran, J. D., Greenberg, L. S., & Rice, L. N. (1988). Integrating psychotherapy research and practice: Modeling the change process. *Psychotherapy, 25,* 1–17.

Safran, J. D., Crocker, P., McMain, S., & Murray, P. (1990). Therapeutic alliance rupture as a therapy event for empirical investigation. *Psychotherapy, 27,* 154–165.

Salvio, M., Beutler, L. E., Wood, J. M., & Engle, D. (1992). The strength of the therapeutic alliance in three treatments for depression. *Psychotherapy Research, 2,* 31–36.

Scarr, S. (1985). Constructing psychology: Making facts and fables of our times. *American Psychologist, 40,* 499–512.

Shoham-Salomon, V. (1990). Interrelating research processes of process research. *Journal of Consulting and Clinical Psychology, 58,* 295–303.

Shoham-Salomon, V. (1991). Studying therapeutic modules precedes the integration of models. *Journal of Psychotherapy Integration, 1,* 35–41.

Sloane, R. B., Staples, F. R., Cristol, A. H., Yorkston, N. J., & Whipple, K. (1975). *Psychotherapy versus behavior therapy.* Cambridge, MA: Harvard University Press.

Smith, M. L., Glass, G. V., & Miller, T. I. (1980). *The benefits of psychotherapy.* Baltimore: Johns Hopkins University Press.

Stiles, W. B., & Shapiro, D. A. (1989). Abuse of the drug metaphor in psychotherapy process-outcome research. *Clinical Psychology Review, 9,* 521–543.

Stiles, W. B., Shapiro, D. A., & Elliott, R. (1986). "Are all psychotherapies equivalent?" *American Psychologist, 41,* 165–180.

Stiles, W. B., Shapiro, D. A., & Firth-Cozens, J. A. (1988). Verbal response mode use in contrasting psychotherapies: A within-subjects comparison. *Journal of Consulting and Clinical Psychology, 56,* 727–733.

Strupp, H. H. (1980a). Success and failure in time limited psychotherapy: A systematic comparison of two cases (Comparison 1). *Archives of General Psychiatry, 37,* 545–603.

Strupp, H. H. (1980b). Success and failure in time limited psychotherapy: A systematic comparison of two cases (Comparison 2). *Archives of General Psychiatry, 37,* 708–716.

Strupp, H. H. (1980c). Success and failure in time limited psychotherapy: With special reference to the performance of a lay counselor (Comparison 3). *Archives of General Psychiatry, 37,* 831–841.

Strupp, H. H. (1980d). Success and failure in time limited psychotherapy: Further evidence (Comparison 4). *Archives of General Psychiatry, 37,* 947–954.

Strupp, H. H. (1989). Psychotherapy: Can the practitioner learn from the researcher? *American Psychologist, 44,* 717–724.

Strupp, H. H., & Hadley, S. W. (1979). Specific vs. nonspecific factors in psychotherapy. *Archives of General Psychiatry, 36,* 1125–1136.

Wilson, G. T., & Evans, I. M. (1977). The therapist-client relationship in behavior therapy. In A. S. Gurman & A. M. Razín (Eds.), *Effective psychotherapy: A research handbook* (pp. 544–565). New York: Pergamon Press.

Wolfe, B. E., & Goldfried, M. R. (1988). Research on psychotherapy integration: Recommendations and conclusions from an NIMH workshop. *Journal of Consulting and Clinical Psychology, 56,* 448–451.

Yalom, I. D. (1985). *The theory and practice of group psychotherapy* (3rd ed.). New York: Basic Books.

Zetzel, E. R. (1956). Current concepts of transference. *International Journal of Psychoanalysis, 37,* 369–376.

CHAPTER 4

Common Factors in Psychotherapy

Joel Weinberger

DEFINITIONS AND TERMINOLOGY

The term *common factors* refers to effective aspects of treatment shared by diverse forms of psychotherapy. Theorists and researchers interested in them argue that they may be more important than are factors unique to specific treatments and hailed by advocates of these treatments to be the important change agents (see e.g., Frank, 1973). This argument is bolstered by the fact that whereas psychotherapy has been shown to lead to beneficial effects, rarely has any specific type of treatment been shown to be superior to any other (Lambert, Shapiro, & Bergin, 1986; Luborsky, Singer, & Luborsky, 1975; Smith, Glass, & Miller, 1980; Stiles, Shapiro, & Elliot, 1986). If the multitude of different systems examined in these reviews can legitimately claim equal success, and it seems that they can, then maybe their diversity is illusory and they share core features which, in fact, are the curative elements responsible for therapeutic success (cf. Lambert, 1986).

Some writers have referred to what I have just termed common factors as "nonspecific" effects, probably to tie them in with the placebos studied in medical research (see e.g., Rosenthal & Frank, 1956). In such research, investigators are only interested in effects that are unique or specific to the procedure or medication they are testing. Any effects not directly attributable to these variables are of no interest. They test for this via placebo control groups. Differences between the experimental and the placebo groups are attributed to the medication or procedure. Similarities in the two groups are attributed to psychological variables and are termed *placebo* or *nonspecific effects* and indicate that the procedure or medication is ineffective. (For reviews of the placebo literature see Shapiro & Morris, 1978; and Turner, Gallimore, & Fox-Henning, 1980). In psychotherapy, however, the picture is quite different. It is exactly the psychological aspect of treatment that is of interest (cf. Parloff, 1986). Further, the term *specific* has come to be used to refer to technique variables, whereas *nonspecific* most often means the therapeutic relationship (Strupp, 1970, 1974; Strupp & Hadley, 1979). This usage would preclude discussion of common therapeutic techniques. Finally, the term *nonspecific* is actually a misnomer (cf. Kazdin, 1979; Wilkins, 1979, 1984). So-called nonspecific effects are actually quite specific; they

Joel Weinberger • Derner Institute of Advanced Psychological Studies, Adelphi University, Garden City, New York 11530.

Comprehensive Handbook of Psychotherapy Integration, edited by George Stricker and Jerold R. Gold. Plenum Press, New York, 1993.

can be identified and empirically investigated as Frank (1973, 1982) has done. For these reasons, the term *common factors* is employed throughout this chapter (cf. Critelli & Neumann, 1984).

EARLY EFFORTS TO IDENTIFY COMMON FACTORS

The idea that common factors exist and that they are activated in diverse treatments is not a new one. The first serious treatise on this subject was a paper published by Rosenzweig (1936) who wondered whether the factors alleged to be operating in particular types of therapy were, in fact, the relevant ameliorative factors. He pointed out that, in addition to these identified factors, unrecognized events exist that may be even more critical to therapeutic progress. Moreover, he suggested that these factors may be common to different forms of therapy.

The factors identified by Rosenzweig as cutting across the various schools of therapy were:

1. The *therapeutic relationship*, conceptualized as a means of socially conditioning (or reconditioning) the patient.
2. Provision of a *systematic ideology or rationale* to help explain the patient's condition and the means for improving it. This functions to replace a possibly confused state of mind with a plausible understanding of the problems that brought the person in for treatment. Rosenzweig even suggested that the objective truth or falsity of this rationale was not as important as its believability and systematic nature.[1]
3. *Change may be initiated from any of a number of starting points* and alteration of any one area of functioning can have a synergistic effect on other areas. That is, an approach need not be comprehensive. As long as it can affect some aspect of the personality, the interdependence of the personality subsystems would communicate this effect to each other and to the personality as a whole.
4. The *therapist's personality* may have an important influence that is independent of

treatment modality. A stimulating, inspiring therapist may be able to effect change regardless of what form of treatment is practiced. That is, some therapists are simply good and no type of therapy has a monopoly on them.

All of Rosenzweig's ideas remain relevant today. His identification of the therapeutic relationship and rationale were taken into the influential model developed by Frank (1973, 1982) discussed below. The ideas about the therapist's inspiring qualities and interrelationships within the patient's personality have not been followed up as much as they should have been (although recent work on the self is beginning to get at the latter issue—see Curtis, 1991). Even the quote from *Alice in Wonderland* with which Rosenzweig opened his paper: "At last the Dodo said, 'Everybody has won and *all* must have prizes.'" (p. 1), has served as a metaphor for therapy outcome research (Luborsky *et al.*, 1975), as well as for Jerome Frank's (1973) influential common factors model, and has been termed the "Dodo Verdict" (Stiles *et al.*, 1986).

Rosenzweig's (1936) intriguing ideas lay fallow for years. In 1940, the results of a meeting held to ascertain areas of agreement among therapeutic systems were reported by Watson. The participants (Rosenzweig was one) concluded that support, interpretation, insight, behavior change, a good therapeutic relationship, and some therapist characteristics were common features of successful treatment across different schools (see Sollod, 1981). But nothing much more came of this.

The next major step may have been a paper by Alexander and French (1946) wherein they coined the term "corrective emotional experience" (CEE). This referred to having the patient behave in ways that he or she may have previously avoided so that he or she could realize that feared consequences do not occur. Originally, the CEE was placed within a psychoanalytic context. Alexander (1963) later explicitly expanded the notion of the CEE to learning theory. Thus, it was put forth as a factor common to both psychoanalysis and learning theory-based treatments.

In Dollard and Miller's (1950) attempt to combine psychoanalysis with learning theory—to be more accurate, they tried to translate psychoanalysis into learning theory terms—they saw

[1]This parallels the notion of narrative versus historical truth described by Spence (1982).

therapist factors as critical to therapeutic success. They identified such factors as differential approval, the calm and general permissiveness conveyed, and the support given to the patient to confront his or her fears. Also in 1950, Fiedler found greater similarity among experienced therapists of different schools than among beginners. He concluded that with increased practice, therapists became more alike. That is, they discovered for themselves what was effective and changed their approach to be more in line with their experiences. In the terminology being used here, they independently gravitated toward increased use of common factors. Fiedler's findings reflect what has come to be called the "therapeutic underground" (Klein, Dittman, Parloff, & Gill, 1969; Wachtel, 1977). This is a reference to the possibility that there are informal, perhaps unspoken, observations on what is clinically effective that never reach the literature, which continue to espouse other, more theoretically "pure," techniques.

Work on common factors continued to appear sporadically throughout the 1950s. Heine (1953) compared psychoanalysis, nondirective client-centered therapy, and Adlerian therapy. He concluded that psychotherapeutic progress was attributable to factors common to all three schools. He recommended that research should attempt to identify and describe the nature of these factors, but this challenge was not immediately taken up. Garfield (1957) identified a sympathetic non-moralizing healer, a supportive therapeutic relationship, catharsis, and an opportunity to gain an understanding of the problems besetting the patient as critical factors that cut across the different treatment modalities.

THE WORK OF JEROME FRANK

The work described thus far was sporadic. Articles by various authors were rarely followed up. There was no systematic, programmatic research on common factors. This scene changed with the pioneering and extremely influential work of Jerome Frank and his colleagues (Frank, 1973—first published in 1961, 1982). In his classic book "Persuasion and Healing" (Frank, 1961, revised ed., 1973), Frank defined treatment as any attempt to enhance a person's sense of well-being. The manner in which this is done is societally and technologically determined. Treatment always involves a personal relationship between a healer and a sufferer. This healer is usually socially trained and sanctioned. When the treatment relies primarily on the healer's use of psychological means to mobilize healing forces in the sufferer, it may be termed *psychotherapy*.

Frank further defined psychotherapy as having the following three characteristics. As stated above, there is a trained socially sanctioned healer whose healing powers are accepted by the sufferer and by his or her social group (or at least an important segment of it). Next, there must, of course, be a sufferer who seeks relief from the healer. Finally, there is a circumscribed, more or less structured, series of contacts between the sufferer and the healer. Through these contacts, the healer tries to produce certain changes in the sufferer's emotional state, attitudes, and behavior. These efforts at inducing change are primarily exercised through the use of words, acts, and rituals in which both the healer and the sufferer participate. The healer, the sufferer, and society at large all believe that these procedures will lead to helpful changes.

Frank avers that when a person enters psychotherapy he or she is in a "demoralized" state. Because the person believes that the therapist can be of service, he or she has "hope." This sets up an "expectation" that things will improve. This expectation, in and of itself, is ameliorative. Frank, Gliedman, Imber, Stone, and Nash (1959) provided support for this notion. They showed that patients improve *prior* to administration of a placebo. Similarly, Frank, Nash, Stone, and Imber (1963) found that patients expecting treatment showed improvement on mood measures before treatment took place. And Friedman (1963) found that patients improved following an evaluation interview. Presumably, these findings are attributable to expectations of or hope for improvement. Hope also makes it easier for a sufferer to enter previously avoided situations and to try out new ways of dealing with problems; self-exploration may also be encouraged by hope (Brady et al., 1980). In these ways, hope may lead to a corrective emotional experience (CEE).

Investigators working independently of Frank have also demonstrated the importance of expectancies. Marcia, Rubin, and Efran (1969) and

Leitenberg, Agras, Barlow, and Oliveau (1969) found that expectancies played a role in behavioral treatments. A review by Gomes-Schwartz, Hadley, and Strupp (1978) concluded that expectancy plays a major role in psychodynamically oriented psychotherapy outcome. Going even further, Shapiro (1981) has argued that psychotherapy effects are *entirely* due to the arousal of expectancies. Kirsch (1985) has developed a model of what he calls "response expectancy" which says pretty much the same thing. He also provides a great deal of supporting evidence from the placebo, phobia, and hypnosis literatures. Recent work by Bandura (1977, 1982, 1986, 1989) on what he termed "self-efficacy" also underlines the importance of expectancies. Bandura's work is reviewed in more detail later in this chapter.

By 1982, Frank had identified four common factors that he felt led to improved morale, presumably by strengthening hope. These are:

1. An intense, confiding *relationship* with a helper. The core of this relationship, according to Frank (see, e.g., Brady *et al.*, 1980), is the therapist's ability to inspire the patient's confidence in him or her as competent and as concerned with his or her welfare. This serves to increase expectations or hope of success, which, in turn, improves morale. Frank has gone so far as to aver that without a good relationship, any procedure will fail; with it, on the other hand, most patients and probably any procedure will succeed. Thus, Frank attributes enormous importance to the therapeutic relationship. Later in this chapter, I review recent evidence that supports this view.
2. A *healing setting*.
3. A *rationale* which includes an explanation of the person's difficulties and a method for relieving it. Frank (1973, 1982) has referred to this rationale as a "myth" to highlight the fact that its objective reality is less important than its believability. The explanations embodied in the rationale or myth are held to provide the patient with a framework through which he or she can better understand his or her personal distress. That is, such a framework can confer meaning to previously inexplicable ex-

periences. This new framework carries with it the implicit understanding that change is possible and even likely. This then enhances hope.
4. A set of *prescribed treatments* or "rituals," as Frank often calls them, for alleviating the problem. This takes the myth or rationale out of the hypothetical to provide concrete prescriptions derived from the myth for alleviating the difficulties. Participation in such rituals, if believed, enhances expectations of relief because the patient is actually doing something about his or her problems. To the extent that the experiences provided by these techniques lead to actual mastery or success experiences, self-esteem and morale are further enhanced.

Frank's model has much in common with and serves to support the thoughts of Rosenzweig that were reviewed earlier. That is, like Rosenzweig, Frank places great importance on the therapeutic relationship and on the inspiring qualities of the therapist. Additionally, both theorists espouse a systematic ideology, rationale, or myth for explaining and alleviating the patient's suffering. The difference is that Frank has expanded on and operationalized the constructs set forth by Rosenzweig and has cited empirical data in support of them. Moreover, he has proposed a dynamic through which these factors achieve their success, namely, through expectation of success or hope which then leads to improved morale. He has provided evidence supportive of his views here as well. In summary, Frank has argued that people seek treatment because they are demoralized. He has proposed a common structure for treating such people psychologically. It consists of a close relationship, a rationale or myth that makes sense of suffering and improvement, and a set of prescribed rituals for alleviating suffering. All of these work by instilling hope which then improves morale.

Frank did not limit his model to psychotherapy. He also applied it to attitude change, political indoctrination, and even to so-called primitive and religious healing. Colijn and Sollod (1990) offered a dramatic example of this latter application. They compared traditional healing in Sri Lanka, which involves demonology, with psychoanalytic psychotherapy. They showed that all of the factors identified by Frank were formally present in both, even though the content and procedures of the two forms of healing were radically different. Frank's model therefore represents a set of common factors that must be taken quite seriously.

THE EMERGENCE OF COMMON FACTORS AS A MAJOR TREND IN THINKING ABOUT THERAPY

Despite the work of Frank and others (see Goldfried, 1982, for a reprinting of many articles referring to common factors), the features shared by all treatments were still relatively neglected through the mid-1970s (Frank, 1976). Just a few years later, however, Bergin (1982) could state that the identification of common factors across therapeutic perspectives was one of the most significant trends in therapy research and thinking to emerge in the 1980s. Similarly Arkowitz (1989), Beitman, Goldfried, and Norcross (1989), and Norcross (1986) could hail the common-factors approach as one of the major thrusts of the psychotherapy integration movement.

I believe that two sets of events account for this change. They are the emergence of efforts at rapprochement between diverse schools of psychotherapy and the findings of various well-conducted psychotherapy outcome reviews. The two are intimately related. I briefly discuss psychotherapy outcome research first.

As stated at the beginning of this chapter, psychotherapy outcome studies generally show that no form of therapy is superior to any other. Probably the most influential such review was the comprehensive meta-analysis conducted by Smith *et al.* (1980). On the basis of analyzing 475 studies, these investigators came up with an average effect size of .85. This means that the average person who undergoes psychotherapy is better off than 80% of untreated controls. More germane to the issue of common factors, Smith *et al.* also found no real differences between different treatment approaches. This led them to conclude that the evidence greatly favors a general factor interpretation of psychotherapeutic effectiveness. Subsequent meta-analyses supported this conclusion (e.g., Shapiro & Shapiro, 1982). This lent credence

to earlier non-meta-analytic reviews that also found no substantive differences between different modes of treatment (e.g., Luborsky *et al.*, 1975) and to well-conducted individual studies (e.g., Sloane, Staples, Cristol, Yorkston, & Whipple, 1975) reporting the same result.

Parallel to this development and partly fueled by it is the fact that in the 1970s, the issue of rapprochement between different therapeutic modalities had gained momentum and had begun to develop into a clearly delineated area of study (Goldfried, 1982).[2] Interest became so widespread that an organization, termed the Society for the Exploration of Psychotherapy Integration (SEPI), was formed to focus on issues related to such rapprochement. In such an atmosphere, it is not surprising that attention to common factors has expanded. In short, the Zeitgeist has changed and the time is ripe for exploration of these issues. This development is not an unmixed blessing, however. Different writers have focused on different domains or levels of treatment. This has led to diverse conceptualizations of how these commonalities should be thought of as well as to different lists of common factors (Karasu, 1986; Lambert, 1986). As a result, there has been a veritable explosion in proposed common factors (cf. Patterson, 1989). Moreover, the trend is expanding. There is a positive relationship between year of publication and number of commonalities and change processes being proposed (Grencavage & Norcross, 1990).

Unfortunately, this embarrassment of riches is not usually based on empirical research. In most cases, a writer reports what he or she does or observes in the treatment session. Although gathering all of these ideas is fine for the discovery phase of the scientific enterprise, there must be some way of winnowing them down so that the justification part of science can determine their truth or falsity (see Reichenbach, 1938, for the philosophy of science view on discovery and justification). Two papers have offered partial solutions to this winnowing process. The first is a theoretical paper (Goldfried, 1980); the second employs a purely empirical approach (Grencavage & Norcross, 1990).

Goldfried (1980) conceptualized the task of

[2]Wachtel's (1977) classic book on integrating psychoanalysis and behavior therapy was a major force in this movement.

looking for common factors as best thought of in terms of *levels of abstraction* from what is directly observable. Furthest removed from actual observation is the theoretical framework and accompanying philosophical stance that seeks to explain how and why change takes place, in the context of a model of human functioning. Goldfried concluded that rapprochement at this level is not yet possible because we do not yet have an agreed upon model of personality or human functioning. The lowest level of abstraction, the one closest to actual observations, involves the therapeutic techniques actually employed in treatment. Goldfried rejects this as well because he feels that the similarities yielded at this level would be trivial.

Between these two extreme levels of abstraction lies the level favored by Goldfried, which he calls the level of *clinical strategies*. He argues that any such strategy that emerges across varying orientations is likely to be robust and genuine since it survived the distortions imposed by clinicians' varying theoretical biases. These strategies can then function as clinical heuristics that implicitly guide the therapist's treatment efforts.

Goldfried goes on to say that such strategies need to be investigated empirically. Studies would focus on tactics best suited to providing the relevant experiences, the optimal nature and number of such experiences, and their interactions with other relevant variables. When a particular strategy receives this kind of empirical support, it would be upgraded to a *principle of change*.

An example of efforts to describe common factors at the intermediate level of abstraction recommended by Goldfried is the work of Orlinsky and Howard (1987). They argued that any theory of psychotherapy must include an explication of five components (see below) as well as their interrelationships. Moreover, their comprehensive review of psychotherapy process research (Orlinsky & Howard, 1986) indicated what the extant research had to say about each of these components.

The first component identified by Orlinsky and Howard is the therapeutic *contract*. This defines the purpose, format, terms, and limits of psychotherapy. The most effective therapeutic contract calls for collaboration between patient and therapist. More specifically, this translates into therapist encouragement of patient initiative

and patient assumption of an active role in resolving his or her problems.

The next component is termed therapeutic *interventions*. These comprise the official "business" of therapy, carried out under the terms of the therapeutic contract. Therapeutic interventions found to be effective include confrontation, immediacy of affective expression (together these sound like the aforementioned CEE), and therapist skillfulness.

The therapeutic *bond* is next. This is said to be an emergent aspect of the relationship that forms between the patient and therapist as they become involved with each other and perform their respective roles in treatment. Orlinksy and Howard attribute a great deal of importance to this factor. Empirical findings related to this variable are discussed in some detail later in this chapter. Orlinsky and Howard's findings are also reviewed there.

Orlinsky and Howard also discuss what they term *patient-self relatedness*. This refers to the manner in which the patient experiences and manages his or her thoughts, feelings, and self-definitions in treatment. It can be boiled down to openness versus defensiveness. The research shows that openness (or lack of defensiveness) is strongly and positively related to outcome.

Finally, Orlinsky and Howard discuss therapeutic *realizations* which are the helpful impacts generated within the therapeutic sessions. Not surprisingly, these within-session positive changes turn out to be associated with outcome.

The scheme proposed by Orlinsky and Howard makes intuitive sense. Moreover, they have reviewed empirical evidence that fills in some of the critical factors that make up these components. A caveat must be offered, however. Their 1986 review is in box-score rather than meta-analytic form. That is, it consists of a simple count of positive and negative findings with no regard for effect sizes. Bergin (1971) pointed out the potential problems of such box-score reviews. Most of these were resolved with the advent of meta-analysis which provides an objective and statistically valid way of determining the reliability and strength of effects (cf. Weinberger, 1985). Until such time as a meta-analysis confirms the Orlinsky and Howard review, their conclusions cannot be considered to have been conclusively demonstrated.

Grencavage and Norcross (1990) had a different approach to the multiplicity of common factors being proposed. They collected articles concerned with common factors and then simply counted the number of times each common factor was discussed. The most consensually agreed upon commonalities were, in order of their frequency:

1. The development of a *therapeutic alliance*.
2. The opportunity for *catharsis* or ventilation of problems.
3. The *acquisition and practice of new behaviors*. This involves patients' attempting behaviors that they heretofore feared or never thought of. It parallels the CEE originally proposed by Alexander (1963; Alexander & French, 1946).
4. Patient positive *expectations* and hope for improvement.
5. Beneficial *therapist qualities*, particularly the therapist's ability to cultivate hope and enhance the patient's positive expectancies.
6. Provision of a *rationale* that provides a plausible explanation for the patient's problems as well as procedures for resolving them.

As Grencavage and Norcross (1990) realize, all they have established is consensus. For the most part, authors merely asserted, on the basis of their clinical experience, that these variables were critical. There was little empirical research to back up these claims. Until such research is conducted, these factors must be considered tentative or in the language of the philosophy of science (Reichenbach, 1938), not yet justified. In Goldfried's terminology they are clinical strategies rather than principles of change. Nonetheless, this work helps tell the researcher where to look in the welter of proposed common factors. Moreover these factors support Goldfried's (1980) notion that the most fruitful level of abstraction for common factors is somewhere intermediate between global theories and specific techniques.

EMPIRICAL RESEARCH

In this section, I review some of the empirical work supporting the common factors identified by Grencavage and Norcross (1990). There is vir-

tually none that looks specifically at provision of a therapeutic rationale, although Frank makes a good case for it. There is, however, some suggestive work on interpretation that provides indirect support for this notion. Thus, Mendel (1964) offered the same six general interpretations to four patients. In 20/24 instances, the patients showed a decrease in anxiety level following one of these interpretations. If all that is necessary for an interpretation to work is that it be plausible, then perhaps the same can be said for psychotherapy as a whole. Nonetheless, this remains to be supported for an overall therapeutic rationale.[3] That leaves the therapeutic relationship, expectations for change, therapist qualities, catharsis, and practice of new behaviors. Included in the section on expectation, I review the relatively recent and highly influential self-efficacy model of Albert Bandura (1977, 1982, 1986, 1989). I combine the factors of catharsis and the acquisition and practice of new behaviors because they seem to form the CEE discussed by Alexander. I also add an additional variable not discussed by Grencavage and Norcross (1990) because its systematic investigation has begun very recently, although it has long been mentioned in the literature (see e.g., Strupp & Hadley, 1979). This is the area of *values*.

The Therapeutic Relationship

The therapeutic relationship was the variable that came up most often in the Grencavage and Norcross (1990) survey, specifically in the form of the *therapeutic alliance* (sometimes referred to as the "working alliance"). All views of the therapeutic alliance, despite some differences, see it as a collaboration between therapist and patient (Gaston, 1990). The alliance is often thought to be activated through therapist manifestations of some variant of the Rogerian (Rogers, 1951, 1957b) triad of unconditional positive regard, accurate empathy, and genuineness. But reviews of research (e.g., Beutler, Crago, & Arizmendi, 1986; Orlinsky & Howard, 1986) have found that it is the *patient's* sense that these variables are operative rather than the therapist's or an objective ob-

---

[3]Even the idea that interpretations are interchangeable has not been definitely shown to be true. Thus, Weiss, Sampson, and the Mount Zion Research Group (1986) have demonstrated differential effectiveness of different kinds of interpretation. (Also see Silberschatz, Fretter, & Curtis, 1986.)

server's that is critical to their effectiveness. So Rogers's notion of therapist offered conditions needs to be amended to add, in effect, "as perceived by the patient."[4]

The empirical data support the importance of the therapeutic alliance (Bordin, 1979; Gaston, 1990). Whatever else they may mean, for example, the Vanderbilt I studies (Strupp & Hadley, 1979) clearly demonstrate the critical value of a positive relationship to psychotherapeutic improvement. There is also now a large body of data that shows that the alliance is an excellent predictor of therapeutic outcome (Alexander & Luborsky, 1986; Horvath & Greenberg, 1986). And Gaston's (1990) review of the alliance literature indicates that it is directly related to outcome. Similarly, there are data that show that in successful therapy there is an increase in the strength of the therapeutic bond as treatment progresses, whereas no such increase occurs in less successful treatments (Klee, Abeles, & Muller, 1990).

The empirically answerable question critical to this aspect of treatment is *what kind (or kinds) of relationship best fosters therapeutic effectiveness?* There is as yet no empirically proven answer to this question, although psychodynamic and humanistic writers have offered clinical and theoretical guesses. Depending on whom you read, psychoanalysts have implicated a sense of being

provided for (the therapist will take care of me), a safe haven (the therapist will protect me), a solid base (life is predictable here) and/or an opportunity to merge with a nurturing parenting figure (Lachmann, 1971; Silverman, 1979). Humanists have referred to safety, absence of threat, and complete freedom to make choices and decisions (Rogers, 1957a, 1958). Of course, these are not mutually exclusive. Any combination of these may be operative in treatment. Moreover, different patients may fare better in different types of therapeutic relationships (cf. Blatt, in press). Future empirical research must address these issues.

Expectancy

I reviewed some of this evidence earlier in this chapter when discussing Frank's work. Here I discuss the more recent work of Albert Bandura (1977, 1982, 1986, 1989) on self-efficacy.

Self-Efficacy. Bandura (1977) defined self-efficacy as the belief or expectation that one is able to execute a behavior upon which reinforcement is contingent. It is concerned with judgments of how well a person can execute the actions required to deal with prospective situations. In line with the common factors we have been discussing, it is an *expectation* that the person holds that he or she can successfully perform some behavior(s). These expectations are held to be a function of direct and vicarious experiences, social influences, and logical thinking (Bandura, 1982, 1986, 1989). There are two major differences between the types of expectations discussed earlier and Bandura's self-efficacy expectations. First, the former were typically global, concerning generally favorable therapeutic outcomes, whereas the latter involved detailed assessments of expectations concerning specific behaviors. Second, the expectations discussed earlier were assessed (or inferred) before therapy began, whereas self-efficacy expectations were measured at both the beginning and end of treatment so that changes in them could be mapped.

Research (see Bandura, 1982, 1986, 1989) has revealed that a person's judgments concerning his or her self-efficacy determine whether he or she will initiate a behavior, how much effort he or she will expend on it, and how long he or she will persist at it in the face of obstacles or aversive

---

[4]This notion that patient perception is more important than actual therapist behavior brings to mind transference, an aspect of the therapeutic relationship not identified by Grencavage and Norcross (1990) as a common factor. Transference does not accurately reflect the actual ongoing relationship-oriented events occurring in treatment, as does the therapeutic alliance. It is rather a misconstrual of these events. The patient misunderstands the present in terms of the past and "transfers" past attitudes to the present (Fenichel, 1945). The distortions inherent in the transference provide the therapist with the opportunity to directly observe the past of the patient as it manifests itself in the present and thereby to understand the development and expression of the patient's conflicts.

Even though the Grencavage and Norcross review did not find transference to be a frequently discussed common factor, there is now solid empirical work on this phenomenon. Thus, Luborsky and his associates (Luborsky, Crits-Christoph, & Mellon, 1986) have developed a measure for assessing transferential issues which they term the "core conflictual relationship theme" method. Similarly, Strupp and Binder (1984) have employed the structural analysis of social behavior (Benjamin, 1984) for assessing transferential issues in their short-term dynamic psychotherapy. Examination of transference phenomena might prove fruitful for those interested in common factors (cf. Weinberger, 1990a,b, 1991).

experiences. The higher the level of self-efficacy, the higher the performance accomplishment and the lower the emotional arousal associated with performance efforts. Self-efficacy also predicts relapse of maladaptive behaviors like smoking (e.g., Candiotte & Lichtenstein, 1981). Investigations supporting the self-efficacy model have been conducted in the areas of social behavior, phobia, stress responses and physiological arousal, self-regulation of addictive behaviors, achievement striving, physical stamina, and career choice and development (Bandura, 1982, 1986, 1989). In all of this work, perceived self-efficacy was shown to be a better predictor of subsequent behavior than actual performance attainment. This supports the notion advanced by Bandura that people are more influenced by how they read their performance than by the performance itself. That is, the expectation set up by a performance is more critical to predicting subsequent performance than is the actual level attained.[5]

Bandura has specifically identified self-efficacy as a common factor (if not the *sine qua non*) of psychotherapy. That is, different modes of therapeutic influence are said to alter coping behavior partly by creating and strengthening self-perceptions of efficacy. Behavior then corresponds closely to the level of self-efficacy change, regardless of the method by which self-efficacy is enhanced (be it through direct experience, vicarious experience, social influence, and/or logical thinking). The higher the level of perceived self-efficacy, the greater the performance accomplishment. The patient will successfully execute tasks that fall within his or her range of perceived self-efficacy and shun or fail those that exceed his or her perceived coping capabilities.

Corrective Emotional Experience

As stated above, confrontation and immediacy of affective expression were identified by Orlinsky and Howard (1986) as related to positive outcome in psychotherapy. The Menninger Foundation Psychotherapy Research Project (Horwitz, 1974, 1976), which examined psychodynamic psychotherapy, found that corrective experiences

[5]Bandura's interpretation of his work has not been universally accepted. Some have argued that his studies have focused on too limited a domain of behavior to justify the wide-ranging relevance attributed to it (e.g., Brody, 1983).

resulted in long-lasting therapeutic changes. The largest and most systematic number of empirical investigations of this variable, however, has been undertaken by behaviorally oriented researchers in their investigations of *exposure*. Exposure can be seen as providing a CEE because the patient faces the issue troublesome to him or her and learns that it is not as devastating as imagined or feared. This work shows that the emotional component of the CEE may not be necessary, however. Exposure in and of itself seems to be ameliorative (Boudewyns & Shipley, 1983; Emmelkamp, 1986; Wilson & Davison, 1971). That is, neither increasing nor deadening anxiety altered the effectiveness of exposure (e.g., Hafner & Marks, 1976). Moreover, the trappings that often accompany exposure and that exist to control affective arousal like relaxation, graduated scenes, and so forth seem to be of lesser importance (Emmelkamp, 1982; Wolpin & Raines, 1966). This suggests that affective arousal may not be necessary for a corrective emotional experience. This result does not jibe with Orlinsky and Howard's finding that immediacy of affective expression is a positive correlate of outcome, however. It may be that affect has usually covaried with confrontation but is not necessary to its effectiveness or it may be that it has beneficial effects independent of exposure. Clearly, more research is required. Whatever the underlying means whereby the CEE works, however, it seems clear that patient's practicing of new behaviors and/or confronting fears, especially through techniques like exposure, is ameliorative.

The Therapist's Personality

Surprisingly, there is little of substance that has been empirically demonstrated as regards therapist personality attributes. In their authoritative review of therapist variables, Beutler *et al.* (1986) state: "Collectively, the influence of the therapist's personality on psychotherapy is inconclusive" (p. 271). There are some relatively well-established findings discussed by the aforementioned authors, such as that therapists with the lowest levels of emotional disturbance produced the best outcomes. Similarly, therapist expertness or competence was found to be positively related to outcome. Neither finding is particularly surprising, although they may be reassuring. Moreover, as stated earlier, the traditional Rogerian triad of therapist-provided conditions (genuineness, accurate empathy, and unconditional positive regard) has not turned out to be related to outcome unless the patient perceives that these qualities are present (Beutler *et al.*, 1986; Orlinsky & Howard, 1986). Clearly, a great deal of work is necessary in this area. As of now, very little is known.

Values

Although not identified by Grencavage and Norcross (1990), values may be something that therapists have in common and teach to their patients (London, 1986). This has only come under systematic study lately so that its investigation may have been somewhat uncommon at the time of the Grencavage and Norcross paper. In a relatively comprehensive survey study, Jensen & Bergin (1988) empirically demonstrated that therapists share a common set of values. They found this to be supported (with some exceptions, of course) across a range of helping professions, theoretical orientations, and demographic variables. Other research has shown that convergence of therapist and patient values may be associated with positive therapeutic outcome (Beutler *et al.*, 1986; Kelly, 1990). If therapists, in fact, share a common set of values, this convergence is probably toward that common set and therefore to a common outcome. In this view, common outcome is partly attributable to a shared set of values. Any common-factors model of psychotherapy will probably have to tackle the issue of values (cf. Bergin, 1983, 1985; Garfield & Bergin, 1986; Strupp & Hadley, 1977).

CREATING A COMMON-FACTORS MODEL OF PSYCHOTHERAPY

The data are inconclusive so that no definitive common-factors model can be proposed at this time. But certain features of therapy seem to come up again and again and are supported by empirical research. These can be grouped together and would have to be incorporated into any proposed common-factors model. It is apparent that the *therapeutic alliance* is a critical aspect of therapy that cuts across different treatment modalities (Gaston, 1990). *Expectations* both of outcome generally (Frank, 1973) and of specific behaviors (Bandura, 1982, 1986) are also factors that seem to be effective in different clinical contexts. The *corrective emotional experience* (CEE) generally and *exposure* particularly are clearly ameliorative, although the role of affect remains unclear.

A further issue concerns the relative importance of these factors. There are several possible ways of addressing this matter. I offer four (also see Weinberger, 1991). They fall under the headings of necessity, sufficiency, interaction, and separate roads to the same end.

First, the factors can be thought of in terms of *logical priority*. In such a conceptional scheme, the therapeutic relationship would assume the greatest importance. This is so because the relationship is necessary before the CEE can occur and possibly even before therapeutic expectancies can form (cf. Frank, 1973). This seems to be the perspective taken by those who stress the relationship as the *sine qua non* of psychotherapy (e.g. Bordin, 1979; Gaston, 1990; Strupp & Binder, 1984).

If on the other hand, the factors are looked at from the point of view of *sufficiency, expectancy* assumes the greatest importance. This is so because some research has shown that expectations can lead to improvement even in the absence of other factors. Moreover, the work of Bandura (1982, 1986, 1989) shows that expectations of success or failure (particularly when they are attributed to the self) are sufficient for lasting therapeutic change. Without positive expectations, change was shown to be ephemeral, if it occurs at all. This emphasis on sufficiency is the perspective taken by those who see expectancy and/or self-efficacy as the key to psychotherapeutic success (e.g., Bandura, 1982, 1986, 1989; Shapiro, 1981).

When the factors are seen as *interacting reciprocally*, no factor stands out as primary. All interact with one another (cf. Bandura, 1978). No one aspect of the model is more important than any other in principle; all should occur for therapy to be maximally effective. Such a view has been taken by Appelbaum (1978). He suggests that there is an interaction of factors which contribute to therapeutic effectiveness in a synergistic manner. In this conception, no factor assumes the mantle of cause or effect or even of necessity or sufficiency because all operate as part of a total configuration.

Finally, it is conceivable that any or all of the factors could operate in a particular treatment to similar effect. This was the position taken by Rosenzweig (1936) when he suggested that as long as a factor impacts on some aspect of the personality, the interdependence of the personality subsystems would communicate this effect to the personality as a whole. Thus, similar change could be initiated by any of the different common factors, either alone or in combination.

Weinberger (1990a,b, 1991) has offered a tentative common-factors model based on the extant empirical findings. He also deals with the relative importance of the common factors he proposes. The model is termed *REMA* because the proposed critical factors are the *r*elationship, *e*xposure, *m*astery, and *a*ttribution. In this model, all of the factors interact and are of equal importance. All must operate for positive change to occur and to be maintained. Thus, this model follows Appelbaum's (1978) ideas of therapeutic causation. The relationship is ameliorative in its own right but insufficient in and of itself. Exposure to critical issues is only effective in the context of a therapeutic relationship and only works if it leads to mastery experiences, which together make up a corrective emotional experience. That is, trying out a new behavior (exposure) can potentially lead to failure rather than mastery. This could then retraumatize the individual. Only when exposure leads to mastery is it therapeutically beneficial (cf. Appelbaum, 1976; Wachtel, 1975). Finally, change will last only if the patient attributes improvement to himself or herself (as opposed to the therapist and/or the treatment).

SUMMARY

A great deal of work, beginning with Rosenzweig (1936), has been conducted on common factors in psychotherapy. The most influential is probably that of Frank (1973, 1982). In recent years, this work has burgeoned. This has led to a profusion of proposed common factors. Goldfried (1980) has suggested a way to fruitfully conceptualize these factors and Grencavage and Norcross (1990) have winnowed them down to those most often written about. This chapter has indicated that there is adequate empirical support for the proposed factors of expectancies, the thera-

peutic relationship, corrective emotional experiences, and values. Provision of a rationale makes sense but there is as yet no empirical work specifically focused on it. Similarly it seems evident that the therapist's personality must be important, but this has yet to be empirically demonstrated in any meaningful way. Frank has proposed that all of these factors work through arousing hope, but this too has not yet been demonstrated. Four different ways to conceptualize the relationship of common factors to one another and to therapeutic success were offered. Finally, a tentative model of common factors based on the extant literature (Weinberger, 1990a,b, 1991) was proposed.

REFERENCES

Alexander, F. (1963). The dynamics of psychotherapy in the light of learning theory. *American Journal of Psychiatry, 120,* 440–448.

Alexander, F., & French, T. M. (1946). *Psychoanalytic psychotherapy: Principles and applications.* New York: Ronald Press.

Alexander, L., & Luborsky, L. (1986). The Penn helping alliance scales. In L. Greenberg & W. Pinsof (Eds.), *The psychotherapeutic process: A research handbook* (pp. 325–366). New York: Guilford.

Appelbaum, S. A. (1976). The dangerous edge of insight. *Psychotherapy, 13,* 202–206.

Appelbaum, S. A. (1978). Pathways to change in psychoanalytic therapy. *Bulletin of the Menninger Clinic, 42,* 239–251.

Arkowitz, H. (1989). The role of theory in psychotherapy integration. *Journal of Integrative and Eclectic Psychotherapy, 8,* 8–16.

Bandura, A. (1977). Self-efficacy: Toward a unifying theory of behavioral change. *Psychological Review, 84,* 191–215.

Bandura, A. (1978). The self system in reciprocal determinism. *American Psychologist, 33,* 344–358.

Bandura, A. (1982). Self-efficacy mechanism in human agency. *American Psychologist, 37,* 122–147.

Bandura, A. (1986). *Social foundations of thought and action.* Englewood Cliffs, NJ: Prentice-Hall.

Bandura, A. (1989). Human agency in social cognitive theory. *American Psychologist, 44,* 1175–1184.

Beitman, B. D., Goldfried, M. R., & Norcross, J. C. (1989). The movement toward integrating the psychotherapies: An overview. *American Journal of Psychiatry, 146,* 138–147.

Benjamin, L. S. (1984). Principles of prediction using structural analysis of social behavior (SASB). In R. A. Zucker, J. Aaronoff, & A. J. Rabin (Eds.), *Personality and the prediction of behavior* (pp. 121–174). New York: Academic Press.

Bergin, A. E. (1971). The evaluation of therapeutic outcomes. In A. E. Bergin & S. L. Garfield (Eds.), *Handbook of psychotherapy and behavior change* (pp. 217–270). New York: Wiley.

Bergin, A. E. (1982). *Comment on converging themes in psychotherapy.* New York: Springer.

Bergin, A. E. (1983). Values and evaluating therapeutic change. In J. Helm & A. E. Bergin (Eds.), *Therapeutic behavior modification* (pp. 9–14). Berlin, Germany: VEB Deutscher Verlag der Wissenschaften.

Bergin, A. E. (1985). Proposed values for guiding and evaluating counseling and psychotherapy. *Counseling and Values, 29,* 99–116.

Beutler, L. E., Crago, M., & Arizmendi, T. G. (1986). Research on therapist variables in psychotherapy. In S. L. Garfield & A. E. Bergin (Eds.), *Handbook of psychotherapy and behavior change* (pp. 257–310). New York: Wiley.

Blatt, S. J. (in press). The differential effect of psychotherapy on anaclitic and introjective patients. The Menninger Psychotherapy Research Project revisited. *Journal of the American Psychoanalytic Association.*

Bordin, E. S. (1979). The generalizability of the psychoanalytic concept of the working alliance. *Psychotherapy, 16,* 252–260.

Boudewyns, P. A., & Shipley, R. H. (1983). *Flooding and implosive therapy: Direct therapeutic exposure in clinical practice.* New York: Plenum Press.

Brady, J. P., Davison, G. C., Dewald, P. A., Egan, G., Fadiman, J., Frank, J. D., Gill, M. M., Hoffman, I., Kempler, W., Lazarus, A. A., Raimy, V., Rotter, J. B., & Strupp, H. H. (1980). Some views on effective principles of psychotherapy. *Cognitive Therapy and Research, 4,* 269–306.

Brody, N. (1983). *Human motivation.* New York: Academic Press.

Candiotte, M. M., & Lichtenstein, E. (1981). Self-efficacy and relapse in smoking cessation programs. *Journal of Consulting and Clinical Psychology, 49,* 648–658.

Colijn, S., & Sollod, R. N. (April 1990). *The relevance of traditional healing for psychotherapy: Content and/or context?* Paper presented at the meeting of the Society for the Exploration for Psychotherapy Integration, Philadelphia, PA.

Critelli, J. W., & Neumann, K. F. (1984). The placebo: Conceptual analysis of a construct in transition. *American Psychologist, 39,* 32–39.

Curtis, R. C. (Ed.). (1991). *The rational self.* New York: Guilford.

Dollard, J., & Miller, N,. E. (1950). *Personality and psychotherapy.* New York: McGraw-Hill.

Emmelkamp, P. M. G. (1982). *Phobic and obsessive-compulsive disorders: Theory, research, and practice.* New York: Plenum Press.

Emmelkamp, P. M. G. (1986). Behavior therapy with adults. In S. L. Garfield & A. E. Bergin (Eds.), *Handbook of psychotherapy and behavior change* (3rd ed., pp. 385–442). New York: Wiley.

Fenichel, O. (1945). *The psychoanalytic theory of neurosis.* New York: W. W. Norton.

Fielder, F. E. (1950). The concept of an ideal therapeutic relationship. *Journal of Consulting Psychology, 14,* 239–245.

Frank, J. D. (1961). *Persuasion and healing.* Baltimore, MD: Johns Hopkins University Press.

Frank, J. D. (1973). *Persuasion and healing* (rev. ed.). Baltimore, MD: Johns Hopkins University Press.

Frank, J. D. (1976). Restoration of morale and behavior change. In A. Burton (Ed.), *What makes behavior change possible?* New York: Brunner/Mazel.

Frank, J. D. (1982). Therapeutic components shared by all psychotherapies. In J. H. Harvey & M. M. Parks (Eds.), *The master lecture series (Vol 1): Psychotherapy research and behavior change* (pp. 9–37). Washington, DC: American Psychological Association.

Frank, J. D., Gliedman, L. H., Imber, S. D., Stone, A. R., & Nash, E. H. (1959). Patients' expectancies and relearning as factors determining improvement in psychotherapy. *American Journal of Psychiatry, 115,* 961–968.

Frank, J. D., Nash, E. H., Stone, A. R., & Imber, S. D. (1963). Immediate and long-term symptomatic course of psychiatric outpatients. *American Journal of Psychiatry, 120,* 429–439.

Friedman, H. J. (1963). Patient expectancy and symptom reduction. *Archives of General Psychiatry, 8,* 61–67.

Garfield, S. L. (1957). *Introductory clinical psychology.* New York: Macmillan.

Garfield, S. L., & Bergin, A. E. (1986). Introduction and historical overview. In S. L. Garfield & A. E. Bergin (Eds.), *Handbook of psychotherapy and behavior change* (3rd ed., pp. 3–22). New York: Wiley.

Gaston, L. (1990). The concept of the alliance and its role in psychotherapy: Theoretical and empirical considerations. *Psychotherapy, 27,* 143–153.

Goldfried, M. R. (1980). Toward the delineation of therapeutic change principles. *American Psychologist, 35,* 991–999.

Goldfried, M. R. (Ed.). (1982). *Converging themes in psychotherapy.* New York: Springer.

Gomes-Schwartz, B., Hadley, S. W., & Strupp, H. H. (1978). Individual psychotherapy and behavior therapy. *Annual Review of Psychology, 29,* 435–471.

Grencavage, L. M., & Norcross, J. C. (1990). What are the commonalities among the therapeutic factors? *Professional Psychology: Research and Practice, 21,* 372–378.

Hafner, R. J., & Marks, I. M. (1976). Exposure in vivo in agoraphobics: Contributions of diazepam, group exposure, and anxiety evocation. *Psychological Medicine, 6,* 71–88.

Heine, R. W. (1953). A comparison of patients' reports of psychotherapeutic experience with psychoanalytic, nondirective, and Adlerian therapists. *American Journal of Psychotherapy, 7,* 16–23.

Horvath, A. D., & Greenberg, L. S. (1986). The development of the working alliance inventory. In L. Greenberg & W. Pinsoff (Eds.), *The psychotherapeutic process: A research handbook* (pp. 529–556). New York: Guilford.

Horwitz, L. (1974). *Clinical prediction in psychotherapy.* New York: Aronson.

Horwitz, L. (1976). New perspectives for psychoanalytic psychotherapy. *Bulletin of the Menninger Clinic, 40,* 263–271.

Jensen, J. P., & Bergin, A. E. (1988). Mental health values of professional therapists: A national interdisciplinary survey. *Professional Psychology, 19,* 290–297.

Karasu, T. B. (1986). The specificity versus nonspecificity dilemma: Toward identifying therapeutic change agents. *American Journal of Psychiatry, 143,* 687–695.

Kazdin, A. E. (1979). Nonspecific treatment factors in psychotherapy outcome research. *Journal of Consulting and Clinical Psychology, 47,* 846–851.

Kelly, T. A. (1990). The role of values in psychotherapy: A critical review of process and outcome effects. *Clinical Psychology Review, 10,* 171–186.

Kirsch, I. (1985). Response expectancy as a determinant of experience and behavior. *American Psychologist, 40,* 1189–1202.

Klee, M. R., Abeles, N., & Muller, R. T. (1990). Therapeutic alliance: Early indicators, course, and outcome. *Psychotherapy, 27,* 166–174.

Klein, M., Dittman, A. T., Parloff, N. B., & Gill, M. M. (1969). Behavior therapy: Observations and reflections. *Journal of Consulting and Clinical Psychology, 33,* 259–266.

Lachmann, F. (1971). A recent development in the technique of psychanalysis: The therapeutic alliance. *Clinical Psychologist, 25,* 10–11.

Lambert, M. J. (1986). Implications of psychotherapy outcome research for eclectic psychotherapy. In J. C. Norcross (Ed.), *Handbook of eclectic psychotherapy* (pp. 436–462). New York: Brunner/Mazel.

Lambert, M. J., Shapiro, D. A., & Bergin, A. E. (1986). Evaluation of therapeutic outcomes. In S. L. Garfield & A. E. Bergin (Eds.), *Handbook of psychotherapy and behavior change* (3rd ed., pp. 157–212). New York: Wiley.

Leitenberg, H., Agras, W. S., Barlow, D. H., & Oliveau, D. C. (1969). Contribution of selective positive reinforcement and therapeutic instructions to systematic desensitization therapy. *Journal of Abnormal Psychology, 74,* 382–387.

London, P. (1986). *The modes and morals of psychotherapy* (2nd ed.). New York: Norton.

Luborsky, L., Crits-Cristoph, P., & Mellon, J. (1986). Advent of objective measures of the transference concept. *Journal of Consulting and Clinical Psychology, 54,* 39–47.

Luborsky, L., Singer, B., & Luborsky, S. (1975). Comparative studies of psychotherapies: Is it true that "Everyone has won and all must have prizes"? *Archives of General Psychiatry, 32,* 995–1008.

Marcia, J. E., Rubin, B. M., & Efran, J. S. (1969). Systematic desensitization: Expectancy change or counterconditioning? *Journal of Abnormal Psychology, 74,* 382–387.

Mendel, W. M. (1964). The phenomenon of interpretation. *American Journal of Psychoanalysis, 24,* 184–189.

Norcross, J. C. (Ed.). (1986). *Handbook of eclectic psychotherapy.* New York: Brunner/Mazel.

Orlinsky, D. E., & Howard, K. I. (1986). Process and outcome in psychotherapy. In S. L. Garfield & A. E. Bergin (Eds.), *Handbook of psychotherapy and behavior change* (3rd ed., pp. 283–330). New York: Wiley.

Orlinsky, D. E., & Howard, K. I. (1987). A generic model of psychotherapy. *Journal of Integrative and Eclectic Psychotherapy, 6,* 6–26.

Parloff, M. B. (1986). Placebo controls in psychotherapy research: A sine qua non or a placebo for research problems? *Journal of Consulting and Clinical Psychology, 54,* 79–87.

Patterson, C. H. (1989). Foundations for a systematic eclecticism in psychotherapy. *Psychotherapy, 26,* 427–435.

Reichenbach, H. (1938). *Experience and prediction.* Chicago: University of Chicago Press.

Rogers, C. (1951). *Client-centered therapy.* Boston: Houghton Mifflin.

Rogers, C. (1957a). A note on "the nature of man." *Journal of Counseling Psychology, 4,* 199–203.

Rogers, C. (1957b). The necessary and sufficient conditions of therapeutic personality change. *Journal of Consulting Psychology, 21,* 95–103.

Rogers, C. (1958). The characteristics of a helping relationship. *Personnel and Guidance Journal, 37,* 6–16.

Rosenthal, D., & Frank, J. D. (1956). Psychotherapy and the placebo effect. *Psychological Bulletin, 53,* 294–302.

Rosenzweig, S. (1936). Some implicit common factors in diverse methods of psychotherapy. *American Journal of Orthopsychiatry, 6,* 412–415.

Shapiro, A. K., & Morris, L. A. (1978). The placebo effect in medical and psychological therapies. In S. L. Garfield & A. E. Bergin (Eds.), *Handbook of psychotherapy and behavior change* (2nd ed., pp. 369–410). New York: Wiley.

Shapiro, D. A. (1981). Comparative credibility of treatment rationales: Three tests of expectancy theory. *British Journal of Clinical Psychology, 21,* 111–122.

Shapiro, D. A., & Shapiro, D. (1982). Meta-analysis of comparative therapy outcome studies: A replication and refinement. *Psychological Bulletin, 92,* 581–604.

Silberschatz, G., Fretter, P. B., & Curtis, J. T. (1986). How do interpretations influence the process of psychotherapy? *Journal of Consulting and Clinical Psychology, 54,* 646–652.

Silverman, L. H. (1979). The unconscious fantasy as therapeutic agent in psychoanalytic treatment. *Journal of the American Academy of Psychoanalysis, 7,* 189–218.

Sloane, R. B., Staples, F. R., Cristol, A. H., Yorkston, N. J., & Whipple, K. (1975). *Psychotherapy vs. behavior therapy.* Cambridge: Harvard University Press.

Smith, M. L., Glass, G. V., & Miller, F. I. (1980). *The benefits of psychotherapy.* Baltimore, MD: Johns Hopkins University Press.

Sollod, B. (1981). Goodwin Watson's 1940 conference. *American Psychologist, 36,* 1546–1547.

Spence, D. P. (1982). *Narrative truth and historical truth: Meaning and interpretation in psychoanalysis.* New York: Norton.

Stiles, W. B., Shapiro, D. A., & Elliot, R. (1986). Are all psychotherapies equivalent? *American Psychologist, 41,* 165–180.

Strupp, H. H. (1970). Specific versus nonspecific factors in psychotherapy and the problem of control. *Archives of General Psychiatry, 23,* 393–401.

Strupp, H. H. (1974). On the basic ingredients of psychotherapy. *Psychotherapy and Psychosomatics, 24,* 249–260.

Strupp, H. H., & Binder, J. L. (1984). *Psychotherapy in a new key: A guide to time-limited dynamic psychotherapy.* New York: Basic Books.

Strupp, H. H., & Hadley, S. W. (1977). A tripartite model of mental health and therapeutic outcomes. *American Psychologist, 32,* 187–196.

Strupp, H. H., & Hadley, S. W. (1979). Specific versus nonspecific factors in psychotherapy: A controlled study of outcome. *Archives of General Psychiatry, 36,* 1125–1136.

Turner, J. L., Gallimore, R., & Fox-Henning, C. (1980). An annotated bibliography of placebo research. *JSAS Catalog of Selected Documents in Psychology, 10,* 33 (Ms. No. 2063).

Wachtel, P. L. (1975). Behavior therapy and the facilitation of psychoanalytic exploration. *Psychotherapy, 12,* 68–72.

Wachtel, P. L. (1977). *Psychoanalysis and behavior therapy: Toward an integration.* New York: Basic Books.

Watson, G. (1940). Areas of agreement in psychotherapy. *American Journal of Orthopsychiatry, 10,* 698–709.

Weinberger, J. (1985). Is the meta-analysis/placebo controversy a case of new wine in old bottles? *Behavioral and Brain Sciences, 7,* 757–758.

Weinberger, J. (April, 1990a). *Application of the REMA model to psychodynamic psychotherapy.* Paper delivered at the Society for the Exploration for Psychotherapy Integration, Philadelphia, PA.

Weinberger, J. (April 1990b). *The REMA common factor model of psychotherapy.* Paper delivered at the Society for the Exploration for Psychotherapy Integration, Philadelphia, PA.

Weinberger, J. (1991). *The REMA (relationship, exposure, mas-*

tery, attribution) common factor model of psychotherapy. Unpublished manuscript, Derner Institute, Adelphi University.

Weiss, J., & Sampson, H., and the Mount Zion Research Group. (1986). *The psychoanalytic process*. New York: Guilford.

Wilkins, W. (1979). Expectancies in therapy research: Discriminating among heterogeneous nonspecifics. *Journal of Consulting and Clinical Psychology, 47,* 837–845.

Wilkins, W. (1984). Psychotherapy: The powerful placebo. *Journal of Consulting and Clinical Psychology, 52,* 570–573.

Wilson, G. T., & Davison, G. C. (1971). Processes of fear reduction in systematic desensitization: Animal studies. *Psychological Bulletin, 76,* 1–14.

Wolpin, M., & Raines, J. (1966). Visual imagery, expected roles and extinction as possible factors in reducing fear and avoidance behavior. *Behavior Research and Therapy, 4,* 25–37.

PART II

Individual Approaches

CHAPTER 5

Cyclical Psychodynamics

Jerold R. Gold and Paul L. Wachtel

INTRODUCTION

In this chapter, we will present an overview of the cyclical psychodynamic approach to psychotherapy integration (Wachtel, 1977). The cyclical psychodynamic method of psychotherapy was one of the first systems to achieve a good measure of true conceptual and methodological integration (Norcross, 1984). This approach to psychotherapy integration is based upon a theory of personality and psychopathology which is rooted in the tradition and concepts of psychodynamic theory but takes it in new directions. The cyclical approach to psychodynamics allows concepts from behavioral, cognitive, and systems approaches to be included in a contextually oriented dynamic theory and therapy.

Theoretical and Conceptual Position

Cyclical psychodynamics has at its heart key modifications of traditional psychoanalytic concepts and concerns. Chief among these are the notions of the *contextual unconscious* (Wachtel & Wachtel, 1986), the *vicious circle* (Wachtel, 1977), and the *ironic vision of neurotic conflict and behavior* (Wachtel & Wachtel, 1986). Cyclical psychodynamic theory retains from traditional psychodynamic theories emphases upon unconscious processes, motivations and conflicts, anxiety and defense, and a concern with the dynamic roots of behavior. The person's behavior is considered to be influenced significantly by these factors, which are derived from past learning and developmental experiences. However, unconscious wishes and motives are as likely to be considered *dependent variables* or to be the results of other psychological and behavioral processes as they are to be the driving forces of the personality. Such a viewpoint contrasts with the traditional psychodynamic insistence on wish and fantasy being the primary (if not only) causal factors in behavior (Wachtel, 1978a). The influence of childhood experience and motivation is understood to be mediated by a host of later experiences as well as by the developing individual's evolving character structure and the distorting effects of neurotic anxieties. Anxiety and the efforts by the patient to avoid it are placed in a central position in the development and maintenance of disturbed behavior (Wachtel, 1977).

Past and present, unconscious conflict and overt behavior, and individual and interpersonal

Jerold R. Gold • Doctoral Program in Clinical Psychology, Long Island University, Brooklyn, New York 11201. Paul L. Wachtel • Department of Psychology, City College of the City University of New York, New York, New York 10031.

Comprehensive Handbook of Psychotherapy Integration, edited by George Stricker and Jerold R. Gold. Plenum Press, New York, 1993.

context are mutually influencing and influenced. From the vantage point of cyclical psychodynamics, it is incorrect to look for simple linear causation in personality functioning and in psychopathology (Wachtel, 1977, 1978a,b, 1982). Cyclical psychodynamic theory is based upon a contextually oriented, circular model of multiple causality. The repetition of painful experiences and relationships figures heavily in this model, but, as will become apparent, is again understood from a perspective that modifies the traditional psychodynamic viewpoint.

Developmental Considerations

Traditional psychoanalytic theories hold that childhood motives, conflicts, and ties to relationships (fixations) remain present in the adult mind in their original form and exert an unmodified and powerful influence on the personality. These archaic layers of the psyche are considered to be causal in the development and maintenance of psychopathology. This has been described as the "woolly mammoth" approach to psychodynamics (Wachtel, 1977). Its image of archaic forces preserved in their original form by splits and layers of repression is reminiscent of those archaic creatures, so preserved in their original form under the protective layers of the Arctic ice.

In contrast, the prevailing cyclical psychodynamic metaphor is the circle (Wachtel, 1977, 1978a,b; Wachtel & Wachtel, 1986). In the cyclical psychodynamic view of development, the influence of the past is felt in the skewing, misshaping, or deficits of adult character, cognition, perception, and interpersonal behavior. These difficulties are derived indirectly from experiences in childhood which were anxiety laden or otherwise dysphoric. The sources of anxiety and developmental distress are interpersonal in nature. Children feel anxiety when they lose or anticipate the loss of their sense of security, well-being, and self-esteem. Such anxiety occurs in response to a real or imagined action or reaction on the part of a significant adult. Any internal experience (wish, motive, thought, or fantasy) or any way of behaving on the part of children which meets with negative consequences, such as adult disapproval, abandonment, or withdrawal of love, may become a *cue* or personal signal of impending loss of security. Such experiences and behaviors are

avoided, repressed, or disavowed by children to prevent the anticipated adult reactions, and to ward off the inner experience of anxiety. Anxiety is an interpersonal experience. Motives, wishes, and fantasies become cues for anxiety because of the *relational meaning* associated with the experience or expression of those intrapsychic states. The childhood experiences and relationships which caused anxiety do not live on in an unaltered but repressed manner impervious to new experiences. To be sure, styles and modes of perceiving, thinking, feeling, and behaving which were learned in the face of early experiences of anxiety and pain do frequently become characteristic of the person even after the original source and context of that anxiety have disappeared. However, these mental structures and contents are thought to persist only as long as the person's experience and behavior provide continuing input and reinforcement for them (Wachtel & Wachtel, 1986). Old dynamic issues, and the character structures which develop around them, remain potential sources of anxiety because the ways the person lives his or her life, and the responses to that way of life from others, make change impossible or provide new confirmation of the presence of potential losses of security.

In sum, early experience is important when the person is then disposed by current factors, and by the evolving character structure to repeat such experiences.

Vicious Circles and the Irony of Psychopathology

The ironic vision of cyclical psychodynamic theory (Wachtel, 1979, 1985) replaces the predominantly tragic vision of classical psychoanalysis (Schafer, 1976), which describes individuals as being at the mercy of forces unknown to them, and over which they have little or no control. The tragic view is most apparent in psychoanalytic theory in the concept of the repetition compulsion (Freud, 1926), which posits an instinct aimed toward death and disintegration as the inevitable and impersonal motive behind the repetition of traumatic experiences by an individual. Cyclical psychodynamics assumes that many of the most troubling effects are unintended. These unforeseen consequences become a primary reason why the person's pathology continues in an unchanged way. The patient's attempts at establishing satisfying relationships and at achieving the gratifications of what he or she experiences as a need result in consequences unforeseen and unwanted. Frequently, the patient is successful in creating an unwitting repetition of past maladaptive relationships and traumatic experiences in the very search for new and productive interactions.

Characterologically based anxiety is considered by cyclical psychodynamic theory to be at the center of this ironic and maladaptive repetition. Such anxieties are understood to be the result of the perceived threat to the patient's security which is posed by particular thoughts, images, motives, and other inner states. The person's methods of disavowing or narrowing experience to avoid feeling anxious will yield a temporary escape from anxiety and a restoration of a sense of safety. But such efforts also have the ironic result of confirming the attitudes and perceptions which caused the anxiety, placing the person in a vicious circle of vulnerability, anxiety, avoidance, security operations, and a quick return of the original sense of vulnerability. These unforeseen consequences reflect the person in conflict: consciously he or she seeks to find new and different partners and modes of interacting. Unconsciously, the person's paramount goal is the avoidance of anxiety through the disavowal or dissociation of intentions, ideas, behaviors, and self or object representations which have been linked with the loss of security. The patient's unconscious security operations will compromise or distort his or her thoughts and perceptions, as well as the overt manner of interaction, with frequently ironic results.

Security operations can produce confirmation of anxiety-generating thoughts, perceptions, and representations of self and other in at least several ways (Wachtel, 1977). Patients suffer from what Dollard and Miller (1950) call "neurotic stupidity": gaps and distortions in both conscious and unconscious thinking and problem-solving which result from the need to avoid certain ideas and areas of experience. The frequent and insistent avoidance of anxiety-generating mental contents produces a narrow, rigid, cognitive style (cf. Shapiro, 1965), which prevents persons from learning from experience. The patients repeat because they know no other course of action, and consciously believe that each new interaction or

effort will be unlike other experiences. They remain unaware of their security-seeking efforts. As a result, they are bewildered, hurt, and defeated when finding themselves in a new version of a maladaptive interaction.

The avoidance of anxiety perpetuates its existence by preventing the individual from having new experiences. New experience may demonstrate that the fearful meaning connected with any mental event is no longer accurate (Wachtel, 1977, 1978a,b). Lacking new experiences, the patient continually interprets certain inner states in the same fearful ways, ensuring that an old sense of vulnerability is renewed and reinforced without current objective reasons.

Psychopathology occurs within an interactional context in which "every neurosis requires accomplices" (Wachtel, 1977; Wachtel & Wachtel, 1986). Part of the responsibility for the maintenance of pathological vicious circles lies with the people with whom the disturbed person interacts. Other people in the patient's life usually are unwitting participants in his or her repetitive patterns, and (at least initially) do not intend to reinforce the patient's psychopathology. There are many ways in which the patient finds or creates accomplices who will provide confirmatory responses for anxiety-generating cues. Frequently, patients select others who will not require them to change, or who do not require them to interact in ways which they find anxiety-provoking. The irony, of course, is that the result of such selections is often precisely the maintenance of the anxiety which the patients wish to avoid.

Often, the partner's response to an issue which threatens the patient's sense of security is ambiguous or conflictual. In such circumstances the neurotic person is likely to imbue such ambiguity with the meanings from the past which were the source of the anxiety. At other times the accomplice's response to security operations is complementary, and the person behaves in the way that the patient feared. Such interactions confirm for the person the reality of his or her fears, and confirm also the need for the security measures which inspired the complementary response. Finally, as described in the family therapy literature (see Wachtel & Wachtel, 1986), significant persons in the patient's life often have an unconscious investment in keeping the patient from changing. In such instances, accomplices will respond to the patient's new patterns of action and experience in discouraging ways, while offering much reinforcement for older and maladaptive behavior.

The Contextual Unconscious

Cyclical psychodynamic theory places great importance on the role of unconscious mental processes in understanding psychopathology and in the conduct of psychotherapy. However, from this perspective, unconscious fantasies, wishes, and motivations are often viewed as the consequences of the person's current behavior and manner of interacting with others. Chiefly, unconscious processes are thought to be the end products of anxiety and of its narrowing of intrapsychic and interpersonal experience. Unconscious processes, therefore, can be understood to be either *independent* variables (the cause of other events) or *dependent* variables (the outcome of other processes). Unconscious mental processes and contents can be located at any of several points on the vicious circle of maladaptive interactions. The decision to view a wish or fantasy as a cause or a consequence of other interactional processes depends on its role and position in the person's immediate interaction, and on the focus of the therapy at that point. When unconscious processes are viewed as the symbolic outcome of ongoing relationships and behavior patterns, they inform the patient and the therapist of the unacknowledged aspects and qualities of those interactions. It is those pieces of the person's dealings with others which, unknown to the patient, may be central in causing and maintaining a sense of vulnerability. Such fantasies and desires show how and when the person's security operations interfere with his or her ability to obtain interpersonal satisfactions and successes.

CLINICAL AND THEORETICAL ANTECEDENTS

Freud's work is an obvious predecessor of this system as it would be for any student of unconscious mental life. More than most psychodynamic theories, however, cyclical psychodynamic theory is rooted in Freud's (1926) revi-

sion of his theory of anxiety. This significant and underestimated reworking by Freud included his conclusion that repression and other defenses were efforts to diminish anxiety about wishes and motives. This revised theory of anxiety has been expanded upon in the work described in this chapter.

The interpersonal psychoanalytic theories of Horney (1939, 1945) and Sullivan (1953) have been mentioned earlier as major influences upon the development of cyclical psychodynamics. These writers understood anxiety to be an interpersonal phenomenon which had unforeseen consequences in the form of self-perpetuating modes of relatedness and narrowing of experience. Horney (1939, 1945) and Sullivan (1953) both added significantly to Freud's (1926) signal theory of anxiety. The impact of their newer concepts can be found in the discussions in this chapter of the developmental origins of anxiety, of interactional vicious circles, and of the ironic and self-maintaining character of security operations and defenses.

Two radical revisions of classical psychoanalysis have also been important influences. The experiments of Alexander (Alexander & French, 1946) in clinical psychoanalysis were important in establishing that action and new experiences were as important as insight in treating neurosis. The integration of psychoanalytic concepts into a learning theory perspective by Dollard and Miller (1950) was a significant antecedent of the cyclical theory of conflict and anxiety and of the contextual nature of unconscious wishes.

Of the many emerging positions in psychotherapy integration, resemblances may be found between cyclical psychodynamics and the integrative positions of Ryle (1990, and Chapter 7 in this volume), Safran and Segal (1990), and Beutler (Chapter 12 in this volume). Each of these systems shares with this one a theoretical integration of interpersonal, intrapsychic, and behavioral constructs and an emphasis upon the ways in which maladaptive patterns are maintained in the here and now of experience. There are technical similarities between this approach and the "broad-spectrum" or eclectic behavioral approaches such as Lazarus' multimodal therapy (1981), though cyclical psychodynamics differs greatly in its theory.

THE TECHNIQUE AND PRACTICE
OF PSYCHOTHERAPY

The integrative psychotherapy which is based on cyclical psychodynamic theory is an evolving method. Its major technical components are psychodynamic exploration and active, behaviorally oriented exercises and interventions. Cyclical psychodynamically based therapy includes interventions from other models, including gestalt therapy and family therapy (Wachtel, 1985).

Assessment and the
Conceptualization of
Psychopathology

The focus of assessment and intervention in psychotherapy is on the patient's anxiety-based disturbances and distortions of character and relatedness (Wachtel, 1977, 1985). The patient's patterns of interaction are studied carefully with the goal of identifying all points on the vicious circles: the inclination which may be arousing anxiety, the meanings which predict a loss of security, the interpersonal context of the desire, the ways in which the person interacts with others to keep threatening experiences unacknowledged and anxiety minimized, the reactions of others to the person's security operations, and the ways in which this last event feeds back to maintain the same anxieties, meanings, and defenses. The ways the patient keeps himself or herself from finding out what he or she is afraid of, (and the way others assist in this task) are at the center of both assessment and intervention. The anxiety-reducing techniques are selected following an assessment of the patient's vicious circles. Anxiety which is maintained by behavior or experience occurring at different points on the circle will require different interventions.

The above description notwithstanding, another critical feature of patient assessment from the cyclical psychodynamic perspective is the identification of strengths in the patient. Clinical theories have an unfortunate tendency to pathologize in their descriptions of personality, and therapists practicing from the cyclical perspective are careful to balance descriptions of maladaptive patterns with appreciation of the patient's adaptive assets. Unless one understands the strengths

of the patient, there is little for the therapy to build on.

Mechanisms of Change
and Choice of Intervention

Inquiry. Psychotherapy from a cyclical psychodynamic perspective proceeds in a manner which in many of its features is indistinguishable from other psychodynamic psychotherapies. The therapist listens, inquires, seeks clarification and additional data, and invites and assists the patient in the task of speaking as comfortably and as completely as is possible. Nonetheless, the conceptual framework through which the therapist listens and formulates differentiates this aspect of the psychotherapy from other seemingly very similar approaches.

The patient is not required to free associate as a normative part of the participation, nor is the therapist expected to be largely silent or inactive (Wachtel, 1977). Free association in the presence of a continuously silent therapist can create a situation akin to a stimulus deprivation experiment. While the response elicited in such a situation can be revealing and interesting, the patient's communications also can be construed as consequences of an abnormal interpersonal interaction. Much is missed and much is misunderstood if this is the only source of data about the patient's experiences.

The detailed inquiry which typifies much of the therapeutic work is one source of change in itself, as it may lead to the expansion of self-knowledge and of experience (Wachtel, 1977). However, the role and value of inquiry far surpass this use. As patient and therapist explore a specific vicious circle, multiple possibilities for intervention are suggested. Active intervention is based on the formulations which are derived from a period of inquiry (Wachtel, 1977, 1985). This activity may be dynamically oriented, be based upon behavioral exercises, include techniques from gestalt therapy (Wachtel, 1985) or family therapy (Wachtel & Wachtel, 1986), or may be an amalgam of techniques from the dynamic, behavioral, and systems positions (Wachtel, 1985, 1991). These last mentioned interventions may take the manifest form of a technique which is drawn from one of the therapies to be integrated, but their use is frequently modified or expanded by concepts and data from one of the other positions. For example, interpretation can be used to impart insight (its traditional psychodynamic role) but also can be an aid in exposing the patient to warded off sources of anxiety, or as a reinforcer of new behaviors (Wachtel, 1985). The therapist is free to use any technique or procedure which would usefully interrupt a vicious circle or assist the patient to be rid of a particular anxiety.

Once any period of active intervention has been completed successfully, inquiry and exploration often will resume until another repetitive interaction pattern or symptom becomes the focus. At times, a period of active work will elicit new data which modify both the patient's and the therapist's image of the appropriate targets for change. This therapy is marked by its own rhythms of activity and repetition; the work moves back and forth between the exploration of inner states and experience and the application of new understanding to action and behavior in daily life. In turn, these changes in living influence and inform the insight-oriented work.

The issues identified through dynamic inquiry, or as consequences of active intervention can be approached through several proposed change mechanisms (Wachtel, 1977, 1985; Wachtel & Wachtel, 1986), to be discussed below.

Exposure. A central component of anxiety reduction is exposure to those ideas, desires, behaviors, and situations which have been avoided because of the anxiety-generating meanings associated with each. The patient needs to suspend his methods of avoiding fearsome situations, persons, and interactions, and also must face the inner states which are warded off by defenses and security operations. The therapist may use a number of techniques to promote such exposure. *Interpretation* and *confrontation* of anxiety-generating inner states and of defenses is a standard technique drawn from dynamic therapies. Such interventions are used to expose the patient to thoughts, feelings, and desires which are the sources of anxiety. Repeated exposure through interpretation allows the anxiety-generating meanings of these intrapsychic states to be modified. Interpretation and confrontation are effective in aiding efforts toward exposure when such communications are formulated and worded so that the behavioral goal of *response prevention* is achieved

(Wachtel, 1977). This is accomplished when interpretations interrupt the patient's defenses and avoidances or make them less effective in constricting or distorting the person's experience.

The counterparts to interpretation in facilitating exposure to *external* sources of anxiety are the familiar behavioral methods of *systematic desensitization* and *flooding*, whether in imagination or *in vivo*. These techniques are particularly useful when the person suffers from a phobia or an inability to enter specific situations, but they are not limited to such applications. Desensitization often can be used hand in hand with dynamically oriented intervention. As patients change their avoidant behavior in confronting a source of external anxiety, they often become more aware of the unconscious anxiety-cueing meanings of that external stimulus (Wachtel, 1977). These insights can promote further exposure to cues newly recognized to be relevant to the patients' difficulties.

Desensitization and other behaviorally oriented exposure techniques may also serve as a framework for creating a dynamic-behavioral amalgam, in which patients are exposed to a hierarchy of feared inner states (Wachtel, 1985). For example, patients who avoid the open expression of intimate feelings because they have learned to anticipate rejection from others at such moments could be helped to construct an imagery-based hierarchy of scenes in which they expressed these feelings.

Any technique which appropriately enables persons to experience a part of their life which they have avoided, and thus to interrupt the repetitive and ironic maintenance of anxiety, and of problematic interpersonal relations is of potential use to the cyclical psychodynamic therapist. The original psychodynamic and behavioral integration in this model has been enhanced by techniques drawn from gestalt therapy and from family systems approaches (Wachtel, 1985; Wachtel & Wachtel, 1986). Such techniques, including gestalt exercises which refocus the person toward progressively more intense and private aspects of experience, and family therapy methods, such as reframing, paradoxical interventions, and structural interpretations, have their place. All of these interventions are useful in bypassing, inhibiting, modifying, or disabling intrapsychic and interactional methods of avoiding anxiety and feared experiences. As therapeutic experience continues within this framework, it is likely that exposure techniques from other therapies will be further assimilated both in their original forms and in transformed ways.

Insight. Although insight is not the only mechanism of change in this model, it is considered to be an important contributor to progress. Insight is important in allowing persons to name and confront what they have feared. Discriminations between perceptions from the past and of the present are made more easily when understanding of experience is expanded. Such discriminations enable persons to try new behaviors and ideas, and are an aid in overcoming anxiety (Dollard & Miller, 1950; Wachtel, 1977; Wachtel & Wachtel, 1986).

Insight develops through dynamic exploration, utilizing clarification and interpretation. Insight also may be the unexpected consequence of behavioral change. Generated either way, such expansion of the self paves the way for further exposure, and can be equivalent to exposure in nudging patients to experience an internal state which they have strenuously avoided. Insight also serves to consolidate behavioral changes and to assist persons in generalizing such changes from one source of anxiety to another. Awareness of the developmental similarities between symptoms and security operations often is a basis for greater willingness to expose oneself to anxiety. This awareness of connections is reassuring and therefore a limiting factor upon the intensity of anxiety (Wachtel & Wachtel, 1986).

The nature of the insights which are considered to be useful in cyclical psychodynamic psychotherapy differs somewhat from the self-knowledge valued in traditional dynamic therapies. The content of interpretive work is expanded to include explanation of the persons' embroilment in a vicious circle. Cyclically oriented interpretation will point out to patients the ways they and other people promote, stimulate, and maintain, unconscious fantasies and inclinations (Wachtel, 1977). The interpretations usually also are action oriented; the insights sought are particularly those that enable patients to act differently (Wachtel & Wachtel, 1986).

Gradualism. Gradualism is a guiding principle for therapeutic planning in the cyclical psycho-dynamic method (Wachtel, 1985). We refer here to the advantages offered the patient in changing slowly and with small steps. This principle can be applied to imagery-based and *in vivo* techniques which are aimed at exposure, to exercises which are meant to modify or build new behavioral skills (see below), and to interpretive work. In each type of procedure, the patient's anxiety level can and should be monitored carefully. Learning and change are unlikely to take place when severe anxiety is present. The extremely anxious patient is likely to try out new behaviors in such an awkward and uncomfortable way that other people will respond negatively or with hostility, thus perpetuating a maladaptive vicious circle (Wachtel & Wachtel, 1986). Such ironic interference is avoidable by grading exposure-oriented exercises into small units, by working toward manageable and modest additions to a patient's behavioral repertoire, and by offering interpretations which go just beyond the patient's current state of self-awareness.

Reinforcement and New Behavioral Consequences

The therapist often must assess and change the intrapsychic and interpersonal consequences of neurotic behavior. Cyclical psychodynamic therapy integrates consideration of reinforcement into a dynamic framework (Wachtel, 1977, 1985) which stresses the nonconscious and conflictual nature of most reinforcers. People often are unaware of the reactions which they seek from other people. They frequently are unaware as well of the gratifications (reinforcements) which these responses bring to them. Patients also typically disavow their multiple and contradictory intentions toward others, which can result in interactions which are consciously distressing to them, but which fulfill an unconscious desire. For example, the patient who consciously feels guilty about not living up to his wife's expectations may unconsciously be reinforced and gratified by her distress and anger, but must repress the latter. It is important to note, however, that from a cyclical psychodynamic perspective, if such motives are discovered, they are generally not assumed to constitute a kind of dynamic bedrock, reflecting basic drives or powerfully embedded internal objects, but rather are themselves examined as consequences of the frustrations inherent in the patient's problematic patterns of living.

Significant others frequently will continue to offer feedback to patients which is reinforcing of old and pathological behavior. New behavior and experience will emerge fully and be maintained by the patients only when they find such behavior worthwhile. It is often necessary to assist the patients in altering the behavior of accomplices (Wachtel & Wachtel, 1986). This can be accomplished in several ways. With patients who are aware of the need for change in their own behavior and that of others, new skills and behaviors can be shaped and practiced (see below), or strategies and exercises for eliciting new reactions from others can be planned. Such planning may include helping patients to selectively reinforce desirable behavior and extinguish unwanted interactions.

Interpretation can be a positive or negative reinforcer as well as a vehicle for insight (Wachtel, 1977). The therapeutic relationship is not considered to be a neutral interaction in this model. Therapists' comments frequently, if not always, will be perceived by patients to have an evaluative and reinforcing component, and this component may be used to shape new skills and behaviors, as well as to interrupt or extinguish others. Therapists who are operating from a cyclical psychodynamic perspective will be especially alert to those meanings and implication and the ways in which interpretations can have punitive implications (Wachtel, 1980; Wile, 1982, 1984). As best they can, they will attempt to nurture and encourage emerging adaptive trends and expansions of awareness, and will reinforce efforts in this direction. The further exploration of ways in which therapists typically make other kinds of comments to either encourage or discourage growth in the patients' self-esteem and readiness to accept and explore new material is one of the most important directions in which work from this perspective is going (see Wachtel, in press).

Overcoming Skill Deficits

A life which has been marked by anxiety and its consequent narrowing of experience is also a life in which the opportunities to develop a full range of social skills have been constricted. While the persons are enmeshed in their neurotic patterns, such deficits will go unremediated. Sometimes, interruption of a vicious circle will result

in the patient's spontaneously capitalizing upon new possibilities and potentials, but often direct assistance is needed.

Variants of such techniques as assertiveness training frequently are incorporated into treatment (Wachtel, 1977, 1985). Modeling, role playing, and graduated homework are incorporated in the therapy when instruction and practice in new modes of behavior are necessary. However, the content and style of these techniques are transformed. Often, instruction and interpretation are blended in a comment about a latent desire and its behavioral expression: "Sounds like you'd like to get closer to John. Is there a way of spending time with him alone?"

A series of such interpretations may lead to changes in social behavior and in the dynamic components of that behavior. When more direct instruction is indicated, new behaviors are shaped, modeled, and practiced hand in hand with new ways of dealing with the thoughts, feelings, and desires which prompt and are stimulated by those behaviors. Much skill building is aimed at the acceptance and expression of affective states and needs (closeness, anger, sadness, sexuality). Patients who have avoided the expression of these issues will initially express them in awkward ways which could lead to unfacilitative feedback from others. The therapist must recognize that patients will not find the same acceptance for such crude changes outside of therapy as they do from the therapist. Therefore, behavior rehearsal is a critical technique in assisting the patient to generalize new learning from the relative safety of the therapy to the broader world.

THE THERAPEUTIC RELATIONSHIP

The therapeutic interaction is considered to be a critical source of therapeutic data, and a frequent and important locus of learning and change (Wachtel, 1977, 1985, 1987). We will discuss next the unique cast given to this interaction in cyclical psychodynamic psychotherapy.

Active Participation and Support

The therapist is an active participant in the therapeutic relationship. Befitting the integrative nature of this therapy, the therapist serves as a catalyst for exploration and understanding, and directs the person toward new actions and experiences. Therapist activity is of many types: questioning, interpreting, suggesting active exercises and homework assignments, giving advice, offering encouragement when the patient is frightened or discouraged, and offering feedback and information about in-session and out-of-session behavior. This list is meant to be illustrative rather than exhaustive. Such involvement with the patient is prescribed by the contextual point of view of this therapy, which holds that a neutral therapist is an impossibility. Silence, anonymity, and inaction do not yield a pure culture of the patient's psychology, but instead are stimuli for circumscribed and stereotyped behaviors, perceptions, and fantasies (Wachtel, 1977). The "truth" of the patient's experience and his or her psychological structures is contextually determined. Therefore, there is not one privileged way of relating or behaving with the patient which will yield uniquely accurate or useful therapeutic data. Opportunities to experience the patient from multiple perspectives in relation to a varied range of interactive situations will enhance the therapist's grasp of the patient and the patient's opportunity to understand himself or herself more fully. Active interventions thus do not have to be avoided due to their potential for distorting or diluting the transference. In fact, the patient's transference reactions are often observed and explored most effectively when he or she is engaged in active change processes.

The patient's responses to the therapist's participation are considered to be significant and useful in understanding and interrupting security operations. The patient's ways of fleeing or compromising authentic interpersonal engagement, of rationalizing the avoidance of anxiety, and of repressing affects and wishes, will be most apparent when therapists are willing to participate in an affective and engaged manner. The therapists' observation of their own behavior will inform them of the overt and subtle ways in which the patient has caught them in a vicious circle. Once involved in and aware of such a repetition, the therapist can assist the patient to see how the therapist was made into an accomplice. This knowledge can then become the source of insight, exposure, and the acquisition of new interactional skills.

The state of the therapeutic relationship is a major variable in assessment when determining whether to use an active technique. Such techniques cannot be introduced in isolation from the patient's history, dynamics, cognitive style, and interpersonal perceptions. The meaning of an intervention will also reflect what has happened between patient and therapist up to the point at which the technique is proposed (Wachtel, 1977). Heightened anxiety and security measures may follow the suggestion of a new procedure. When that occurs, the sources and nature of the anxiety and the meaning to the patient of the intervention chosen must be examined carefully together.

The emotional tone of the therapeutic relationship is that of support and warmth. The therapist attempts to balance involvement and participation with enough reflective distance and reticence to keep the interaction at a clinical level of discourse (Wachtel, 1985). Support and encouragement are viewed as fostering expanded self-awareness as well as the necessary courage for exposing oneself to chronic and severe anxieties (Wachtel & Wachtel, 1986). It is also appropriate and often necessary for the therapist to assume an educative and advisory role. People who have been unable to learn cannot simply teach themselves once the impediments to learning have been corrected. Helping the patient to understand the behavior of others, and to learn to think and interact with them in more beneficial ways, is a significant phase of the therapist's job. The patient's affective, ideational, and behavioral reactions to educative efforts are worked through as would be any data.

Transference and Countertransference

The discussion of the therapist as a participant–observer is especially important in a discussion of transference and countertransference. Much exploration and interpretation of transference takes place in the therapy, and this is considered to be a major source of expanded self-awareness (Wachtel, 1985). Transference is construed as a contextual phenomenon with roots in both past and present experience. It is more than a simple displacement of the past into the current scene. Transference manifestations are a blend, on the one hand, of ways of thinking and of representing the self and others which are products of past experience, and on the other, of perceptions and images which reflect accurately some behavior or attitude of the therapist (Wachtel, 1977). The images and perceptions from the past which are distorted and distorting reflect the assimilative aspects of transference, while its accommodative dimensions are understood in exploring the ways in which the transference perception does accord with something really going on in the room (Wachtel, 1981).

The therapeutic approach to transference interpretation in cyclical psychodynamic therapy is modified according to this contextual definition and its inclusion of attention to the accuracy and fit of the patient's appraisals. To be sure, attention is paid to the ways in which old representations are forced onto the image of the therapist in a distorted manner. However, interpretations as frequently are focused on, and acknowledge the real similarities between past and present. This becomes the basis for further understanding of the ways in which the person transforms the therapist (not only perceptually but in actual behavior) into someone similar to figures from the patient's past. The maintenance of vicious circles and the ironic consequences of the patient's relational style (especially in its unsuccessful self-protective dimensions) are made clear and frequently are resolved through such work on the accommodative aspects of the transference.

Countertransference, too, is understood to be the result of assimilative and accommodative processes: the therapist's reactions to the patient are a blend of his or her character and history and of the specific and unique feelings, thoughts, and behaviors evoked by the individuality of the patient. Such reactions are considered to be an inevitable and unavoidable part of the therapeutic relationship. By observing their participation and the ways in which their experience and behavior are influenced by their patients, therapists can learn much about the patients' style and patterns of relating and of protecting themselves from anxiety. Countertransferential experiences become the silent basis for many interpretations and other interventions. They are communicated to patients when the therapist judges that such feedback would be useful in helping patients to understand how they affect other people and transform them into accomplices. Whenever this is done, great care is taken to assure that this does not become a matter of blaming the patient for the interactional style that is the problem for which they are seeking help (see Wachtel, in press).

Pitfalls and Contraindications

The practice of cyclical psychodynamically based integrative psychotherapy requires the therapist to become fully conversant with its unique theoretical model and with interventions drawn from several technical approaches. Its blend of exploration and activity will be unfamiliar and difficult for those therapists who have been committed to any system which emphasizes either approach exclusively. It is possible that the novice will switch between insight and active technique too rapidly, thus reducing the gains which each has to offer. It is also conceivable that some therapists will linger in the exploratory or the active intervention phases for too long a time. This lack of movement could reflect unresolved theoretical allegiances, but more likely would be a manifestation of some interactionally derived anxiety and avoidances in the therapist. Countertransference issues may thus become apparent in the therapist's use or disuse of certain interventions.

This therapy was developed in an outpatient setting with and for adult patients who suffered from neurosis and character problems (Wachtel, 1977). It has been applied to crises of children and families (Gold, 1988) and to the long-term therapy of children (Gold, 1992). It has not been tested formally with inpatients or with psychotic, sociopathic, and organically impaired patients. As a therapy with a prominent psychodynamic component, successful participation requires certain levels of psychological awareness and reflection, as well as the ability to delay gratification and to work toward change slowly. Patients with very circumscribed problems (e.g., simple phobias or limited sexual dysfunctions), or those who do not wish to undertake a longer and inner directed therapy, may be better served by treatment in a more strictly behavioral model. Similarly, very aggressive, impulsive, and behaviorally disturbed patients may need a more directive and structured therapy, or at least an introductory phase of that type.

CASE EXAMPLE[1]

Judy was a woman in her mid forties who began psychotherapy with complaints of chronic

[1] This patient was treated by the first author (JRG).

depression and severe somatic symptoms, including migraine headaches, gastrointestinal discomfort, and lower back pain. Medical exams had ruled out any overt physiological causes for these problems. Judy came to therapy thinking that her pain and discomfort were stress related.

The first phase of the therapy was devoted to assessment and to the dynamic exploration, from a cyclical perspective, of Judy's interaction patterns, vicious circles, security operations, anxieties, and motivations. These issues were studied through her reports of her activities and relationships, and through the therapist's observation and participation in twice weekly sessions. This phase lasted for about three months. Judy's relationships were marked, almost without exception, by great concern about "being good, being liked, and fitting in." She perceived herself to be unlikable and in danger constantly of losing the affection and good will of her family and friends. As a result, she strained to agree with any opinion or suggestion offered by someone in her circle, and tried to anticipate and gratify any wish or need of theirs, no matter how great the effort or cost to Judy herself. Judy experienced anger, sadness, or disappointment as threats to her security because such emotions were potential indications that she had needs of her own, which would be perceived as unacceptable by others in her life. Any sign of individuality, independence, or an inclination to say no to someone were perceived by Judy to be equally dangerous. As she said of her interactions, "People tell me I'm such a joy to be around because I'm so agreeable and thoughtful. I'm afraid that if I speak my mind, then I won't be thought of in that way, and no one will want to have anything to do with me."

Contained within this statement is an allusion to the ways in which other people served as accomplices in Judy's maladaptive interaction patterns. She consistently chose people who were only too happy to have Judy do for them and who actually were intolerant of her needs and interests. Other people who might have behaved differently toward her were subtly transformed into accomplices by Judy's seeming eager to serve and to please others without regard for her own satisfactions. Judy's relationship with her husband was the most glaring example of this type of interaction. She described him as exceptionally handsome, charming, and self-involved, and as "always on stage." He was interested in her ap-

pearance, her ideas, and of her interests only as they reflected upon him. Judy's spouse constantly reminded her that she was his representative and alter ego at the many business dinners and meetings which they attended. Her two grown children thought nothing of demanding her time, money, and attention whenever they felt in need, and her friends behaved in the same ways. These people reacted to Judy's minute efforts at expressing her own opinions with disinterest or with irritation. Judy summed up the interactional reactions to her occasional revelations of her depression and unhappiness in this way, "My, where did our sunny Judy go? Let's have a smile, and could you go and get me a cup of tea?"

As these interactions were explored, Judy became more aware, spontaneously and through interpretation, of how enraged, exploited, and bitter she felt, and of a sense of helplessness and of being trapped which pervaded most of her dealings with other people. She also learned that her somatic symptoms were the consequences of the resentment which she felt, and inhibited, when she took care of someone else out of anxiety and fear. The interpretations which were offered to Judy were intended as positive reinforcers as well as ways of conveying insight. The therapist attempted to shape and encourage small expressions of assertiveness and anger, while pointing out the anxiety and interpersonal compromises connected with those issues: "It would be much more pleasant if you were able to disagree with your husband, and didn't have to hide your opinions out of worry and then feel sick."

Dynamic work also yielded historical material which helped explain the development of Judy's anxiety and character. She was able to see the ways in which her parents had been self-involved and needy, and that she had felt securely attached and loved most often when she was attentive and admiring with them. In this way, anger, assertiveness, and individuality had taken on their current meanings. Historical data were discussed with Judy in a way which emphasized that her past was being kept alive by current behavior, which, if changed, would allow her to bury old ghosts and feelings.

The initial period of such interpretive work became the basis for more active interventions aimed at breaking Judy's vicious circle of compliance, self-deprivation, and anger. The first exercise was a blend of dynamic insight and system atic desensitization. Judy was asked if she could imagine scenes in which she pleasurably spoke her mind in an angry or irritable way with her husband and friends. She gradually moved from timid and tiny expressions in imagery to scenes where her expressions of rage were violent and powerful. As Judy became more comfortable with these ideas and images, she spontaneously gained insight into her anxiety about anger, and about some of the unconscious factors which reinforced her compliant behavior. Judy reported imagining herself frightening other people, and taking pleasure in the power which that fear represented. She also learned that her caretaking behavior gave her a covert sense of power as well, as it unconsciously provoked fantasies of being better and more capable than the people to whom she acquiesced consciously.

Power and its absence then became the focus of interpretive work and active intervention. Exploration of these fantasies revealed that they were kept active by the absence of a real sense of mastery and power in Judy's life. Her fantasies also were the source of guilt and anxiety (if she were found out, other people would dislike her), and so encouraged the vicious circle of compliance, caretaking, and rage. The therapist used these insights to suggest graded role-playing exercises in which Judy practiced being powerful with others. This took the form of learning to say no, asking for things from others, and disagreeing when her ideas differed from those of her companions. These behaviors were modeled by the therapist, and practiced by Judy in imagery and in behavior in sessions, with the therapist providing feedback and guidance and helping Judy to refine her skills. The meaning of these exercises was discussed as well. The fantasies, anxieties, and affects which were stimulated were explored, and much discussion was devoted to anticipating and planning for the reactions of Judy's family and friends. She was helped to be ready for their puzzlement, negativity, and hostility. A reframing intervention was suggested to Judy to help her with these possible reactions: any resistance to her efforts at change could be interpreted by her to be acknowledgment of her real power.

These exercises were followed by the suggestion that Judy apply in her outside relationships what she had practiced in sessions. At this point, she faltered, had an exacerbation of symptoms,

and found reasons to postpone the completion of homework. Exploration of this stalemate revealed a recreation of Judy's vicious circle in the therapeutic relationship. She perceived the therapist to be more interested in, "your brilliant ideas, and how good a case I am, than in me and what I want." So, Judy had been angry at many points during the therapy, but had repressed it and had behaved compliantly and admiringly. The efforts she would have had to make to change significant relationships were experienced by her as compliance with ideas and initiatives which she perceived to be the therapist's rather than her own. Repeating her inability to assert herself directly, she had become symptomatic.

The exploration of this circle proceeded by studying the roles of both parties in its development and maintenance. Judy came to understand the repetitive and anxiety-generated aspects of her perceptions and behavior, whereas the therapist realized that in some ways he had become an accomplice. Judy's undemanding and "sunny" demeanor, and her steady progress and cooperation, had been pleasing to him and were a boost to his self-esteem. These factors had resulted in both parties avoiding the repetitive and maladaptive features of their interactions, eventuating in resistance and a therapeutic stalemate. When the therapist was satisfied that he had understood his part in the circle, he acknowledged this participation openly. His comments were worded (he hoped) so as to be reinforcing of Judy's refusal to do something she had not wanted to do: "We both were doing the same number we've been talking about. You were afraid that I would be like everyone else, and I slipped into that by being too pleased with what was going on. You really put us back on the track by not doing the exercises. You stood up for yourself in an important way. Let's see if we can get out of this and build on it." Judy found this discussion to be helpful in understanding the ironic consequences of her interactions, and was able to proceed with out-of-session assignments.

These assignments and their consequences dominated the last phase of the therapy. Judy gradually tried out new self-assertive behaviors with her family and friends, and as predicted, received some difficult and hostile feedback from her accomplices. She found the reframing of this feedback helpful (an acknowledgment of her power) and other methods for coping with it were discussed as well, including learning to be inattentive, confronting people with their hostility, and using paradoxical interventions with them: she enjoyed and was good at telling particularly difficult people how they would respond before they could, and so averting that response. She felt a sense of real power and control in her interactions and realized that she was no longer as resentful, trapped, or insecure. She also found that her wish to hurt others, and her secret feelings of being better than other people, had faded.

Judy learned that some of her old friends could not accept "the new Judy" and decided to end these relationships. Her marriage became rocky and she brought her husband into the therapy for several conjoint meetings. He was hurt, angry, and confused, but was able to grasp Judy's need to change in some ways. He also realized that her new strength and diminished symptoms made her more interesting and available socially and sexually.

All these behavioral and interpersonal changes were discussed in sessions from the complementary perspectives of behavioral strategy and dynamic meaning, with each potentiating the other. When the work faltered, the resistance usually was attributable to a transferential vicious circle which had been overlooked. Such issues were worked through by the combination of interpretation and judicious therapist acknowledgement described above. In each instance of resistance, the meaning of an intervention and its place in the interaction cycles was made clear, and opportunities for change in the therapeutic relationship became apparent.

Judy's therapy ended after about two years. She was rarely depressed and her somatic symptoms were mild and infrequent. When she experienced an exacerbation of either type of symptom, she usually was able to trace it quickly to an interpersonal event in which she had been anxiously compliant and unassertive. Such awareness typically led to fast changes in the interaction, which meant that Judy was able to keep her symptoms well under control.

CONCLUDING COMMENTS

Cyclical psychodynamics is a theoretical perspective that is still evolving. Its progress and change come both from the assimilation of new clinical observations and new research findings and from the expansion of its integrative thrust in the direction of other schools of thought. Cyclical psychodynamics does not seek to become still another "school," but rather an evolving framework within which the contributions of therapists and theorists of varying points of view can be examined and integrated. As will be evident to the readers of this handbook, cyclical psychodynamics is but one effort to provide such an integrating framework. As it evolves further, it is to be expected that it will attempt to synthesize ideas deriving not only from the previously existing schools but also from other integrative theories as well.

Cyclical psychodynamic theory has been applied not only in the clinical realm but also in the examination of broader social issues. The most elaborated analysis along those lines is contained in *The Poverty of Affluence* by Wachtel (1989). There the contextually oriented perspective of cyclical psychodynamic theory is utilized to gain an understanding of the consequences of the acontextual individualism that characterizes American society, and to illuminate how that individualism influences how we think about therapy, about psychopathology, and about the "everyday unhappiness" that Freud thought was beyond the impact of psychoanalytic treatment. In particular, the analysis in *The Poverty of Affluence* shows, from a psychological perspective, the illusions and the high cost associated with a way of life organized around economic growth and material possessions. Utilizing a framework similar to that presented in this chapter, *The Poverty of Affluence* analyzes a number of key vicious circles, operating on both individual and social levels, that have been developing in Western society for several hundred years—for example, how the disruption of community and ties to place and family that began with the enclosure laws and the development of factories led to an increased emphasis on the material dimensions of life. This, in turn, led to social policies and individual decisions that still further disrupted such ties, and thus, to still further need to compensate via producing and owning more, and so forth. In this light, certain experiences of stress and frustration in modern life that usually feel attributable to "simply how things are" are understood as part of a historical process whose social and psychological features are potentially in our control; and a way of life which seems inexorably to create accelerating ecological deterioration and social inequality and unrest is seen in a new light that offers alternatives to the course on which we seem to be set.

The further integration of social and historical perspectives into our thinking about the distresses we address as psychotherapists is the next frontier facing our field. For theorists and therapists of an integrative bent, such a further expansion ought to be particularly appealing and exciting. Cyclical psychodynamic theory, with its open ended framework, its emphasis on context, and its focus on vicious circles, seems ideally suited to take up this next task.

REFERENCES

Alexander, F., & French, T. (1946). Psychoanalytic therapy. New York: Ronald Press.

Dollard, J., & Miller, N. E. (1950). Personality and psychotherapy. New York: McGraw-Hill.

Freud, S. (1926). Inhibitions, symptoms, and anxiety. In J. Strachey (Ed. and Trans.), The standard edition of the complete psychological works of Sigmund Freud, Vol. 20. London: Hogarth Press.

Gold, J. R. (1988). An integrative approach to psychological crises of children and families. Journal of Integrative and Eclectic Psychotherapy, 7, 123–137.

Gold, J. R. (1992). An integrative-systematic approach to severe psychopathology in children and adolescents. Journal of Integrative and Eclectic Psychotherapy, 11, 55–70.

Horney, K. (1939). New ways in psychoanalysis. New York: Norton.

Horney, K. (1945). Our inner conflicts. New York: Norton.

Lazarus, A. A. (1981). The practice of multimodal therapy. New York: McGraw-Hill.

Norcross, J. C. (1984). Eclectic psychotherapy: An introduction and overview. In J. C. Norcross (Ed.), Handbook of eclectic psychotherapy (pp. 3–24). New York: Brunner/Mazel.

Ryle, A. (1990). Cognitive-analytic therapy: Active participation in change. Chichester: Wiley.

Safran, J., & Segal, Z. (1990). Interpersonal processes in cognitive therapy. New York: Basic Books.

Shafer, R. (1976). A new language for psychoanalysis. New Haven: Yale University Press.

Shapiro, D. (1965). Neurotic styles. New York: Basic Books.

Sullivan, H. S. (1953). The interpersonal theory of psychiatry. New York: Norton.

Wachtel, E. F., & Wachtel, P. L. (1986). Family dynamics in individual psychotherapy. New York: Guilford Press.

Wachtel, P. L. (1977). Psychoanalysis and behavior therapy: Towards an integration. New York: Basic Books.

Wachtel, P. L. (1978a). On some complexities in the application of conflict theory to psychotherapy. Journal of Nervous and Mental Disease, 166, 457–471.

Wachtel, P. L. (1978b). Internal and external determinants of behavior in psychodynamic theories. In L. A. Pervin & M. Lewis (Eds.), Perspectives in interactional psychology (pp. 58–81). New York: Plenum Press.

Wachtel, P. L. (1979). Contingent and non-contingent therapist response. Psychotherapy: Theory, Research, and Practice, 16, 30–45.

Wachtel, P. L. (1980). What should we say to our patients? On the wording of therapist's comments. Psychotherapy: Theory, Research, and Practice, 17, 183–188.

Wachtel, P. L. (1981). Transference, schema, and assimilation: The relevance of Piaget to the psychoanalytic theory of transference. Annual of Psychoanalysis, 8, 59–76.

Wachtel, P. L. (1982). Vicious circles: The self and the rhetoric of unfolding. Contemporary Psychoanalysis, 18, 259–273.

Wachtel, P. L. (1985). Integrative psychodynamic therapy. In S. Lynn & J. Garske (Eds.), Contemporary psychotherapies (pp. 148–179). Columbus, Ohio: Charles E. Merrill.

Wachtel, P. L. (1987). You can't go far in neutral: On the limits of therapeutic neutrality. In P. L. Wachtel, Action and insight (pp. 176–184). New York: Guilford Press.

Wachtel, P. L. (1989). The poverty of affluence: A psychological portrait of the American way of life. Philadelphia: New Society Publishers.

Wachtel, P. L. (1991). Towards a more seamless integration. Journal of Psychotherapy Integration, 1, 32–41.

Wachtel, P. L. (in press). Principles of therapeutic communication: The therapist's contribution to the therapeutic process. New York: Guilford Press.

Wile, D. (1982). Couples therapy: A nontraditional approach. New York: Wiley.

Wile, D. (1984). Kernberg, Kohut, and accusatory interpretations. Psychotherapy: Theory, Research, and Practice, 21, 315–329.

CHAPTER 6

Behavioral Psychotherapy

Herbert Fensterheim

The behavioral and the psychodynamic perspectives are the two major approaches in psychotherapy. Each perspective provides both strengths and weaknesses in resolving psychopathology. It seems evident that if the proper combination of the two could be found, such a hybrid would yield a more effective psychotherapy than would either taken alone. One major step in formulating this integration of the therapies is to provide some systematic method for determining when the concepts, strategies, and tactics of one perspective should dominate and when those of the other perspective should be the main guide to the therapeutic process. Behavioral psychotherapy (BP) attempts to provide just such a systematic method.

Behavioral psychotherapy describes a way for the therapist to think about the patient rather than attempting to present some theory of the way the patient is. Its goal is to lead the therapist to some action, to some therapeutic intervention, which moves the treatment process toward its ultimate aim of changing the person, resolving problems, and removing psychopathology. To achieve this end, BP takes from the behavioral

perspective the ideas of target behaviors and utilizes the concept of a psychological organization to identify such targets. It takes from psychodynamics the concepts of the unconscious, of defense mechanisms, and of psychodynamic conflict arising from childhood experiences, and it uses variants of the Law of Parsimony to determine when to introduce these concepts into the therapeutic process.

The overall structure of BP does not depend on a specific form of behavioral or of psychodynamic theory. The one limitation to this statement is that the behavioral perspective is nonbehaviorist. Although behaviorists have made major contributions in this area, the philosophy itself has never been an unalienable pillar of behavior therapy. Indeed, one of the early roots of behavior therapy had as its main ingredient the nonbehaviorist Pavlovian physiological processes (Salter, 1949). Save for this limitation, the therapist can fit into the BP model the behavioral and psychodynamic approach in which he or she is most comfortable.

The basic model for BP originally was presented in Fensterheim and Glazer (1983) and summarized by FitzPatrick and Weber (1989). In this chapter, I will first present an application of the Law of Parsimony and the concept of levels as means for determining when to use behavioral and when to use psychodynamic perspectives and techniques. Then I will present the use of behav-

Herbert Fensterheim • Department of Psychiatry, The New York Hospital–Cornell Medical Center, New York, New York 10021.

Comprehensive Handbook of Psychotherapy Integration, edited by George Stricker and Jerold R. Gold. Plenum Press, New York, 1993.

ioral organizations as a guide for conducting the behavioral interventions and also as a means for beginning to allow for the consideration of psychodynamic variables. Next, I will discuss the use of behavioral methods with psychodynamic and unconscious material and with defenses that play so important a role in maintaining psychopathology. Finally, the entire BP approach will be illustrated through a brief case presentation.

LAW OF PARSIMONY

BP makes deliberate use of the Law of Parsimony to help determine the points for therapeutic intervention. This fundamental principle of scientific thinking states that the simpler of two hypotheses, the one making the fewest assumptions, should be preferred if all other things are equal. Lloyd Morgan applied this principle to comparative psychology stating: "In no case may we interpret an action as the outcome of the exercise of a higher psychical faculty if it can be interpreted as the exercise of one which stands lower in the psychological scale" (quoted in Aronson, Tobach, Rosenblatt, & Lehrman, 1972, p. 34). Thus, an act should not be attributed to thinking if the lower order of memory would equally serve. Nor should it be ascribed to memory if the still lower order of a conditioned reflex is an equally probable interpretation.

In BP, the working hypotheses on which treatment is based use Morgan's canon. Working hypotheses framed in terms of conditioned reflex are given preference over those framed in terms of cognitive variables which, in turn, are preferred over motivational-based formulations. An illustration of this approach has already been given by Fensterheim and Kantor (1980). A man has a sexual dysfunction, an erectile impotency. He feels humiliated and his wife feels frustrated. He may have a motive to frustrate his wife or perhaps to frustrate all women. Or he may have a need to humiliate himself. Or he may have more direct residuals of his Oedipal period. These may have initiated or at the very least been active in maintaining his sexual problem. Men are capable of having such motives and of having them influence their behavior. However, it may also be that with this man anxiety, perhaps only the fear of having a dysfunction, has become conditioned to the sexual act. Men are capable of forming such

conditioned reactions and these can also bring about the sexual dysfunctions. The Law of Parsimony requires that, all other things being roughly equal, the conditioned reflex hypothesis be given preference and that this hypothesis be the basis for the first treatment intervention.

The concept of levels is advanced as a useful means for introducing the Law of Parsimony into the treatment formulations. In formulating the treatment approach to a specific patient or problem the therapist thinks in terms of three levels (Fensterheim, 1989):

Level I is the behavioral level. When working at this level, the therapist follows the usual behavior therapy models. After relevant information is gathered, a careful behavioral analysis is conducted for the purpose of selecting target behaviors for change. Behavioral technologies are then used in attempts to change these target behaviors. Evaluation of change is constantly carried out to see whether the target behaviors are indeed changing and, if so, whether the patient's problem under treatment is indeed being ameliorated. If changes are not coming about, the treatment approach must be modified. This approach works a surprising amount of the time—but not always.

Level II is the obstacle level. It concerns those things that keep the behavioral approach from fully working. It can use both behavioral and psychodynamic concepts in helping to identify and to modify these obstacles. Various fears, such as a fear of change or a fear of being dominated by the therapist, may be a major obstacle. It may be a general characteristic of the patient such as a passive orientation that is the obstacle. Or there may be gains/reinforcers from maintaining the problem. At times the obstacle may lie in the therapist–patient interaction or even in the therapist's own problems. In one instance, the therapist's fear of the way that specific patient expressed anger appeared to be the obstacle; desensitizing the therapist to the fear was followed by a marked progress in the patient's treatment. As these obstacles are dealt with, it often becomes possible at that time to implement the Level I treatment program. Jacobson (1983) reported on an obsessive checker who was able to use response prevention for the checking behavior. However, the impulse to check did not extinguish and the patient became severely depressed necessitating his only hospitalization. The obstacle was identified as a phobic reaction to the feelings of helplessness. As this phobia was reduced, the patient himself reinstituted the response prevention procedures, this time with success.

Level III deals with psychodynamic variables. People are capable of functioning at the higher psychological levels and these higher faculties may indeed be the initiators and/or the maintainers of the pathology which brought the patient into treatment. They often are motivational variables or emotional reactions in the present to memories of childhood events. Defenses many times keep these variables from being obvious. At times, the initial evaluation strongly suggests that the critical treatment hypothesis should be framed in such psychodynamic terms. More often, when the first two levels do not yield to successful treatment, this Level III should be systematically investigated. In addition to the usual therapeutic methods for identifying such processes, such behavioral methods as desensitization and satiation, when applied to dreams and to childhood memories, may elicit useful insights. Once identified and once a therapeutic formulation may be framed in psychodynamic terms, both psychodynamic and behavioral therapeutic methods may be used to treat them. The criterion for success at this level is the same as for the other two levels: the emergence in life situations of the therapeutically desired changes.

The choice of levels is not to be rigidly applied. The main aim of the use of levels is to help the therapist keep the Law of Parsimony in the forefront of his thinking about the patient. In this way the Law of Parsimony attempts to integrate the behavioral and the psychodynamic approaches. The rule is that in formulating treatment hypotheses upon which to base therapeutic action, precedent should be given to framing the hypotheses in terms of those faculties that stand lower on the psychological scale. Preference should be given first to framing them in terms of learning and conditioning, then in terms of cognition, and finally, in terms of motivational and purposive variables. However this is not to be taken as a rigid rule but as a way of organizing thoughts about the patient; clinical judgment always predominates.

THE BEHAVIORAL LEVEL

Formulating hypotheses at the behavioral level does not necessitate a behaviorist mode of thinking. It does not demand that behaviors be considered as separate entities, each maintained by its own network of reinforcers. Rather behaviors are seen as being organized, as forming a behavioral organization composed of systems and subsystems. Within each system the behaviors are in functional relation with each other, are in a hierarchical order with some behaviors being central to the organization and some being peripheral, with the organization as a whole possessing characteristics beyond those of the component behaviors, and with behaviors emerging from the organization rather than being maintained by independent reinforcers. There are a number of practical clinical consequences that stem from this perspective.

Phenotypy

A behavior is not a behavior is not a behavior. That is, that no behavior can be taken solely in terms of its overt appearance but must be considered within the context of the underlying behavioral organization. Behaviors may be phenotypically very similar and yet have very different underlying organizations and require very different therapeutic approaches. For example, three hypothetical patients present with a problem of chronic lateness that is sufficiently severe to have caused difficulties in holding jobs and that have been a major disruptive influence in their social relations. In each instance, the behavior appears to be completely out of deliberate control except for the briefest periods of time. In one patient, the behavior was formulated as being a blind habit to be treated through a self-monitoring program with reinforcers built in to maintain persistence. In the second patient, the initial interview led to a formulation in terms of the avoidance of anxiety-provoking situations and treatment centered around tension and phobic reduction methods. Finally, in the third patient, the chronic lateness was seen as a behavior emerging from a psychodynamic conflict concerning authority and power and the problem of chronic lateness would not even be considered during the early phase of therapy.

Fensterheim (1981) presented a similar analysis of depression. He noted that depression may stem from a condition of general tension, a form of phobic reaction to specific stimuli (including thoughts), leading to and being maintained by ruminative obsessions, habitual reactions sometimes being maintained by reinforcers within the family, and by reactions to assertive difficulties which may lead the patient into truly depressing situations, into feelings of loss of mastery, and into lowered self-esteem. Each of these organizations leads to a different treatment strategy. These organizations, as is obvious, are not the only ones possible with depression. Therefore, according to the BP principles, the diagnosis of depression does not automatically lead to a specific treatment but requires that the behavioral organization underlying the depression be considered and serve as the basis for treatment.

Behavioral Organization

It is assumed that behaviors do not exist in isolation from each other but are integrated and interrelated. When faced with a symptom or a problem, the therapist attempts to formulate the behaviors involved in the problem and their relations with each other. It is assumed that in this organization some behaviors are dominant and some are subordinate; that some are more central to the overall organization while others are peripheral. It is also assumed that each organizational system or subsystem has a core behavior, a focal point, around which the main aspects of the system are organized. The core tends to color and to influence the expression of the other (subordinate) behaviors that compose the system. Modification of peripheral behaviors would be expected at best to yield only minor or transient changes in the problem area. Modification of the core behavior leads to a change in the entire behavioral organization and, hence, of the manifestation of each component behavior. Thus, modifying these more important behaviors would be expected to lead to more generalized and more permanent changes in the problem area.

It is also assumed that within the behavioral organization the different component behaviors are in a functional relationship with each other. This goes beyond a mere facilitating or inhibiting of a given behavior by other behaviors serving as reinforcers. Rather the term *functional relationship* is used in its mathematical sense: "a relationship between two or more variables such that the value of one is dependent on the value of others" (Wilson, 1972, p. 394; also see Haynes & O'Brien,

1990). Fensterheim (1975) reported on a woman whose assertive problems were maintained by a subsystem whose core consisted of social fear and social skill deficits. It was predicted that by changing these core behaviors, not only would the assertive problem be relieved but that the central motive of that subsystem would change from self-protection to self-fulfillment.

An example of the concept of behavioral organization guiding treatment is provided by FitzPatrick and Weber (1989). The patient Janet was a 30-year-old woman who presented with problems of managing multiple life stresses and of dealing with people. The formulation of the patient's behavioral organization is shown in Figure 1. The writers placed a passivity–independence conflict at the core of the organization. It was assumed that as this conflict was reduced, assertive behavior would be less inhibited, ability to cope would improve, and the guilt about independence would diminish. Note that the "need to be good" and the "fear of aggression" that fuel the core conflict may be psychodynamic variables. If the original treatment approach had not worked, this eventuality would have been considered.

The core conflict of passivity–independence became the major treatment target and the formulation influenced even the most trivial aspects of the therapy. When Janet was taught relaxation methods, lowering her anxiety level was only the secondary purpose; the primary purpose was to replace a passive orientation to anxiety with an active orientation. Even the choice of the specific relaxation exercise to be used was influenced by the formulation. Rather than to assign the exercise which the therapist believed would be the most effective, the therapist assigned the one Janet preferred in order to encourage her independence.

Behavioral Formulation

Formulating the psychological organization is a clinical art. The organization is formulated as it is functioning in the present. Emphasis is placed on maintenance rather than on genesis, on what keeps the organization going rather than on what led to its original formulation. The conditions under which the organization first formed, the variables or psychodynamic forces then at work, may not be active in the present. The problem organization as a whole, for example, may

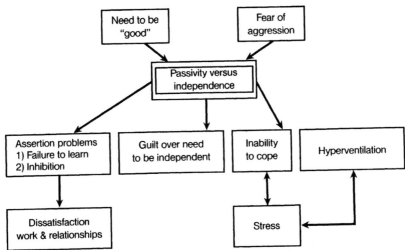

Figure 1. Behavioral formulation with the conflict over passivity versus independence as the core of the problem organization. From "Integrative Approaches in Psychotherapy: Combining Psychodynamics and Behavioral Treatments" by M. M. FitzPatrick and C. K. Weber, 1989, *Journal of Integrative Eclectic Psychotherapy, 8.* Copyright 1989 by Brunner/Mazel. Reprinted by permission.

have become autonomous from other aspects of the patient's organization and may possess characteristics or lead to actions that maintain itself. Some of the sexually variant behaviors seem to be clear examples of this (cf. Maletzky, 1980). Genesis becomes important only as it suggests for investigation characteristics that may be functioning now to maintain that organization.

The main aim of the behavioral formulation is to lead to a plan of action that appears to be promising of change in terms of everything the therapist knows about the patient. The aim is not to verify a hypothesis about the patient; even if the treatment works it does not mean that the formulation upon which it was based was a correct one. The aim is to furnish a blueprint for action leading to a series of planned and integrated therapeutic interventions. The aim of the interventions is to resolve that particular problem. If the expected change does not come about, it is the therapist's responsibility to reformulate and plan a different series of interventions. Also, as new information about the patient is gained, reformulation may also be indicated. One of the main characteristics of BP is a continual process of reformulation.

THE PSYCHODYNAMIC LEVEL

Despite the fact that the Law of Parsimony gives preference to behaviorally oriented formulations, psychodynamic motivational variables often do play an important role in planning treatment. At times, the initial interview leads directly to a formulation in terms of psychodynamic variables. At other times, the need for psychodynamic formulations becomes clear only after unsuccessful attempts at behaviorally oriented treatment. Even simple appearing problem behaviors may be syntonic with motives or with teleologic goals of which the patient is unaware. There are times when "obvious" straightforward behavioral procedures are expected to work, when no technical difficulties in the application of these procedures are present, and yet the expected results do not take place. Unassertive behaviors may be in the service of strong dependency needs. Sexual anxieties may be in the service of controlling unacceptable sadistic impulses or of achieving a masochistic self-humiliation. Social anxieties may not be conditioned responses but may emerge from a Rankian-type goal conflict between conforming and expressing individuality. Although these are not frequent occurrences, they happen often enough that they should be kept in mind.

At times the patient may be at least partially aware of such obstacles. This seems to be particularly true when avoidance of specific feelings is involved. Fensterheim (1983) reported on a woman with a sailing phobia which was important because it disrupted her marital relations with her "sailboat nuts" husband. After the obvious hierarchies involving the sailboat heeling to the wind or rough seas did not work, it was she who suggested the fear of drowning as the correct approach. The core of the fear turned out to be a childhood memory of seeing the body of a friend who had drowned. The need for avoidance was based on the fear of experiencing once again the guilt feeling she remembered from that incident.

Defenses

In the psychodynamic area, BP pays considerable attention to the defense mechanisms. Often when the defenses no longer function in a given area, insights and/or behavioral change come about. It is well known that some psychoanalysts claim that the core of their treatment is the analysis of resistances. Once these protections are no longer necessary, the patient is better. Although defenses, as do other behaviors, may have different underlying organizations, many of them seem to be phobic avoidances. There is some core of feeling, of memory, of fantasy, that acts as phobic stimulus and that the patient strives to avoid. Because these stimuli are internal, the patient cannot escape from them by changing geographic location; the defense mechanisms serve that purpose instead. Should we be able to reduce the phobic reaction, the avoidance behaviors (the defenses) would become less necessary and the original disturbing element will emerge into consciousness to be dealt with therapeutically. Often desensitization or satiation procedures can be used for this purpose. Two examples will be cited.

Dreams, not often but sometimes, respond to such an approach. A young woman being treated for panic reaction brought in a dream. This was a repetitive dream which had been discussed a number of times during two previous (psychodynamically oriented) courses of therapy. In the dream, she and her boyfriend were standing on a deserted train platform. The train came in; it was a half ovoid, opened at the top, and revealed an inside lined with purple plush. Suddenly the platform was crowded with all kinds of people. She was separated from her boyfriend, vainly trying to get to the train. The train closed up and departed. She was all alone on the platform feeling helpless and abandoned, painfully so. She had no idea of what the dream meant except that she felt that it was very important.

Nonsystematic desensitization (Fensterheim, 1972) was used with the dream. The patient was relaxed, was instructed to think about the dream and to signal the first sign of any disturbed feeling, and then relax again. After the seventh such repetition, she suddenly sat up saying that she knew what the dream was about. It was her beloved grandfather's funeral when she was four years old. The inside of the train was similar to the lining of his casket. She remembers the crush of people and the feelings of abandonment when they all left to go to the cemetery and she remained behind with a sitter. Great feelings of sadness filled her at this point and she cried. It would be gratifying to report the major behavioral changes that then took place, but, in actuality, no observable change did occur. However, it did open the area of separation anxiety for further exploration.

Many behaviors may be "fueled" by psychodynamic variables of which the patient is unaware and which can be made conscious through phobic reduction techniques. Fensterheim (1983) presented one such case of a woman with a fear of criticism. The patient presented with many problems including a long history of mild-to-moderate chronic depression and years of only slightly helpful psychotherapy. The problem that brought her into treatment at this time was a work block. Behavioral analysis suggested that the current work block was due to a fear of criticism and a need to avoid the possibilities of such criticism. However, desensitization procedures led to only slight and transient improvement. Discussion of the fears with the patient revealed two other lines of phobias feeding into the fear of criticism (see Figure 2). In one line, the criticism led to self-criticism which elicited strong feelings of self-hate. These, in turn, led to the belief that she was truly "evil" in the moral sense of the word but she could not elaborate on this. The second line led to a fear of rejection which led to a fear of abandon-

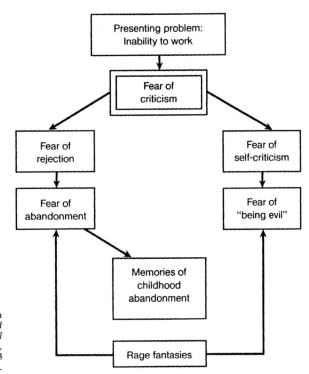

Figure 2. Fueled phobia of criticism. From *Behavioral Psychotherapy: Basic Principles and Case Studies in an Integrative Clinical Model* by H. Fensterheim and H. I. Glazer, 1983, New York: Brunner/Mazel. Copyright 1983 by Brunner/Mazel. Reprinted by permission.

ment, of feeling helpless and alone in a hostile world. These feelings led to memories of her parents abandoning her when she was a child; events such as going off for a day and leaving her with a governess. Recalling these memories in the present elicited feelings of fear.

The abandonment memories had been discussed a number of times in her previous treatments. At that time, they also brought forth the fear feelings but therapy had been unable to take her beyond them. It was these memories that were now made the target for desensitization. With desensitization, over a period of three sessions, other feelings emerged. Fear was replaced by helplessness, depression (fleetingly), guilt, anger, and finally rage. As the feelings of rage diminished, no other feeling replaced it. At that time the patient recalled a series of vindictive fantasies and actual actions where she "got even" with her parents by *her* abandoning *them*. One vivid recollection was of the time when she hid in the woods near the house for the entire day and did not come

out until evening. Her parents had spent all day frantically searching for her and were most distraught. These memories, incidentally, had never come up in her previous therapies. At the time the memories emerged, she had an insight that her feeling of being evil stemmed from these actions and fantasies. In any event, not only did the fear of criticism disappear without any further work, but she was free of her chronic depression for the first time in about 30 years. My own interpretation of this result is that the defense mechanism of isolation was involved. As the core disturbance was reduced through desensitization, this defense was no longer needed, and the originally phobic memories became available.

Fueling Phobias

Experiences such as these has led to the concept of fueling phobias. Childhood memories are considered to be phobic stimuli. Feelings elicited by such memories in the present, or defenses against such feelings, may be major variables in the maintenance of current problems. Once such a fueling phobia is identified, it may be treated with the usual behavioral phobic reduction methods. When this procedure works, it may lead to a general and widespread change in a whole behavioral pattern. In the woman with a work-block problem described above, there came about a major and a general change in a very long-term chronic depression. One common change with successful reduction of fueling phobias is the disappearance of assertion-inhibiting features, the spontaneous emergence of assertive behaviors, and the changes in mood and in self-esteem that come about consequent to the increase in assertiveness. As with the work-blocked woman, the changes in feeling response to the specific memories or the insight into the true phobic area are not uncommon. One woman, while being desensitized to the humiliation-provoking responses to the memories of her father hitting her, suddenly began to experience anger at her mother for not protecting her from her father. Desensitization to this newly recognized fueling phobia led to the spontaneous emergence of assertive behavior as described above.

Often the fueling phobia is not as specific or as clearly defined as in the illustrations. The general memory area having the potential for being a fueling phobia may have been identified but the specific phobic stimuli may remain unknown. Often there may be many different memories that are conditioned to elicit the same feelings. Often, as the phobic quality is reduced, new memories or new perceptions emerge. For such reasons, imagery satiation procedures usually are more productive and flexible than the more structured desensitization scenes. The subject is instructed to recall the general set of situations as vividly as he or she can for a present period of time while avoiding all escapes. Records are kept of the feelings and the intrusions that occur during these exercises when they are performed as homework and these are discussed during the office visit. There are times when this procedure leads to a chain of unexpected and rather complex memories associated with the phobic area.

These and other psychodynamic variables are used in BP. When possible, the behavioral methods are attempted to resolve whatever conflict may be found. At other times, the more standard psychodynamic therapeutic methods are used. The main point is that psychodynamic variables are not automatically called upon. They are used only when no more parsimonious formulation can be derived. Of course all our patients have psychodynamic activity going on within them. However, many times these forces may not be related to the problem under treatment. Even if they are related to the problem, this does not necessarily mean that they have to be incorporated into the treatment plan. Many problems can be resolved without recourse to the Level III concepts. Remember that the aim of BP is not to understand but to cure the patient.

CASE EXAMPLE

Melissa, a 48-year-old woman, presented with a problem in her relationship with Bob, her boyfriend. This is a relationship of some 8 years duration which, after the first beginnings, has always had difficulties. At present there is fighting between them, little pleasure, and she feels exploited and helpless. She is also in a mild to moderate depressive episode, of which she has had several over the years most always connected with her relationship with men. She had some ten years of psychotherapy, both individual and group, for these problems with several different therapists, but received little help from these treatments. The current episode began during the past summer when, instead of the relaxation and enjoyment in their summer house they had both looked forward to, she brought along administrative work from her job. She spent part of each day working on this over Bob's strong objections.

She, along with a younger sister, was brought up in a New England devoutly Catholic home. Her father was a talkative, sociable man who was uncommunicative about his feelings and who drank a lot but was not alcoholic. Her mother was an angry woman, a drudge with few friends. She was judgmental and critical of Melissa and expected her always to be good. One vivid childhood memory was of her mother talking to the principal of the Catholic school where she was trying to have Melissa admitted into first grade and telling the principal that she was a "good, sweet girl." Throughout grade school Melissa felt the burden of living up to this standard. In retrospect, she views her home and her school as restrictive and coercive experiences where she constantly felt helpless and hopeless in the face of negative judgments.

After high school graduation, Melissa joined a convent. Here she tried so hard to do everything right that she became rigid, compulsive, and depressed to the point that the convent sent her for a psychiatric consultation and then expelled her. Following this, she went to a Catholic college where she was an excellent student, led an active social life, but with little dating. Eventually she earned a Ph.D. in one of the humanities from an Ivy League university. She became a college teacher and loves her work. Despite her enthusiasm for her work and her demonstrated scholarly ability, she has too many self-doubts to have published or to have presented professional papers.

First Formulation and Treatment

Following the principles of BP, the first working hypothesis formed was at Level I, the behavioral level (Figure 3). The core of the problem was formulated as being a set of assertiveness difficulties. She does have trouble in saying no, in making requests, in the appropriate expression of all feelings but particularly of the negative ones, and difficulty in handling any kind of criticism. In general, she has great problems in knowing what are her rights in any given situation and in standing up even for those few rights she does acknowledge. These assertive problems are maintained by a social phobia of being disapproved by people which is allied to a more general phobia of being "sinful." There is also a cognitive rule that the way to achieve closeness with others is to be "quiet and good."

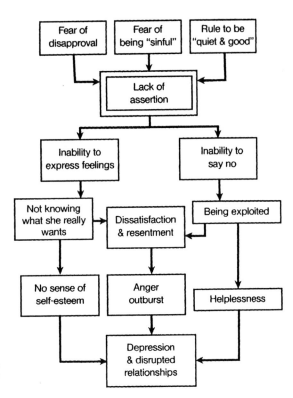

Figure 3. Formulated behavioral organization (Level I) of a woman with depression and relationship problems.

The inability to say no leads her into taking on undesired tasks such as the summer administrative tasks from her job. Also in her relations with Bob she not only cannot say no to his requests but attempts to anticipate them and satisfy them before they are actually made. So if Bob were to ask her what time she wanted to have dinner, she would attempt to figure out what time *he* wanted dinner and would say that time rather than to think of what time she herself would like to eat. This difficulty led to strong feelings of resentment, of dissatisfaction, and of being exploited. It also led to great feelings of helplessness.

A second consequence of her assertive difficulties was her inability to express her feelings. This led to Bob never really knowing what she felt and what she wanted and, even more importantly, to her not knowing these very same things. Therefore she could never truly feel satisfied, and the concept of self-esteem did not even enter her mind. Because of her difficulties in expressing her feelings, the resentments and angers would build up until eventually she would have sullen outbursts. These outbursts would further disrupt the relationship and, when combined with the feelings of helplessness and with the lack of self-esteem, led to depression.

Hence the assertive behaviors became the first treatment target. It was formulated that if her ability to assert herself was increased, then this organization would break up. She would be less depressed, her relations with Bob would markedly improve, and she would truly be more in command of her life. Further, as she practiced assertive behaviors, she would be exposed to her fears of disapproval and of being sinful and these would be extinguished or, at least, lowered. She would also be forced to challenge her rule of the importance of being "quiet and good." Thus, it was predicted that changes in her assertive behaviors would bring about major changes in the entire problem organization.

Assertiveness training was carried out over a period of about 5 months. A number of procedures were used, but the main part of this treatment concerned specific interactions with other people. She kept records for each incident, and these were used to teach her the concepts and principles of assertiveness and to give her specific exercises or assignments to perform. For example:

She wanted work–study students to duplicate some papers right away so that she could get certain work done. She felt intimidated (note that we did not explore why) and instead told them to have it by the next day. Later in the afternoon, she gathered her strength and told them that she wanted it done that day. She realized that her goal was to get her work done as soon as possible and that her desired action was to say "Do it right now" to the students. I taught her how to practice the desired response in imagery. She did use this rehearsal method for a number of similar situations, not only making the desired response more probable in future situations, but also turning a self-flagellation into a constructive exercise.

Over the course of several months there was indeed a change in her feeling of worthlessness, in her general mood, although there were many fluctuations, and a very definite increase in her assertiveness. However, there was still great strain when it came to assertion and an overall feeling of her holding back. It became time to reformulate.

Reformulation and Second Treatment Approach

The reformulation introduced the concept of fueling phobias and a Level III (psychodynamic) approach. The organization described in Figure 3 still appeared to be a useful working hypothesis but some variable not yet depicted seemed to be maintaining this structure. It was now formulated that there were a set of childhood experiences, feelings, or thoughts that Melissa had to avoid, and that it was this need to avoid that inhibited her spontaneous assertive behaviors. According to this formulation if such areas could be identified, if their phobic quality could be reduced, then the need for avoidance would disappear and the inhibition of assertiveness would no longer be a problem.

However, it was not clear what fueling phobia areas might be and we realized that some experimentation would be necessary. We would use the satiation in imagery method where Melissa would recall and dwell on memories in certain parts of her childhood for preset periods of time and note what feelings emerged during this procedure. Discussing it and trying out different images during the office sessions led to a first try of memories concerning her confining home and school environment. She was indeed able to recall a large number of specific memories but there was one difficulty: it was all the memory of feelings; no feelings were stirred up in the present. We tried several different possible phobic areas including fictional ones where she would imagine acting "naughty." With all of these she would have clear memories of how she felt at the time; in the fictional "naughty" scenes she was certain that had she acted that way, she would have felt hopeless and helpless. These last feelings came up in a number of memories, sometimes she remembered feeling great love and attachment toward her mother at the very same time. Again, however, no feelings at all (or very little at best) were aroused during these recalls. We went along on these tracks for about 6 weeks with Melissa doing the satiation at home about 4 times a week and our discussing her experiences at our once a week session. During this time, she was maintaining, even slightly increasing, her assertive behaviors, but no major change was taking place.

Finally we hit on an area that proved to be productive. In our discussions, we decided to try out the fear of her own anger, rage, and violence. She began to satiate to images of beating up her mother and for the first time we began to get very strong and changing feelings. "For example, picking her up and smashing her against the floor until she bled, taking an axe to her, throwing her off a high building. . . . It was very violent, not just slapping her. I also imagined screaming things at her—blaming her for the kind of life I had led. . . . I got into it so much, smashing her against the floor, etc., that my head was bobbing up and down." The subjective units of disturbance (SUD) level was up to 90 with anger and hate and intruding feelings of wild exhilaration.

During one satiation session the feelings of hate toward her mother changed into feelings of self-hate and she went around for a day or two with those fairly strong self-hate feelings. In her next satiation, the imagery of beating her mother did not change these feelings. Then she began to remember how as a very small child she loved her mother and believed her mother loved her. But then she began to doubt whether her mother loved her for the right reasons—whether she was loved for being quiet, pliable, and in agreement with mother. Melissa felt that her mother's love

weakened her in some way. At that point the self-hate came down and she felt better.

The session following that satiation began with Melissa telling me that she suddenly had feelings of great warmth toward me and they frightened her. For one thing she was afraid that the warm feelings would lead to an exploitative, degrading, "enslaving" relationship such as she had with her mother. For another thing, she was afraid that she would get angry with me and our relationship would break up.

Along about this time, too, she brought in several spontaneous changes. At faculty meetings she was generally fairly quiet and stayed in the background. Now, suddenly, she took over several meetings. She felt strong and calm, something she had never felt before. And apparently it was quite appropriate because several of her colleagues thanked her for what she had done and commented on how well she had done it.

We discussed her feelings of warmth toward me and especially her fears of it. This transferential nature of these fears was evident to both of us. However, we decided that the fear of her anger and rage was still most important. Therefore she continued her satiation exercises of being violent as she had been doing with her mother but now she was to do it with either Bob or with me. She had a great deal of difficulty with this; she would fall asleep, or she could not keep her mind from wandering, and she began to avoid doing the exercises (probably the first time in her life she failed to do an assigned task). After working at this for 3 weeks, we decided that it was too difficult an area for her to approach at this time.

She did note during these attempts at satiation that during the day many thoughts about her father began to come to her and that similar thoughts would intrude during the satiation attempts. Satiations to her father's drunkenness led to the realization that she had been frightened that he might touch her or molest her, although he never had. It also led to feelings of contempt for him, centering around thoughts that his drunkenness was a sign of his weakness in relation to her mother.

I believed that her feelings about her father's drunkenness were even stronger than she reported. I wanted to work more directly on them through a desensitization procedure and I did so using the eye-movement method (Shapiro, 1989).

In this instance, it worked well using her father's drunken-sexual acts as the stimuli. The feelings about him came way down during that one session and it had an unexpected result: Earlier in our treatment we spoke of her sexual relations with Bob. One of the things she really and truly hated were his "sloppy kisses" while he was making love. Following this desensitization she saw it in perspective, felt less helpless, and that she could talk to him about it. She did talk with him and whether or not he changed I do not know but it no longer is a problem.

In the weeks following, a number of changes took place. For the first time, she went around feeling strong and feeling good about it but also feeling angry and irritable. It was as if she was going around saying to herself, "I won't let them take advantage of me." Then she had a fight with Bob and instead of her usual outburst of a sullen striking out at him, she actually yelled—the very first time in her life she had yelled at anyone. Since that time she has been feeling bad, hating herself.

Current Status

After this last satiation series, several life problems came up which diverted the treatment into different channels. These were successfully handled. Then summer came on and Melissa was out of the city, coming in only twice. We did assign a number of satiation areas for homework but none aroused much feeling. However, there were a number of definite changes. She was far more aware of the good things Bob did in relation to her. She was able markedly to decrease her constant nagging. Still far from perfect, the relationship was more pleasant that summer than it had been since the early parts of their being together.

Bob was talking with a contractor about a disagreement regarding some work he was doing for them. Usually, Melissa would be aware of every little point where she thought Bob was doing something wrong. She would keep quiet, not say anything, but would feel irritated for several hours afterward. This time she found that she agreed with Bob, spoke up along with him to the contractor, and afterward Bob thanked her for being so much with him.

There have been an increasing number of such spontaneous incidents. However Melissa remains unsure of what constitutes appropriate assertive behavior in many situations and she remains phobic to being "sinful." We both felt that, although not completely resolved, major reductions in the assertion inhibiting fueling phobias had been achieved. So once again we reformulated the approach. This time we went back to the original Level I formulation and attempted to implement it by having Melissa join my integrated assertiveness group. In this group she practiced being "naughty" and doing "sinful" things and she also rehearsed self-respect inducing behaviors. At this time, she has gone for more than a year with no marked depression, her relationship with Bob still has many problems but has greatly improved, and, in general, she is far more able to take her own needs into consideration.

SUMMARY

The case of Melissa illustrates the workings of behavioral psychotherapy. It is primarily a way for the therapist to think about the patient and to organize a vast amount of information. It aims at providing a course of therapeutic action that is at once systematic yet flexible. Using the concept of levels from the behavioral to the psychodynamic, it attempts to apply the Law of Parsimony as a basis for choosing the level of intervention. It uses the concept of psychological organization to identify keystone behaviors that serve as treatment targets. BP is intended to be a hardnosed practical approach to psychotherapy with the criterion always being whether the desired changes in the patient's life are taking place.

REFERENCES

Aronson, L. R., Tobach, E., Rosenblatt, J. S., & Lehrman, D. S. (Eds.). (1972). *Selected writings of T. C. Schneirla*. San Francisco: W. H. Freeman.

Fensterheim, H. (1972). The initial interview. In A. A. Lazarus (Ed.), *Clinical behavior therapy* (pp. 22–40). New York: Brunner/Mazel.

Fensterheim, H. (1975). The case of Marion: Behavior therapy approach. In C. A. Loew, H. Grayson, & G. H. Loew (Eds.), *Three psychotherapies* (pp. 41–59). New York: Brunner/Mazel.

Fensterheim, H. (1981). Clinical behavior therapy of depression. In J. Clarkin & H. Glazer (Eds.), *Depression:*

Behavioral and directive intervention strategies (pp. 205–228). New York: Garland Press.

Fensterheim, H. (1983). The behavioral psychotherapy model of phobias. In H. Fensterheim & H. I. Glazer (Eds.), *Behavioral psychotherapy: Basic principles and case studies in an integrative clinical model* (pp. 22–39). New York: Brunner/Mazel.

Fensterheim, H. (1989). Commentary: Integrating behavioral and psychodynamic therapies. *Journal of Integrative Eclectic Psychotherapy, 8,* 121–124.

Fensterheim, H., & Glazer, H. I. (1983). *Behavioral psychotherapy: Basic principles and case studies in an integrative clinical model.* New York: Brunner/Mazel.

Fensterheim, H., & Kantor, J. S. (1980). The behavioral approach to sexual disorders. In B. B. Wolman & J. Money (Eds.), *Handbook of human sexuality* (pp. 313–324). Englewood Cliffs, NJ: Prentice Hall.

FitzPatrick, M. M., & Weber, C. K. (1989). Integrative approaches in psychotherapy: Combining psychodynamics and behavioral treatments. *Journal of Integrative Eclectic Psychotherapy, 8,* 102–117.

Haynes, S. N., & O'Brien, W. H. (1990). Functional analysis in behavior therapy. *Clinical Psychology Review, 10,* 649–668.

Jacobson, M. E. (1983). Behavioral psychotherapy of obsessional checking: Treatment through the relationship. In H. Fensterheim & H. I. Glazer (Eds.), *Behavioral psychotherapy: Basic principles and case studies in an integrative clinical model* (pp. 91–108). New York: Brunner/Mazel.

Maletzky, B. M. (1980). Assisted covert sensitization. In D. J. Cox & R. J. Daitzman (Eds.), *Exhibitionism: Description, assessment and treatment* (pp. 187–252). New York: Garland Press.

Salter, A. (1949). *Conditioned reflex therapy.* New York: Farrar, Straus and Giroux.

Shapiro, F. (1989). Efficacy of the eye movement desensitization procedure in the treatment of traumatic memories. *Journal of Traumatic Stress, 2,* 199–223.

Wilson, D. G. (1972). Function. In H. J. Eyesenck, W. Arnold, & B. Meili (Eds.), *Encyclopedia of psychology* (Volume 1, p. 394). New York: Herder & Herder.

CHAPTER 7

Cognitive Analytic Therapy

Anthony Ryle and James Low

INTRODUCTION

Cognitive analytic therapy (CAT) evolved as an integration of theory and practice from various sources. In the course of its development a number of particular therapeutic methods have evolved and an underlying theoretical model has been elaborated. The main sources were cognitive psychology and cognitive psychotherapy on the one hand and psychanalytic object relations theory, restated in a more cognitive language, on the other. The method is marked by an emphasis on the process of reformulation of the patient's problems, the resulting descriptions being used as a "scaffolding" within which a range of therapeutic methods may be applied. Cognitive-behavioral methods and the use of transference are combined with the use of these descriptions by both therapist and patient as tools of understanding and change. A full account of the approach will be found in Ryle (1990).

The idea of reformulation can be linked to the following description from artificial intelligence: "learning to learn is like learning to de-

Anthony Ryle and James Low • Psychotherapy Section, Division of Psychiatry, United Medical and Dental Schools, Guy's Hospital, London SE1 9RT England.

Comprehensive Handbook of Psychotherapy Integration, edited by George Stricker and Jerold R. Gold. Plenum Press, New York, 1993.

bug complex computer programmes, to be good at it requires one to be good at describing processes and good at manipulating such descriptions" (Minsky and Pappert 1972). The particular skill required of the CAT therapist is to be good at generating accurate and useful descriptions of the patients' difficulties. The difficulties will be described in terms of patterns of thought and behavior, with an emphasis as how these actively maintain the problems; written description will often be supplemented with diagrams.

Elaboration of these descriptions requires active patient participation. The final written and diagrammatic reformulation will be agreed between the patient and the therapist and provides the basis for therapy, the aim of which will be the revision of these negative or maladaptive procedures. Thus, reformulation is a tool used by the patient for self-monitoring and used by the therapist to understand and guide the process of therapy. Cognitive analytic therapy is normally applied in therapies lasting between 8 and 16 sessions to a wide range of patients, such as are encountered in public service outpatient practice.

THE THEORETICAL BASIS OF CAT

Initially, CAT evolved from outcome research in psychodynamic therapy. It became clear that the kind of target problem descriptions used in behavioral therapy outcome research were not satisfactory for dynamic therapy, where changes in patterns of understanding and of action are sought. Consideration of a number of completed therapies led to the identification of three main patterns through the operation of which maladaptive processes were sustained. These patterns were entitled *traps, dilemmas,* and *snags* (Ryle, 1979). The characteristics of these patterns can be summarized as follows: Traps involve negative assumptions about self or reality, leading to actions which generate consequences evidently confirming the assumptions. Dilemmas represent false dichotomization of the options available for roles or actions. Snags represent the true or false, conscious or unconscious, appraisal of appropriate actions as being forbidden by self or others, leading to the avoidance of, undoing of, or paying for achievement or happiness.

Descriptions of traps, dilemmas and snags, making use as far as possible of the patient's own words and metaphors, proved to be a satisfactory way of focusing upon the particular areas of difficulty or abandoned aims in a given patient. A more general model of how aim-directed activity is normally organized, maintained, and revised, called the *procedural sequence model* (PSM), was then developed. This model offers an account of the regularly recurring sequences of mental processes, actions and environmental events which are concerned in the maintenance of intentional behavior. Understanding why patients fail to revise maladaptive behaviors requires that the full

sequence of both internal and external processes be described. The normal sequence is described in Figure 1 and can be summarized as follows: Environmental event; perception; appraisal (involving memory, beliefs and systems of value and meaning); formation of aim; consideration of the capacity to achieve the aim and of the consequences of so doing; the choice of means (subprocedures) and action. The evaluation of the effectiveness of the act and of its consequences will lead to the reinforcement, revision, or abandonment of the means or of the aim.

Such a sequence will normally be maintained through a process of continuing anticipation and feedback. In terms of this model, neurosis consists of the persistent use of unrevised procedures and the aim of reformulation in therapy is to identify these procedures and demonstrate how it is that revision has been prevented. Relating this model to the description of traps, dilemmas and snags, it is clear that these can be located upon it as follows:

1. Traps involve the full circle: negative beliefs and assumptions underlying appraisal generate actions which produce consequences which serve to reinforce the underlying assumptions.
2. Dilemmas occur at the point at which alternative subprocedures or means are being considered and essentially represent the narrowing down of possible means (actions or roles) to two polarized alterna-

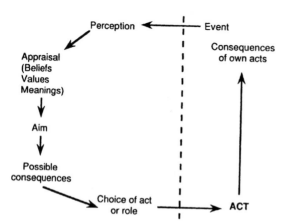

Figure 1. The procedural sequence model: A circular sequence of mental and behavioral processes maintained by *anticipation* and *feedback*.

tives, the enactment of one or other of which seems to confirm the fact that there is only one alternative.

3. In the case of snags appropriate aims are abandoned because of the anticipation (true or false) that to achieve the aims would be "forbidden" or would evoke negative consequences of some sort.

A fuller description of these patterns, with examples, is given in the appendix to this chapter in the "Psychotherapy File," a document normally given to patients at the start of their treatment (see below).

Descriptions of this sort are a satisfactory way of identifying key neurotic procedures, and patients are frequently quick to recognize which ones apply and quick to learn to use that recognition to halt and replace unsatisfactory procedures. However, it is not a fully satisfactory account of the whole process of neurosis, and some consideration must be given to questions of personality structure. One aspect of this structure can be seen to be simply hierarchical, insofar as a normal procedure will be carried out through the operation of subprocedures and may itself represent a subprocedure for a higher order one. For example, cleaning one's teeth could be a subprocedure, part of the general procedure of maintaining one's health, itself part of the existential procedure of living one's life. Beyond this hierarchical structure, however, lie some other complexities best understood in terms of a developmental and structural model of personality such as is provided by *object relations theory* (ORT). In particular, this clarifies the origins of the appraisal mechanisms which are part of the procedural sequence and suggests how different procedures may be efficiently or inefficiently articulated together. The resultant model may be labeled the *procedural sequence object relations model* (PSORM).

The developmental origins of personality structure in terms of a modified object relations theory, free from some aspects of psychoanalytic metapsychology (Ryle 1985), can be summarized as follows:

The newborn infant, equipped with inborn attachment behaviors and using sensorimotor forms of intelligence, is involved actively, for birth, in elaborating *role procedures* for relating to mother and other caretakers. These early role pro-

cedures will initially be concerned with parts of, or aspects of, the mother, and their early development precedes the infant's capacity to discriminate self from other. A role procedure requires one to predict, as the consequences of one's action, the responses of the other; hence, in acquiring a role procedure for interacting with mother, the child, in fact, acquires a model of *two* role procedures, one self-derived and one other-derived (see Ogden 1983). This may be manifest, for example, by the child feeding her mother or mothering a doll or teddy bear. With the development of speech, it becomes clear that, in addition to this, the child begins to enact the maternal role toward herself. The process of internalization of adult "voices" is the basis of the individual's capacity for self-care, self-management, and self-consciousness whereby the self becomes both subject and object. This process of internalization is seen by Vygotsky (1978) as the distinguishing characteristic of the psychological development of humans as opposed to animals and as the basis of our capacity for abstract, unmediated thought. Object relations theorists, however, have been concerned particularly with a reconstruction of the very early phases of development and with problems around this process of internalization. The physically dependent infant can only control the environment by way of communication with the mother, and this communication will have a large affective component. Hence, the individual's sense of the world, of the self, of others, his capacity to express and control feelings and his earliest learning how to manipulate the world are all first acquired within the mutual relationships of infancy.

Early primitive reciprocal role procedures (initially "part object") are the origin of both later whole person reciprocal role procedures and of self-management procedures. A major task of childhood is the integration of these early procedures into complex, whole person ones. Both self-management procedures and reciprocal role procedures can be seen to be derived from the early patterns of "inner parent-inner child" relating formed from the earliest interaction. Successful integration of these will depend upon the reliability and security of the care provided by the parents and is likely to be disrupted by separation, deprivation, or abuse; moreover, more negative childhood experience will often be accom panied by inconsistent or misleading accounts which further damage the process of integration. It is in these failures to integrate that the origin of the more severe adult personality disorders is found.

Persistence of poorly integrated, partial reciprocal role procedures and self-management procedures are manifest in what analysts describe as "splitting" (highly polarized procedures) and in "projective identification" in which one pole of an inner parent-inner child role procedure is elicited from another person. In CAT, these phenomenona are seen as primarily due to failures of integration rather than as having a defensive function.

In producing useful descriptions of more complex personality disordered patients, it becomes necessary not only to identify particular unrevised procedures but also to identify the ways in which different appraisal/enactment systems may be elicited. In this respect, the work of Horowitz (1979) in identifying "state shifts" from psychotherapy protocols was of value in the development of an approach to reformulation called *sequential diagrammatic reformulation* (SDR). Any given neurotic procedure can be seen to originate from one particular aspect of personality. This can be regarded as a subpersonality and as being defined by a characteristic interaction between "internalized parent" and "inner child" roles derived from the developmental process described above. In verbal reformulation one is normally concerned with procedures generated by a single characteristic internal parent-internal child configuration, or by the subjective state associated with one or other pole, usually the child pole (e.g., low self-esteem). In more disordered patients, however, there may be two or more quite recognizable, distinct patterns, occurring discontinuously. In such cases, a diagram is the most effective way of conveying understandings of the structures and sequences involved. A typical example would be that of a borderline personality disorder with a major split between one part characterized by seeking ideal fusion, and the other part characterized by a highly conflictual inner parent-inner child relationship (see Figure 2). From the former may be generated an idealizing transference, the loss of self in "fusion" relationships, or powerful identifications with beliefs or organizations, usually leading in due course to disillusion and a switch into the alternative state.

In this conflicted state there may be attacks upon the self (e.g., parasuicide, drug abuse, alcoholism) or others may be attacked or may be induced to attack the self (abusing-abused, sadomasochistic type relationships). None of these procedures are able to correct the underlying, unmet needs nor do they allow integration of the disparate aspects of the self to take place. More complex models where there are three or four distinct "internal parent-inner child" configurations may require even more complex diagrams, in which the different states or subpersonalities are each characterized by particular internal parent-internal child roles, and in which the sequence between them is traced. Each of these states can generate both self-management procedures and particular patterns of relationship procedures and will be characterized by particular moods or defensive (affect-avoiding) patterns.

Such diagrams, developed to an adequate level of complexity, provide for the therapist an accurate guide with which to make sense of the patient's reported experience and of the therapeutic relationship and, for the patient, a basis for self-understanding and control. Only when the self-maintaining sequences of subpersonalities and the self-reinforcing neurotic procedures derived from these are identified can the patient and the therapist avoid collusive repetitions and initiate recognition and revision.

TECHNIQUE AND PROCESS OF THERAPY

The selection criteria of patients for CAT are broad; provided patients are not currently abusing heroin or alcohol and have not any evidence of active psychosis, most of those referred are taken on, including those suffering from personality disorders of some severity. Over 90% of patients referred to our unit from general practitioners or from psychiatrists are offered individual CAT.

Three phases of therapy may be recognized, namely (1) assessment, leading to reformulation, (2) active therapy, and (3) termination, but in reality in time-limited therapy (CAT is usually given over 16 sessions but shorter interventions have been used) changes will often begin during the first phase and termination will be on the agenda all the way through. The first three or four sessions combine a largely unstructured exploratory

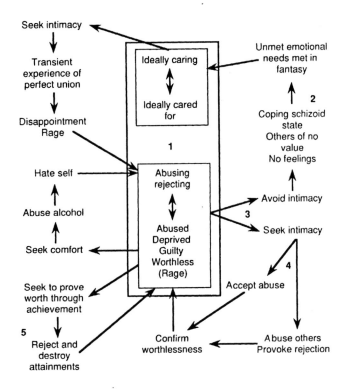

Figure 2. The technique of sequential diagrammatic reformulation: a case of borderline personality.

1 = Split core state
2 = "State of Mind"
3 = Dilemma: Either painfully involved or cut off
4 = Dilemma: Either abuse or accept abuse
5 = Snag

interview technique with the use of certain specific devices, the aim being, at the end of this period, to present the patient with a draft reformulation for modification and agreement. Usually patients are given the Psychotherapy File at the end of their first meeting (see Appendix) and are invited to identify the descriptions which apply to them and bring these back to discuss with their therapist. The file contains instructions in self-monitoring, and any patient with variable mood or other psychologically determined symptoms will carry this out. Some other paper-and-pencil procedures may also be incorporated. At the fourth session, in most cases, the therapist will offer an account drawing upon these sources

and upon observation of the patient in the interviews to date. Normally, this will be in the form of a letter which will rehearse the main difficulties in the patient's life, will describe how these were coped with, and will offer descriptions of their current maladaptive target problem procedures (TPPs). These TPPs represent descriptions of the processes generating and maintaining the patients target problems (TPs), which will also be listed. At the end of this letter, target problems and target problem procedures are listed in abbreviated form and these provide the agenda for the rest of the therapy. Diagrams, where used, will usually be constructed after the written reformulation has been discussed and modified as necessary. Thereafter, at subsequent sessions, either the diagram or the list of TPPs will be on the table and the patient will be invited to rate progress in relation to the material discussed at the end of each session. It will be apparent that these descriptions reflect very directly the theoretical assumptions underlying the approach.

The main use made of the reformulation in the subsequent course of therapy is as a new instrument through which the patient learns to recognize and in due course modify his or her TPPs. This is done through homework assignments (for example, keeping a "placation diary") and will also be used in sessions to make sense of reported behavior and experience and of transference-countertransference interactions in the room. Most patients respond very positively to the reformulation process and subsequently consult their diagrams or TPP lists frequently. At the meeting at which the reformulation letter is read, it is common for patients to cry, indicating that the explicit understanding and acceptance of their pain has been an important experience to them. The therapeutic alliance is cemented at this stage. Where patients make only limited progress other techniques may be introduced in relation to particular procedures; for example, small-scale behavioral programs, the use of role play or gestalt techniques, or whatever other particular skill the therapist may have, but all such interventions will be clearly linked to the overarching understanding offered by the reformulation. At the penultimate session, the therapist will read to the patient a draft "goodbye letter" outlining the work which has been done and indicating areas where further work and vigilance are necessary, and patients are also invited to write their own assessment of what they have achieved. This writing serves to hold the work of therapy actively in the patient's mind during the follow-up period. A review is usually offered at 3 months at which point the patient may be discharged, offered further follow-up, or, in a proportion of cases, offered further sessions. Patients requiring time to work through what they have learned and lacking the social context in which to do it will be referred to group therapy.

This way of working includes, therefore, a range of techniques, especially those drawn from cognitive psychotherapy, but considerable attention is paid to the manifestation of the patients' procedures in their relationship with the thera-pist. All methods are applied in relation to the reformulation, which is the basis upon which patients acquire greater accuracy and skill in self-observation and control. Most psychoanalysts would feel that the use of active techniques would rule out the use of transference interpretations but, in fact, transference manifestations are marked and provoked early in CAT, perhaps by the activity of the early sessions. Such transference manifestations, however, are seldom of a deeply regressive nature. Perhaps the most striking feature of CAT is the way in which patients suffering from brittle, fragmented personality structures feel "held" by reformulation and are able to develop quite rapidly a greater degree of integration and the capacity to cooperate with the therapeutic process. Parallel to this, therapists, who are commonly confused and perturbed by patients with unstable personality structures, are able, with the help of their reformulations, to contain and make sense of, rather than collude with or be confused by, the shifts and vagaries shown by such patients.

Most CAT therapists who have worked in other modes are particularly struck by the speed and depth of work that is achieved within the time frame. Therapy in this mode is hard work for therapists and involves some anxiety, particularly around termination, but experience with over 1,500 patients over the past 8 years suggests that intervention along these lines is safe. There have been no suicides which appeared to be therapy provoked; of the five occurring between assessment and follow-up, three were in severe long-standing personality disorders and two were in patients with bipolar affective disorders; three of these patients were currently inpatients. It may well be that for the more severely disturbed patients this integrative, time-limited, explicit approach is particularly suitable.

CASE EXAMPLE

An Eight-Session Therapy
(by James Low)

Jean was seen for an eight-session CAT from June to September, 1990. There were several breaks because of holidays but apart from that her attendance was regular.

Jean was referred by her physician because of her temper tantrums which were getting her into trouble at work. They were occurring on a daily basis and lasted about half an hour. During the tantrums, Jean shouted at people, threw things about, hit herself, and cried uncontrollably. Jean has a lifelong history of such tantrums and related feelings of low self-esteem and worthlessness.

In the first interview, Jean was very quiet, closed in on herself, offering no eye contact. The silence felt highly charged, as if I was in the presence of a volcano ready to erupt. She said her angry outbursts and mood swings were "not ladylike" and that they got in the way of her being the nice person she wanted to be. I felt pulled into activity, asking too many questions. She was either too placating, answering all my questions, or else she filled the room with paralyzing hostility. Both transference and countertransference seemed to swing from feelings of compliant impotence to a terrifying omnipotence.

Jean, aged 19, lived with her parents and an older sister who had mild neurological damage resulting from a traffic accident. Jean was jealous of the attention her sister received and felt that she was excluded from the family. In fact, she refused all their invitations to shared activities and lived as if in a bed-sit. She had another sister who was married with young children and lived in the flat above her parents. Jean had no memories of her life before she went to school. The first experience she could remember was getting into trouble at school for disobedience and she said, "I've never respected authority. I do what I like." When she was 11 she tried to strangle a boy in her class who had annoyed her and had to be prized off by her sister.

Jean described life at home as a child as relaxed and friendly, but also reported her parents constant arguing largely because of her father's heavy drinking. When she was 12, he encouraged her to drink at home with him and for the next 2 years she regularly got drunk with him, sitting on the sofa watching television. She has little memory of what occurred when she was drunk and while clearly angry at him for starting her on alcohol also felt pleased to have had this special relationship.

Since leaving school at the age of 16, Jean had worked as a sales assistant in a souvenir shop and then in a jewelers. From 15 to 17, she drank a lot, getting out of control and being sexually exploited by men. She had kept friends from that period and felt drawn toward periodic binges of drunkeness with them. From the age of 17, most of her behavior had been dominated by her conversion to Evangelical Christianity. This had become a support for her strong urge to take care of others, putting herself out for them to the point of self-abuse.

By the end of the first interview, which had been marked by extreme mood swings, I had identified at least six out of the eight DSM-III-R criteria for borderline personality organization; namely, unstable relationships, impulsiveness, unstable affect, loss of control anger, identity disturbances, and feelings of emptiness.

It was clear that Jean felt herself to be dangerously omnipotent, always able to get her own way, and was terrified of this. At the same time she repeatedly stated, "I have no right to be here, I don't know what to do."

Jean took away the Psychotherapy File and brought it to the second session. She had double ticked most items and was interested to know what I made of her "condition." I drew a diagram (Figure 3) illustrating how her version of the placation trap seemed to underlie so many of her difficulties. She said, "I'm like my mother, I'll do anything for anybody." She was verbally very grateful for the diagram but put it on the floor under her feet. There followed an angry silence which I broke, out of a need to offer some containment. I asked how she felt and she demanded, "Why do you hate me?"

I felt intimated by the vehemence of her question but sensed it was important not to pull back. I said I felt that it was she who was full of anger and hate due to her difficulty in allowing me to offer her care and attention. A minute of eye balling followed and then she relaxed and said, "I almost walked out, you know." That seemed to be the first turning point in the therapy, with Jean experiencing containment as non-annihilating—but still very threatening.

In the third session, Jean and I worked on a second diagram together. In order to do this we had to sit side by side and this really helped to lower the confrontation atmosphere; it seemed that co-operation, sharing, and mutual adjustment in order to promote clarity were experiences

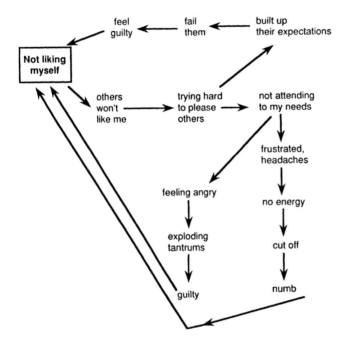

Figure 3. Jean: Preliminary sequential diagram.

Jean responded well to. When I commented on this at the end of the session, she was angry, feeling that I was being patronizing, and laughing at her. I asked her to look at me, not stare at me, and tell me if she really believed it. She smiled and said, "No, its okay." I was unsure if this was just her flipping into the placation trap, but sensed that she was allowing herself to receive something positive before she split into her aggressive or placatory modes.

At the start of the fourth session, I presented her with the completed sequential diagrammatic reformulation (Figure 4). She said, "That's me, that's just how it is." The splitting of the core state made perfect sense to her and she was able to express deep yearning for the two halves to come together. That felt like the first real statement she had made from a position of an integrating center of self, the aspiration holding the basis of its own fulfillment.

Part of the power of the diagram seemed to lie in the absence of ways out, pushing the focus toward the center. As we went round it together,

Jean's attention was drawn again and again to the basic split in her core state. The depiction of the two halves allowed her to see how and why her mood flipped from limitless placation and selfless generosity to a fierce abusive resentment.

The effectiveness of the diagram appeared to lie in its accessibility, its immediate containing effect, and its power as a symbol of the fact of her being understood within a meaningful human relationship.

From the third session, Jean had been monitoring her target problems and target problem procedures; these were finally presented in the reformulation letter at the fifth session. Monitoring these shifts was important because Jean had not wanted to keep a written diary of mood swings and temper outbursts—largely because she feared being controlled by me. But the cumulative effect of the Psychotherapy File, diagrams, monitoring chart, and then the reformulation letter given in the fifth session seemed to constellate a new sense of nonoppressive containment.

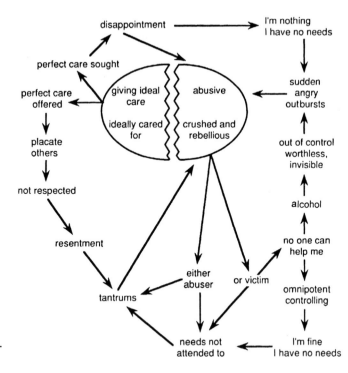

Figure 4. Jean: Diagrammatic re-formulation (final form).

REFORMULATION LETTER

Dear Jean,

You have come for therapy because you are worried about your stormy temper and the trouble it brings you. Your strong desire to change has helped you to make good use of the therapy so far and you have been able to recognise the problematic patterns and procedures which underlie your behavior.

When you were a young child your parents were often fighting and this seems to have been provoked by your father's heavy drinking. You felt that they were too absorbed in their own problems to give you the attention you needed. Rather than helping you to find yourself, they behaved in a way that made you feel angry and isolated, but also unable to express yourself. You became like your mother in not being able to say no to anyone. You feel that your two sisters received more love and attention than you did; not being able to

discuss this in the family you have withdrawn from them more and more, so that although you still live in the same house you find excuses to avoid doing things together.

In the sessions so far, we have looked at the problems that have arisen from your experience and seen that though these responses may have been useful at one time you are now ready to move on to a more easy way of being with yourself and with others. Not being able to express what you feel when you feel it and not being able to recognize and assert your own needs seem to be the principal difficulties underlying your outbursts of violent temper.

Your wild mood swings and feelings of being out of control arise from your basic split; much of the time you feel you must either be an abused victim or an abuser. This is supported by the dilemma concerned with expressing feelings, where it is as if you must either keep feelings bottled up or you risk being rejected, hurting others, and making a mess.

This dilemma has been the focus of our work so far and, as you report, you are starting to experience the possibility of other choices. You have more sense of your own needs, and of the fact that telling others of your needs will not drive them away. Learning to negotiate the middle ground of mutual satisfaction is not easy but it is in that open area that you will find relief from the pressure of either all for others, with a feeling of exhaustion, or all for self, with a feeling of guilt. I note also that you are enjoying the changes that are starting to occur for you. Let's use the rest of therapy to consolidate your growing sense of an appropriate self-confidence.

Yours sincerely,

James Low

The usual procedure in CAT is to provide the prose reformation before developing the sequential diagrammatic reformulation (SDR). However, with patients who exhibit severe mood swings and other borderline symptoms the visual representation of the conflicted aspects of the personality, or of the sequence of personality states, appears to have an immediate containing effect. The "whole picture" of the person is presented and this encourages the development of a more complete sense of self, since the part selves cannot make sense of the whole.

In the fifth session, Jean was able to report more instances of being able to set realistic limits at work and with friends. Thus, she was able to tell a woman for whom she regularly baby sat till 4 A.M. that she would be available from 8 P.M. till 11 P.M. but would then leave whether the woman had returned or not. Jean made a great show of being guilty about this but there was a real twinkle in her eye and she gradually allowed herself to celebrate the sense of identity and reality in the world that it gave her.

The final three sessions were spread out because of holidays but the focus on the SDR as a means of illuminating what was happening in Jean's life gave a sense of continuity. It also encouraged her in the confidence that her new perspective was one which she would be able to develop and sustain after the end of therapy. For example, while on a coach tour in Italy, the first such holiday she had ever taken, Jean fell in love with the coach driver. They had an emotionally intense but nonsexual relationship and she was able to recognize the point when she rejected his care as too threatening and to talk about it with him. In this way, she allowed herself, through the focus of the SDR, to acknowledge her fear of intimacy and avoid abusing someone important to her because of her fear of being abused. She was also able to hang on to the notion of "good enough" care as opposed to her previous consuming fantasy of total perfect care.

Working with Jean became increasingly easy and pleasurable as her sharp intelligence learned to play with the insights that were generated in therapy. She became expert at analyzing options and in assessing which choices would satisfy her various needs. I felt I was witnessing the birth of a self, a real person arising out of the wild maelstrom of uncontrollable moods which she had previously existed as.

Jean's goodbye letter, given to me in the last session, gives some indication of the clarity she developed and how she was able to make the SDR and the CAT experience a part of her life. Ending was very moving because the loss was explicit and yet tempered by a very present sense of the gain, manifest as a definite ability to consciously experience the loss without deflection into tantrums or compensatory caring.

JEAN'S "GOODBYE LETTER"

James,

Since we met some weeks ago, I feel I have grown a lot in maturity and logic. When I first met you I was very unsure of having someone to listen to me for a whole hour but I feel I have learnt to build up a trust with you and a few other people. I feel that our sessions of counseling have been of great value to me both mentally, in the way I think, and emotionally. I have finally realized that I do have a value as a human being and also I have a choice, both with my time and energy. I also recognise I have the right to say *"No"* to people.

I am beginning to feel more secure in myself and now know that there is an in-between, a level balance of my moods. I am also beginning to believe in myself and my abilities as a person not just a bitch or a waste of time.

I am slowly beginning to understand that

people could and do want to know me and be with me, not a false person who is always acting. I can now relax and take time out to do things for myself not just other people.

Thank you for being so understanding in your work,

From,

Jean

THE THERAPIST'S GOODBYE LETTER

Dear Jean,

You have worked really hard with this therapy, recognizing your patterns of thought and behavior and struggling to be aware of the other options that are available. You have been very excited to see how you can exercise choice and live with the uncertain feelings of the area between the extremes that you were so familiar with in the past.

In the first few sessions you often experienced me as a hostile figure and felt you had to struggle with me for control. When you accepted that I would not be destroyed by your anger you were able to step out from behind it and expose some of your vulnerability, loneliness, and neediness. This allowed you to relax your role as universal savior and gave you a bit of space to start taking care of yourself. In this way you have found ways out of the dilemma we identified at the beginning; "either I keep feelings bottled up or I risk being rejected, hurting others, and making a mess."

Letting others know that you have needs yourself and that there is a limit to what you can give has not been easy. You have experienced guilt and confusion but your keen intelligence has helped you to understand that the old patterns were at work and you have pursued your new goals. In doing this you have been able to tell your friends and colleagues that you are changing and that they too must change their expectations of you.

I am very impressed by your understanding and your diligence; by turning your stubborn streak to good advantage you have resisted the power of the old procedures.

Jean I have very much enjoyed getting to

know you and sharing your changes. I'm confident that you have the capacity to keep changing and growing as you further relax your fixed positions and allow yourself to blossom in the dance of life.

With Best Wishes,

James Low

FOLLOW-UP

At the follow-up session 2 months later, Jean was initially withdrawn and rather hostile, once more experiencing me as a threatening authority figure. After a silence of several minutes near the beginning of the session I asked her how she was. "Fine!" she growled. When I smiled at that, she was able to laugh and for the rest of the session was relaxed and forthcoming.

She had had a fight recently with her father and had been able to tell him of some of her disappointment in him. This felt very scary for her, "I've no right to attack him just because he attacks me." But by referring back to SDR she was able to see that standing up for herself was not actually the same as attacking someone else. The session ended with Jean experiencing a sense of being a survivor—and that others near to her would both survive her strength and survive without needing her to rescue them.

I felt that the clear skeletal structure of CAT provided Jean with a meaningful containment, one that she was able to recognise as being on her side. Without such a structure the work would have been both less successful for her and much more painful and confusing for me. The fact that she had tangible mementos of the therapy in the form of the reformulation, SDR, and goodbye letter also made it easier for Jean to end her therapy and for me to end working with this engaging young woman.

DISCUSSION

Jean was treated in a research program comparing 8- and 16-session interventions. At follow-up, she could have received a further 8 sessions had these been indicated. Her treatment illustrates most of the "technical" features of CAT including the verbal reformulation, the joint construction of a sequential diagram, and the use of transference and countertransference both as a source of understanding and as one arena within which the identified procedures were enacted and understood. The powerful effect of reformulation in enabling this patient to take over self therapy is also apparent.

In the current movement toward integrated approaches in psychotherapy, many of the individual features of CAT are utilized by other workers but we believe that the level of practical and theoretical integration achieved and the close integration of theory with practise are unique. Thus, while cognitive therapists are paying increasing attention to implicit structures and are willing to discuss transference, these models of personality structure seem inadequately developed. At the theoretical level, Liotti (1987) proposed the model closest to that of CAT. From the psychoanalytic world a recognition of the need to identify the patient's own "plan" is emphasized by Curtis and Silberschatz (1986); this represents a move toward joint reformulation and is linked with a flexible approach to therapy and with a particular focus upon what in CAT would be called *snags*. We are clearly a long way from reaching any final conclusions in this field but the lessening gulf between psychoanalysis and the rest of psychology is encouraging. In this atmosphere, we hope that CAT will continue to evolve, elaborate, and evaluate its theory and practice.

APPENDIX

The Psychotherapy File

An aid to understanding ourselves better

We have all had just one life and what has happened to us, and the sense we made of this, colors the way we see ourselves and others. How we see things is for us, how things are, and how we go about our lives seems "obvious and right." Sometimes, however, our familiar ways of understanding and acting can be the source of our problems. In order to solve our difficulties we may need to learn to recognize how what we do makes things worse. We can then work out new ways of thinking and acting.

These pages are intended to suggest ways of

thinking about what you do; recognizing your particular patterns is the first step in learning to gain more control and happiness in your life.

Keeping a diary of your moods and behavior

Symptoms, bad moods, unwanted thoughts or behaviors that come and go can be better understood and controlled if you learn to notice when they happen and what starts them off.

If you have a particular symptom or problem of this sort, start keeping a diary. The diary should be focussed on a particular mood, symptom, or behavior, and should be kept every day if possible. Try to record this sequence:

1. How you were feeling about yourself and others and the world before the problem came on.

2. Any external event, or any thought or image in your mind that was going on when the trouble started, or what seemed to start it off.

3. Once the trouble started, what were the thoughts, images or feelings you experienced.

By noticing and writing down in this way what you do and think at these times, you will learn to recognize and eventually have more control over how you act and think at the time. It is often the case that bad feelings like resentment, depression, or physical symptoms are the result of ways of thinking and acting that are unhelpful. Diary keeping in this way gives you the chance to learn better ways of dealing with things.

It is helpful to keep a daily record for 1–2 weeks, then to discuss what you have recorded with your therapist or counselor.

Patterns that Do Not Work, but Are Hard to Break

There are certain ways of thinking and acting that do not achieve what we want, but which are hard to change. Read through the list that follows and mark how far you think they apply to you. Applies strongly + + Applies + Does not apply 0

Traps

Traps are things we cannot escape from. Certain kinds of thinking and acting result in a "vicious circle" when, however hard we try, things seem to get worse instead of better. Trying to deal with feeling bad about ourselves, we think and act in ways that tend to confirm our badness.

Aggression and assertion

People often get trapped in these ways because they mix up aggression and assertion. The fear of hurting others can make us keep our feelings inside, or put our own needs aside. This tends to allow other people to ignore or abuse us in various ways, which then leads to our feeling, or being, childishly angry. When we see ourselves behaving like this, it confirms our belief that we shouldn't be aggressive. Mostly, being assertive—asking for our rights—is perfectly acceptable. People who do not respect our rights as human beings must either be stood up to or avoided.

Examples of traps

1. AVOIDANCE

We feel *ineffective* and *anxious* about certain situations, such as crowded streets, open spaces, social gatherings. We try to go back into these situations, but feel even more anxiety. Avoiding them makes us feel better, so we stop trying. However, by constantly avoiding situations, our lives are limited and we come to feel increasingly *ineffective and anxious*.

2. DEPRESSED THINKING

Feeling *depressed*, we are sure we will manage a task or social situation badly. Being depressed, we are probably not as effective as we can be, and the depression leads us to exaggerate how badly we handled things. This makes us feel more *depressed* about ourselves.

3. SOCIAL ISOLATION

Feeling *underconfident* about ourselves and anxious not to upset others, we worry that others will find us boring or stupid, so we don't look at people or respond to friendliness. People then see us as unfriendly, so we become more isolated from which we are convinced we are boring and stupid—and become more *underconfident*.

4. TRYING TO PLEASE

Feeling *uncertain about ourselves* and anxious not to upset others, we try to please people by doing what they seem to want. As a result (1) we end up being taken advantage of by others, which makes us angry, depressed or guilty, from which our uncertainty about ourselves is confirmed; or (2) sometimes we feel out of control because of the need to please, and start hiding away, putting things off, letting people down, which makes other people angry with us and increases our uncertainty.

Dilemmas (False Choices and Narrow Options)

We often act as we do, even when we are not completely happy with it, because the only other ways we can imagine, seem as bad or even worse. These false choices can be described as dilemmas, or either/or options. We often don't realize that we see things like this, but we act *as if* these were the only possible choices.

Do you act as if any of the following false choices rule your life? Recognizing them is the first step to changing them.

Choices about yourself: I act as if:

1. Either I keep feelings bottled up or I risk being rejected, hurting others, or making a mess.

2. Either I feel I spoil myself and am greedy or I deny myself things and punish myself and feel miserable.

3. If I try to be perfect, I feel depressed and angry. If I don't try to be perfect, I feel guilty, angry, and dissatisfied.

4. If I must, then I won't (other people's wishes, or even my own, feel too demanding, so I constantly put things off, avoid them, etc.).

5. If other people aren't expecting me to do things, look after them, etc., then I feel anxious, lonely, and out of control.

6. If I get what I want, I feel childish and guilty; if I don't get what I want, I feel angry and depressed.

7. Either I keep things (feelings, plans) in perfect order, or I fear a terrible mess.

Choices about how we relate to others

Do you behave with others as if:

1. If I care about somebody, then I have to give in to them.

2. If I care about somebody, then they have to give in to me.

3. If I depend on someone, then they have to do what I want.

4. If I depend on someone, then I have to give in to them.

5. Either I'm involved with someone and likely to get hurt, or I don't get involved and stay in charge, but remain lonely.

6. As a woman, I have to do what others want.

7. As a man, I can't have any feelings.

8. Either I stick up for myself and nobody likes me, or I give in and get put on by others and feel cross and hurt.

9. Either I'm a brute or a martyr (secretly blaming the other).

10. Either I look down on other people, or I feel they look down on me.

Snags

Snags are what is happening when we say "I want to have a better life, or I want to change my behavior but. . . ." Sometimes this comes from how we or our families thought about us when we were young; such as "She was always the good child," or "In our family we never. . . ." Sometimes the snags come from the important people in our lives not wanting us to change, or not able to cope with what our changing means to them. Often the resistance is more indirect, as when a parent, husband, or wife becomes ill or depressed when we begin to get better.

In other cases, we seem to "arrange" to avoid pleasure or success, or if they come, we have to pay in some way, by depression, or by spoiling things. Often this is because, as children, we came to feel guilty if things went well for us, or felt that we were envied for good luck or success. Sometimes we have come to feel responsible, unreasonably, for things that went wrong in the family, although we may not be aware that this is so. It is helpful to learn to recognize how this sort of pattern is stopping you getting on with your life, for only then can you learn to accept your right to a better life and begin to claim it.

You may get quite depressed when you begin to realize how often you stop your life being happier and more fulfilled. It is important to remember that it's not being stupid or bad, but rather that: (a) We do these things because this is the way we learned to manage best when we were younger, (b) we don't have to keep on doing them now we are learning to recognize them, (c) by changing our behavior, we can learn to control not only our own behavior, but we also change the way other people behave to us, (d) although it may seem that others resist the changes we want for ourselves (for example, our parents or our partners), we often underestimate them; if we are firm about our right to change, those who care for us will usually accept the change.

Do you recognize that you feel limited in your life:

1. For fear of the response of others,
2. By something inside yourself.

Difficult and Unstable States of Mind

Indicate which, if any, of the following apply to you:

1. How I feel about myself and others can be unstable; I can switch from one state of mind to a completely different one.

2. Some states may be accompanied by intense, extreme, and uncontrollable emotions.

3. Others by emotional blankness, feeling unreal, or feeling muddled.

4. Some states are accompanied by feeling intensely guilty or angry with myself, wanting to hurt myself.

5. Or by feeling that others can't be trusted, are going to let me down, or hurt me.

6. Or by being unreasonably angry or hurtful to others.

7. Sometimes the only way to cope with some confusing feelings is to blank them off and feel emotionally distant from others.

REFERENCES

Curtis, J. T., Silberschatz, G. (1986). Clinical implications of research on brief dynamic psychotherapy: 1. Formulating the patient's goals and problems. *Psychoanalytic Psychology*, 3(1), 13–25.

Horowitz, M. J. (1979). *States of mind: Analyses of change in psychotherapy*. New York: Plenum Press.

Liotti, G. (1987). The resistance to change of cognitive structures: A counter proposal to psychoanalytic meta psychology. *Journal of Cognitive Psychotherapy*, 1, 87–104.

Minsky, M., & Pappert, S. (1972). *Artificial intelligence*. (Progress report). Cambridge: Massachusetts Institute of Technology.

Ogden, T. H. (1983). The concept of internal object relations. *International Journal of Psychoanalysis*, 64, 227–241.

Ryle, A. (1979). The focus in brief interpretive psychotherapy: Dilemmas, traps and snags as target problems. *British Journal of Psychiatry*, 134, 46–64.

Ryle, A. (1985). Cognitive theory, object relations and the self. *British Journal of Medical Psychology*, 58, 1–7.

Ryle, A. (1990). *Cognitive-analytic therapy: Active participation in change*. Chichester: Wiley.

Vygotsky, L. S. (1978). *Mind in society: The development of higher psychological processes*. (Ed. by M. Cole et al.). Cambridge: Harvard University Press.

CHAPTER 8

Existential Psychotherapies

James F. T. Bugental and Richard I. Kleiner

INTRODUCTION

What is *is* what *exists*. Existential perspectives attend to existence, to what is. Rather than postulating some other basic drive—for example, sexuality, power—an existential orientation sees the fact of being itself as the central issue of our lives. How shall we be alive? What are we making of the miracle of our conscious being? How are we to be more fully, more truly realizing (i.e., recognizing and making actual) that which is latent within our nature? This is the outlook and the challenge of existentialism.

In this chapter, we will briefly sketch the postulates which guide our thinking and our clinical applications of this outlook. Obviously, there is an ocean of literature addressing these questions, and, equally obviously, we can offer but a few cupfuls in this setting. Nevertheless, these samples will likely gain in communication potency by the fact that we are living beings, and thus we are all existentialists in some measure.

James F. T. Bugental • Saybrook Institute and California School of Professional Psychology, Berkeley, California 94949. Richard I. Kleiner • Bay Counseling and Consulting, 201 San Antonio Circle, Mountain View, California 94040.

Comprehensive Handbook of Psychotherapy Integration, edited by George Stricker and Jerold R. Gold. Plenum Press, New York, 1993.

About Naming This Orientation

Unlike many schools of psychotherapy, the existential perspective—which is basically a philosophical stance—informs a range of therapeutic approaches. It is a viewpoint or meaning context within which to conduct psychotherapy. Frequently one will find therapists who view themselves as "existential" and who also see themselves as psychoanalytic, Jungian, gestaltist, object-relations, or humanistic (Ofman, 1985). In this chapter, we will try to identify the conceptual position that most of these therapists share, and when doing so will use the unqualified term, *existential*. When we come to discuss clinical applications—the zone in which the differences within this family are most evident—we will use the adjective "humanistic" to make clear that this is our own practice and to recognize that not all existential therapists may share these views (Hoeller, 1990).

CONCEPTUAL POSITION

The existential-analytic approach to psychotherapy developed from the literature of existential philosophy and in contrast to reductionistic and deterministic approaches to psychotherapy. These orientations characteristically put the primary focus of psychotherapy on various sub-aspects of persons and insist on a deterministic (causal) outlook. Thus, approaches as divergent as psychoanalysis and behaviorism agreed in viewing people as best understood by objective analysis. Existentialism shifts the emphasis back to the whole human being: "Man supersedes the sum of his parts" (Bugental, 1965, p. 11).

Existential psychotherapy recognizes the usefulness of attending at times to part-units of humans, such as drives and stimulus-response patterns, but places them in a more appropriate context—specifically the total "beingness" of the human. This brings the focus to the client's inner sense of being and provides an overall framework within which therapy may occur (May, 1958a). The therapist attends to the person as a whole, the actual immediate person, and regards that person's distress as related to the client's overall being in the world, not solely as some inner disease or injury which is to be objectively studied and cured.

The fact of being alive and thus of having to confront ultimate existential questions creates anxiety. Bugental (1965) described the sense of contingency and uncertainty which we must all live with, the inability ever to guarantee completely our security or the outcomes of our efforts. This inherent awareness of being subject to fate is the source of existential anxiety. May and Yalom (1984) asserted that, "anxiety arises from our personal need to preserve our being and to assert our being" (p. 354), and May (1983) highlighted existential anxiety as distinct from other emotions. It is characteristic of humans—rooted in our very existence—thus it is not something to be overcome, eliminated, or outgrown. "Anxiety is the experience of the threat of imminent non-being" (p. 109).

Despite this anxiety of our natural condition, we must also find a way to be in the world. Accordingly, we structure our world, make a "map" of the world, to provide some sense of order or "knowness." To create this structure, however, we must limit our world and ourselves to knowable proportions. When this constriction process becomes too fixed or rigid, when our attempts to ward off existential anxiety too severely limit our sense of beingness or aliveness, we experience emotional distress. Psychotherapy attempts to aid clients' attempts to relieve this constrictive misery. By fostering explicit awareness of the

limits we put on our worlds, it becomes possible to reduce these distortions and to risk confronting the existential givens of being alive (Bugental, 1965).

Human beings are, so far as we know, the only organisms with the capacity to be conscious and to be aware of our consciousness at the same time. It is this capacity for reflexive self-awareness that is at the root of the approach we are here describing. Our reflexive awareness gives us the possibility of diminishing or transcending the blocks to authentic living. Therapy of this orientation puts this task in its center.

CLINICAL AND THEORETICAL ANTECEDENTS

Existential philosophy developed in Europe in the nineteenth and twentieth centuries through the work of Binswanger, Heidegger, Husserl, Jaspers, Kirkegaard, and others. It began to have a psychotherapeutic offshoot following World War II (and particularly the Nazi occupation of France). Ellenberger, Angel, Sartre, and Camus are among those who especially advanced this movement in its early form, an emergence which coincided with a growing dissatisfaction with the deterministic philosophies. Existential thinking remained largely a European phenomenon, however, until the publication in 1958 of *Existence: A New Dimension in Psychiatry and Psychology*, edited by Rollo May, Ernest Angel, and Henri Ellenberger. In this book, May (1958, p. 11) defines existentialism as "the endeavor to understand man by cutting below the cleavage between subject and object which has bedeviled Western thought and science since shortly after the Renaissance."

This widely influential book had a marked impact on many in the American psychological community. Today the existential approach continues as a growing influence in American psychotherapy, but so far this has been chiefly a matter of individual contributions rather than a basis for the development of formal training programs or institutes.

Closely related to the growth of existentialism in psychology was the rise of humanistic psychology, often known as the "third force" (in contrast with psychoanalysis and behaviorism). This orientation shared with existential psychology an impetus to go beyond the reductionistic, overly objectified view of humans characteristic of classical psychoanalysis and behaviorism (Bugental, 1965). Among the leading proponents of humanistic psychology were Maslow, Rogers, Buhler, Moustakas, Jourard, Bugental, and Kelly. This movement stressed the need in understanding human experience for more humanistic concepts, such as choice, values, love, creativity, self-awareness, and human potential.

Although the terms *existential* and *humanistic* are not synonymous, there is considerable overlap, and the area of their overlap is rich in potential for greater understanding of human experience. Yalom (1980) acknowledged the overlap but also emphasized that there is a fundamental difference in some regards. While the European existential tradition emphasized human limitations and the tragic dimensions of existence, humanistic psychology in the United States developed in an atmosphere of expansiveness and optimism, emphasizing development of potential, enhancing awareness, peak experiences, and self-actualization.

Our "Thrown Condition"

When I consider the brief span of my life swallowed up in the eternity before and behind it, the small space that I fill, or even see, engulfed in the infinite immensity of spaces which I know not, and which know me not, I am afraid, and wonder to see myself here rather than there; for there is no reason why I should be here rather than there, now rather than then. (Pascal, 1946, p. 36)

This eloquent statement of the nature of existential anxiety also portrays what is referred to as our human "thrown condition." It is out of this recognition that we confront the "givens" of being. Each of these conditions of being or givens brings with it an inescapable circumstance or "confrontation" which must be dealt with in some manner. Various theorists have presented their own lists of these fundamental concerns. Yalom (1980) suggests four, and Bugental (1987) offers five with a confrontation identified to each. Table 1 demonstrates the similarities between the two views:

Underlying existential psychotherapy is the belief that all human life is ultimately concerned with these conditions of our being, that the patterning we give to our lives is so derived, and that the symptoms or distresses we bring to psycho-

Table 1. Two Views of the Existential "Givens"

Yalom (1980)	Bugental (1965, 1987)	
Given	Given	Confrontation
	Embodied	Change
Death	Finitude	Contingency
Freedom }	{ Action-able	Responsibility
Meaninglessness }	{ Choiceful	Relinquishment
Isolation	Separate-but-related	A-part-from and apart-of

therapy have their ultimate—even if not conscious or explicit—roots in how we have dealt with these givens.

Embodiedness—Change. We experience life chiefly through the medium of our bodies. Whatever one's metaphysical stance may dictate, this also means that our corporeality is continually present and influencing much that is not material. Our bodies are living metaphors for the continual changefulness of being. Just as they mature, sicken and heal, age, and eventually die, so all aspects of living are transitory and evolving. Indeed, life *is* process.

This impermanence permeates our views of ourselves and our worlds, and the efforts we make to deny or overcome changefulness are a frequent source of psychological distress. Of course, our embodiedness interacts with each of the other givens in important ways, and that interactivity is another manifestation of the fundamental unity of our being.

Death—Finitude. Human life is limited in all experienced dimensions (although our vision may seek infinity). We know we will only live so long, can only do so much, may learn much but not everything, and are limited in our strength. Finitude lays us open to contingency, to circumstance, to chance benefits or harms, to fate.

The awareness of death is the most prominent aspect of finitude and is an inescapable aspect of being. For many it is a core inner conflict which plays a major (if not always conscious) role in their lives. The awareness of the certainty of one's death coupled with the uncertainty as to

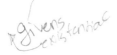

when and in what manner that end will arrive colors experience powerfully.

Yet the influences of our finitude are matters of daily experience, not simply of morbid reflections. We continually seek certainty, save our money, protect our homes, support police and armies, buy "insurance" (as though it were really purchasable), and obey driving laws to try to be safe and avoid unwanted contingencies. Similarly, we buy lottery tickets, take risks in the stock market, engage in hazardous sports, and in a dozen other ways court favorable fortune.

Freedom—Action-able and Meaninglessness—Choiceful. Compared to other species, human beings enter the world with little inherent structure or design. There can be a pervasive terror in confronting such inexorable groundlessness.

Life means the inexorable necessity of realizing the design for an existence which each one of us is. . . . The sense of life . . . is nothing other than each one's acceptance of [this] inexorable circumstance and, on accepting it, converting it into [one's] own creation. (Ortega y Gasset, cited in May, 1981, p. 93)

If we have lives with meaning and purpose, or if our lives lack all such value, we are ultimately responsible for so creating them.[1] Thus we are not passive observers of what is; we are active participants in its creation. Thus, our ability to act and to not-act makes for our having a significant part in the creation of actuality. Thus, it is a root of the dignity of being human, but one that is gained at the price of confronting the emptiness of existence, the lack of any overarching value to which all adhere.

To be the authors of our being, not merely actors carrying out a predetermined script, is a heavy responsibility which we often attempt to shift. When we accept it, we recognize that we are always creating meanings and values by our actions and our non-actions.

Isolation—Separate-but-Relatedness. We enter the world and depart from it ultimately alone; yet our lives between these two events are inextricably joined with others. Humans are always

---

[1]This hard recognition implies no blame for those who due to circumstances are forced into meaningless and futile living. It simply faces the reality that ultimately the individual is the final arbiter of her or his own life and that some few incredibly escape from such destinies.

paradoxically pressed and pulled by the need for relation with others, the sense of being unchangeably separate from them, the threat of being abandoned, and the revulsion of sensing connection with those we abhor. Our very lives depend on how we handle these conflicting impulses. Moreover, what fulfillment or distress we experience derives from the response we make to this need to be at once *apart from* all others and yet still *a part of* all humankind. Existential isolation recognizes that full and complete connection between human beings can never be attained; there will always remain an unbridgeable chasm. Yet existential relatedness, ironically, insists we are inextricably tied to our fellow humans and deeply in need of a sense of connectedness.

In no part of our lives are the effects of this given absent, whether it be the much focused on relations between the sexes or the dangerous and momentous realm of international competition, cooperation, and struggle.

Other Existential Concepts

Beingness—I-Process. The human experience of "being" or "existence" is, of course, central to the existential-analytic viewpoint. However, this is not as simple a matter as might be thought. At any given moment we may think ourselves aware of our own being, but reflection will often reveal that that awareness is of the self as an object—that is, of our body, our observed thoughts, our experienced emotions, and so on. It is important to recognize that these are all objectifications of our living; they are not the living process itself.

Indeed, it is—by its very nature—impossible to observe our living process, for it is that process *which is the observing.* Just as we cannot see our own eyes, only their reflections in mirrors, so we cannot see the process of our subjectivity, only its objectification in various forms.

Nor is this a minor philosophic issue. It underlies the paradox of failed intention: We seek to have charge of our lives, but in a very real way, we are seldom able to make significant changes in established patterns. So we decide that psychotherapy is needed, but psychotherapy that concerns itself solely with the objectified self is limited and dependent on outer influences—authority, force, or mechanical enforcement.

In contrast, therapy which leads to the discovery of one's own subjecthood, a much less usual experience, can have lasting and powerful results, for such therapy addresses our loss of centered consciousness of our own true identity.

In those rare moments which supersede objective knowledge of oneself, one is filled with awareness of the naked fact of being. Such a time may be referred to as an "I-am" experience (May & Yalom, 1984). These are times of "knowing" rather than "knowing about."

Bugental (1965) used the term "I-process" to distinguish the truly subjective and experiencing aspect of our being, the unseen seer and the vital knowing back of what is known. It is in crucial contrast with the objective aspects, "me" and "self." Obviously, it is the task of truly life-changing psychotherapy to arouse this consciousness in the client; only then will lasting and deep changes be possible.

Manifestly, these are matters of critical importance to therapists as they relate with their clients: "When we seek to know a person, the knowledge about him must be subordinated to the overarching fact of his actual existence" (May, 1958a, p. 38).

Existential versus Neurotic Anxiety. Earlier we noted the significance of existential anxiety to our underlying theoretical perspective. It is useful to contrast it with neurotic anxiety. Whereas existential anxiety is inherent in our existence, resulting from the threat of nonbeing and the experience of contingency, neurotic anxiety results from distorting the existential realities of life in an attempt to diminish or avoid existential anxiety.

Neurotic anxiety is nearly always what is presented in the first therapeutic encounters. Existential anxiety may never be openly or explicitly identified as such in the work. Yet the therapist recognizes that it lies beneath the surface like the skeleton below the surface of the skin. A patient's anxiety about a particular life issue will often be the form in which deeper existential issues such as finitude or meaninglessness are clothed.

THE TECHNIQUE AND PROCESS OF PSYCHOTHERAPY

The basic existential approach to psychotherapy provides a perspective more than a spe-

cific series of techniques or directives about how to perform such work. Accordingly, there are wide variations in procedures among psychotherapists regarding themselves as "existential." In this section, we will present one way of carrying out psychotherapy that is consonant with an existential perspective. Manifestly, this cannot claim to be *the one way*. However, what is largely shared among therapists of this orientation can be identified through setting forth a set of basic tenets:

1. *An existential orientation recognizes that psychological distresses overlie deeper (and often implicit) existential issues.*

We reviewed these "existential issues" in the previous section. Here we need only recognize that existential therapists gradually develop an "existential ear" which senses these life concerns underlying the more obvious problems and complaints of their patients. The point is the enrichment (by an awareness of these existential concerns) of the therapist's organismic appreciation for what the client presents.

2. *An existential orientation maintains primary regard for the unique individuality and humanness of each client.*

As significant as are one's understanding of existential tenets, one's grasp of psychotherapeutic doctrine and practice, and one's personal commitment to his or her profession, the overriding value for the therapist always needs to be the client's own integrity. The client's welfare and autonomy as a unique individual transcend any theories or hypotheses held by the therapist.

3. *An existential orientation gives central attention to the client's own beingness, awareness, or subjectivity.*

As we saw above, the site of the most important psychotherapeutic work is the subjectivity, the inner stream of experience, of the client. Therapists of this perspective generally foster greater inner awareness of clients, increased sensing of their own powers, emotions, and intentions, meanwhile developing recognition of how clients are self-impeding.

This tenet makes evident why the loss of connection to one's sense of inner being is regarded as a primary source of psychological distress and as a barrier to vitality and satisfaction in living.

4. *An existential orientation emphasizes the atemporality—the lived present—of subjective life, and thus all other time frames are seen chiefly in their relation to the immediate.*

Without negating the role of past experience in influencing present emotions and actions, the existential therapist regularly attends to that which is in fact "alive" or current in the client's subjectivity. It is for this reason that such therapists often attend to *how* the client speaks about the past or the future as much as to what the client says about these other life phases. Life concerns take on full meaning only in the context of the person's current being-in-the-world.

Accordingly, for existential thinking as here summarized, resolution of distress is only possible in the present. Similarly, for example, it is deemed impossible to "go back to" an earlier trauma. The fundamental principle is that growth or change may be had only by way of the route through confronting present perceptions and emotions.

Importance of Subjectivity. Having sketched the theoretic foundation of the existential orientation, we now address the actual processes of such therapy when conducted from an existential-humanistic stance. What does such a psychotherapist actually do—insofar as generalizations about the answer to this question are possible?

Our third tenet above emphasized the importance of the clients' inner sense of their own being. Much therapeutic attention is focused on aiding clients in recognizing, bringing into focus, and valuing work with this always present but often disregarded realm. May (1958a) says,

The central task and responsibility of the therapist is to seek and understand the patient as a being and as a being in his world. All technical problems are subordinate to this understanding. . . . With it the groundwork is laid for the therapist being able to help the patient recognize and experience his own existence, and this is the central process of psychotherapy. (p. 77)

To sense one's own being is to be regularly aware of the range, depth, and unending stream of subjective experience. Bugental (1987) defines subjectivity as,

That inner, separate, and private realm in which we live most genuinely. The furnishings or structures of this realm are our perceptions, thoughts, feelings and emotions, values and preferences, anticipations and apprehensions, fantasies and dreams, and all else that goes on endlessly night and day, waking and sleeping, and so determines what we do in the external world, and what we make of what happens to us there. . . . Subjectivity is the seedbed of the concerns which impel us to undertake therapy, and it is the root system of our intentionality, which must be mobilized if our therapeutic quest is to succeed. (p. 7)

Existential-humanistic therapy gives particular attention to clients' patterns of response to the questions life poses: What and who are you? What is this world? What brings satisfaction? What is hurtful and disappointing? What sources of power can you draw on to aid you in your life?

Client confrontations with these questions may produce satisfaction and aliveness or frustration and emptiness, but it is through the examination of client subjectivity that the basic patterns which structure their worlds and ultimately account for their experience of being in the world are best revealed and worked with.

When one's existing pattern of life fails to bring sufficient gratifications and yields too much pain, it must be reexamined and amended. This, however, is a demanding and often frightening and painful process. The therapist must support the client's courage and be steadfast through the trials of relinquishment and tentative change.

It is this exploration of subjectivity and the continuing attempt to access the experience of being which comprise the basic task of existential-humanistic psychotherapy.

Presence. For therapeutic work to go forward effectively, it is essential that both client and therapist be as fully engaged in that work as may be possible for them. To describe life concerns from an inner subjectively alive and experiencing place is a crucially different process for the person engaged in doing so than is talking about those same matters in an objective, detached manner in which the actual experience or substance of the concern is barely experienced and remains abstract and impersonal. Clients, particularly at the start of therapy, may present their lives and concerns in just such a detached way; they appear to be observing rather than experiencing their lives.

Clients demonstrate lack of presence in myriad ways. They may minimize the importance of the therapy itself by their attitude toward frequency of sessions, promptness, and missed appointments. They may avoid presence by their attitude toward themselves in the session (e.g., sarcasm, belittling, detachment), or they may resist presence by maintaining a cool, analytical intellectual approach to their concerns. All of these ways of avoiding full presence are forms of resistance and must be addressed by the therapist.

Not only must the therapist monitor the client's presence, but the therapist's own presence must be maintained and must match or even lead the client's. For example, at times the therapist may manifest deeper presence than the client as a way of calling forth or deepening the client's immersion.

It is essential that therapists regard their patients' concerns with genuine respect. Although this may seem obvious, it is sadly evident that some therapeutic approaches encourage therapists to adopt a casual, detached, or investigative attitude toward such issues. It is our belief that such an approach plays into clients' resistances, reduces their genuine presence, and fosters a counterproductive dependence on therapists.

Client concern, in short, is an essential element in the therapeutic process as it provides both motivation and guidance to the therapeutic work.

Locus of Therapeutic Change

By emphasizing the importance of the exploration of the client's subjectivity and by relying on the client's concern as a source of guidance in that process, a very particular assumption is being made with regard to the locus of therapeutic change—namely that the locus of therapeutic change resides within the client—*and only within the client*. This is in stark contrast to medical models and therapies that view the therapist as the primary agent of change.

Existential-humanistic (and other "inner search" oriented) therapies insist that access to the change potential residing within their clients is to be via those clients' exploration of their own inner subjective experiencing. Therapists facilitate this inner exploration in a variety of ways, knowing that only by this route do significant and lasting changes in life structures become possible.

Herein lies a truly important but often overlooked point: *Therapists cannot give insight to clients.* Our ultimate separateness from other individuals is clearly demonstrated by our limited capacity to access another's inner subjective world. Therefore the "whodunit" approach of many schools of psychotherapy which attempt to teach or infuse the patient with a particular theory or interpretation has little place in an existential-humanistic framework. A possible insight is only valuable to the extent that it emerges from and is consistent with the client's inner subjective experience. Without this, the therapist's theories, despite their possible abstract brilliance, are futile and empty.

Seeing matters in this way does not prohibit therapists from making observations and interpretations, analyzing patterns of behavior, or giving feedback, but the purpose of such interventions is always to access or deepen the client's own inner sight (Bugental, 1978).

The therapist's role therefore is not to cure, fix, or change clients but to help clients to manifest that capacity which already exists within themselves but which is blocked. It is this blocking—or interference with clients' inner exploration that in the existential view is regarded as *resistance*; resistance to full, centered awareness—be it noted—not to the therapist or the therapeutic process only.

Phases in the Therapeutic Process

Developing the Alliance. As in most systems of psychotherapy, the beginning phase of an existential-humanistic approach is primarily concerned with developing the therapeutic alliance. Bugental (1978) described this relation as,

the bridge over which the client will travel from a present way of life to a reborn way of being. It will have to provide support in times of enthusiasm and times of despair, in periods of struggle and conflict, and through the dark days when the client may need to attack the bridge itself and me as well. . . . This relationship is not immediately comparable to any other in life. It is a friendship; it is a love affair; it is a partnership; it is a blood bond; it is a duel; it is all of these and none of them and yet something more. (p. 72)

Fostering an effective therapeutic alliance is not a discrete step in the therapy process, but a development which is occurring simultaneously with other functions. Along with the obvious business of getting acquainted in the early sessions, therapists must also assess their clients' available inner resources which motivate them toward growth (Bugental, 1978) and their readiness and ability to explore the subjective realm. Instilling in clients a belief in and a valuing of the need to expand their inner awareness is intrinsic to this whole work.

Deepening the Client's Concern. As the therapeutic alliance is gradually being developed and intensified, therapists must help their clients deepen and expand their initial understanding of their concerns. This often calls for encouraging a link-up between the client's conscious awareness of a particular symptom or problem and deeper, more significant underlying conditions. It is at this phase that the existential approach differs sharply from behavioral or other short-term systems of therapy which emphasize symptom relief and would accept the symptoms at face value. In contrast, problems are regarded as indications of the clients' crippled inner awareness, and symptoms are used as springboards to address this. Critically important here is the recognition that this inner division of symptoms from their deeper lying sources is a form of resistance, and that, in turn, holds suggestions of the manner in which clients have structured their own identities and that of their worlds.

So, as early as possible in the therapy, clients are introduced to an experience-based appreciation that presenting problems have deeper meanings, that they themselves are the only ones able to discover these meanings, and that to do so they must begin to explore their subjective inner worlds. Soon they discover that their capacity to perform this inner exploration is handicapped (i.e., the resistance), and so the client begins to develop an experiential and cognitive understanding of the need for greater subjective self-awareness (Bugental, 1978).

Inner Exploration. The major portion of the therapeutic process is involved in helping clients discover their capacity for inner discovery. This capacity is often unfamiliar to them, but it is psychologically an important part of our native endowment. When we do not have well established pathways for dealing with situations, we spontaneously begin a subjective process which has been variously called "searching," "unfolding" (Buber), "focusing" (Gendlin), "trial and error," and "free association" (Freud).

We prefer to call it *searching* since that term has a long history in American psychology. As clients learn to access this process, they allow various thoughts, impulses, emotions, and other subjective material to emerge—without criticism or editing—into their consciousness. This is, of course, the basis of imagination, discovery, and creativity. It is a powerful vehicle for life direction, once one learns to use it and to set aside the many constrictions we have learned to put on it (i.e., the resistances).

Disclosing and Working through the Resistance. Having developed a working therapeutic alliance and aided clients in deepening their concern and curiosity about the need to explore their inner worlds while recognizing their limited capacity to do so, the next task is to assist clients in actually confronting their blocked access to this subjective experience. This is a painstaking and time-consuming disclosing and working through of the client's resistances, a process central to most dynamic schools of therapy but one which has particular meaning in the existential-humanistic view.

Freud saw resistance as manifested in the patient's failure to follow "the basic rule" of free association and in the refusal to accept the analyst's interpretations (Freud, 1916/1917). Currently many psychotherapeutic systems continue to regard resistance as the client's defense against therapist interpretation. The existential-humanistic view of resistance accepts this view as relevant and useful but expands upon it. Bugental defined resistance from the existential viewpoint as,

the impulse to protect one's familiar identity and known world against perceived threat. . . . Resistance is those ways in which the client avoids being truly subjectively present—accessible and expressive—in the therapeutic work. The conscious or unconscious threat is that full immersion will bring challenges to the client's being in her world. (1987, p. 175)

It is useful to distinguish between the purpose or meaning of the resistance and the way in which it is manifested. The purpose of the resistance is to protect against threat. Ultimately clients protect against the threat of nonbeing, but at varying levels they may be avoiding confrontation with other existential issues as well. To avoid confrontation with this threat, they have constructed ways of being in the world which at the same time shrink their aliveness in the world. As psychotherapy attempts to address this constriction process, the patient's basic sense of being is experienced as under assault—thereby creating a need for resistance or, as manifested in the therapeutic hour, a blocked access to inner awareness.

Resistance is generally thought to occur in many layers and at many levels and to present itself in a variety of ways. In brief, the working through of the resistance involves a three-step process: (a) identifying the resistance pattern as it is displayed in the therapeutic hour, (b) repeatedly presenting this pattern to the client as it continues to occur, and (c) encouraging the client's discovery of the need or purpose served by maintaining the particular resistance pattern which has been presented. This may stimulate the client's curiosity and encourage seeking for the source of the resistance pattern. As the client begins to recognize the purpose of the particular resistance pattern, its underlying function will usually become clearer (Bugental, 1978).

The work of identifying and disclosing resistance patterns is one of the major phases of intensive existential-humanistic psychotherapy. By maintaining a consistent focus on facilitating the client's inner search process, and expanding one's subjective awareness, the varying layers of resistance will continue to be confronted.

Although a more thorough discussion of resistance is beyond the scope of this chapter, the reader is referred to Bugental (1965, 1987) for a description of the varying dimensions of resistance and a detailed and systematic approach to working through the resistance.

The Therapeutic Relationship

Although some psychotherapeutic systems posit the therapeutic relationship as the primary agent of client change, in an existential-analytic approach the relationship between client and therapist is not seen as the change agent, but rather it is recognized as the medium in which change occurs (Bugental, 1965). This in no way minimizes the importance of the therapeutic rela-

tionship to the support of client endeavors. May and Yalom (1984) have described existentially oriented therapists as striving toward honest, mutually open relationships. Typically (but not always) therapist and client address one another by first names, therapists try to demystify the therapy process, they answer questions (with attention to timing and implications) as openly and fully as possible, and avoid a posture of passivity.

The existential approach regards the therapeutic relationship as more than just a vehicle through which to analyze transference issues. The patient's relationship with the therapist is regarded as real, and, despite the fact that it is temporary, the experience of intimacy and the other emotions which occur in the relationship are permanent, and remain in the patient's inner world as a lasting reference point. The therapist expresses deep, genuine concern for the patient's life, and cares about his or her growth. The above description presents the personal qualities, style, or demeanor of the existential-humanistic therapist.

Viewed in another way, the function of therapists within the therapeutic relationship may well be described as that of consultant (Bugental, 1965). Here the relationship is one in which therapists act as consultants-guides to their clients who always retain the place of being principal agents and focuses. While therapists remain inexorably external to the ongoing inner process and exploration ("searching") of their clients, their interest, and genuine caring for their clients support, sustain, and encourage that work.

Occasional and measured self-disclosure by the therapist is not off-limits, and may help to convey an existential universality to the patient's struggles. Finally, one must acknowledge the fact that despite the therapists' "consultant" role, they are not unmoved or unaffected by these relationships. The therapeutic relationship converges around a mutually shared enterprise in which the therapist gains and is affected as well as the patient.

Psychopathology, Diagnosis, and Assessment

For the most part an existential-humanistic orientation does not focus on psychopathology as conceptualized in a traditional medical model.

Assessment

Existential psychotherapy generally tends to be more a philosophical venture than a medical procedure. Hence diagnostics in the style of DSM-III-R descriptions are rarely relevant (except as required by insurance companies).

However, a form of assessment is used, its purpose being twofold: (a) to assess the suitability of the client for an existential-humanistic, depth therapy approach and (b) to begin to assess or conceptualize the client's problems and concerns within an existential framework. With regard to the former, it is manifest that an existential-humanistic perspective is not suitable to all clients. For some it is inappropriate because the nature of their problems is situation-specific. Others may lack motivation or resources for a deep explorative type of psychotherapy. Accordingly, our assessment focuses on the following two areas:

Does the patient exhibit such extreme emotional distress or inadequate ego functioning as to suggest inability to tolerate a deep, explorative style of therapy?

For patients with a high potential for acting out, likely need for hospitalization, or presence of an organic syndrome an existential approach would be contraindicated (Bugental, 1965).

Do the patient's emotional, financial, and logistical resources permit sufficient availability to pursue a deep, long-term, explorative psychotherapy experience?

It is highly desirable to see clients two or more times per week, with an expectation of therapy continuing two years or more. Clearly, the client must have the financial resources, emotional depth, and willingness to commit the time to such an endeavor.

Undertaking a full course of existential-humanistic psychotherapy is regarded as a major life endeavor—on a par with college or graduate education, marriage, parenthood, and similar lastingly life-significant commitments. As they are experientially ready to understand this reality, it is presented to prospective clients as a part of the assessment of their willingness and suitability for this kind of work.

Insofar as external conditions (legal and insurance requirements) permit, assessment is limited to the procedure described above. This is because a more formal, traditional assessment (e.g., psychological testing, or DSM-III-R diagnosis) tends to support clients' tendencies to objectify themselves and their problems and to see them as separate from their actual being in the world.

Furthermore, traditional psychodiagnosis may interfere with the development of the therapeutic alliance for both patients and therapists. For patients, it reinforces the notion of the therapist as doctor or authority, and for therapists, it is likely to over-objectify their clients and obscure the unique human being who is being encountered.

From initial interviews through to the final meetings, the task of conceptualizing the patient's concerns in an existential framework is a shared endeavor. It is this which continually provides a way of thinking about how patients constrict their awareness, avoid full presence in their lives, and the relationship of their presenting problems to these broader aspects. It also involves listening with an "existential ear"—maintaining an awareness and acceptance of emergence of the existential issues which are underlying or related to the clients' conscious focus.

CASE EXAMPLE

Barbara, 34, a junior high school teacher, comes for therapy with the complaint that she has lost her appetite, her interest in social activities, and her motivation at work. She describes a life of very limited range, chiefly centered around her work and only occasionally involving men friends. Her manner is listless, detached, and apparently fatigued.

Early in her twice-a-week therapy, Barbara reveals a failed romance but insists that she never had high hopes for it anyway. She also begins to express a smoldering resentment toward some of her fellow teachers who have families and friends but who never invite her to share their activities.

The therapist experiences Barbara as distant, subtly angry, and even more subtly pulling for agreement with her feelings of the unfairness of her life. Therapist activity is largely confined to pointing out how Barbara keeps her experience at an "arm's length," denying that any of it really matters, and holding off any direct statement about her needs. At first, the client is fully in agreement with these observations, but as time passes, she becomes annoyed at their repetition and questions the value of this process.

A first crisis occurs when the therapist continues to insist that Barbara is avoiding letting her life really matter and she for the first time lets her anger find direct expression: "You keep telling me I'm not doing things right here, but you—damn you—you don't ever help me to do them any better!" After this outbreak, the client slumps in tears into her chair and avoids meeting the therapist's eyes. He waits quietly, and eventually Barbara, still tearful, talks about her desperate feelings of having "failed life," as though it were a course or examination.

Now a period of more productive work ensues in which Barbara increasingly risks emotional and subjective expression. She finds it hard to engage in the needed inner "searching" because of her continual concern to check on the therapist's approval, but in time this lessens. Her searching reveals a deep resentment that others have always seemed to have things better than she—in intelligence, in attractiveness, and in the opportunities that opened to them.

This phase of the work goes on for some time and brings out a number of interrelated themes, mostly centering around the sense of having lost out so often in her life. In this way, she reviews her family of origin conflicts with an attractive and successful younger brother, her too early sexual initiation which left her guilty and confused, her vain attempts to make study and learning the whole of her life, and her yearnings for a love relationship and a family of her own.

Well over 18 months after beginning therapy, Barbara begins to lose the momentum that she had achieved for the work. Once again there is the sense of slow-burning resentment, of a pulling away from her immediate inner experience, and of repeated efforts to involve the therapist in some way. At times the last of these takes the form of very modest seductive efforts; at other times it is manifested as an attempt to provoke a fight with the therapist. Then Barbara misses two appointments without cancellations.

When the therapist calls to confirm that he is expecting Barbara at her next scheduled time, she is evasive and petulant. At his insistence, she comes in for a special session. She is unkempt,

with large circles under her eyes, and a restless, troubled air. The therapist feels shocked at her manifest regression. Without much difficulty, an account is elicited of another failed (and largely imagined) love affair and, interwoven with this, anger that the therapist is "just like all men—looking for physical beauty only."

Barbara's heretofore repressed fantasy of winning the therapist as her lover or even husband now becomes available, and rather readily yields to further awareness of primitive yearnings to be cherished, protected, and relieved of adult responsibilities for herself.

The final stage of the work involves repeated workings-through of Barbara's fantasies which have substituted for emergence out into the world, carefully measured support for her tentative ventures from her separateness into relations with her fellow-teachers and some dating with eligible men, and balanced recognition and companionship in her grief-work for the years that are irretrievably lost.

Barbara ends therapy a little over two years after she began it. She is making better relationships, has begun dating and some mild sexual activity, and is looking toward returning to graduate school to upgrade her professional qualifications. Far from living "happily ever after," she still has occasional depressed moods and is often fearful just before a date or a special social occasion. However, she expresses an underlying confidence that she will be able to handle these times on her own.

CONCLUDING COMMENTS

Our knowledge of our own nature as human beings is at a very early stage—at a guess, at about the level of the invention of the steam engine, in other words at about the beginning of the industrial revolution. We know so much more about inanimate nature, than about conscious nature. Our methods for controlling our fellows are very much the same as those of Neolithic men—the use of threat and force. Our methods of guiding our own lives are not a great deal more advanced. The connection between these two global problems is not happenstance.

Psychotherapy is, when viewed from a certain angle, a species research tool. We seek to learn to help each other to attain more of the kind of lives we all can imagine but all too few ever live. What we can learn in this way may have significance for other aspects of our lives as well. Within the broad span of psychotherapies, the existential and humanistic strains are gambles on a particular viewpoint—one that emphasizes human subjectivity. It is not at all certain that this gamble will pay off. It is only reasonably certain that it represents something of a fresh avenue of exploration after centuries of emphasis on the objective.

Time alone will render the verdict.

REFERENCES

Bugental, J. F. T. (1965). *The search for authenticity: An existential-humanistic approach to psychotherapy.* New York: Holt, Rinehart & Winston.

Bugental, J. F. T. (1978). *Psychotherapy and process: The fundamentals of an existential-humanistic approach.* New York: McGraw-Hill.

Bugental, J. F. T. (1987). *The art of the psychotherapist.* New York: Norton.

Freud, S. (1916/1917). Introductory lectures on psychoanalysis. Part III. General theory of the neuroses. (Lecture XIX: Resistance and Repression) In *The complete psychological works of Sigmund Freud* (Vol. 15). New York: Norton.

Hoeller, K. (1990). An introduction to existential psychology and psychiatry. In K. Hoeller (Ed.), *Readings in existential psychology and psychiatry* (pp. 3–19). Seattle: Review of Existential Psychology & Psychiatry.

May, R. (1958a). Contributions of existential psychotherapy. In R. May, E. Angel, & H. F. Ellenberger (Eds.), *Existence: A new dimension in psychiatry and psychology* (pp. 37–91). New York: Basic Books.

May, R. (1958b). The origins and significance of the existential movement in psychology. In R. May, E. Angel, & H. F. Ellenberger (Eds.), *Existence: A new dimension in psychiatry and psychology* (pp. 3–36). New York: Basic Books.

May, R. (1981). *Freedom and destiny.* New York: Norton.

May, R. (1983). *The discovery of being.* New York: Norton.

May, R., Angel, E., & Ellenberger, H. F. (Eds.), (1958). *Existence: A new dimension in psychiatry and psychology.* New York: Basic Books.

May, R., & Yalom, I. (1984). Existential psychotherapy. In R. J. Corsini (Ed.), *Current psychotherapies* (pp. 354–391). Itasca, Il: Peacock.

Ofman, W. D. (1985). Existential psychotherapy. In H. I. Kaplan & B. J. Saduck (Eds.), *Comprehensive textbook of psychiatry IV* (pp. 1438–1443). Baltimore: Williams & Wilkins.

Pascal, B. (1946). *Pensées of Pascal.* New York: Peter Pauper Press.

Yalom, I. D. (1980). *Existential psychotherapy.* New York: Basic Books.

CHAPTER 9

Toward an Integration of Cognitive, Interpersonal, and Experiential Approaches to Therapy

Jay Reeve, Thomas A. Inck, and Jeremy Safran

INTRODUCTION

Background to the Approach

In this chapter, we will outline and illustrate some of the central principles of the integrative approach to psychotherapy being developed by Safran and colleagues (Safran 1984a,b, 1990a,b; Safran, Crocker, McMain, & Murray 1990; Safran & Segal 1990). This approach draws heavily on the cognitive therapy tradition. For example, a central emphasis consists in helping clients to examine their perceptions and to treat them as hypotheses to be tested. The approach, however, is also strongly influenced by both experiential and interpersonal frameworks.

Traditional cognitive therapy presents the therapist's task as helping the client develop a

more accurate or objective view of reality by relying on such tools as logic and empirical evidence. The assumptions are that psychological problems result from distortions of reality, and that it is the correction of these distortions, on a rational, cognitive level, that promotes change. However, given the growing evidence that logical computation is only a small component of our complex information-processing system and the integral role of emotions in the change process (Greenberg & Safran 1987), the position that equates psychological health solely with rationality seems clearly untenable. Moreover, as Coyne and Gotlib (1983) have argued, when the client lives in a dysfunctional interpersonal situation, the assumption that psychological problems result from cognitive distortions can have potentially pernicious effects because it can lead the therapist into condoning an unhealthy status quo. Much empirical evidence suggests that in many circumstances, depressed individuals are actually more accurate in their perceptions and assessments than nondepressed individuals (Taylor and Brown 1988).

The approach that will be outlined in this

Jay Reeve, Thomas A. Inck, and Jeremy Safran • Derner Institute of Advanced Psychological Studies, Adelphi University, Garden City, New York 11530.

Comprehensive Handbook of Psychotherapy Integration, edited by George Stricker and Jerold R. Gold. Plenum Press, New York, 1993.

chapter stresses that the therapist must accept the client as the final arbiters of his or her own reality and that the therapist must be genuinely open to the possibility that the patient knows something about reality that the therapist does not. This facet of the approach is grounded in the experiential tradition, which emphasizes that only the client can be the expert on his or her own reality (Perls 1973; Rice 1974; Rogers 1961). Moreover, rather than subscribing to the rationalist assumptions of more traditional cognitive therapy, the current approach emphasizes a developmental constructivist approach (Guidano 1987; Guidano & Liotti 1983; Mahoney 1990). We are not interested in teaching our clients an objective view of reality, but rather in helping them understand how they construct reality and the effect that this construction has on their lives. Our framework for exploring how clients construct reality is the therapeutic relationship as it unfolds over the course of therapy.

Overview of the Approach

From the integrative perspective we are presenting, the central mechanism of change is conceptualized as the disconfirmation of the client's maladaptive interpersonal schemata and the modification of associated dysfunctional strategies for maintaining relatedness. The interpersonal schema construct can be viewed as an elaboration of the self-schema construct commonly employed in cognitive and social cognitive theory (e.g., Beck, Rush, Shaw & Emery, 1979; Kuiper and Olinger, 1986; Markus, 1977).

Beck and his associates (1979), for example, theorize that the self-schema is a tacit rule which guides the process of self-evaluation. For them, the self-schema is essentially an internal rule or standard employed to evaluate and guide one's own behavior.

An interpersonal schema is conceptualized as a *generalized representation of self–other relations*. Although this model incorporates Beck's emphasis on self-evaluation (1979), it assumes that implicit in one's self-evaluation is an evaluation of one's potential for interpersonal relatedness (Safran, 1990a; Safran & Segal, 1990). Interpersonal schemata shape and are maintained by dysfunctional cognitive-interpersonal cycles through which maladaptive strategies for maintaining relatedness pull for complementary behaviors from

others (Carson, 1969; Kiesler, 1982a; Leary, 1957; Safran and Segal, 1990; Strupp and Binder, 1984; Wachtel, 1982).

By attending to their own internal processes as well as their clients', therapists generate hypotheses about the maladaptive relational pulls, or hooks, that their clients display in other interpersonal interactions. They engage in a collaborative process with the client in which both parties' contributions to the interaction are explored, and the details of the client's interpersonal schema are elucidated. Through this exploratory process therapists gradually unhook themselves from the client's interpersonal pull, thereby disconfirming and challenging the beliefs underlying the maladaptive pattern. This is the work of our psychotherapy.

A key factor in this task is "the inner discipline of the therapist," that is, the ability for therapists to look at the therapeutic relationship from the empathic yet detached stance of what Sullivan (1953) referred to as the participant-observer. This ability is particularly important when working with clients who produce particularly powerful interpersonal pulls.

In this chapter, we will discuss the basic theory behind the interpersonal schema and the cognitive interpersonal cycle. We will then discuss the therapeutic techniques of metacommunication and unhooking and the resulting client experience of disconfirmation and decentering. These concepts are illustrated in a transcript from therapy sessions with a difficult client. Finally, we will examine the inner discipline of the therapist.

THEORETICAL AND CONCEPTUAL POSITION

The Interpersonal Schema

Freud asserted that the human infant is like an embryo within a closed, self-sustaining psychic shell (Freud, 1964). However, innumerable psychological theorists and empirical investigators have convincingly challenged this assertion. Realms of psychology as disparate as Bandura's work on modeling (1971), psychodynamic object relations theory (Greenberg and Mitchell, 1983), and mother–infant research (Stern, 1985) converge on the idea of the centrality of interpersonal interaction in human development. The development of the self occurs within and through an interpersonal context (Stern, 1985). It is through relationships with others that humans develop understandings of themselves and models of relationship.

Bowlby argued that the development of the self is largely achieved through attachment behavior. All infants have a propensity for proximity to a significant care giver, or attachment figure; it is as basic a need as food or water (Bowlby, 1969, 1973). This propensity for attachment is a universal aspect of the human condition; it is "hard-wired" into the basic constitution of each individual (Safran and Segal, 1990).

Each infant expresses this universal need for proximity to an attachment figure within a specific cultural context and, more narrowly, within the unique interpersonal context created by each infant–caretaker dyad. Each of these interpersonal contexts are shaped by numerous interacting parts, for example, the caretaker's interactional style, the caretaker's expectations of the infant, the unique personality dispositions of the infant, and so forth. Within this interpersonal context the infant forms consistent strategies for maintaining relatedness, that is, the infant forms attachment patterns.

Each individual infant develops attachment patterns to an *individual* caretaker—a caretaker who is optimally approached and related to in a particular way. Some of the infant's relational behaviors will be reinforced because of their efficacy in attaining the goal of relatedness with their caretakers, while others will not. Thus, each infant's attachment patterns reflect the uniqueness of the interpersonal context in which it was formed.

Based on these patterned infant–caretaker interactions, the infant forms cognitive/affective representations of self/other interactions (Bowlby, 1969). These representations can be conceptualized as interpersonal schemata, which function as programs for maintaining relatedness (Safran, 1986; 1990a). Interpersonal schemata represent the kinds of behaviors that the individual can use to attain relatedness with different kinds of people in different situations. Likewise, the schema contains information about how certain thoughts and feelings can be threatening to maintaining interpersonal relations.

An individual with consistent relationship problems is likely to have a maladaptive interpersonal schema which represents relatedness as be-

ing contingent on thinking, feeling, and acting within a constricted and narrowly defined range. An interaction which calls for the individual to access thoughts, emotions, or behaviors which fall outside of this range arouses anxiety. The individual with a maladaptive interpersonal schema likewise expects others to behave in stereotypical ways, and as cognitive theory suggests, tends to interpret others' actions in a schema consistent fashion.

How do interpersonal schemata become maladaptive? If a significant other repeatedly interacts with an individual in a particular manner, the individual will encode a representation of that behavior embedded within a specific interpersonal context and, in the future, will expect the same context and significant other to produce the same behavior. When the individual's relationships change, the individual's interpersonal schema should ideally adapt to the new situation. Unfortunately, internal interpersonal schemata do not change as easily as external relationships, particularly if the interpersonal schema was formed in childhood within an interpersonal context where the child's emotional needs were not being adequately met by a significant caretaker.

Let us take for example a mother who feels suffocated by her male child's need for attention. She is unable to adequately attune to the child's attempts at interpersonal relatedness, and instead prematurely encourages the child to become independent. The child will form an interpersonal schema that represents emotional neediness as threatening to relationships. The child will believe that significant others are unable or unwilling to meet his needs, and will believe that the only route to achieving interpersonal relatedness is to not be too needy but rather to be independent and autonomous. As the child becomes an adolescent and the adolescent an adult, this individual is still likely to believe that his significant others will not meet his emotional needs. The interpersonal schema will not have changed.

The Cognitive Interpersonal Cycle

Maladaptive interpersonal schemata are maintained through both cognitive and interpersonal processes (Carson, 1969; Kiesler, 1983; Strupp & Binder, 1984). The individual who believes that others will ignore his or her emotional needs may react to this expectation by interacting in an overly demanding way, thus creating a real situation where the significant other is forced to be unable or unwilling to meet the individual's needs. The individual is thus trapped within his or her own dysfunctional cognitive-interpersonal cycle.

Kiesler (1982b, 1983, 1988) and other interpersonal theorists (e.g., Benjamin, 1974; Leary 1957) elucidate the working mechanism of dysfunctional cognitive-interpersonal cycles through the concept of complementarity. The theory of complementarity, or what Sullivan (1953) referred to as the theorem of reciprocal emotions, states that all interpersonal acts are designed to pull, elicit, evoke restricted types of reactions from those with whom we interact, particularly from significant others. Other's range of reactions to our behaviors are thus shaped and constrained by our own interpersonal repertoires. Our actions are designed to get others to confirm our self-definitions and our view of the interpersonal world; that is, our actions are designed to validate our interpersonal schemata. In the example above, the individual is likely to act in such a way that elicits non-caretaking behaviors from his or her significant other, thus confirming the belief that others cannot or will not fulfill his or her needs. Finally, we are largely unaware of how we actively pull others to react within a restricted range; the process is played out on a mostly automatic level (Kiesler, 1988).

THE TECHNIQUE AND PROCESS OF PSYCHOTHERAPY

Unhooking

In order to avoid perpetuating clients' dysfunctional cognitive interpersonal cycles, therapists must disconfirm clients' maladaptive interpersonal schemata through their relationship stance and provide what Balint (1935) referred to as "a new beginning." This requires therapists to be able to react in a noncomplementary manner toward clients, when clients are engaged in a dysfunctional cognitive interpersonal cycle.

The therapeutic stance which enables this is that of the participant-observer (Sullivan, 1953). As a participant-observer, the therapist allows him or herself to feel the client's interpersonal pull while at the same time observing the interaction that he or she is participating in with the client.

Only through participating in client's characteristic cognitive interpersonal cycles can therapists generate hypotheses about these cycles and explore the interpersonal schemata which fuel these cycles.

The therapist's first step in unhooking involves turning his or her attention inward to detect the perhaps subtle feelings and thoughts that one experiences during the interaction. If the therapist begins with preconceptions about his or her true feelings, they may well impede the process of discovering what the true feelings actually are. The process of clarifying and articulating tacit feelings that result from the therapeutic interaction can be slow, and the therapist should be prepared to devote a considerable amount of time to this process. As we discuss below, it is necessary for the therapist to observe his or her inner experience for an attitude of nonattachment. Once the therapist has made some progress in understanding his or her own feelings and thoughts in a dispassionate, nonattached manner, the therapist begins to monitor and identify which of the patient' nonverbal behaviors and communications his or her feelings appear to be linked to. If the therapist's feelings are consistently linked to specific client behaviors, the therapist will metacommunicate about this interaction.

Metacommunication

The topic of countertransference disclosure is a hotly debated theme in the current psychoanalytic literature. The theoretical emphasis has clearly shifted in a more interpersonal/relationally oriented direction, with a strong technical focus of the explanation of transference/countertransference dynamics. As Bollas (1989) suggested, however, there continues to be an almost "phobic avoidance" of countertransference disclosure.

Our approach to this topic has been strongly influenced by the experiential tradition (Perls, 1973; Rogers, 1951), which places great emphasis on the importance of therapist genuineness, and by Kiesler's (1982b; 1983; 1988) excellent and systematic articulation of the principles of therapeutic metacommunication.

We will discuss four types of metacommunication separately, though in practice, often two or more of these types are combined in a single therapist's turn of speech (Safran & Segal, 1990).

In the first type of metacommunication, therapists disclose their own feelings with an eye to helping clients become more aware of the impact that they have on others and thus their role in the interaction. For example, a therapist who becomes aware of a tendency to behave nurturantly toward a patient might say: "I feel like protecting you right now." A therapist who becomes aware of feeling insulted by a patient might say: "I'm feeling put down right now." It is particularly helpful to couple this type of feedback about the specific actions or communications of the client which caused these feelings in the therapist (Kiesler, 1982b; 1988).

In the second type of metacommunication, therapists convey their own feelings in order to probe for or further facilitate the unfolding of the client's inner experience. A therapist may say, "I'm feeling very cautious with you right now . . . as if it would be easy for me to say or do the wrong thing. Does that relate to anything you are experiencing?" Or: "I'm feeling like I'm playing a game of chess. Does that connect to anything that you are feeling right now?" A therapist who realizes that he or she has been feeling irritable may say, "I feel like I have been attacking you in little ways. Does that fit your experience?" A therapist who becomes aware of feeling helpless and may say: "I feel really powerless right now—like nothing I could add would be helpful. Does that connect to your experience at all?"

In both of these types of self-disclosure, it is vital that the therapist convey his or her feelings in an inviting, exploratory manner. The aim is never to blame the client but rather to invite the client to further investigate his or her feelings.

In the third type of metacommunication, the therapist identifies particular client actions or communications, called *interpersonal markers*, and tries to help clarify their contribution to the interaction. For example: "I feel patronized right now and I think it's connected with the tone of your voice and the smile on your face."

In the fourth type of metacommunication, the therapist uses the identified interpersonal marker as a springboard for further cognitive/affective exploration. For example: "I'm aware of a sudden easing in your manner of speech? Are you aware of that?" Or: "I'm aware that you began to nervously tap your foot. What's going on for you?" By drawing attention to nonverbal behavior that the client is not aware of, the therapist aims to facilitate client awareness of associated internal

experience. The client whose speech begins to flow easily may become aware of an inner experience of increased trust in the therapist; the client who nervously taps his foot may become aware of feelings that he or she is being judged by the therapist.

In all four types of metacommunication, it is important that therapists emphasize the subjective nature of their perceptions and accept full responsibility for these perceptions, rather than treating these perceptions like objective reality. The subjective nature of a perception can be conveyed by linking the perception to one's own feelings, but other ways of conveying one's subjective perspective are acceptable as well. By conveying subjectiveness, the therapist implicitly acknowledges that his or her perception may be wrong and creates a space where the client can use the therapist's inaccurate perception as a stimulus for exploration. A failure to leave room for an incorrect therapist perception will undermine the client's confidence in his or her own perceptions. Our understanding of metacommunication is guided by the principle that the client is the expert on his or her own reality, and that an important goal of therapy is to help clients become more trusting of their own experience.

Metacommunication allows therapists to bring a previously covert interactional pattern to the attention of their clients, and to unhook themselves from cyclical interactions in which they feel trapped. In the unhooking stage, clients' expectations around therapists' responses to their presentation are thwarted—therapists do not act the way everybody else does in response to client's characteristic interpersonal gambits. Therapists do not provide complementary responses which reinforce the beliefs underlying their client's interpersonal schemata.

Disconfirmation and Decentering

By unhooking from the client's maladaptive pull through metacommunication, the therapist activates two interdependent change mechanisms; *experiential disconfirmation* and *decentering* (Safran & Segal, 1990).

Unhooking shifts the interaction. The client is faced with an other that does not fit into his or her expectation for interpersonal interaction. The therapist provides the client with a concrete, emotionally immediate experience of a new, healthier way of interacting. Through the therapist's very actions, he or she can experientially disconfirm the client's automatic thoughts and expectations about relationships.

Likewise, through empathically exploring the client's inner experience as it unfolds in the therapeutic relationship, therapists help clients to understand how their expectation, beliefs, and appraisals help create the immediate interaction. Clients are encouraged to decenter, that is, to see their own role in constructing the present interaction. Clients begin to regard perceptions about relationships as hypotheses to be tested. As therapists provide their own subjective emotional feedback and pinpoint specific client behaviors that foster these reactions, clients move from experiencing themselves as passive participants in unfulfilling, incomprehensible interpersonal interactions to a position of agency where they can see and choose active contributions to interactions.

Experiential disconfirmation and decentering thus begins within the context of the therapeutic relationship. However, clients have formed generic representations of self–other interactions from a lifetime of experience; it is unlikely that the new experiences with the therapists alone will be enough to change these generic representations. Therefore, once the therapists and client have begun using the therapeutic relationship to identify beliefs and expectations that shape the client's maladaptive interpersonal cycle, the client is explicitly encouraged to experiment with out-of-session interactions to test these same expectations and beliefs. Paying special attention to the issue of generalizability and continually encouraging clients to test their beliefs in both the therapeutic and "real-world" relationships plays a vital role in providing the range of interpersonal experience necessary to gradually change the client's interpersonal schemata. This type of intervention provides a good example of the way in which interpersonal and cognitive approaches can be fruitfully integrated at a technical level.

CASE EXAMPLE

In the following excerpt from a therapy session transcript, the cognitive interpersonal cycle which the client utilizes to maintain feelings of security and personal worth also serves to alienate and distance others. The client is a 46-year-old, white woman who entered therapy in order to address feelings of depression and difficulties in interpersonal relationships. All excerpts are taken from her third therapy session. This client has an interpersonal schema that represents others as hostile, insensitive to her needs, and devaluing. She also views relatedness as contingent upon being special. She feels assaulted, slighted, and angry much of the time, and responds to these feelings with angry counterattacks.

These counterattacks tend to elicit anger, rejection, and/or withdrawal from others, thereby perpetuating a dysfunctional interpersonal schema. This is particularly true when the client generalizes the interactions which she elicits through her attacking style to be typical of all people.

We present her interaction with her therapist as an example of a dysfunctional cognitive interpersonal cycle. Her therapist verbalizes his sense of the interaction in a good example of unhooking through metacommunication.

The following excerpt occurs approximately 5 minutes into the session. The client began the session by briefly and cryptically expressing anger that there was a broken water fountain in the bathroom, but quickly moved to another topic. The second topic is followed by a pause, where the therapist points out an interpersonal marker:

THERAPIST: Hm. I'm aware of your smile right now, are you aware of it at all?

CLIENT: Yes.

THERAPIST: What's your experience, behind the smile?

CLIENT: I'm telling you where it's at and putting you down at the same time. I'm letting you know you're not going to get the better of me.

THERAPIST: So you're pissed off at me right now?

CLIENT: Oh it's just people in general, that nonsense downstairs and everything else. That was a put down of you, the fact that I said the thing about the toilet, and it was also a put down of you about the other cause I get fed up with people. I don't take shit like that. Sure I was, that's what the smile was, I was saying like, you know.

THERAPIST: I'm feeling kind of lumped in with everybody else right now.

CLIENT: Well, why not, you're a person. You're part of humanity, why shouldn't you be lumped in with everybody else.

THERAPIST: But I feel that I'm not being treated as a person. That you're just lumping me in with everybody else.

CLIENT: Well, look at you! You're just like everybody

else. You deserve it. You act like everybody else and as far as that goes, you don't deserve to be lumped in with everybody else. You've known that thing [the water fountain] hasn't worked for ages and what the hell did you do about it. Nothing, the same thing that everybody else did, so you deserve to be lumped in with everybody else.

THERAPIST: I'm feeling really hesitant about saying anything else. I'm concerned that anything I say will provoke you further.

CLIENT: [Pause] Well, I guess it's kind of difficult to talk with me when I'm in the midst of one of my tirades.

In this passage the client is angry with her therapist because she believes he mistreats her the way everyone she interacts with does. She perceives his failure to have the water fountain fixed as yet another instance of others ignoring her needs and treating her poorly. This perception that this is just another instance of a recurring theme in her life leads her to express her anger in a generalized way, rather than toward this specific person in this specific situation. At the same time, this generalized response serves a self-protective function by helping her avoid the risk of expressing her anger directly and specifically toward her therapist. The therapist begins by commenting on the most salient aspect of his experience at the moment, that is, a sense of not really being related to directly as a unique person, a sense of being "lumped in with everybody else." This initial feedback evokes a more intense and personalized expression of anger from the client. The effect of her angry response is to render the therapist cautious about saying anything else—possibly a reaction commonly elicited by this client. The therapist becomes aware of his cautiousness and metacommunicates his experience to her. This allows the therapist to unhook from the maladaptive interpersonal cycle created.

Were the therapist to react to the client by being muted or hostile, he would confirm the client's world view and feed into her maladaptive cognitive interpersonal cycle. By verbalizing his feelings in the session, the therapist unhooks from the cycle and allows both himself and eventually his client to disengage from the dysfunctional interchange in which they are caught. By keeping the focus of the session specifically on the here and now of their relationship, the therapist provides the client with an experientially alive opportunity to explore and test her interpersonal expectations.

The following segment of transcript shows the therapist assessing the interaction and offering disconfirming and perhaps novel responses to the client's standard interpersonal stance. Before this section, the client has just expressed her nervousness after her angry outburst. The therapist encourages her to attend to her experience of anxiety and to explore the associated fears and beliefs.

THERAPIST: Uhum. Now, what I'm encouraging you to do is to take a look at what you're doing, and slow it down. Are you willing to do this with me? Can you get a sense of what your rears are?

CLIENT: It goes back to my playing God, and thinking I'm the only one that's right, it's all part of my basic philosophy. I can show a little bit of it, but it goes much further than that. Right now I'm sort of bothered by how many people there are in the world and boy!, what I'd do to them if I had my wish.

THERAPIST: What would you do to me if you had your wish?

CLIENT: (looking away) I don't know, it's not the specific people in the world. Well, of course, if I could do what I wanted with you, I'd hit you over the head and make you present things to me the way I wanted you to.

THERAPIST: (The therapist notes that she is looking away.) Are you willing to actually make contact with me as you're saying this?

CLIENT: Instead of the camera over there, which is impersonal and safe?

THERAPIST: It's safer looking over there for you.

CLIENT: Yeah.

THERAPIST: What's happening for you right now?

CLIENT: Now I'm back to being nervous again. I wasn't nervous a few minutes ago. I wasn't paying attention to myself.

THERAPIST: Okay, so you're in contact with your nervousness again.

CLIENT: Yeah.

THERAPIST: And when I ask you to really make contact with me, you say, "I want to hit you over the head." What's the risk, if you say this while you're in contact with me—if you're really direct with me?

CLIENT: If I dealt with you as a person, I couldn't act the way I do. If I actually thought of people as people, and put myself in their position then I couldn't do what I do. I have to put a barrier and distance them and make them into entities or I couldn't act the way I do.

The therapist clears a space to stay with the client with an invitation. He respectfully asks her if she is willing to look at what she fears. The client responds by articulating her rage at the number of people in the world. The therapist consistently responds to this and subsequent abstract, depersonalized client speech by asking about the client's anger in the here and now, that is, her anger specific to the therapist, and by asking the client to try and engage directly with him. He moves the client away from abstractions, toward the concrete experience of the here-and-now relationship. By drawing her attention to the way in which she avoids contact (by turning away) as she expresses her anger in a concrete, direct way, he paves the way for exploring fears, beliefs, and expectations that prevent her from expressing her anger in a more personalized way. By encouraging her to experiment with expressing her anger in a direct, contactful way, the therapist sets the stage for testing her belief that she will not be accepted if she shows her true feelings.

By staying present in the interaction and collaborating with the client, the therapist has provided a concrete example that begins to disconfirm the client's expectation that others will withdraw or respond in anger. It is upon this expectation that a major and debilitating theme of her life is built, that is, no one can fulfill her needs nor tolerate her anger. The therapist has given his client the opportunity to clearly test out her belief that others are always hostile toward her and "out to get her." By testing this belief, the client is able to begin assessing the validity of her ingrained view of interpersonal interactions.

By responding to his "gut" feeling that he was caught in a cyclical interaction, disengaging himself from his more reactive response, and staying with the client through metacommunication, reflective listening, and questions crafted to focus the client on her immediate inner experience, the therapist provides a novel experience for the client—that of a relationship that survived even the ferocious storm of her anger. Had the therapist become defensive or angry, or fell mute in the presence of the client's anger, her underlying sense of her intolerability, and the intolerability of her feelings, would have been confirmed. Only by sensing feelings of being under attack in himself was the therapist able to verbalize these feelings, disengage from them, and unhook from the client's maladaptive cycle.

THE INNER DISCIPLINE OF THE THERAPIST

The therapist's ability to unhook from a dysfunctional cognitive-interpersonal cycle—the ability to function as a participant-observer—requires an inner discipline (Safran & Segal, 1990).

To the extent that the therapist has a flexible interpersonal schema, that is, to the extent that the therapist has access to a full range of internal experiences, he or she can potentially attune to a full range of client emotions. In contrast, therapists with rigid self-definitions may have difficulties dealing with feelings which fall outside of their internal boundaries, and this may cause real difficulties in treatment.

Therapists who believe that it is not permissible for them to feel angry toward their clients may have difficulty listening to a provocative or sadistic person in treatment. They may keep their angry feelings out of their own awareness. However, this anger will inevitably leak into and pollute the therapeutic interaction in the form of subtle hostile gestures.

Therapists who believe it to be wrong to feel sexually attracted to their clients may be unaware of their own flirtatiousness in sessions. If their clients notice this flirtatiousness but elicit reactions of shock or surprise when they try to discuss it, therapists will convey the message that there are certain things which the client cannot discuss. More likely, clients in this situation will conclude that they are imagining the flirtatiousness, or that they are at fault for somehow provoking it. This will tend to restrict clients' range of acceptable thoughts and feelings even further, and further confirm dysfunctional cognitive interpersonal cycles.

The success of therapy is thus dependent in a crucial way upon the degree to which therapists are willing to fully attend to their *own* thoughts and feelings while in the session. Such attention reduces the possibility of therapists of failing to recognize when they are hooked into maladaptive cognitive interpersonal cycles.

The inner discipline which must be cultivated in order to facilitate this process is akin to Freud's concept of evenly suspended attention. Despite the fact that the importance of this type of stance is either explicitly or implicitly acknowledged in many psychotherapeutic writings, there has been little systematic attention to the nature of the relevant internal processes in the literature. One striking exception was Reik's (1948) *Listening with the Third Ear*.

A useful body of relevant knowledge falling outside of traditional psychotherapeutic writings can be found in the Buddhist practice of insight meditation. In insight meditation, one of the important goals is the acquisition of self-knowledge through disciplined and dispassionate observation of one's inner experiences. All phenomena, whether occurring intra- or extrapsychically, whether pleasant or painful, are to be accorded the full attention of the meditator. At the same time, it is important for the meditator not to remain attached to these phenomena after new ones have arisen to supplant them. In this way, attention and concentration on immediate sensory, cognitive, and emotional input are developed, and the meditator grows increasingly rooted in real, current experience.

A widely used metaphor in this tradition is that of the mind as the sky, and thoughts as clouds. In both meditation and psychotherapy, it is important to acknowledge and attend to the clouds as they pass, and to attend fully to each newly passing cloud. The emphasis here is on rootedness in immediate experience, rather than nostalgia for old thoughts or feelings, anticipation of new thoughts or feelings, or discriminatory preference for one thought or feeling over another.

In order to achieve this sort of free-floating attention, it is important that there be no forbidden areas within practitioners' thoughts. Blocking certain "bad" or unacceptable thoughts results in negative attachments, just as dwelling on pleasant or "edifying" ones produces positive attachment. In both cases, attention is diverted from what may be arising at the moment.

Therapists can utilize this type of meditative discipline to unhook from dysfunctional cognitive interpersonal cycles. To do so, they must fully attend to their own feelings as well as those of their clients. Once therapists have accurately identified their own feelings, whatever they are, they may then label the interactions in which they arise, metacommunicate their perception of the interaction to their clients, and thereby unhook from the maladaptive cycle.

The inner discipline of the therapist is also useful beyond the primary therapeutic task of assessing, metacommunicating, and disengaging from the cognitive interpersonal cycle. Dysfunctional cognitive interpersonal cycles are generated by the belief that there are a limited number of acceptable relational modes. The more dysfunctional a belief system, the more limited that

number is. By approaching psychotherapy as, in some senses, a meditative task calling for free-ranging, evenly hovering attention, therapists attend to all thoughts and feelings that arise both in themselves and in their clients, without becoming negatively or positively attached to any of them. In so doing, therapists disconfirm their clients' belief that there are certain thoughts or feelings which are necessarily forbidden.

This disconfirmation is accomplished, in part, through therapists' modeling their own acceptance of any thought or feeling that arises. Demonstrating a high degree of self-acceptance and nonattachment provides an example which clients can emulate. Therapists provide a model for attending to any and all thoughts and feelings by not treating any thoughts or feelings as bad or forbidden, and by continually grounding interventions in the immediate interaction between themselves and their clients. Such modeling may provide a helpful tool for clients whose interpersonal relationships are impeded by narrowly constrained and rigid cognitive interpersonal cycles.

Attending to the whole of their clients' experience, therapists ensure that they do not covertly endorse one or the other of their clients' thoughts or feelings as the "correct" one to gain therapist approval. By practicing this nonattached style, therapists may keep from subtly reinforcing a narrow and constricted view of what constitutes "acceptable" thinking and feeling.

The discussion of feelings and thoughts that have traditionally been neglected (or positively forbidden) as inimical to the maintenance of relationship calls for considerable courage from both patient and therapist. The discipline required is the willingness to attend to all thoughts and feelings, whether or not they have been stigmatized within the mores of our culture. Only by doing so can therapists be responsive to the whole of their clients' experience throughout treatment.

CONCLUSION

Summary of Central Principles

The field of cognitive therapy continues to evolve at a rapid pace. The chapter represents our attempt to foster this evolution by broadening cognitive therapy's theory and technique through the incorporation of principles from a number of different traditions, including interpersonal therapy, client-centered therapy, gestalt therapy, and Buddhist psychology. The central principles of our approach are summarized below:

1. This approach emphasizes phenomenological exploration rather than interpretation. We assume that clients are the experts on their experience and that interpreting their experience for them changes the nature of that experience and deprives the client of the important opportunity of articulating it for themselves.

2. It emphasizes accessing and modifying cognitive processes in an emotionally immediate way. It assumes that cognitive processes that are cut off from the corresponding affective component do not adequately represent the full organismic experience.

3. It emphasizes using the therapeutic relationship as a laboratory for exploring maladaptive interpersonal cycles and challenging interpersonal schemata. However, it does not assume that the patterns that emerge in the therapeutic relationship necessarily parallel other patterns in the clients life and therefore advocates that therapists must take full responsibility for their role in the relationship.

4. The client's construal processes are first explored within the experientially immediate context of the therapeutic relationship. After the therapeutic interaction has been explored in depth and the therapist has acknowledged his or her own contribution to the interaction does the therapist instruct the client to monitor for similar experiences between sessions.

5. It advocates formulating and continually reformulating understandings of the client's interpersonal schemata.

6. It advocates the skillful use of the therapist's own feelings to generate hypotheses about interpersonal patterns that are characteristic for the client.

7. It emphasizes using interpersonal markers as junctures for cognitive/affective exploration.

8. It advocates understanding the client as an active collaborator, who explores and tests his or her beliefs and expectation, both in and outside of the therapeutic relationship.

9. It emphasizes maintaining a therapeutic focus by paying careful attention to what is emotionally alive for clients and by using accurate empathic reflection to facilitate a deepening of experience.

Future Directions

As summarized in the previous section, this particular blend of traditions has a distinct bias in the direction of a noninterpretive, here and now, emotionally immediate focus. Important questions to consider in the future will be issues, such as (1) Are there specific points at which interpretation is more helpful than empathic exploration? (2) Are there specifiable indications for focusing on the past versus the present? And (3) are there times when working in a less emotional immediate fashion is more helpful? Exploring questions of this type in a differentiated way will be an important step in the direction of moving toward the development of a systematic, context sensitive body of knowledge about human change which is truly integrative in nature.

REFERENCES

Balint, M. (1935). Pregenital organization of the libido. In *Primary love and the psychoanalytic technique.* New York: Liveright, 1965.

Bandura, A. (1971). Psychotherapy based upon modeling principles. In A.E. Bergin & S.L. Garfield (Eds.), *Handbook of psychotherapy and behavior change: An empirical analysis* (pp. 621–658). New York: Wiley.

Beck, A. T., Rush, A. J., Shaw, M., & Emery, G. (1979). *Cognitive therapy of depression.* New York: Guilford.

Benjamin, L. S. (1974). Structural analysis of social behavior. *Psychological Review. 91*, 392–425.

Bollas, C. (1989). *Forces of destiny: Psychoanalysis and human idiom.* London: Free Association Books.

Bowlby, J. (1969). *Attachment and loss: Vol. 1. Attachment.* New York: Basic Books.

Bowlby, J. (1973). *Attachment and loss: Vol. 2. Separation, anxiety, and anger.* New York. Basic Books.

Carson, R. C. (1969). *Interaction concepts of personality.* Chicago: Aldine.

Coyne, J. C., & Gotlib, I. H. (1983). The role of cognition in depression: A critical appraisal. *Psychological Bulletin 94,*472–505.

Freud, S. (1964). *New Introductory Lectures on Psychoanalysis.* New York: W. W. Norton.

Greenberg, L. S., & Safran, J. D. (1987). *Emotion in psychotherapy*. New York: Guilford.

Greenberg, J. R., & Mitchell, S. A. (1983). *Object relations in psychoanalytic theory*. Cambridge: Harvard University Press.

Guidano, V. F. (1987). *Complexity of the self: A developmental approach to psychopathology and therapy*. New York: Guilford.

Guidano, V. F., & Liotti, G. (1983). *Cognitive processes and emotional disorders*. New York: Guilford.

Kiesler, D. J. (1982a). Interpersonal theory for personality and psychotherapy, In J. C. Anchin & D. J. Kiesler, (Eds.), *Handbook of interpersonal psychotherapy* (pp. 3–24). Elmford, NY: Pergamon Press.

Kiesler, D. J. (1982b). Confronting the client-therapist relationship in psychotherapy. In J. C. Anchin & D. J. Kiesler (Eds.), *Handbook of interpersonal psychotherapy* (pp.). Elmford, NY: Pergamon Press.

Kiesler, D. J. (1983). The 1982 interpersonal circle: A taxonomy for complementarity in human transactions. *Psychological Review 90*, 185-214.

Kiesler, D. J. (1988). *Therapeutic Metacommunication: Therapist impact disclosure as feedback in psychotherapy*. Palo Alto, Calif.: Consulting Psychologists Press.

Kuiper, N. A., & Olinger, L. J. (1986). Dysfunctional attitudes and a self-worth contingency model of depression. In P. C. Kendall (Ed.), *Advances in cognitive-behavioral research and therapy* (pp. 115–142). Orlando, FL: Academic Press.

Leary, T. (1957). *Interpersonal diagnosis of personality*. New York: Ronald.

Mahoney, M. J. (1990). *Human change processes*. New York: Basic Books.

Markus, H. (1977). Self-schemata and processing of information about the self. *Journal of Personality and Social Psychology 35*, 63–78.

Perls, F. S. (1973). *The gestalt approach: An eyewitness to therapy*. Palo Alto, Ca: Science and Behavior Books.

Reik, T. (1948). *Listening with the third ear*. New York: Farrar, Straus, & Giroux.

Rice, L. N. (1974). The evocative function of the therapist.

In D. Wexler and L. N. Rice (Eds.), *Innovations in client-centered therapy*, (pp. 289–312). New York: Interscience.

Rogers, C. R. (1951). *Client-centered therapy*. Boston: Houghton Mifflin.

Rogers, C. R. (1961). *On becoming a person*. Boston: Houghton Mifflin.

Safran, J. D. (1984a). Assessing the cognitive-interpersonal cycle. *Cognitive Therapy and Research, 87*, 333–348.

Safran, J. D. (1984b). Some implications of Sullivan's interpersonal theory for cognitive therapy. In M. A. Reda & M. J. Mahoney (Eds.), *Cognitive psychotherapies: Recent developments in theory, research and practice* (pp. 251–272). Cambridge, MA: Ballinger.

Safran, J. D. (1986, June). *A critical evaluation of the schema construct in psychotherapy research*. Paper presented at the Society for Psychotherapy Research, Boston, Massachusetts.

Safran, J. D. (1990a). Towards a refinement of cognitive therapy in light of interpersonal theory: I. Theory. *Clinical Psychology Review, 10*, 87–105.

Safran, J. D. (1990b). Towards a refinement of cognitive therapy in light of interpersonal theory: II. Practice. *Clinical Psychology Review, 10*, 107–121.

Safran, J. D., & Segal, L. S. (1990). *Interpersonal process in cognitive therapy*. New York: Basic Books.

Safran, J. D., Crocker, P., McMain, S., & Murray, P. (1990). The therapeutic alliance rupture as a therapy event for empirical investigation. *Psychotherapy, 27*(2), 154–165.

Stern, D. N. (1985). *The interpersonal world of the infant*. New York: Basic Books.

Strupp, H. H. & Binder, J. L. (1984). *Psychotherapy in a new key: A guide to time-limited dynamic therapy*. New York: Basic Books.

Sullivan, H. S. (1953). *The interpersonal theory of psychiatry*. New York: W.W. Norton.

Taylor, S. E., & Brown, J. D. (1988). Illusion and well being; A social psychological perspective on mental health. *Psychological Bulletin 103*, 193–210.

Wachtel, P. L. (1982). *Resistance: Psychodynamic and behavioral approaches*. New York: Plenum Press.

CHAPTER 10

Unified Psychotherapy

David M. Allen

INTRODUCTION

Unified therapy (Allen, 1988, 1991) is an eight-stage approach to the treatment of neurologically intact adults between the ages of 21 and late midlife who exhibit repetitive self-destructive behavior, chronic affective symptomatology, or long-term overt family discord. These three phenomena are seen as three separate manifestations of the same underlying process. All three are assumed to be present and occurring simultaneously, even if one or two of them are covert and/or unacknowledged at the time patients first present themselves for therapy. Therapy is done with one individual, but aims to impact both the individual and his or her family system in such a way as to make any divergence between the interests of the two converge. The theory behind unified therapy can be adapted for use in family and couples therapy, as well as for other age groups; that will not be discussed here.

The therapy incorporates ideas from most of the major schools of psychotherapy including psychodynamic, family systems, cognitive-behavioral, and existential, and aims to avoid the

reductionism inherent in intrapsychic, family systems, and sociological explanations for maladaptive behavior. The conceptual framework derives from a non-Marxist version of dialectic philosophy and epistemology (Basseches, 1986). The unifying notion is that of a dialectical relationship between human individuals and all larger social groups or *collectives* that can create an intrapsychic conflict in set goals (Weston, 1985) within the individuals comprising the group.

This chapter will outline the theory behind unified therapy, its theoretical antecedents, and the technique and process of therapy. Key concepts will be italicized.

THEORETICAL AND CONCEPTUAL POSITION

Perhaps the most significant theoretical controversy in modern psychotherapy is the one between family systems therapists, who see maladaptive behavior as a reaction to systemic social forces, and individual therapists, who often see it as a deficit within individuals. Humans are indeed the most social of organisms, so it is hardly surprising that much of our behavior is reactive to our social environment. From an evolutionary standpoint, individuals count for little; in order for the genes of the species to survive, what is important is the survival of the herd, or in

David M. Allen • Department of Psychiatry, University of Tennessee, Memphis, Tennessee 38105.

Comprehensive Handbook of Psychotherapy Integration, edited by George Stricker and Jerold R. Gold. Plenum Press, New York, 1993.

human terms, the tribe or family. The idea that one should, under certain circumstances, be willing to die for one's country is a good example of our genetic programming to sacrifice ourselves for the good of the many.

It is also true, however, that we can have individual interests that diverge from those of the groups to which we belong. We have strong inclinations toward self-survival and self-expression. We possess the capability of processing external information through our own unique perceptual apparatus, and to independently manipulate this information through thinking in order to generate idiosyncratic ideas that may benefit none but ourselves. In modern times, as time devoted to basic survival needs decreases because of technology, we have more time to think about "self-actualization."

We are at once individuals and a functioning part of various groups. As group members, we have specific *role functions* to fulfill which may run counter to our own natural inclinations. Unified therapy posits a *dialectic relationship* between self and system that is characterized by the following:

1. Self and system exist in a relationship which makes both of them what they are. Each is defined by its relationship to the other; neither can exist without the other, yet each exists separately.

2. The relationship is never static but continuously evolves over time in a unidirectional manner.

3. The evolution of the relationship is characterized by the increasing development of the individual members of the system. That is, a process of separation and individuation occurs so that the members of the system become progressively more unlike one another and less dependent on any specific group for survival. They interact with an increasingly larger number of individuals, so that no two individuals belong to the same relationship system.

The forces of separation and individuation operate on both individuals and groups at all levels, forcing upon groups a continuous need to restructure themselves. This need for restructuring conflicts with another need of the system: the need for predictability and smooth functioning known as *family homeostasis* in systems theory. These conflicting needs lead to a constant state of tension between the needs of individuals to

evolve and individuate and the need of the entire system for stability. In particular, the larger culture demands more and more individuated, flexible, and less role-driven behavior from family members—particularly the younger members—in a process known as *cultural evolution* (Fromm, 1941/1969). Cultural evolution is spearheaded by the advance of technology and the explosion of information, and is the source of the so-called generation gap. In an attempt to maintain family homeostasis in this changing environment, family members provide various "services" for one another as described below.

Dialectic theory shows how individuals within a system interact. They influence each other neither in a linear fashion in time, as individual therapies often assume, nor in a circular manner, as systems theory predicts. Instead, individuals continuously and simultaneously influence one another. Individuals form *schemata* or mental images of self, others, and relationships which are, as long as the others are living, continuously updated through the twin processes of assimilation and accommodation (Ivey, 1986). In particular, family members engage in the process of *motive reading* in order to better ascertain the needs of other family members. Reactions to others are based upon both the schemata themselves and specific set goals. The goals of behavior must at some level remain conscious, although much behavior becomes so habitual that it takes place without conscious deliberation. We are all adept at tuning in to specific cues which trigger behavior automatically in familiar-appearing situations; novelty serves as a flag to signal us to give the matter more thought (Edelman, 1989). Language serves as one of the most important cues which tell us how to respond in interpersonal situations.

One set goal to which we are genetically programmed to give highest priority is the maintenance of family homeostasis. We are all perfectly willing to sacrifice other goals—such as self-actualization—if our families seem to require it. Many analytic formulations contain the concept of a false self or *persona*. From the unified perspective, the persona is a role that we play in order to maintain the equilibrium within our families. In order to play this role, we must often deny, repress, and denigrate our own natural inclinations. This process is termed *mortification*. We must be, to varying degrees, self-destructive. The process of mortification leads to the irrational thoughts catalogued by cognitive therapists (Ellis & Grieger, 1977). We must rationalize away our tendencies to act in ways contrary to our role. The role that we play literally becomes an act. In order to play the role well, we must often come to believe that we really are the character whom we are playing (the *actor's paradox*).

Of course, our real selves never disappear. Any appearance of "fixation" or "regression" to a less individuated state represents a false self. As we progressively *differentiate* from one another as we mature, a war begins to develop within each of us between our own personal wishes and the needs of the larger social systems. Freud had the right idea: self-destructive behavior is generated by *intrapsychic conflict*, not a defective ego. However, the war is not between libidinal drives and conscience, but between the forces of individuality and the forces of togetherness (Kerr & Bowen, 1988).

A well-known example of the effects of cultural evolution is the changing status of women in the United States. Settling into the well-defined role of wife and mother to the exclusion of other interests is no longer even possible, let alone fashionable. As mores change, men and women no longer seem to know what to expect from one another. Developments such as this begin to tear apart group cohesion at all levels. In our own time and place, the nuclear family has begun to come apart at the seams. Two career families, step families, latchkey children, emotional distance, and single parent homes have become epidemic.

Because we are all genetically programmed to concern ourselves with the group before we think of ourselves, the dissolution of the family is extremely anxiety-provoking. This leads within the individual to what an analyst might call a *reaction formation*. In order to counter our tendencies to split from our old roles, we sometimes begin to cling ever more tightly to them. Our role behavior becomes more compulsive and more *polarized*.

Now let us return to the subject of the "services" family members provide for one another within this context. When the needs of individuals and the system converge, members support the individual needs of other members by *mirroring* (Kohut, 1977) or consensually validating the others' thoughts, perceptions, and behaviors.

Mirroring helps us to feel "at home" in the world and helps us to believe that what we know is valid and real. Without such validation, our individual perceptions continue to exist, but they cause a severe form of anxiety known as *existential groundlessness*: a sense of unreality and defamiliarization which leads to panic. Unmirrored activities are unlikely to be expressed overtly.

When the interests of the system and the individual are perceived to diverge—that is, when a significant threat to family homeostasis results from individuated behavior—family members refuse to mirror such behavior. In fact, they begin to actively undermine one another through the use of reverse mirroring, *disqualification* (Watzlawick, Beavin, & Jackson, 1967). (Examples will be given later.) Threats to family homeostasis fall roughly into two categories: internal and external. External threats are those which physically endanger the survival of the group. A good example is the threat of external racism whenever a black family member attempts to advance socially. Internal threats are those posed by an emotional breakdown of the leaders of the family system, most likely the parents, due to anxiety, depression, or self-destructiveness.

The most central cause of internal threats derives from parental *role function ambivalence*. Older family members also hear the siren song of individualism, but as mentioned, are apt to try to cling to old, outmoded ways of functioning. This sets up a situation in which they appear to need help from other family members to maintain their roles. Others are induced to find ways to mirror role behavior and disqualify individuation. In actuality, conflicted parents give off mixed messages about what sort of behavior they would like to have mirrored. However, other family members are apt to pay more attention to the parental role behavior and discount contradictory signals (Allen, 1991).

An attempt to mirror role functioning is termed *role function support*. Often, in order to provide such support, other family members must develop a role of their own. This takes place because younger family members often induce role function ambivalence in their parents by the example of their own individuated behavior, which has been partially mirrored by the larger culture. The parents see that such behavior is possible, and become envious and regretful over their pasts. In order to avoid causing an existential crisis in the parents, the younger family members will voluntarily sacrifice any such aspect of themselves and develop a role which helps the parent to remain "in character." Here are examples of what they may do:

1. They may act out repressed desires of the parent so the parent can receive vicarious satisfaction of suppressed impulses. They may act out the parents' repressed ambition (the "savior" role) or anger (the "avenger" or "sociopath" role) (Slipp, 1984).

2. They may sacrifice their own potency and become hostile and dependent on their parents (the "spoiler" or "borderline" role) so that the parents are forced to continue parenting but are provided with a convenient target ("lightning rod") for their anger over being so burdened. If parents are themselves functioning in a spoiler role, younger family members may become "narcissists" who attempt to take care of the parents but always fail.

3. They may become loathsome in some way to help parents feel justified in having been abusive.

4. They may become "defective" in such a way as to force a parent to maintain a gender-specific role, such as "caretaking mom" or "provider dad." The "defect" (examples: hypochondria, bulimia) causes the "defective" to be unable to function in some specific area, such as love or work, thereby requiring help from the parent.

Naturally, these roles are also played ambivalently, thus creating a situation in which the younger family members also give off mixed messages. All the family members in this situation begin to experience a great deal of discomfort because their attempts to mirror one another are rejected. Each one is rejected by the other because the roles being "supported" are not those which the other enjoys, but which are being performed solely for the supposed benefit of the supporter! Each individual is basing his or her appraisal of the other on the basis of the persona of the other, not the true self. Their mutual devotion is therefore driving everyone to distraction, a phenomenon known as the *altruistic paradox*. Attempts to sacrifice for the other backfire and in fact harm the other. The other would, covertly, like to receive mirroring for the true self, not disqualification. This mutual discomfort actually drives family members away from one another in a process which is termed *distancing*. Distancing behavior causes family bonds to loosen and speeds up the destruction of the collective.

When it becomes time for "adult children of an ambivalent parent" to marry, they will usually pick someone who mirrors their own role functioning. They need such support because of their ambivalence. They would like to give up the role, but if they did, they would suffer two consequences: an existential crisis for the family of origin and, therefore, an existential crisis for themselves. They therefore look for someone who seems to need them to continue the role. If the role of the spouse is complementary, which it almost always is, they can mirror one another's role (*mutual role function support*). This forms the basis of the so-called marital quid pro quo. Each spouse instinctively knows what behavior the other expects. What they do not know is *why* such behavior is expected. They cannot ask such a question for reasons to be addressed shortly, and instead make some sort of guess, usually inaccurate. Because psychoanalytic concepts have become part of our culture, the guess is often a bad version of a psychoanalytic interpretation, such as "He needs to abuse me so he can have an outlet for his repressed hostility toward his mother."

Of course, because all roles are held ambivalently, each spouse will create tension in the other because of the role function support. All such problems in both marital couples and family of origin could be easily solved if only family members could discuss the factors leading to their ambivalent role function behavior (*metacommunication*). They would then understand one another and mirror one another for devising alternative strategies for solving the original threat to family homeostasis. Unfortunately, such conversations are not often held in dysfunctional families. The reasons are twofold: the tendency of family members to protect one another as well as themselves from uncomfortable feelings, and the *game without end* (Watzlawick et al., 1967).

The "protection racket" develops in families because confrontations about ambivalence, distancing, and confusing motives lead to a number of negative reactions that serve both to raise doubts about the wisdom of talk and to disqualify attempts at metacommunication. A parent may begin to become depressed and regretful about his choices in life, envious of the younger member who had more choices, anxious about the possibility of change, or ashamed of past inability to solve the problem. Seeing this, the individual making the confrontation worries that the parent will become dysfunctional, and backs away. Of course, the parent will continue to experience the bad feelings anyway. Moreover, appearances to the contrary, we are all strong enough to face these feelings. We often feel that we are not, ironically, because everyone around us acts as though we are not. If others back away from a confrontation, we begin to think they believe we "cannot take it." We then begin to doubt ourselves.

Additionally, if the confrontation sounds like a criticism, the other naturally reacts with defensiveness and denial. This causes the "confronter" to be less sure of his position and feel groundless. The confronter backs off.

The second problem, the game without end, develops because individuals tend to be suspicious when others around them suddenly change or ask for change. After only one or two conversations, participants may feel better about acting differently, but not completely comfortable. New behaviors will be performed tentatively, as if to test the waters, and therefore come across as ambiguous. Each person may then begin to question the desires of the other and come to believe that the old rules still hold. This then becomes a self-fulfilling prophecy, and further discussion may seem pointless.

The therapy to be described is designed to help the client to get over these hurdles and push forward with the metacommunication process so that family members may learn to mirror more individuated behavior from one another, and to solve through rational means problems concerning family homeostasis. Once our true selves have been mirrored by our families, and our old roles have become obsolete, we become free to give up the self-defeating persona.

CLINICAL AND THEORETICAL ANTECEDENTS OF UNIFIED THERAPY

As the reader may be aware, the key concepts listed above derive from, but are not identical with, a variety of conceptualizations from the major schools of psychotherapy and philosophy. To summarize: Dialectics from Hegel; separation-individuation, intrapsychic conflict, and reaction formation from psychoanalysis; cultural evolution from Fromm; persona or false self from Jung and Winnicott; mirroring from Kohut; groundlessness from existentialism; family homeostasis and marital quid pro quo from family systems theory; disqualification and the game without end from Watslawick; differentiation of self from Bowen; mental schemata from Piaget; mortification through the use of irrational thoughts from Ellis and Beck; and the altruistic paradox from Rand.

Murray Bowen's (1978) school of therapy comes the closest to the dialectic view of self and system. He envisioned a "differentiation of self scale" by which he measured the degree to which individuals in a family system are enmeshed with one another. That is, less differentiated family system members are more reactive to one another, and less flexible in their role function behavior. Bowen's therapy is to send his patients back to their family of origin in order to learn how to behave in a less enmeshed fashion, and if they are successful, this behavior seems to carry over into all aspects of their lives and relationships. Other family members seem to have the power to help one another behave less self-destructively. From a unified perspective, they have the power to mirror—and far more of such power than does a therapist.

Unified therapy is a variation of Bowen therapy based upon a criticism of Bowen by Daniel Wile (1981). In therapy sessions with his patients, Bowen uses education, logic, and collaboration to coach them in how to deal with their families. What he teaches them, however, has far more in common with strategic family therapy than it does with Bowen therapy. Unified therapy believes that clients can be more successful if they, too, use logic, education, and collaboration when it comes to dealing with their families.

THE TECHNIQUE AND PROCESS OF PSYCHOTHERAPY

The goal of the therapy is to help patients give up self-defeating role function behavior, while maintaining contact with those family members who have in the past reinforced it. The client learns to solve problems of cultural change through the use of empathic metacommunication and rational discussion. Ultimately, the client must learn about how role behavior within the family affects him or her, and confront the parents or other family members with this knowledge. Although not ultimately responsible for changing anyone's behavior outside of the client–other relationship (the behavior within the relationship *must* change if the client's responses change), the client can help the entire family to behave in a more individuated way. First and foremost, however, the client must stop the parental behavior which serves to trigger the client's destructive role.

The attitude of the therapist is all important in determining whether or not the patient will provide an accurate description of the goings on within his or her family and participate in homework assignments. Important principles of attitude include the following: First, the therapist must convey the belief that the patient and other family members are not defective. They have no cognitive deficits; they have all matured into adults. No matter how heinous their behavior, they are not inherently evil. Clients come to therapy not because they *are* a problem, but because they *have* a problem. Second, the problem can be solved if both client and therapist are persistent. Third, the problem is best solved within the existing family system. The therapist and client alone can only do so much, and effectively "divorcing" one's family of origin is next to impossible. Divorcing a spouse is also considered less satisfactory than working out the relationship, unless the marriage would be life-endangering during the period in which the working out is done.

The therapy can be conceptualized as a series of stages, although the various stages overlap and are at times handled concurrently. I will now discuss the nature of each stage, as well as characteristic interventions.

Stage I: Assess the need for therapy and involve the patient. The therapist takes a good history and intrigues the patient into continuing therapy. History taking follows the medical model of presenting complaints, history of present illness, past psychiatric/psychological history and treatment, and an extensive social history. During history taking and during all subsequent stages, therapists boldly go where others fear to tread. They

feel free to ask *any* question, on the principle that the answer may be relevant, and the therapist cannot know if it is in advance. They are matter of fact when it comes to matters of physical, emotional, and sexual abuse. They know that a client can cope with the most disturbing aspects of existence, no matter how unpleasant the process. Most importantly, they ask *follow-up questions.*

Patient descriptions of family process often are disguised judgments; patient explanations for their motivation are often disguised descriptions. For example, a client may say, "My father contradicted everything I said." The therapist would then follow by asking for specific examples. A patient may say, "I overeat because it relieves my anxiety." The therapist would then ask, "Anxiety over what? And exactly how does eating help that particular problem?" A client may say, "My husband always tries to control me." The therapist then asks, "Exactly what is he trying to make you do?" When client statements appear to be illogical, exaggerated, or contradictory, the therapist politely asks the patient to clear up the confusion. When a client gives an explanation for his behavior that seems too cut and dried, the therapist says, "I think there might be more to it than that." For instance, if a patient attributes her depression to a single incident of having been molested as a child by a stranger, the therapist might say, "Well that certainly must have been traumatic, but I wonder why you are so depressed about it now, so many years later. What was the reaction of the people around you when this happened?"

Statements such as "I do not remember anything that happened when I was between six and ten," are countered with specific questions designed to jog the patient's memory. Patients always recall something about the period in question that can give the therapist a lead. When therapists pursue history taking with the proper attitude, all is eventually revealed, and additional testing or hypnosis is rarely necessary.

Symptomatic treatment, such as the use of medication or desensitization, is encouraged in cases in which it is indicated, and can be used as a lever to involve the client in treatment. Clients are unable to focus on their problems during severe depressions, obsessional states, or panic attacks. If clients do not comply with prescriptions, the therapist inquires as to the good reason behind their fears of giving up their symptoms.

Involving the patient in the therapy involves two goals which are processed concurrently: offering an initial frame for treatment, and reducing transference reactions and transference resistances. In unified therapy, transference is conceptualized as an *acting out of the client persona within the therapy session* ("acting in"). Clients come to therapy not knowing if the therapist will be like their family and reinforce their persona, or help them to find better ways to behave. They will offer up role function behavior in order to find out. An analyst fosters transference so as to gain power over it, while a unified therapist undermines it so that clients can concentrate on family dynamics. (The unified therapist does not ignore transference.) A *transference resistance* is conceptualized as an attempt to disqualify the therapist when the therapist attempts to see the client's true self. It involves transference because it is a replay of the way in which the clients themselves have been disqualified by other family members.

The basic frame offered to clients is that they must have a very good reason for behaving in a self-defeating manner, because they are obviously not enjoying the "fruits" of such behavior, and the therapist does not believe in masochism or sadism. Since clients usually expect to be told what is wrong with them, such a statement is a refreshing surprise and tends to hook them in. A few patients come to therapy only for confirmation of their own deficiencies; they will be frightened away by this type of statement, because they are not really coming for help. Fortunately, those clients who hold not a glimmer of hope for change and yet come to therapy are quite rare.

As mentioned, pop psychoanalysis is omnipresent in our culture, and clients will often have a negative explanation about their own behavior derived from such ideas. Therapists can both involve the client and reduce transference by bringing up the explanation themselves, and then discounting it. For example, a narcissistic husband obsessed with a borderline spouse can be told, "You know, some people might say that you are domineering and controlling your wife because you are all wrapped up in yourself and think of no one else. I don't believe it for a minute. I can see how much you care about her; no one would put up with the way she acts who didn't."

A second transference reducing technique is the *paradoxical prediction*. Patients are told that,

since they have had certain experiences in the past, they are likely to reexperience them within the context of therapy. Should that happen, the therapist adds, it is important that the client bring it up for discussion. For instance, if a client mentions in an early session that his family never believes anything he says, and that he withdraws in response, the therapist might say, "There may be times in here when you think *I* don't believe you. I sounds as if you might get quiet or leave therapy if that happens. I would hope that instead you might let me know, so we can discuss it." Usually, patients will respond that they do not think this will happen, since they are primed for therapy and feel good about the therapist. After this exchange, the problem, in fact, rarely does come up.

A third method by which transference is reduced involves countering client remarks which disqualify the therapist. The ways in which this is done are very similar to those taught to the patient later in therapy for use in patient–family metacommunication. Empathy is central to the process—the therapist acts as if the client's behavior is understandable without agreeing that it is all right for the client to act in such a manner. Attempts by clients to distance the therapist are turned around and used to move closer to the client. The therapist looks for something valid in what the client is saying and tries to avoid defensiveness, lectures, or "accusatory" interpretations. If a therapist makes a mistake in this regard, he or she apologizes for the offending behavior, but not for the feeling that generated it.

The following is a list of some of the disqualifications used by clients with a borderline personality disorder, and possible countermeasures: If the patient uses hyperbole or makes wild accusations, the therapist looks for any kernel of truth in the statements with which to agree and ignores the rest. If the patient demands immediate solutions to his or her problem, or tries to make therapists feel guilty or incompetent, therapists reply that they honestly wish they could do more for the patient right then. If the patient makes illogical-sounding statements, therapists look for alternate meanings that make more sense. If the client makes vague suicide threats, therapists reply, "If you really think you might do something like that, then you need to be in the hospital, but only for your own protection. I'd hate to have you go because I'd be concerned that you would feel even worse about yourself." (Usually, clients will then stop making the threats.) If a patient uses a hostile tone of voice, the therapist responds only to the lexical content of what is said, not the tone. If the client complains about a referral source, the therapist replies, "I wasn't there to see what happened, and I have had a better impression of him from before, so it would be hard for me to comment." If a client becomes more and more hostile for no apparent reason, the therapist inquires, "Why are you picking a fight?" If the patient makes an abrupt switch from a discussion of a hot transference issue to a discussion of his or her family dynamics, therapists go along with the switch without comment.

Other types of patient disqualifications include withdrawal, changing the subject, pleading amnesia, denial, double binds, blame shifting, nitpicking, overgeneralizing, and becoming overly fatalistic.

Stage II: Elicit the nature of the problem. The nature of the problem includes the role the patient's self-destructive behavior plays in the family homeostasis, the roles and role-function ambivalence of other significant family members, and, if available, the historical evolution of these family characteristics. The client must learn to what family cues he or she is responding, and why such cues occur. Stage II is an expansion of the history-taking process that began in Stage I. The therapist aims to construct a *genogram* (McGoldrick & Gerson, 1985) in order to provide the client with a context for the problem. Family history which may be important includes cultural background, experiences with death or disease, emigration, business failures, and family attitudes toward gender roles, education, and family size. The relationships between parents, between parents and their siblings, and between parents and grandparents are explored in detail. If patients are uninformed, they are sent back to any available older relative who can provide information. This often serves as the first step in the process, taught later on in therapy, of family metacommunication.

Stage III: Establish the client's altruistic motives. Clients should be convinced that their motives are pure; they hurt themselves not because they are defective, but to further the ultimate good of the family—even if superficially their behavior seems destructive. The basic form of the interpretation

is, "When you do such and such, other family members appear to be (less envious, depressed, or anxious; stop fighting with one another; and so forth). Clients are praised for being caring people, willing to make sacrifices for those they love. The only selfish motive they might have is the wish to avoid the anxiety they feel when they neglect their families. If clients become angry as they become more aware of their sacrifices, the therapist helps them to become more empathic with the rest of their family. After all, they are all in the same boat.

Stage IV: Discuss how the patient's attempts to solve the family problem backfire. This involves demonstrating how the client, by attempting to protect the parents from depression and anxiety, is instead helping to prevent the parents from learning how to get over their depression and anxiety. An interpersonal problem that cannot be discussed cannot be solved. The therapist emphasizes that other family members only seem to require the patient's self sacrifice—they really want what is best for the client, and are only reacting negatively to individuated client behavior because of their own internal conflicts.

Stage V: Offer and describe an alternate solution. The alternate solution consists of the client making contact with living family members—usually the parents—and initiating metacommunication about the nature and origin of the problems with role functioning that all the members of the family share. Significant family members are generally seen one at a time. The client must also warn in advance any peripheral family members who may interfere about what is to come, and address their concerns so they will stay clear. This is done in order to avoid "triangulation" (Bowen, 1978). If all important family members are deceased, the alternate solution can be done as a psychodrama within the therapy session. The goal of the alternate solution is for family members to learn how and why they trigger negative behavior from one another, and to decrease those negative interactions in the future.

The client does not usually begin with a direct confrontation about the parents' ambivalence and its effects. Rather, he or she begins with a discussion about how the problem existed in prior generations or earlier in the parents' lives. Such discussions of "ancient history" are metaphors for the current difficulties and are generally less threatening. They also help set the stage for empathic discussions of the current situation. The client is coached to avoid sounding overly critical of any relatives from earlier generations, as the targeted family member may become angry and jump to their defense. Gradually, the client moves the discussion from the past into the present.

Stage VI: Explore the difficulties the client might encounter with the alternate solution. The difficulties in metacommunication fall into two categories: the mistakes that the client will make, and the numerous ways by which the targeted family members will attempt to disqualify the client's efforts.

Client errors consist of problems with the use of the two keys to effective metacommunication: empathy, and respect for the potency and integrity of other family members. Empathy means that the client attempts to understand negative or destructive behavior without agreeing that the behavior was right or productive. If instead the client begins to blame or attack, the targeted family member will naturally become defensive and counterattack. Instead of discussion of a mutual problem, the conversation will quickly degenerate into a shouting match, or will be unceremoniously cut off. Avoiding angry or defensive behavior in the midst of a charged discussion is not easy, and is practiced using role playing, which is described in Stage VII. Respect for the potency of the other means that the client should not give up on talking about family interactions just because the parent seems to become depressed or anxious in response. Even if the parent acts out in a self-destructive manner in response to metacommunication, the client must look for ways to press forward.

The types of disqualifications used by family members on patients are the same as those that the patient uses on the therapist. The client and the therapist attempt to anticipate exactly which maneuvers the other might use to derail the conversation, so that the client will be prepared with a countermove. This is also accomplished through the use of role playing, which brings us to stage VII.

Stage VII: Role playing. Each step of the metacommunication process—getting past history out of a reluctant relative, the discussion of family dynamics in the past, and the actual confrontation over the current problem—is practiced in advance. The client gets a chance to try out various techniques within the safe confines of the therapy session. Once clients get out into the field, they are told to go as far as they can until they come up against an unanticipated roadblock or find that they cannot avoid emotional reactivity. When either problem occurs, they are told to back off immediately and return to the therapist for further strategy planning and practice. After each conversation, clients are instructed to write down as much as possible about what transpired for review with the therapist. This will help client and therapist to plan the next step.

Role playing is divided into two parts. The first is a role reversal in which the therapist plays the client's part and the client plays the role of the targeted other. Role reversal allows the therapist to try out, and to model, possible approaches, and to find out experientially what the client is up against. The therapist gets a chance to feel what clients feel when they are disqualified. The therapist also learns how to play the targeted other when the roles are exchanged during the second act of the role play. Patients, meanwhile, learn to put themselves in the shoes of the person whom they are about to confront. This helps the client to be more empathic. Role reversal may be particularly tough for clients with a borderline personality disorder because it breaks a family rule: parents are never supposed to be given the gift of empathy. The therapist nonetheless prods them to try it out in the session.

After the role reversal, client and therapist trade places. The client can then practice the strategy that is agreed upon during the role reversal. The therapist, meanwhile, presents the client with worst case scenarios. The other is played by the therapist to be as vicious, aggravating, and disqualifying as can be, consistent with the past behavior of that person. This is done both to prepare the client for the worst, but also to make the initial experience with the actual family member more successful. If the therapist and client are on target with their strategy, the family member will be easier to deal with than the therapist playing the family member.

The therapist will design the strategy in accordance with the descriptions furnished by the patient of troublesome interactions in the past. In addition to teaching specific countermeasures for the various disqualifications, the following general principles of assertiveness are taught: The patient should imagine himself an observer of the conversation as well as a participant. Others are always given the benefit of the doubt when it comes to evaluating their motivation; their motives are praised while only the effects of their behavior are questioned. The client should tactfully verbalize anger and disappointment, not act them out. When the motives of the other seem questionable, the client should assume nothing and puzzle over the motives aloud.

Stage VIII: Terminate therapy and arrange follow-up. After the client has successfully confronted those family members who have been reinforcing his or her self-destructive behavior, the family can often go on to discuss alternate ways to solve any remaining problems for family homeostasis. If not, the family will at least stop cuing the client in their usual way. Clients then find that they can more easily give up their roles, or at least tone them down considerably. They can give up self-defeating behaviors, and begin to experiment with new ones. They can try out different types of interpersonal relationships with peers and lovers. Often behavior change is accomplished without any further input from the therapist. With some clients, however, the therapist must work to prod the client to start doing new things. *In vivo* behavioral techniques can be very effective at this stage, since new behavior is no longer subject to family disqualification.

When the client is doing well, termination is quickly suggested. Reactions to termination are expected to be realistic; if the client has a negative transference reaction to the suggestion of termination, more work may need to be done. The client should be able to acknowledge both his or her own and the therapist's contribution to the solving of the problem. The therapist should then bring up the idea that both clients and their families will be expected to revert to former behavior from time to time. The therapist then expresses confidence that the client can use newly learned skills to handle such a situation quickly. This intervention is not meant as a paradoxical prediction of a relapse as in strategic therapy, but as a realistic assessment of the way people normally do behave. After termination, the therapist suggests that the client come back again after three months, and again after a year, to see if the new behavior and attitudes have taken root.

CASE EXAMPLE

Samuel was a single, 38-year-old, Jewish accountant who came into therapy with a history of self-destructive behavior on the job and in his relationships. At a new job, he would at first be a "rising star" showing much promise, and quickly advance, but then later get himself fired through absenteeism and frequent, inexcusable errors. He had a series of live-in relationships with women that followed a set pattern. The women would often be nurses or other caretakers who would attempt to get Samuel to get to work every day and make fewer mistakes. Eventually he would tire of their nagging and would suddenly move out.

In therapy, the patient at first described himself as a person with a fear of failure. Whenever he was doing well, he would start to fear that he would begin to do poorly, and become so anxious that he would in fact do poorly. When I brought up the self-fulfilling nature of this prophecy, he admitted that he knew he had a lot of talent, but he nonetheless insisted that he thought of himself as inadequate. I made the observation that his fear of failure was but half the story. He did in fact fear failure—when he lost one job, he would do whatever it took to get another. However, he also seemed to be anxious about success. He had just admitted how talented he was; there must be a good reason why he would tell himself otherwise just as he was about to make big money. I added, "This may seem like an off-the-wall question, but what would be the downside if you became more successful?"

He said that he could not imagine any downside. I wondered aloud if some one else he cared about might be adversely affected if he did well. At first confused by my question, he did recall hearing his father tell him on frequent occasions, "You'll never amount to anything." He added that he always felt that no matter how well he did, his mother never seemed pleased with his performance. Before following up on these leads, I made the following transference-reducing prediction: "It sounds as though there may be a time where you feel that I'm not pleased with your progress; if that happens, it would be important to let me know."

Further questioning revealed that both parents would seem threatened if he was too successful. His father would become depressed and withdraw from the patient. For example, the father would actively avoid social functions celebrating his son's promotions. The mother, on the other hand, would begin to make more demands on the patient's time for favors and errands as if he should put her needs before job considerations. When the patient would complain, the mother would reply, "I guess you're just too busy for me; go lead your own life." She would then turn to the patient's younger brother for favors. The patient would try to ignore this, but would always feel guilty.

I asked for more information about this whole process, and some further interesting facts emerged. The mother had often acted helpless and scatterbrained, when in fact she was a bright and capable woman. (At first, the patient did not believe she was bright and capable. I mentioned that since he himself was quite bright, it was hard for me to believe that he had come from such a poor gene pool. He gradually remembered incidents in which the mother showed her real capabilities.) The mother demanded much from her husband. The father felt overburdened by these demands and criticized her mercilessly for being so helpless, but he would usually comply. As the patient became more successful at work and began putting in more time, his father would do less and less for the mother, who would then turn to the patient for more and more help.

Gradually we began to construct a genogram. The father had been a major source of financial support in his own family of origin for many years, having quit school in order to do so. The paternal grandfather had immigrated from Russia during a pogrom, having been forced to give up a promising education. In the United States, he had lost a business and had considered himself a failure. The paternal grandmother had always been in poor health, but would in reality be the strength in the family when the grandfather became depressed. The relationship between father and grandfather paralleled the relationship between the patient and his father. The grandfather would withdraw from the father when the father would win awards and promotions.

The maternal grandmother had been one of two daughters in a Jewish Orthodox household. She had received a double message from her parents: be a good Jewish mother, but we really wish that you had been a boy so you could have been a scholar. She dropped out of high school to marry and began having a lot of children. The maternal grandfather was also a poor immigrant, whom the rest of the family considered a failure. The mother and all of her siblings quit school early and began working and sending the money home. Grandma was never appreciative and would ask for more and more. Even after the mother had married, she sent money home to grandma, until her husband stepped in. He made himself the object of his mother-in-law's scorn so that the latter would be angry at him instead of at his wife.

When the patient's parents married, the mother immediately wanted more and more children; the patient was the third of five children and the eldest boy. Father always managed to support this large brood, but had himself been swindled out of a business and was barely able to make ends meet with his current job. Because of a lack of education, he was unable to get a better paying job.

The mother had treated the children like servants—especially the patient, who moved out as soon as he was old enough. When Samuel first started living with a woman, the mother acted very angry and upset, and told the patient that he no longer cared about her. This type of comment was repeated each time the patient struck up with someone new, and would serve as one direct trigger to the patient's doing poorly at work. Predictably, the work problem would alarm the new girlfriend, who would start to nag the patient until he left the relationship.

I praised the patient for being such a devoted son that he would be willing to give up his success to keep things harmonious in his family. He never really agreed that he was doing this, but was able to see how his family's behavior led to guilt and anxiety which interfered with his functioning at work. He tended to blame his girlfriends for the relationship difficulties, attributing their nagging to their innate need for domination and control, but was eventually able to admit that he knew he was feeding into their anxiety with his own behavior.

The next step was convincing Sam that his parents really did want him to succeed, but that his success served as a passive reminder to them of their own conflicts and ambivalence. His father withdrew when the patient became successful, not out of mean-spirited envy, but for two other reasons. First, the father would become depressed at his own failings, and second, he would begin to get in touch with repressed rage toward his own father, which he would just as soon keep repressed. His statement, "You'll never amount to anything," was more a fear than a wish, as the family had in the past been prevented from being successful by forces beyond its control.

The mother, on the other hand, was conflicted about two role functions she was serving. She had given up her own ambitions to have children so as to prevent her own mother from becoming envious and depressed, and to keep her husband burdened down. He appeared to need such a burden in order to continue serving in the role he had played in his own family; if he were not tied down, he would want to bolt. The mother seemed to need the children around to keep this whole process going, but really did not want them to feel as burdened as she had felt with her own mother. When she said, "You're too busy for me; go lead your own life" to the patient, she would do so with an annoyed tone. Nonetheless, no value judgment is contained in the statement. She *admired* the patient for wanting to lead his own life, but could not say so directly without admitting her rage toward her own mother. The angry tone was meant to distance the patient so he *would* live his own life. The mother seemed to be negative regarding the patient's female relationships because she feared he would tie himself down with lots of children just like the rest of the family had.

The patient could readily see how continuing to sacrifice his success could never really solve the problem. Actually, the mother's constant demands pushed him to succeed at the same time they held him back. This accounted for the cycles of success and failure and the fear associated with *either* polarity. We role played possible approaches to discussing these patterns. Luckily, both parents were unusually receptive to discussions of their own backgrounds. The father, however, refused to admit to any anger at the grandfather for the latter's demands or apparent envy. The patient then tried to use the relationship between his father and himself as a parallel to get the father to open up, but unfortunately began the process with the statement, "I never felt any love from you." The father became angry. "I never felt much love from you, either," was the retort.

The patient reported back to the therapist what had happened, and was coached to apologize for accusing the father of not loving him. Sam was coached to add that what he meant was, "I know now how much you did care about me, but at the time I thought you were jealous of my success and wanted me to fail. I can now see how you were just reacting to the success that *you* missed out on." The father then was able to discuss many of his own disappointments. The patient was sure to express empathy for the paternal grandfather as well, who also must have been reacting to his own disappointments.

The patient made a similar error when it came time to have a discussion with his mother. He started talking about the mother's need to dominate and control the children, instead of bringing up the fact that she really wanted him to be free of family burdens. Again the patient was coached to apologize, and talk to the mother empathically about why she had had so many children.

After the process of metacommunication was complete, the patient started a new job. He was quite anxious but managed to press on, and he felt more confident. We then went on to deal with the relationship he had with his current girlfriend; this will not be described here.

CONCLUDING COMMENTS

The dialectic between self and collective seems to be built into almost all facets of human existence, and dialectical thinking may yield additional insights into many other aspects of human behavior, both social and individual. I believe the basic concepts of unified therapy may find application in other psychiatric conditions and social units than the ones described above.

Our knowledge of the neurophysiology of schema formation, and of how schemata change, remains in its infancy. The question of the effect of the deaths of important family members on both schema maintenance and environmental cues to social behavior remains unanswered. Answers to these questions will in the future provide us with clues as to how to help people change their habitual maladaptive behavior more quickly.

REFERENCES

Allen, D. (1988). *Unifying individual and family therapies*. San Francisco: Jossey-Bass.

Allen, D. (1991). *Deciphering motivation in psychotherapy*. New York: Plenum Press.

Basseches, M. (1986). Dialectical thinking and young adult cognitive development. In R. Mines and K. Kitchener (Eds.), *Adult cognitive development* (pp. 33–56). New York: Praeger.

Bowen, M. (1978). *Family therapy in clinical practice*. New York: Jason Aronson.

Edelman, G. (1989). *The remembered present*. New York: Basic Books.

Ellis, A., & Grieger, R. (1977). *Handbook of rational emotive therapy*. New York: Springer.

Fromm, E. (1969). *Escape from freedom*. New York: Avon Books. (Originally published 1941.)

Ivey, A. (1986). *Developmental therapy*. San Francisco, Jossey-Bass.

Kerr, M., & Bowen, M. (1988). *Family evaluation*. New York, W.W. Norton.

Kohut, H. (1977). *The restoration of the self*. New York: International Universities Press.

McGoldrick, M., & Gerson, R. (1985). *Genograms in family assessment*. New York: W. W. Norton.

Slipp, S. (1984). *Object relations: A dynamic bridge between individual and family treatment*. New York, Jason Aronson.

Weston, D. (1985). *Self and society*. Cambridge: Cambridge University Press.

Watzlawick, P., Beavin, J., & Jackson, D. (1967). *Pragmatics of human communication*. New York: Norton.

Wile, D. (1981). *Couples therapy: A nontraditional approach*. New York: Wiley.

CHAPTER 11

An Anxiety-Reduction Modification of Short-Term Dynamic Psychotherapy (STDP)

A THEORETICAL "MELTING POT" OF TREATMENT TECHNIQUES

Leigh McCullough

INTRODUCTION

The focus of this chapter is a modification of the conventional models of short term dynamic psychotherapy (STDP) (McCullough, 1991, 1992). Although this approach retains the fundamental components of its short-term precursors (Davanloo, 1980; Malan, 1979; Mann, 1973; Sifneos, 1979); it differs in three ways: (1) the use of supportive and self-psychological approaches to *reduce* rather than *provoke* anxiety; (2) the intentional incorporation of behavioral, gestalt, psychodynamic, and self-psychological techniques to achieve treatment goals; and (3) the concrete operationalization of treatment techniques.

This integrative modification will also be

shown to encompass Weinberger's (1990) model in which it has been hypothesized that the effective ingredients of psychotherapy are captured in four main components: exposure, alliance, mastery, and attribution. *Exposure* refers to the patient's facing of unpleasant stimuli or the experiencing of previously avoided thoughts, feelings, or behaviors. *Alliance* typically refers to the quality of the relationship bond between the patient and the therapist. In this model, alliance will refer also to how that bond is used to facilitate treatment goals. *Mastery* is the patient's gaining of control over maladaptive responses. *Attribution* is the alteration in the patient's world view that allows the behavioral changes achieved in treatment to be maintained.

To begin, a brief overview of short-term dynamic psychotherapy will be given. Next, a brief discussion of the major clinical and theoretical antecedents to this integrative approach will be provided. This will be followed by a more detailed discussion of the specific techniques involved, and finally a case example.

Leigh McCullough • Department of Psychology in Psychiatry, University of Pennsylvania, Philadelphia, Pennsylvania 19104.

Comprehensive Handbook of Psychotherapy Integration, edited by George Stricker and Jerold R. Gold. Plenum Press, New York, 1993.

THEORETICAL AND CONCEPTUAL FRAMEWORK OF STDP

Short-term dynamic psychotherapy, as the name implies, evolved from a psychodynamic framework. The fundamental ingredients of STDP are the essential elements of psychoanalytic treatment; that is, analysis of defenses and the working through of previously conflicted feelings in large part through the analysis of the patient–therapist relationship.

The pioneers in short-term dynamic therapy incorporated various techniques to decrease the length of time in treatment. Most of these techniques served the function of increasing the patient's anxiety in order to break down resistance to the exploration of "unconscious feeling." In these short-term approaches, heightened therapist activity and a clear focus were two fundamental mechanisms (Flegenheimer, 1982). For example, Mann (1973) set a time limit of 12 sessions, which compelled the patient to work rapidly, and focused on the experience of loss. Sifneos (1979) used rapid and intense interpretation in high-functioning patients to effect a quicker resolution of conflicts. Davanloo (1980) used strong confrontation to heighten anxiety and break down resistance to the working through of conflicts. Malan (1979) used a heightened focus (i.e., focal interpretations involving the "two triangles") to shorten the length of dynamic therapy.

The revised model of STDP that I present in this chapter will incorporate many aspects from each of these pioneering short-term approaches; especially Malan's focus in the two triangles, the reducing of defensiveness, and the experiencing of conflicted feeling. My revised model differs in its attempt to reduce or regulate anxiety, guilt, and shame, rather than to provoke it, and by my intentional rather than chance inclusion of cross-theoretical techniques.

Because Malan's schema of the two triangles forms the basis of the present model, an overview will be given. Malan refers to this schema as the "Universal Theme" in dynamic therapy (1979, p. 94). The first triangle he calls the "triangle of conflict"; work in this triangle involves analysis of defensive behavior, anxiety, and impulse or feeling. The second triangle he calls the "triangle of person"; work in this triangle of interpersonal relationships involves analysis of relationship patterns with the therapist, current persons, and past persons.

An interpretation that includes all six points of Malan's two triangles will provide an example of this theoretical approach. The therapist might say, "When I asked you about your feelings of sadness (impulse/feeling) around your mother's (past person) death, I noticed that you lowered your eyes and became very quiet." (Pointing out the defensive responses used to avoid conflicted feeling.) "I wonder if there is some discomfort for you about those feelings?" (anxiety). "And I wonder if there are some feelings toward me (therapist–patient relationship) for asking you?" "Certainly, you disliked your neighbor (current person) when she brought this up." This sequence illustrates a typical example of interpretation and clarification of defenses in short-term dynamic treatment. I begin with this example because use of Malan's two triangles forms a fundamental component of the model that is being described in this chapter.

CLINICAL AND THEORETICAL ANTECEDENTS

In part, the alteration of psychodynamic treatment from a long-term to a short-term model has been accomplished through the incorporation of techniques from other theoretical orientations than the psychodynamic. It was the inclusion of these "active" and "focused" clinical techniques which originally gave STDP its integrative quality. Generally, the integrative features evolved less from a formal intention toward eclecticism or integration, than from an acute clinical sensitivity regarding "what works" (e.g., Mann's time limits, Sifneos' interpretations, Davanloo's confrontation of defenses, and Malan's focus on the triangles). Nevertheless, aspects from other orientations can be observed in these psychodynamic models. For example, the heightened activity and focus on specific problems used by Mann, Malan, and Sifneos are techniques also used in behavioral and cognitive therapies. Davanloo's use of confrontation is, in part, similar to a behavioral exposure technique. Aspects of gestalt techniques can also be observed in Davanloo's exploration of intense emotion.

The anxiety-reducing modification of STDP that I present here, as well as my previous analysis of STDP (McCullough, 1991) is a more conscious attempt at integration of STDP with other therapeutic orientations. This modification has evolved, in part, from the research on STDP conducted at Beth Israel Medical Center in New York City (McCullough & Winston, 1991), where the STDP treatment approach began to incorporate clarification and support to assist the patient in the difficult assimilation of the confrontation of defenses (Laikin, Winston, & McCullough, 1991). Since that time, more and more cross-theoretical techniques have been purposely incorporated into various steps of the STDP treatment package to enhance the patient's *exposure to and mastery of goals* at each stage of the treatment.

In my revised model of STDP, cognitive and behavioral therapies contribute techniques which make possible the rapid (i.e., short-term) analysis of the observable behaviors which are hypothesized to be representative of ego defenses. Gestalt techniques (e.g. Perls, 1969, 1976) enhance the rapid and intense experiencing of emotion.

Self-psychological techniques (Baker and Baker, 1987; Kohut, 1971, 1984) are utilized throughout to enhance the therapeutic alliance and to provide support, encouragement, and reassurance for the difficult tasks undertaken by the patient in STDP. Most importantly in this approach, techniques, such as an empathic stance and what has been called an "experience near" position to the patient by the therapist are utilized to *reduce* rather than *provoke* anxiety. This particular modification incorporates Luborsky's (1984) supportive-expressive continuum of psychodynamic techniques to determine in what stages and under what conditions various interventions should be implemented.

In summary, the major *foci* in this anxiety-reduction version of STDP come from the psychodynamic orientation. It is in the *activity* of the therapist (i.e., the clinical techniques utilized by the therapist) where the incorporation of cross-theoretical mechanisms takes place. Put differently, the *goals* of this model follow the main principles of psychodynamic theory, while the *methods* used to achieve those goals are drawn from a diversity of techniques from the major theoretical schools.

Because of the convergence of techniques, this anxiety-reducing modification of STDP can be seen as a "melting pot" of theoretical orienta-

tions. Also because of this convergence, not just one or two aspects, but all four aspects of Weinberger's goals model (alliance, exposure, mastery, and attribution) are thoroughly and repeatedly incorporated. The convergence of these techniques will be discussed in detail below.

THE TECHNIQUE AND PROCESS OF PSYCHOTHERAPY

Patient Selection

The prerequisite for undertaking any short-term dynamic psychotherapy approach is a careful assessment to ensure that the patients have sufficient ego strength, sense of self, coping skills, and interpersonal skills to be able to tolerate the demands placed on them in this rapid uncovering form of therapy.

Contraindications include the following: (1) symptoms sufficiently severe that functioning is impaired; (2) lack of impulse control (e.g., alcohol, drugs, eating disorders, loss of temper, etc.); or (3) no close relationships. Patients must have sufficient sense of self and interpersonal skills to be able to form a strong alliance (i.e., evidence of at least one close personal relationship), and have good control over impulses (i.e., no history of acting out of anger, or substance abuse within the past year.

Overview of Treatment

In this model, the specific focus of treatment and the activities utilized are the bases of a two-stage treatment approach. These two stages carefully monitor Luborsky's supportive and expressive aspects of therapeutic interventions. In Stage One, the therapeutic focus is on the analysis and alteration of defenses; this is called the *defense restructuring stage*. In Stage Two, the focus is the experiencing and integration of conflicted feelings; this is called the *affect restructuring stage*.

All four facets of the Weinberger goals model can be seen to occur in both stages of treatment (see Table 1). The activity in Stage One has the goal of restructuring the defenses; that is, alteration of maladaptive patterns of thinking, feeling, or behaving to patterns which are more adaptive. During the defense analysis, learning principles,

Table 1.   Cross-Theoretical Mechanisms in Short-Term Anxiety-Reducing Psychotherapy

Weinberger's goals	Theoretical orientation	Techniques and processes
Defense restructuring stage		
Exposure	Behavioral	Behavior analysis
Alliance	Supportive and self-psychology	Empathy "Experience-near" stance
Mastery	Behavioral principles	Negative consequences
	Psychodynamic	Syntonic to dystonic
Attribution	Psychodynamic	Interpretation
	Behavioral	Discrimination learning
Affect restructuring stage		
Exposure	Gestalt	Physiological awareness; guided affective imagery
Alliance	Supportive and self-psychology	Empathy Experience-near therapist stance
Mastery	Behavioral principles	Desensitization
	Psychodynamic	Working-through
Attribution	Behavioral	Stimulus generalization
	Psychodynamic	Interpretation
	Behavioral	Discrimination learning

behavioral analysis, and cognitive theory are applied to a psychodynamic focus in order to *expose* the patients to (1) an intellectual awareness or *recognition* of the defensive behavior, and the (2) the emotional awareness or feeling of the destructive consequences of what they are doing.

When necessary to maintain optimal patient functioning, the *alliance* can be enhanced through the use of supportive, empathic, and self-psychological interventions (Baker and Baker, 1987; Luborsky, 1984; Pinsker, Rosenthal, & McCullough, 1991). Such modifications reduce the patient's anxiety, guilt and shame about facing such difficult insights.

Mastery might be seen as the demonstration of the change, that is, the replacement of maladaptive defensive behavior with more adaptive expression of emotion. Mastery can be conceptual-

ized as the process in the defense analysis by which the ego-syntonic defenses become ego-dystonic. In this process, the patient having seen his or her defenses, wants to give them up. Mastery is achieved through experiential exposure of the patients to the grief-laden feelings of how they are hurting themselves or maintaining destructive patterns of response, as well as through more directly encouraging the giving up of such behavior.

Finally, the shifts in *attribution* are achieved by patients' arriving at an explanation for the change which gives them a sense of efficacy or control; for example, how the patients view the world before and after the defense analysis—as helpless, victimized persons or persons able to take full responsibility for their actions. A change in attribution in this model is attained through interpretation of the defenses, anxieties, and hidden feelings to alter the patients' view of themselves and their unconscious behavior.

The focus in the Stage Two/Affect Restructuring Phase is the exposure to feeling rather than to defensive behavior. Here the therapist incorporates gestalt techniques to encourage the patient to experience, as intensely as possible, the previously warded-off emotion. This process can be seen as "working through," where, ideally, a patient would be "exposed" to conflicted feeling in a range of interpersonal relationships.

In Stage Two, alliance is strengthened through mechanisms from the self-psychological orientation. These supportive and empathic interventions are woven into treatment as needed in order to ease and reduce anxiety, guilt, and shame around the exploration of these conflicted feelings. Such reduction of guilt and shame by "holding" ensures that defensive avoidance does not block the process.

In the affective experiencing phase, *mastery* can be seen to occur through the "desensitization" of the conflicted emotion. That is, by the experiencing of feelings in a safe, accepting environment (heightened through self-psychological mechanisms), patients no longer attach anxiety, guilt, or shame to such feelings as anger, grief, sexual desire, tenderness, or joy. Mastery can be said to be achieved when the patient demonstrates the capacity to appropriately and joyfully express formally conflicted and defended feelings in a wide range of interpersonal relationships.

Attribution occurs through the interpretive process which provides an explanation for the patients' behavior and clearly places the responsibility within the patients for recognition and alteration of maladaptive patterns.

Table 1 outlines the multiple theoretical processes in each stage, and the goal (identified in Weinberger's model) that activities in each stage are utilized to achieve. Each of the sections in this table will be discussed more fully in the following discussion. The reader is also referred to the *Treatment Manual for Short-Term Anxiety Reducing Therapy* (McCullough, 1992) for a still more detailed description of techniques.

DEFENSE RESTRUCTURING STAGE

Exposure in Defense Restructuring

It is intensely painful for individuals to begin to recognize their defensive behavior. Patients often feel foolish, stupid, or destructive and generally need to muster a great deal of courage to face these vulnerable aspects of themselves. While "exposure" in a behavioral treatment helps an individual face *external* stressors, "exposure" in a psychodynamic treatment involves individuals facing *internal or intrapsychic* stressors (for example, either maladaptive defenses or conflicted feelings). In the initial phase of defense restructuring, the exposure process takes the form of the patients "seeing" or recognizing their defensive behavior. This is an exposure on a cognitive level; that is, defensive behaviors are verbally labeled and thus brought into conscious awareness. There is an affective response to this dawning awareness (i.e., sorrow over the destructive quality of the defensive behavior), but the task is primarily cognitive (i.e., recognition or awareness) in this stage. Intense affect is not elicited until the second stage of treatment when the patients have demonstrated the capacity to see the relationships between their defenses and their feelings.

The therapist might say: "So, you're telling me that you have trouble with your boss. It seems that whenever there is a conflict, you feel very anxious and become withdrawn. Is this how you see it?"

Thus, the therapist reflects back rather than confronts the defenses. This is done in a collaborative "experience-near" style (the therapist's stance is "near" to the patient's), encouraging the patient to join in a noncritical analysis of his or her behavior. Later the therapist might ask, "Do you think you might have some anger toward the boss?" Instead of challenging the patient, or making depth interpretations, the therapist explores various possibilities until the patient is able to see it the same way or explain a different pattern. "Yeah, I do see how I get angry underneath but don't show it. But I don't just withdraw. Sometimes I get real stubborn and passive aggressive, too." Thus, in this first phase of defense restructuring, there is a collaborative effort between the patient and therapist, in preparing the patient to recognize defensive behavior and the hidden feelings.

In a preliminary examination of research cases, I have noted that this anxiety reduction method of analysis of defenses, although much gentler, appears to be just as rapid in reaching the deep emotion of Stage Two as the more confrontational and anxiety-provoking models. In anxiety provoking approaches, especially that of Davanloo, the therapist might say, "Can we look at your feeling toward me right now? Now you smile when I say this. Can we see what that smile is? And, now you look away, and then you're looking out the window. Do you notice you're tapping your finger?" This relentless confrontation provokes a great degree of defensiveness in most patients, but has the potential to subsequently elicit a tremendous amount of feeling which can be "desensitizing" (i.e., the patient learns to express strong emotion without punishment). However, this technique is not one that has been applied consistently. Not many patients can be confronted heavily without much introductory work to help them respond in a constructive manner. (I have noted that only about 10% of research patients can respond easily to strong confrontation; the majority of patients need some degree of preparatory and/or supportive assistance.) In addition, many therapists have great difficulty learning and implementing confrontational techniques. Indeed, the raising of anxiety in the exposure phase of treatment may create unnecessary obstacles for both patient and therapist.

I believe that anxiety-reducing techniques can achieve similar goals more consistently. In the same amount of time, they may provide a more parsimonious approach. Of course, this is an empirical question and must be experimentally validated. In self-psychological terms, one could compare the effectiveness of the "experience far" position of the confrontationist therapist to an "experience near" position of the empathic therapist in the degree of affect experienced by the patient in the exposure phase.

Alliance in Defense Restructuring

The therapist–patient alliance is maintained because empathy and support are used to decrease anxiety levels and an empathic stance allows the patient to move as painlessly as possible toward the recognition of defensive behavior. Although this process is never pain-free, the therapist should be vigilant that the patient should be guided toward grief (i.e., "I feel tremendous sorrow for the losses I have incurred by behaving like this), rather than self-attack (i.e., "I'm stupid or bad for having behaved like this"). In other words, the therapist assists the patient in feeling *compassion* rather than shame or guilt.

Mastery in Defense Restructuring

In behavioral terms, I have hypothesized that mastery, or change in behavior, is accomplished through (1) the therapist's pointing out *negative consequences of defensive behavior and positive consequences of adaptive alternatives,* and (2) the patient's recognizing and feeling the effects of these behavioral patterns (McCullough, 1992). From a psychodynamic perspective, one could say of this same process that mastery is acquired through making the ego-syntonic defenses ego-dystonic. The dynamic and behavioral labels might differ, but the underlying operations are the same. For example, some patients come to each session smiling a lot. When the therapist points out, "You seem to smile whenever you mention some negative thought," an ego-syntonic response would be, "Well, that's the way I am. Isn't it good to smile in the face of difficult feelings?" But, once the patient recognizes the negative consequences of the smiling (i.e., the falseness, the inability to express feelings directly), he or she might begin to say, "I don't like this smiling, compliant person that I am." In this manner, defenses become ego-dystonic by becoming aversive to the patient, and

by the patient gradually wishing to behave differently. Patients begin by identifying how their defenses have hurt them. "Oh, I see what I've been doing. I see the years that have been wasted. I see how I've lost closeness to people in my life, through my passive compliance and denial." Thus, mastery begins to be attained when the patient feels the negative consequences of the defensive behavior sufficiently to catch themselves in action and stop their almost "reflexive" response. Patients can be observed doing this in the treatment session (e.g., "Oh, there I go smiling again. I guess I'm trying to lighten up our discussion and avoid how difficult it is for me"). Patients also demonstrate mastery through their report of catching and stopping themselves outside the session (e.g., "I felt the urge to smile, and avoid the confrontation, but I caught myself and spoke firmly, instead. My boss seemed to respect me for it").

Attribution in Defense Restructuring

In behavioral terms, attribution can be seen as discrimination learning. Patients begin to make distinctions regarding who is the person responsible for their own behavior. The discrimination that is crucial is for the patients to recognize that a maladaptive pattern is being enacted by them. The patients are not helpless, victimized human beings, but rather, they are active participants due to defensive reactions chosen either consciously or unconsciously. In psychodynamic terms, such a shift in attribution occurs through the process of interpretation; the therapist's explanatory statements have shown the patients links between their defensive behavior and impulse, and how such behavioral patterns are played out *by the patients* in various interpersonal relationships. Thus, interpretations are the vehicle by which patients learn vital discriminations and gain mastery over changes in defenses. Generally, mastery is maintained through an attribution that the patients are responsible for their current behavior patterns and emotional responses.

A patient might say, "I see what I've been doing all my life and I can't bear it. I don't want to do this anymore." There is grief associated with such insight and there may be tears at this point. Thus I might say, "Well, you know, you've always avoided the grief over your father's death. Do you think that now we can look at it and see how, in the past, you've run away? We can see that you felt guilt and anxiety. Can we look at this together now?" If patients are ready to collaborate, then I can go into Stage Two of affect restructuring very rapidly.

On the one hand, the more severely disordered the patient, the more restructuring of defensive behavior is necessary before affective restructuring can begin. On the other hand, if patients begin therapy already aware of the negative consequences of their behavior and already voicing an intense desire to change, then less time needs to be spent in the defense analysis. An example might be a patient who says, "I know I've been acting like a compliant, good girl all my life, and I can't stand to do it any longer. I want to be able to say what I really feel, but I can't. I would give anything to be able to stand up for myself and say no when I need to." When the patient's stance is this "ego-dystonic" the therapist can move more rapidly into Stage Two work of affect expression and integration. In this example, the patient already acknowledges her defensive avoidance and might be able to move rapidly into the experiencing and practicing in imagery of angry or assertive feelings.

STAGE TWO: AFFECT RESTRUCTURING

Exposure in Affect Restructuring

In Stage Two, the process of exposure takes the form of encouraging the patient to experience previously conflicted feelings or wishes. The intense experiencing of emotion proceeds most smoothly when the patient has been "prepared" in Stage One with a careful and supportive restructuring of defensive behavior (i.e., the patient no longer wants to maintain the destructive defensive patterns and is motivated to explore troublesome feelings).

Such exposure to the feeling is similar to the desensitization of behavior therapy. Analysis of the transference provides *in vivo* desensitization just as imaginal desensitization would occur from looking at past figures in Malan's interpersonal triangle. Davanloo (1983) has quipped, "If dreams are the royal road to the unconscious, the transference is the super highway." He believes that by focusing on the transference, the greatest level of

desensitization is achieved. I would agree that the more intense affect that is expressed in the transference, the more effective the therapy.

Alliance in Affect Restructuring

As noted in the section on selection of patients, a prerequisite for short-term treatment is a ready capacity for alliance. In addition, that capacity should have been strengthened by the therapist's support and encouragement of the patient during the defense analysis and restructuring. Certainly, in the affect restructuring stage, the alliance should be on a firm foundation; for the alliance must be strong to support the rapid uncovering that will ensue. The optimal implementation of the alliance in this phase is reflected in the use of accurate empathy to deepen and intensify the affective experience, and in the therapist's sensitivity to return to the defense restructuring and/or support when there is a block in the affective working through.

Mastery in Affect Restructuring

In Stage Two, I have hypothesized that mastery, or change in behavior, is accomplished through (1) the patients' increasing ability to experience a wide range of feelings without concomitant anxiety, guilt, or shame, and (2) when appropriate, to express these feelings in a constructive manner to the individual with whom they are interacting. Mastery is a result of what I hypothesize to be the pairing of previously conflicted feelings with positive rather than negative consequences. This can be seen as a process of "desensitization."[1] In other words, patients learn to experience and share (through imagery, not acting-out) the intense experiences of anger, sorrow, sexual desire, or tenderness without experiencing negative consequences. In this first step toward the experiencing of previously shameful or guilt-ridden feelings, the therapist's acceptance and understanding is often a dramatically different response—or consequence than the patient has ever before experienced. In behavioral terms, the

[1] I want to thank Herb Fensterheim for helping me make clear this distinction; that is, that one does not "desensitize" the primary feeling itself but rather the negative experience or feelings associated with it (which typically fall into the categories of anxiety, guilt, or shame).

result of such expression of feelings with the therapist is that the patient's reactions of anxiety, guilt, or shame begin to be "extinguished." Thus, unhampered or unconflicted expression of feeling begins to be possible.

This same pattern of the freeing up of emotional expression in the patient–therapist relationship can be seen as "*in vivo* desensitization." When a patient experiences feelings or wishes of any sort, nowhere will these feelings be more intense than in the face-to-face relationship with the therapist. Two examples of expression of feelings will illustrate this point. The therapist might ask the patient to describe in imagery the angry feeling toward the boss. The patient might reply, "Oh, sometimes I'd like to punch him in the face and knock him flat." The process of expressing such negative feelings to an understanding therapist aids in the "desensitization" process (i.e., the elimination of feelings of guilt, anxiety, or shame associated with primary feelings). Then the therapist can ask, "What are your feelings toward me right now?" and the patient can learn to be spontaneous, look the therapist in the eye, and say, "Oh, I'd like to smash you right now, you're making me so mad." Expression of personal feeling directly to the therapist at the moment is qualitatively more intense than telling the therapist about anger at the third party. Furthermore, if the therapist's response is one of accurate empathy and understanding, the patient who might have formerly felt a great deal of guilt for feeling anger toward a caring person, will come to feel less guilt, and more acceptance of such feelings. Thus we might see this direct interpersonal expression of emotion as *in vivo desensitization*; that is, the reduction or elimination of anxiety, guilt, and shame associated with the face-to-face expression of feelings, which results in mastery over previous conflicts.

Attribution in Affect Restructuring

In behavioral terms, attribution in the affect restructuring stage means that a stimulus which has been identified (i.e., an expression of previously conflicted feelings) should generalize to a wide range of situations outside of therapy. The attributions take the form of self-provided psychodynamic interpretations which provide explanatory propositions for behavior across a range of interpersonal relationships.

The therapist might say: "We see that first you avoided your anger toward your father because you were so guilty about those murderous feelings toward him. And then you cut off all expression of anger with your wife, or at work, or even here with me, because you felt so bad about yourself. Now you know how exploited and taken advantage of you have been as a result of the passive responses you learned."

Thus, recognition of the behavior pattern in many instances, and turning the responsibility over to the patient should lead to a stimulus generalization; the patient can catch himself or herself repeating these behaviors in many different situations, and attribute that to his or her own personal choice whether or not to continue it. However, it is important to note that insight without control over conflicted emotions would be ineffective in changing behavior. Attribution by itself would not change behavior if old affective patterns are still in place. Mastery in experiencing and appropriately expressing feelings must have been acquired first for this final stage of cognitive shifts in attribution to be effective.

CASE EXAMPLE

Tracy, a female college senior, came to treatment because of severe distress over the fear of her boyfriend's leaving her. Her distress was so intense that she was in danger of not completing her course work and thus not graduating. Although she had felt more in control when the relationship began over one year before, she had become increasingly needy and clinging toward him as they became closer. She also became so depressed and anxious whenever they had a fight that she had increasing trouble over functioning in the weeks prior to starting therapy.

Assessment revealed Axis I, major depression and Axis II, borderline and histrionic traits but did not meet criteria for diagnosis. She manifested no history of acting-out or impulse control problems. Typically, she was organized and disciplined in her daily life, and was a good student, without alcohol or drug problems. She had several close friends.

Defense Restructuring Stage

Exposure. Treatment with Tracy began with a gentle exploration of her defensive behavior patterns in relation to criticism from her boyfriend, John. The pattern that emerged revealed that when John criticized her (which he was increasingly doing) she would either become severely depressed and self-critical (masochism) or, when she could take it no longer, she would lash out at him in a rage (displacement), which, of course, would leave her terrified of abandonment by him. In general, she felt incapable of being firm or setting limits with John because of her fear that he would leave her, and because of her feelings of shame that she was basically unlovable and had no right to ask for better treatment.

Tracy quickly recognized that her defensive behaviors of masochism and displacement were her means of avoiding the feelings of anger toward John because of her fear of losing him. The fights with John and her intense emotional reactions continued for a few more weeks.

Alliance. Tracy was deeply embarrassed that though she could see what she was doing, she could not stop it. She also felt a great deal of shame that she was showing me this inadequate part of herself. Our relationship was gently explored until she could see how, in her mind, she made her therapist into a person who judged her rather than supported or understood her. This realization helped reduce her anxiety about opening up to me and helped her stop this projection that I would judge her harshly. As she saw more fully how harshly she judged herself, she became more compassionate toward herself.

Mastery. As Tracy saw the painful consequences of her masochistic behavior she began to feel more compassion than shame for her position. She began to want to be gentler with herself, but she still was so angry with John that she did not want to be gentler with him! During this time, it became apparent that her reactions to John were very similar to her reactions to her father who had been constantly critical of her. She had always felt inadequate and unlovable, though she never had dared to stand up to him. The awareness that she was overreacting to John because he reminded her of her father helped her gain mastery over her reactions, and the fights began to decrease. Through a process of uncovering the types of feelings that she was using the defenses to avoid, she began to attribute her lashing out to unexpressed anger or assertion. Her masochism was her self-attack which helped her avoid the desperate longings to be loved, and displaced anger (defensive feeling). Tracy was able to talk with John about some of these insights and the conflicts between them. Although the fights still occurred, they were less intense and more often came to a resolution that improved their relationship.

Attribution. The attribution that helped Tracy the most, and one about which she emphatically told me many times thereafter, was that *she* was responsible for the form of her reaction toward John. Before therapy, she had seen herself only as the passive victim of angry, critical men. Now she saw she had a range of options in terms of reactions, and that some options were more constructive and helpful than others.

Affect Restructuring

Exposure. When Tracy felt more stable in her relationship again (after about 10 sessions), we began to explore the feelings that she had such trouble expressing; appropriate forms of anger or assertion, asking for what she wanted, and grief over the neglect from her depressed mother and distant father. The anger toward her boyfriend, John, was the first and the easiest for her to experience. In therapy, she was *exposed* to angry scenes of beating up her boyfriend, or throwing things at him, though it was made clear that the imagery was not to be acted out. She felt anxious and guilty about these images at first; but with several repetitions of the angry scenes she became desensitized and could tolerate the feeling of anger at him. This made it possible for her to be as assertive as she needed to be in asking John to be less critical.

The deeper and more intense emotional work involved her grief over her parents' emotional distance, and the longing for their love and attention. Because Tracy's father had forbidden her to cry, she was very blocked in experiencing grief.

Alliance. A strong, supportive therapeutic relationship was crucial to the working through of these conflicted feelings. Tracy's fundamental stance vis à vis me was shame over opening up and showing me these feelings. Her father had told her that "she was not to cry until she was ready to die." As a result, she had cut off all show of emotion in front of him or anyone. She laboriously had to learn to be comfortable crying in front of me, but that took many weeks to master.

Mastery. Mastery was gained over anger, grief, and longing, though Tracy experienced much struggle in doing so. Her increasing ability to tolerate the thought and feeling of anger allowed her to take more of a stand with John. Her experience of anger allowed her to maintain an appropriate stance of assertion that he not thoughtlessly criticize her but that he talk to her in a reasonable way about the things that were bothering him. John was initially resistant, but over time he responded well to her more rational responses and their relationship improved dramatically. This stabilization in her life helped Tracy face the deeper and more painful issues with her parents.

As Tracy allowed herself to trust that I would not judge or condemn her, she slowly allowed herself to cry in my presence. The acceptance and understanding she received calmed her fears, and she was able to proceed with the grieving of the painful memories of her childhood. As she did so, she was able to see how much emotional support she had missed, and how much in her present life these old longings were driving her reactions. By continuing to experience these feelings, she felt less shameful about having them. However, many times in this process, I had to return to defense restructuring because Tracy's desire to avoid painful feelings was very strong. Thus, this exposure phase did not proceed in a linear fashion. There was a cyclical process of both reducing defensiveness and experiencing of conflicted affect.

Attribution. The main changes in Tracy's world view were twofold. First, she could see that lack of appropriate expression of her needs in all her relationships (either to set limits or to ask for what she wanted) kept her isolated and feeling desperately longing inside. She also saw that she had alternatives. The second attribution that was crucial for Tracy's character change was that she no

longer saw herself as shameful or disgusting for having these feelings. Instead, she was a lovable child whose parents had had their own difficulties and were thus unable to respond to her as she had so needed. She thus was able to take a much more compassionate and care-taking role toward herself.

Outcome. At termination, Tracy was a very different person. She and John had a much more mature relationship, and were facing some months of being apart without fear of the relationship breaking up. Tracy felt particularly proud that she not only could tolerate the separation without anxiety, but that also she could look forward to the plans she had made in the interim. She had spoken with both parents at length about the issues that had emerged in treatment. Her mother was understanding and truly sorry that her own lengthy depression and her subsequent divorce had so impacted upon Tracy. Tracy's father was initially hostile and rejecting, but later apologized. At termination he and Tracy were in a tenuous reconciliation. Although her father initially refused, Tracy asked him repeatedly to help her to move and get her car fixed. When he finally complied with her requests, he appeared pleased that he had helped her, and Tracy was extremely proud that she had been effective in repeatedly asking him.

Six months after termination, Tracy called me and asked to come in. She was bright and happy. She reported that she and John were getting along wonderfully and planning to marry, but that she had asked for a long engagement. She also reported that she and her father had worked on their relationship and were beginning to really enjoy each other. She was very pleased in her current job, but was looking forward to graduate school in a couple of years. She was able to tell me how the working through of her fears of closeness to me had helped her in all of her relationships. She had been too shy to say all this to me at termination, but now, after 6 months, she not only felt comfortable but eager to tell me.

CONCLUDING REMARKS

The interventions that are outlined above represent only the main ingredients of this short-term approach. Space does not permit a full discussion of techniques with all indications and contradictions. The treatment manual mentioned above provides a more detailed discussion of specific techniques.

REFERENCES

Baker, H., & Baker, M. (1987). Heinz Kohut's self psychology; An overview. *American Journal of Psychiatry, 114*, 1–9.

Davanloo, H. (Ed.). (1980). *Short-term dynamic psychotherapy*. New York: Jason Aronson.

Davanloo, H. (1983). Personal Communication. New York, NY.

Flegenheimer, W. (1982). *Techniques of brief psychotherapy*. New York: Jason Aronson.

Kohut, H. (1971). *The analysis of the self*. New York: International University Press.

Kohut, H. (1984). *How does analysis cure?* Chicago: University of Chicago Press.

Laikin, M., Winston, A., & McCullough, L. (1991). Intensive short-term dynamic psychotherapy. In P. Crits-Christoph & J. Barber (Eds.), *Handbook of short-term dynamic psychotherapy* (pp. 80–109). New York: Basic Books.

Luborsky, L. (1984). *Principles of psychoanalytic psychotherapy: A manual for supportive expressive treatment*. New York: Basic Books.

McCullough, L. (1991). Davanloo's short term dynamic psychotherapy: A cross-theoretical analysis of change mechanisms. In R. Curtis and G. Stricker (Eds.), *How people change: Inside and outside psychotherapy* (pp. 59–81)

McCullough, L. (1992). *Treatment manual for short-term anxiety reducing psychotherapy*. Unpublished manuscript. Study for Adult Development, Brigham & Women's Hospital, 75 Frances St., Boston, MA 02115.

McCullough, L., & Winston, A. (1991). The Beth Israel Psychotherapy Research program. In L. Beutler & M. Crago (Eds.), *Psychotherapy research: An international review of programmatic studies*. Washington, DC: American Psychological Association Press.

Malan, D. H. (1979). *Individual psychotherapy and the science of psychodynamics*. London: Butterworth.

Mann, J. (1973). *Time-limited psychotherapy*. Cambridge: Harvard University Press.

Perls, F. S. (1969). *Gestalt therapy verbatim*. Moab, UT: Real People Press.

Perls, F. S. (1976). Gestalt therapy verbatim: Introduction. In C. Hatcher & P. Himelstein (Eds.), *The handbook of Gestalt therapy* (pp. 21–80). New York: Jason Aronson.

Pinsker, H., Rosenthal, R., & McCullough, L. (1991). Dynamic Supportive Psychotherapy. In P. Crits-Christoph & J. Barber (Eds.), *Handbook of short-term dynamic psychotherapy* (pp. 220–247). New York: Basic Books.

Sifneos, P. E. (1979). *Short-term dynamic psychotherapy: Evaluation and technique*. New York: Plenum Press.

Weinberger, J. (April, 1990). *The goals model of psychotherapy*. Paper presented at the Annual Convention of the Society for the Exploration of Psychotherapy Integration. Philadelphia, PA.

CHAPTER 12

Prescriptive Psychotherapy

Larry E. Beutler and Amy B. Hodgson

INTRODUCTION

Since Luborsky, Singer, and Luborsky (1975) tagged comparisons among psychotherapies with Lewis Carroll's verdict, "all have won and all must have prizes," there has been a decided reluctance among psychotherapy researchers to contradict this conclusion. Luborsky *et al.* based their verdict upon the relatively small group of "horserace" comparisons of global outcome main effects that were available at that time. They neither inspected nor drew conclusions regarding the more interesting and clinically appealing possibility that therapy types interacted with client characteristics to effect certain gains.

Since the landmark but now dated review and conclusions of Luborsky and his colleagues, whether from low regard for subsequent evidence or simple rigidity, purveyors of the literature in the past decade have persisted in reiterating the conclusion that outcomes are indistinguishable among different psychotherapies. Yet virtually all

of these reviews base their conclusions on an assessment of treatment main effects, consistently omitting an analysis of how clients with different characteristics might respond differentially to different psychotherapies. Indeed, the perpetuation of the conclusion of "no differences" ignores an accumulating body of research indicating that all psychotherapies may have indeed won, but they have done so with different types of clients (Beutler, 1991).

This chapter presents some prescriptive guidelines advocated by Beutler and Clarkin (1990) for matching psychotherapeutic procedures and treatment packages with client needs. These guidelines have been developed with three major considerations in mind: (1) they should reflect empirical knowledge when it is available and consensual clinical opinion when it is not; (2) they should be driven by practical and empirical validity rather than by a narrow theoretical framework; and (3) they should incorporate, as much as possible, the collective wisdom of widely diverse investigators who have addressed the problems of matching treatments and clients.

The systematic treatment selection model outlined by Beutler and Clarkin (1990) is presented as a protypical prescriptive procedure. This approach eschews treatment decisions that are derived from narrow theoretical frameworks in favor of basing treatment prescriptions on empirically observed relationships between client

Larry E. Beutler • Counseling/Clinical/School Psychology Program, Department of Education, University of California, Santa Barbara, California 93106. Amy B. Hodgson • Department of Education, University of California, Santa Barbara, California 93106.

Comprehensive Handbook of Psychotherapy Integration, edited by George Stricker and Jerold R. Gold. Plenum Press, New York, 1993.

needs and the efficacies of specific treatment procedures. Beutler and Clarkin's (1990) model introduces the second generation of "technical eclectic" (Norcross, 1986) approaches, drawing heavily on several, independent first generation efforts to derive empirical and pragmatic relationships between patient and treatment characteristics.

THEORETICAL AND CONCEPTUAL POSITION

"Technical eclecticism" (Norcross, 1986; Lazarus, 1981) holds that therapeutic procedures are not inseparably wed to the theories which spawned them, asserting that specific procedures can be matched to clients, not on the basis of therapist's theories of psychopathology and psychotherapy, but on the basis of empirically demonstrated relationships between these matches and treatment outcomes. That is, the empirical value of the procedures for certain conditions and clients may guide their use rather than the validity (or invalidity) of the theories from which the procedures initially arose. This position is distinguished both from "theoretical integration" (the effort to integrate approaches to psychotherapy at the level of theoretical constructs rather than at the level of applications), common factors approaches (the assumption that all psychotherapies exert their effects through the same principles), and haphazard eclecticism (the well-intentioned but unsystematic effort to "do what's best" for the client).

The distinctiveness of technical eclecticism is, first, in its focus on the value of specific procedures rather than on the value of broad treatment packages or theories and, second, in its effort to find specific rather than common contributors to efficacy among therapies. This is not to say that technical eclectic approaches generally, or the systematic treatment selection procedures of Beutler and Clarkin specifically, are either atheoretical or prone to discredit the importance of therapeutic qualities that are common to all schools.

With respect to the value of theory, Beutler and Clarkin (1990) emphasize that each therapist's professional theory of psychotherapy is in part dictated from idiosyncratic experience, rendering it inevitably different from every other therapist's theory. This variability provides an unstable basis from which to seek a cohesive set of guidelines for treatment planning and inevitably defeats the hope that theoretical integration is possible. Even if theoretical eclecticism were a realistic goal, the low correspondence between theory and technical applications of procedures would not result in the development of procedures that can be applied consistently and independently of a given therapist. However, asserting that psychotherapy includes a process of teaching clients a functional life view, Beutler and Clarkin (1990) maintain the therapist's personal theories of psychological functioning and change constitute samples of workable philosophies that may be beneficially adopted by clients as they seek meaning and stability in their lives.

Systematic treatment selection does not attempt to pass judgment on the "truth" of those philosophies that are transmitted to clients by therapists, seeing them as useable life views rather than scientific truths. Instead systematic treatment selection concentrates on defining the methods that will most efficaciously result in the client's being persuaded to adopt the philosophy that the therapist believes will help in adapting to new and stressful experiences. For this task, theories of interpersonal influence and persuasion are considered to be of more value than theories of the etiology of pathology. However, Beutler and Clarkin (1990) emphasize the importance of selecting and training therapists whose personal and professional philosophies are demonstrably functional, as evidenced by the quality and flexibility of adjustment maintained by the therapist.

Acknowledging the role of inherently helpful therapist factors that are common to all effective psychotherapies, the model of systematic treatment selection advocated by Beutler and Clarkin (1990) recognizes that the preponderance of psychotherapeutic benefit is the product of a caring and respectful attitude of listening, support, empathy, and acceptance on the part of the therapist rather than of technical procedures. These common qualities of good therapy form a foundation on which can be added the effects of specific procedures, however. Hence, common and specific factors contributing to change are considered to be interactive and facilitative of positive therapeutic response. These therapist facilitative qualities exert their effects through the therapeutic or working alliance and, in turn, are conveyed by sensitivity to the forces of interpersonal persuasion. Therapists who use these principles of interpersonal influence effectively will convey the empathic support that serves as the foundation for building treatment plans that utilize specific therapeutic procedures to induce specific treatment effects among specific clients within specific environments.

In integrating these various principles, Beutler and Clarkin (1990) emphasize that effective treatment planning entails a sequence of increasingly fine-grained decisions. Four temporally related classes of variables must be considered when making these decisions:

1. *Predisposing client variables*—those characteristics that are brought into treatment and that relate to selecting a diagnosis, determining problem severity, evaluating clients' coping styles, determining client expectations, and assessing supports and obstacles in the client's living environment and background;

2. *Treatment contexts*—those qualities of the setting, treatment format, modality of treatment (medical vs. psychosocial), and planned intensity (frequency and length) that characterize the treatment environment available to the client;

3. *Relationship variables*—those qualities of the treatment which are designed by the clinician either to prepare the client for the type of treatment to be used or to adjust treatment to meet client expectations (including efforts to selectively assign clients to compatible therapists); and

4. *Specific strategies and techniques*—those specific procedures selected to focus the client on the problem, to manage levels of client motivation, to overcome obstacles to successful resolution of problems, and to achieve treatment objectives.

Selecting strategies and techniques occurs as the last step in the sequence and is both the most specific and the most reliant upon situational, moment-to-moment experiences occurring within the psychotherapy session. In turn, the selection of specific strategies and techniques progresses through four levels of specificity: (1) selection of a focal objective by which to define outcome efficacy; (2) selecting the level at which changes are initiated; (3) working toward specific short-term goals that mediate the achievement of final objectives; and (4) conducting work within individual sessions.

1. *Focal objectives* are defined as the outcome goals of treatment, and are broadly classified as either symptom or conflictual in nature. A decision between these two objectives, in turn, is determined by at least two predisposing qualities of the client's problems—the complexity and severity of the problem. The more complex the problem presentation, the more a conflictual outcome objective is indicated; the more distressful the manifestation, the greater the need to work toward some immediate symptomatic relief. Faced with various combinations of these qualities, one may select between symptomatic and conflictual goals as both short-term and long-term outcome objectives (e.g., one may select a symptomatic initial focus on the basis of severity and a conflictual long-term focus on the basis of complexity). The client's history, formal test performance, and current level of impairment are used to assess severity and complexity.

2. *The level of intervention* is selected at the second step of the decision process. The level of change that might be appropriate for a given patient may range from uncovering unconscious wishes or events, to enhancing awareness of sensory and emotional states, altering dysfunctional cognitive patterns, and changing overt behavior. Although change in all of these four levels may ultimately be desired for a given client, the initial level of entry and subsequent patterning of levels are determined by an assessment of how the patient copes with distress and fear.

3. *Mediating goals* are determined by the nature of the long-term objectives, the severity of the patient's dysfunction, and the patient's progress at solving problems. Conflictual goals entail a different set of intermediate steps and require a different level of intervention than symptomatic goals. The stages of therapy outlined by Beitman (1987) offer some guidelines about how the subgoals of treatment might be prioritized and distinguished.

4. *Therapeutic work* is managed from moment-to-moment by an ongoing effort to manage the level and focus of a client's motivation. Motivation, in turn, is a function of arousal and distress (Mohr *et al.*, 1990), and the therapist must select

strategies depending on whether these procedures are likely to reduce or increase arousal and distress levels and/or redirect their focus to a new target. These decisions require the selection of interventions which match with client needs along three dimensions: (1) the internal to external focus of the intervention is matched to the client's method of coping with the threat of change within the session; (2) the amount of directiveness used by the therapist and required by the procedure is matched to the strength of the client's resistance; and (3) the focus upon external events or in-session experience is matched to the client's phase of problem resolution and the stage of therapy achieved.

CLINICAL AND THEORETICAL ANTECEDENTS

The concept of "prescriptive psychotherapy" was originally outlined by Goldstein and Stein (1976) who proposed that patient symptoms and problems, rather than the therapist's theory, should dictate the selection of interventions. This proposal reflected frustration with the proliferation of theories of psychotherapy and the relatively low relationship between adherence to any of these theories and the therapeutic cprocedures utilized. Similarly, Arnold Lazarus (1981) is credited with originally distinguishing technical eclecticism from less systematic and more theory dependent forms of clinical eclecticism.

Building upon these foundation stones of technical eclecticism, and adding the contributions from common factors theorists (Frank, 1987; Garfield, 1980; Parloff, 1980), the systematic treatment selection model outlined by Beutler and Clarkin (1990) adds the individual eclectic approaches to which each of the authors have been identified. The breadth offered by differential therapeutics (Francis, Clarkin, & Perry, 1984) for, first, deciding if treatment is needed and thereafter for selecting treatment settings, modes, and formats combines well with the specificity of systematic eclecticism (Beutler, 1983) for the application of specific psychotherapy procedures.

To these two approaches, Beutler and Clarkin (1990) incorporated concepts from the individual psychotherapy of Beitman (1987) and transtheo-

retical psychotherapy of Prochaska (1984; Prochaska & DiClemente, 1982) to address the problem of the *stages of change*. Beitman's theoretical assertions were used to define the phases of therapy, and concepts from Prochaska's transtheoretical psychotherapy were extracted for defining the stages through which people proceed in changing behaviors.

Furthermore, Beutler and Clarkin (1990) refined the themes that characterize complex problems by incorporating concepts of *core conflictual relationship themes* from the writings of Strupp and Binder (1984) and of Luborsky (1984). The methods offered by these latter authors are used to define reliable qualities of the client's relationship by which to direct therapeutic work. Similarly, concepts were borrowed from numerous behavioral theorists to identify methods for selecting symptomatic targets of change. Hence, the usefulness of these methods for defining the target of change was applied to the general principles of treatment selection to identify the elements of focused treatment.

Beutler and Clarkin's model for treatment selection is a selective integration of these various models, emphasizing the inadequacy of single dimension systems to cope with the complexity of the treatment enterprise. Their model is an acknowledgment of the complexity of those people and problems which are presented for treatment. The goal of this model, therefore, is not to provide a new theory or even new information, but to apply integrative theory and research to the task of making explicit the processes that effective clinicians use intuitively. Such explication, it is hoped, will facilitate the systematic training of clinicians to maximize effective treatment selection.

THE TECHNIQUES AND PROCESSES OF PSYCHOTHERAPY

A growth-producing and safe therapeutic relationship or alliance is virtually essential to psychotherapy progress. The formation of a collaborative treatment relationship begins with the client's first contact with the therapist or the therapeutic environment. Usually, the client initiates therapy with a set of attitudes and expectations about what will take place, and it is important for the therapist to elicit and meet at least some of these expectations in order to cement the client's commitment, remembering that the client has lost a precious sense of balance in his or her life and is likely to be struggling to protect a sense of control and self-esteem. As clients enter the turf of the helping professional, they are at once, anticipating, seeking and wanting. Therefore, in response, to begin the therapeutic process the clinician seeks to determine the compatibility between the client's presentation of predisposing characteristics and (1) the context of treatment, (2) the nature of the relationship to be developed, and (3) the work of specific therapeutic procedures.

Treatment Context

The initial phase of establishing the therapeutic relationship is one in which the therapist seeks to gather data and to evaluate a plan regarding the setting, intensity, modality, and format through which treatment will occur. Dimensions associated with formal diagnosis as well as issues related to problem severity and available environmental support and stress systems are most directly involved at this stage. The decisions reached at this entry point of the process include the degree of restriction required to ensure the client's safety, the degree to which medical interventions are needed to ensure adherence to the treatment plan, and the frequency or duration of intervention needed. Beyond these decisions, issues of treatment format (i.e., specific drugs and use of combinations of group, individual, and family intervention) are often made, but these decisions are frequently less pressing and are revisited throughout treatment as a function of the changes the client makes.

In the initial evaluation process, the client presents the most pressing and logical reasons among many to explain why he or she has had to come to therapy at this moment. The therapist listens, probes, conducts tests, and formulates. Ultimately, an agreement regarding what will transpire must be reached in order to establish a common ground for working together. The evaluation process, while focused on making initial pressing decisions regarding the maximal protection and safety of the client, provides the foundation for the relationship which must support these decisions.

Relationship Development

Recognizing that the therapeutic relationship is central to all treatment decisions, Beutler and Clarkin (1990) identified two areas in which influence may be exerted to enhance the development of an initial therapeutic relationship: (1) role induction, and (2) in-therapy environmental management.

Role induction concretizes the usually implicit terms of the therapy agreement. Before treatment formally begins, the roles of client and therapist are operationalized through various educational techniques. Written or verbal instructions can facilitate symptomatic change, foster role appropriate attitudes, and nurture positive feelings about treatment. Observational and participatory learning methods, such as videotapes or role plays, can provide modeling and develop skills. Therapeutic contracting is a technique which allows the therapist and client to mutually specify the responsibilities of each and the nature of the relationship. In turn, this specification may have an important impact on client motivation. Contracting may occur spontaneously during any role-induction procedure, and may emerge as either a written or verbal agreement. The ingredients of the contract include the delineation of time limits and treatment goals, as well as the consequences for noncompliance with the contract. While the contract addresses some of the client's expectations, it is important to remember that the contract is always in renegotiation and subject to change.

In-therapy environmental management is a procedure whereby the therapist controls her or his styles of communication and establishes the parameters of the ensuing interaction. The work of therapy is largely a matter of managing levels of client motivational arousal—reducing it when arousal interferes with productivity and increasing it when motivation for change drops off. Clients entering therapy seek comfort, safety, and reassurance of personal control. External cues indicative of stability decrease levels of subjective discomfort where needed, while therapist managed cues also may increase client levels of motivational arousal when indicated. Therapy becomes the art of providing selective frustration as clients are brought to face feared material, where the therapeutic alliance provides the commitment and trust to proceed through difficult areas.

Arousal levels can be measured by biofeedback, biochemical analyses of blood samples, formal psychological assessment instruments, and by careful observation of client non-verbal cues. Therapist nonverbal styles, such as forward posture, mutual gaze, and responsive facial expressions can open clients to influence and reduce premature termination. Characteristics of the clinician's practice environment, such as the physical layout, attitude and appearance of the support staff, and the nature of office procedures, can either support or impede these influences. Therapist verbal styles, voice tone, vocabulary, and expressed emotion can be managed in ways that strengthen or weaken the therapeutic relationship.

Beyond these inaugural efforts to engage the client in therapy, what binds the client and therapist together? The client looks for many things in the therapist's role—a new and different perspective on problems, permission for feelings and behavior, and authoritative informant on life's dilemmas, someone who can master what the client has not. The therapist must somehow be enough like the client to be credible as someone who is capable of understanding the influences that affect the client, and at the same time he or she must be sufficiently different to provide an alternative and meaningful view of the situation. Clients bring with them preexisting attitudes about therapy, therapists, and objectives that are born of their unique history of previous professional encounters. These unique attitudes can work either to the advantage or disadvantage of the psychotherapy process. The patient's perceptions of the therapist's credibility and persuasiveness may initially be positive, as a reflection of a history of positive relationships with prior therapists and authorities, but this view may change with time and interaction with a given therapist.

Positive attributes which are both communicated in the foregoing ways and which facilitate the client's commitment to the therapy process, appear to reflect patterns of personal similarity and dissimilarity existing between client and therapist (Beutler & Bergan, 1991). Effective matching and balancing of at least two key dimensions se-

cures the therapeutic bond: (1) demographic similarity and (2) interpersonal response disposition dissimilarity.

Demographic similarity has been posed by Beutler and Clarkin (1990) as being conducive to the development of a therapeutic alliance. Similarity along such dimensions as gender, age, ethnic background, and socioeconomic status may precipitate a sense of trust and twinship that is therapeutically beneficial. These observed relationships, particularly for the dimensions of age and gender, suggest that there may be advantages to matching therapists with given clients (Beutler, Crago, & Arizmendi, 1986). However, actual matching for demographic variables is seldom possible in either public or private clinics. Beutler and Clarkin (1990) suggest that under these circumstance, the development of the necessary trust may be facilitated, when client and therapist backgrounds are dissimilar, by the use of empathic listening skills, by reinforcing areas of viewpoint similarity, and by placing relatively less emphasis on the use of directive and instructional interventions.

Interpersonal response patterns are posed by Beutler and Clarkin (1990) as areas in which clients my benefit from having models for new responses available to them from their therapists. Among the potentially relevant aspects of interpersonal response on which dissimilarity between client and therapist may be conducive to the development of new behavior, two general areas have been singled out: (1) interpersonal striving or needs, and (2) beliefs and values, especially those relating to personal ideals and attributions of causal influence.

Interpersonal striving reflects common life themes of emotional conflict arising in social involvements. Beutler and Clarkin (1990) have focused particular attention on the striving or needs for autonomy and affiliation. They suggest that a discrepancy between client and therapist on this interpersonal dimension, not only facilitates client change, but that very close similarity might threaten some clients with the loss of autonomy (i.e., engender reactance or resistance to influence). Millon (1969; Millon & Everly, 1985) observes that people have needs both for dependency/attachment and autonomy/self-sufficiency. These patterns are reflected in the development of four basic personality styles: Those who are ambivalent because of high needs for both dependency and autonomy, those who are detached from both need systems, those who are principally attachment seeking, and those who are principally autonomy seeking. If therapists represent or present contrasting need systems to those expressed in the relationship themes of their clients, these clients are likely to find models by which to contrast their own behavior and to explore new response systems.

Values and attributional beliefs represent cognitive elements of social functioning that also facilitate client modeling if disparity of style exists between the client and the therapist. Beutler and Clarkin (1990) acknowledge that values and attributions are probably related to demographics and family histories of interpersonal relationships. There are likely to be areas, therefore, on which similarity of beliefs is facilitative of compatibility. Research (Bergin & Jensen, 1989; Beutler & Bergan, 1991; Kelly, 1990) suggests that values related to religious-political philosophies, sexual roles, and social-humanistic attitudes regarding wisdom, knowledge, honesty, and so forth may be among these. On the other hand, compatibility between therapist and client may also involve the facilitative influence of attitudinal and attributional differences regarding the perception of danger and safety in one's environment, the importance of friendship and social recognition, and sexual tolerance.

Although somewhat less clear than value differences, clients' perceptions of causal attribution may benefit from contrasting differences presented by therapists. Couched in the context of a tolerant and supportive therapist, dissimilarities may provide an atmosphere in which clients can explore new ideas in the assurance of the therapist's acceptance of the client's world view and belief system.

Therapeutic Work

The work of psychotherapy is organized around four basic stages (Beitman, 1987): (1) engagement; (2) pattern search; (3) instigation of change; and (4) termination planning. The procedures discussed in the foregoing for initializing the therapeutic relationship and matching client/therapist variables are most closely related to the first two of these stages of psychotherapy. How-

ever, as one begins the work of the second stage, pattern search, additional interventions must be considered. Here, too, one must take into account both the traits and states of the client's presentation.

First in these considerations is the client's readiness for the focus presented in the stage of therapy. Because clients may be unable to do the work of a given therapy stage until they are at an appropriate stage of problem resolution, combinations of the phases of change and the phases of psychotherapy define the intermediate goals of intervention—those goals through which the long-term conflictual and symptom change goals are likely to be reached.

Transtheoretical psychotherapy, as formulated by Prochaska and DiClemente (1986) has offered the clearest insights into this process. Four stages of behavior change are defined, reflecting the types of experience for which the client is ready: (1) precontemplation, (2) contemplation, (3) action, and (4) maintenance. If a client is only at the behavioral change level of precontemplation, relationship enhancement may provide the safety and motivation to move to the stage of contemplation. At the stage of contemplation, a client may be able to engage in a process of self-exploration in search of thematic or symptomatic patterns. As doing so facilitates movement toward action by the client, the therapy may enter a phase of instigating change. And as the change process moves the client to stabilize or maintain gains, therapy moves toward termination and follow-up.

The specific goals that characterize and distinguish clients at each stage of psychotherapy, however, require therapeutic procedures to coincide with both the intermediate and the long-term or outcome goals. The instigation of the personal and interpersonal change process hinges on the collaborative treatment relationship, which has both a healing role and a dynamic nature. Prescriptive psychotherapy functions to adjust approaches and interventions throughout the course of treatment, as the client moves through phases of therapy and change. However, the informed selection and the artful application of techniques that maximally address the client's conflicts and styles are limited by the breadth of the therapist's technical repertoire. Obtaining both training and competence in the use of a wide range of interventions from various philosophical schools advances therapist effectiveness.

In systematic treatment selection, interventions are systematically derived from psychotherapy outcome research and based on client needs. Once the breadth and nature of the focus of treatment and final outcome goals are determined, the therapist can choose specific techniques largely by relying on in-session assessments of moment-to-moment (process diagnoses) variations in the client's motivational arousal (subjective distress), coping style, and resistance level.

Specifically, depending on the client's resistance tendencies or potential, the directiveness and the concomitant intrusiveness of the intervention can be modified. For individuals with high resistance (i.e., reactance) levels, evocative, open-ended, or even paradoxical procedures can be utilized to allow and/or reinforce the client's sense of personal control; whereas for individual with low resistance levels, directive, close-ended procedures are more likely to be successful.

Similarly, the level of intervention, ranging from uncovering unconscious material, to increasing sensory and emotional experience, to modifying cognitive patterns, to changing overt behaviors, can be adjusted to coincide with variations in clients' coping styles. Insight interventions are favored for internalizing patterns of denial and repression, experiential interventions are favored for those with compartmentalized emotional patterns, cognitive interventions are favored for those who experience strong and uncomfortable emotions of anxiety, anger, and depression, and behavioral interventions are favored for undercontrolled externalizing clients. Thus, as clients alter their coping styles around different problems or as personal growth and change occur, the nature of the therapeutic procedures are also altered, contributing to a dynamic process of treatment application.

Beitman's fourth stage of therapy involves preparation for termination. Accordingly, in this stage of therapy the focus changes temporally from past and present, and the client is aided in translating the learning of psychotherapy to interactions in the external, social world. The tasks of termination planning include: (1) activating social support systems, (2) anticipating potential problems, (3) preparing for future stress, and (4) planning for follow-up meetings with the therapist.

Asking clients to anticipate problems following the formal course of treatment begins the shift to independent problem-solving and the reinforcement of natural support networks. Formally applying principles of relapse prevention arms clients with the confidence and skills to manage future stressors and realistically prepares them for the ebb and tide of life. Often, treatment termination is enacted as a final breaking of contact between therapist and client. Continuing maintenance and aftercare, on an extenuated schedule and initiated by the therapist, ensure continued functioning and retention of treatment gains.

CASE EXAMPLE

Thomas is a 33-year-old identical twin who sought personal counseling at a university training clinic. The client presented with concerns about being a twin, a "need to deal with who I am," and difficulties in initiating and sustaining relationships. Thomas was employed part-time at a small local business and reported living alone in a very small trailer. A diagnosis of recurrent major depression and dependent personality disorder was made, based on a 2-hour clinical intake interview and MMPI results. The client reported insomnia, early morning awakening, fitful sleep, procrastination, and recent loss of a love relationship. The MMPI revealed a profile of an individual with low ego strength, social introversion, hypersensitivity to danger, depression, low energy level, and was suggestive of moderate chronicity. The degree of impairment was assessed as moderate.

Thomas was the second-born twin son, first offspring to middle-class parents. When he entered treatment, Thomas had begun reading a collection of over one hundred letters, obtained from his mother, that she had written to the client's grandparents over a 20-year period, telling of her worries about the boys. The letters detailed the client's childhood, and from them he learned that his mother saw him as quiet and shy and his twin as more outgoing. Thomas, his twin, and younger brother and sister attended a rural school with few children where "being a twin didn't matter," until the age of 12 when their family moved to an urban area. Later, Thomas and his twin attended the same four-year college, taking the same major, and living together in an apartment, although with the twin's girlfriend. Thomas and his twin both flunked out of school at the same time as their parents' bitter divorce, following which the client was estranged from his father for ten years, at his mother's request. His twin moved across the state soon after.

> THERAPIST: In what ways would you describe yourself as evolving?
> CLIENT: Well, I had relationships.
> THERAPIST: You hadn't had any before?
> CLIENT: No. I had no friends.

What the client tells the therapist about his or her previous counseling experience and expectations of what will happen now in treatment are indicators of the length and effectiveness of therapy for this individual, in addition to clues about the role the therapist will need to take. Thomas reported one previous counseling experience of four sessions at the college counseling service during the term prior to leaving school. The client remarked that he did not find the counseling helpful because it was too short and he was not willing to work with it. Initially, Thomas expressed ambivalence yet insightful expectations about working in therapy.

> THERAPIST: How would you like counseling to help you?
> CLIENT: Well, I think the twin issue is really the main one. I don't know if it can be gotten into, but I don't know if I can develop relationships that are equal in giving, giving and receiving on some kind of equal level until that's dealt with.

From information gathered in the intake interview and psychometric assessments, a determination of four areas must be made: (1) severity; (2) problem complexity; (3) coping style; and (4) reactance. Excerpts from Thomas's 10-week course of counseling will illustrate these four dimensions. Then, a treatment plan will be introduced that addresses appropriate goals for therapy considering the client's presentation and needs.

Severity

Thomas experienced impairment in most major areas of his life, but was not incapacitated by disturbances to work, relationship, and family. An assessment of problem intensity and coping adequacy points to a long-standing adjustment pattern of moderate severity. Thus, he presented with moderate levels of subjective distress to support and motivate change, mild to moderate levels of impairment in life functions in support of the decision to conduct treatment in an outpatient setting, and a complex of thematic disturbances in support of a thematic rather than a symptomatic focus.

The client had been developing the presenting pattern from a very young age. The complexity of this development came as somewhat of a surprise to him, however. He recalled a single incident related to a family move at age 12 to which he attributed many of his subsequent problems. However, the letters written by his mother and reclaimed by him revealed that a pattern of withdrawal and denial had been established even earlier in childhood and were manifested in his relationship with his twin and family. The observation that the client also experienced distress from current interpersonal relationships confirmed the longevity and recurrence of this pattern and pointed to a complex and long-standing conflict.

Initially in the intake interview, the client disclosed that he had come to counseling at the advice of his former girlfriend, with whom he had split a few weeks prior.

> CLIENT: We'd been together for about a year, two or three years ago, and then broke off because it wasn't going well and she told me that I needed counseling, but I didn't do it. My job improved and I thought I was feeling better about myself, so we got back together. A couple of weeks ago it became clear that it wasn't working and that I really did need counseling.
> THERAPIST: Was it her suggestion this time or did you come to that conclusion?
> CLIENT: I . . . I came to that conclusion and she was very supportive of me.
> THERAPIST: Who broke off the relationship?
> CLIENT: It was kind of mutual. I kind of gave up myself. It was distressing to deal with it, knowing I really need to deal with myself, not put it all on her or pretend that I was all right. And I wasn't. Uhm. And what she said which really sums it up nicely, is you don't really love yourself, you have a hard time expressing your feelings and your needs, and you need to deal with the dependent relationship you have with your—my brother, because you replicate that with other people. I think all those are valid points. Also, my twin brother has been in counseling for a year and has been encouraging me to do it.

Problem Complexity

CLIENT: I remember being shyer than he was. Uhm. But I don't remember the total sense of dependence on him that developed later when we moved to San Diego. Uhm. We moved down here in eighth grade. We were in separate classes. But he, for whatever reason, developed some friendships early on which continued. I never really did. For the most part his friends were my friends, but I never had any relationship with them. He had a couple girlfriends in high school. I remember feeling tremendously threatened by that (cough) and he also started writing poetry, which was something I had wanted to do. He did it first. I remember flipping out in tenth grade as a result of it.

THERAPIST: What happened?

CLIENT: Well, he had gotten a girlfriend and started writing poetry and I felt totally worthless in relationship to him. I don't mean flipping out in terms of being crazy, but internally in relationship to him.

A primary indicator of problem complexity is the thematic repetition across many relationships or situations. Thomas began struggling with separation/individuation issues in therapy, and readily self-identified his issues with dependency with his brother. While Thomas was in therapy, he also enrolled, on his own, in a community college extension course dealing with "Co-dependency." However, midway through the course of therapy, he introduced plans to live with his friend, Arnold, who was physically challenged and an alcoholic.

THERAPIST: Last week you mentioned that Arnold has an alcohol problem.

CLIENT: Yeah, uhmmm.

THERAPIST: And as I was thinking about that during the week, you had also talked about being a victim and a rescuer.

CLIENT: Uhmmm.

THERAPIST: And about the kind of dependent relationship you had with your brother . . .

CLIENT: Uhmmm.

THERAPIST: Do you see yourself recreating that with Arnold?

CLIENT: Oh, yeah I do, but I guess only partly. He's an alcoholic, but he's not drinking. I'm not trying to rescue him in that sense.

THERAPIST: So he's going to AA every week?

CLIENT: Well, he was but he works on into the evening so it's hard for him to go. Uhm. I guess he goes occasionally. Uhm. And he hasn't been drinking for six to eight weeks and he's not likely to. I, yeah, I see it as a dependent relationship to some extent and I do see that I'm trying to rescue him to some extent, partly. But partly, I don't think it is. I mean it used to be that way. I mean there's a tendency to do that,

rescuing, but I think that now that I'm aware that it's a problem, I see myself as being able to work through it. I could be deluded. But, I think in a way it's an opportunity to work through some of those problems with him.

THERAPIST: You see it as a way to work through the problems with your brother, with Arnold?

CLIENT: Yeah.

THERAPIST: I wonder how you see that happening?

CLIENT: Well, to the extent that we're very straight with each other, challenge each other to do things we don't want to do, work through some of our fears, like making phone calls I don't want to make, or writing when he doesn't want to write. But if I just do that and don't deal with my brother, than yeah, I am in the same mold to be sure. So, uhm.

THERAPIST: Do you feel that right now that you've become aware enough of the issues to really get back into that same relationship?

CLIENT: Well, it's a problem. I don't see it . . . well, it is a problem. It's a problem even to the extent that we're straight with each other now and all these . . . I mean, I can see a dependency that could build up over the long term, to the point that it would be hard to move or break it off. It's just that I can't stand living alone. But, when I get into situations with people I don't know, I'm not . . . It's like I'm not living with them anyway. I tend to hide.

Coping Style

The client's coping style is the intrapsychic response to internal and external cues. Coping style is the conscious and unconscious style of responding to uncomfortable internal experiences and/or situational pressures. An individual makes efforts to avoid pain and usually relies heavily on a collection of behaviors which manages contradictions or discrepancies between personal desires or beliefs from outside information.

Four specific categories of coping styles are outlined by Beutler & Clarkin (1990): internalization, repression, cyclic, and externalization. The combination of varying coping styles and reactance levels is important for identifying the individual's defensive pattern and creates a continuum of behavioral responses within each coping style.

In session seven, the therapist introduced a two-chair exercise in which Thomas was asked to talk to his twin brother. Thomas was to allow himself to be angry with his brother and strike a pillow on the chair, building the intensity each time. After several prompts from the therapist,

Thomas stated that he did not wish to continue the exercise, because he felt it was contrived, and the session continued. In session eight, the therapist returned to the exercise of the previous week.

> THERAPIST: I want to switch gears now to talk about what happened last week. I was feeling that you might have gotten angry with me for making you do something so contrived.
> CLIENT: Oh sure. (Laughs) of course. (Laughs)
> THERAPIST: And yet you weren't able to tell me about that.
> CLIENT: Uhhh. No, partly because I thought I should try my best to do it. (Laughs) I must admit, when I came in here I was scared that you were going to make me do that again. (Laughs)
> THERAPIST: Today?
> CLIENT: (Laughs) And I thought I really can't work up much more anger. I just can't.

Thomas's MMPI pattern also suggests an internalizing coping style—high anxiety and introversion. His report also indicates that he manages stressful situations by silently swallowing his anger.

> CLIENT: Well, there were periods that uh . . . that I really hated my brother. Uh, and I still do. We really haven't gotten to the point where we can talk about the twin relationship. I still have a lot of conflicted feelings about it, and so does he I'm sure. I just close up and shut off and feel resentful of him, that he's talking, and then my mother or someone else will notice that I'm being silent. She'll ask me a question. I'll transfer the resentment I'm feeling towards him to the question and try to communicate some anger or something, but it's not very workable as communication.

Not only did Thomas internalize his anger, but he also used denial as a coping process. The following passage illustrates his denial while he is talking about his early family experiences. Here the client is expressing his grief and expectations of his emerging as an individual and the accompanying separation that occurs when one becomes autonomous.

> THERAPIST: Are you still reading those letters from your mother?
> CLIENT: I'm not. I'm going to when I get the time off and I may start reading them.
> THERAPIST: Something happened, you were excited about reading them.
> CLIENT: I just got involved doing other things. I may be a little scared about it. I'm sure that's true.
> THERAPIST: I think that would be terribly frightening.
> CLIENT: Yes, it is. Partly because it's a reminder of this was the family: mother, father, kids. These were the

grandparents. All these people that have been torn asunder, gone their separate ways.

Resistance

Assessment is an ongoing process in therapy. Information about the client's background, as well as problem complexity, coping style, and reactance, may surface as the client–therapist relationship develops. In this case, the client's reactance level was assessed at a moderately high level from the MMPI (Pa and Pd scores) and as the therapist observed intratherapy behaviors. To assess this dimension, the therapist focuses on the client's demands on others in his social network, and his interpersonal style, which might range from passive-compliant to passive-aggressive to aggressive.

TREATMENT PLAN

The treatment modality chosen for Thomas was mediated by time-limited constraints of the counseling clinic in which he was seen. Although this constraint is certainly less than ideal, it is an adaptation many mental health agencies have been forced to make in the face of increasing demands for service, the provisions of managed health care, and limited treatment resources. In the treatment contract developed during the 2-hour intake interview, Thomas agreed to attend individual therapy for 10 weeks. Both his well-developed personal controls and his high level of motivation allowed us to proceed with outpatient therapy on a weekly basis.

One of the first questions a therapist needs to pose at an early point in treatment planning is whether the problems and concerns presented are simple habits maintained by the environment or symbolized expressions of unresolved conflictual experiences. That is, are the symptoms a direct or indirect (symbolic) expression of precipitating events and conflicts? High *problem complexity* was determined by the thematic pervasiveness and duration of the problem. Thomas presented with symptoms indicative of depression and concerns about knowing himself as an individual and relating to others as individuals. A theme of interpersonal dependency was observed in Thomas's relationships with women he had dated, with his brother, and with Arnold. In addition, the problem dated back to a very early age. In the theme selected for Thomas, we conceptualized a conflict in which the client's struggle with separation/individuation was paramount, and was similar to those seen among adolescents with an identity disorder. This conflict was noticeable in Thomas's report of subjective distress and associated his inability to disentangle aspects of his self from his twin brother.

In developing the treatment plan, *problem severity* was the next dimension considered. While we considered Thomas's problem to be quite complex as represented in its recurrence in numerous relationships, there was a need to address and seek relief of his subjective symptoms of distress before thematic aspects of his presentation was addressed directly. Problem severity level was sufficiently high to impede his ability to perceive, evaluate, and cope with his environment, and thus, required direct attention before proceeding to the thematic aspects of his problem presentation.

Thomas's *coping style* of internalization led to the selection of procedures that were designed to intervene at the level of emotional sensitivity and insight. Specifically, the interventions were designed to focus principally on enhancing awareness of feelings and identifying his interpersonal wants and needs.

We evaluated Thomas's *resistance potential* to be moderate. Accordingly, we determined that the directiveness of interventions used should be relatively low and the therapist elected to use techniques that would evoke insights into the motives behind his developing plans. Since Thomas appeared to be in the contemplation stage of change, the general treatment plan was designed with the intermediate goal of moving him to the stage of action.

Early in therapy, Thomas expressed his wish to be both dependent and autonomous, an expression of Millon's (1969) ambivalent personality style. Accordingly, Thomas demonstrated his ambivalence in a pattern of withdrawal and self-isolation. The following passage reflects his childlike or incompetent introject that is at the core of his interpersonal theme.

CLIENT: My sisters have daughters, and they were there that weekend. My brother would play with them and talk with them. Then, I would just fade into the background.

THERAPIST: What were you wanting to do at that time?
CLIENT: Do what he was doing. He was talking with them. Taking them on walks. (Clears throat) I guess there's a sense of competition there that's maybe internal. I don't know that other people think the same thing is going on.
THERAPIST: What do you think was blocking you from going up and talking with them?
CLIENT: I, well, I . . . one of them is my own pass . . . passiv . . . passiveness. He's the active one. I'm passive.
THERAPIST: So it's your view of yourself?
CLIENT: It's my view of myself. And if we're seen as a unit, and often we are, then he can be active and I can be a part of that and I can disconnect. He can kind of be me. I can just sit back. It's also hard for me to deal with kids because they can be very honest and see through you, or so I think.
THERAPIST: So you feel that they might be pointed or reveal something about you.
CLIENT: Right, they assume that you're an adult and you're competent and then you show yourself to be shy.

OUTCOME

Collectively, the treatment plan began with an effort to respond to Thomas's initial request by working directly to alleviate some of his initial discomfort. Increasingly, the treatment focused on a thematic pattern in his relationships, however, and drew upon an analysis of his coping style and resistance potential to design interventions that would direct him toward feeling awareness and insight without violating his need for personal autonomy. This approach was successful and in the final treatment session, Thomas talked about the increased social activity he had engaged in since beginning therapy. These included taking classes and joining a church. He also demonstrated an understanding of his emergence toward autonomy and continued relationship with his twin brother.

CLIENT: I realized that, uhm, while it's real important (cough) for me to express my anger and resentment towards my brother and get all that out in the open, I also realize the other thing that we never really did, was we never told each other that we really loved each other, and what that meant and what that would mean about us becoming individuals. That loving ourselves and being separate and dividing things up would be a way also of saying that we love each other and would like to keep that connection going. And all that makes me much more hopeful about working it through.

REFERENCES

Beitman, B. D. (1987). *The structure of individual psychotherapy*. New York: Guilford.

Bergin, A. E., & Jensen, J. P. (1989). Religiosity of psychotherapists: A national survey. *Psychotherapy, 27*, 3–7.

Beutler, L. E. (1983). *Eclectic psychotherapy: A systematic approach*. New York: Pergamon.

Beutler, L. E. (1991). Have all won and must all have prizes? Revisiting Luborsky *et al.*'s verdict. *Journal of Consulting and Clinical Psychology, 59*, 226–232.

Beutler, L. E., & Bergan, J. (1991). Value change in counseling and psychotherapy: A search for scientific credibility. *Journal of Counseling Psychology, 38*, 16–24.

Beutler, L. E., & Clarkin, J. (1990). *Systematic treatment selection: Toward targeted therapeutic interventions*. New York: Brunner/Mazel.

Beutler, L. E., Crago, M., & Arizmendi, T. G. (1986). Therapist variables in psychotherapy process and outcome. In S. L. Garfield & A. E. Bergin (Eds.), *Handbook of psychotherapy and behavior change* (3rd ed., pp. 257–310). New York: Wiley.

Frances, A., Clarkin, J., & Perry, S. (1984). *Differential therapeutics in psychiatry*. New York: Brunner/Mazel.

Frank, J. D. (1987). Psychotherapy, rhetoric, and hermeneutics: Implications for practice and research. *Psychotherapy, 24*, 293–302.

Garfield, S. L. (1980). *Psychotherapy: An eclectic approach*. New York: Wiley.

Goldstein, A. P., & Stein, N. (1976). *Prescriptive psychotherapies*. New York: Pergamon.

Kelly, T. A. (1990). The role of values in psychotherapy: Review and methodological critique. *Clinical Psychology Review, 10*, 171–186.

Lazarus, A. A. (1981). *The practice of multimodal therapy*. New York: McGraw-Hill.

Luborsky, L. (1984). *Principles of psychoanalytic psychotherapy: A manual for supportive-expressive treatment*. New York: Basic Books.

Luborsky, L., Singer, B., & Luborsky, L. (1975). Comparative studies of psychotherapies. *Archives of General Psychiatry, 32*, 995–1008.

Millon, T. (1969). *Modern psychopathology*. Philadelphia: W. B. Saunders.

Millon, T., & Everly, G. S. (1985). *Personality and its disorders*. New York: Wiley.

Mohr, D. C., Beutler, L. E., Engle, D., Schoham-Salomon, V., Bergan, J., Kaszniak, A. W., & Yost, E. (1990). Identification of patients at risk for non-response and negative outcome in psychotherapy. *Journal of Consulting and Clinical Psychology, 58*, 622–628.

Norcross, J. C. (1986). Eclectic psychotherapy: An introduction and overview. In J. C. Norcross (Ed.), *Handbook of eclectic psychotherapy* (pp. 3–24). New York: Brunner/Mazel.

Parloff, M. B. (1980, April). *Psychotherapy and research: An anaclitic depression*. Frieda Fromm-Reichman Memorial Lecture, Washington School of Psychiatry, Washington, D.C.

Prochaska, J. O. (1984). *Systems of psychotherapy: A transtheoretical analysis* (2nd ed.). Homewood, IL: Dorsey Press.

Prochaska, J. O., & DiClemente, C. C. (1982). Transtheoretical therapy: Toward a more integrative model of change. *Psychotherapy: Theory, Research, and Practice, 19*, 276–288.

Prochaska, J. O., & DiClemente, C. C. (1986). The transtheoretical approach. In J. C. Norcross (Ed.) *Handbook of Eclectic Psychotherapy* (pp. 163–200). New York: Brunner/Mazel.

Strupp, H. H., & Binder, J. L. (1984). *Psychotherapy in a new key*. New York: Basic Books.

CHAPTER 13

The Active Self Model

A PARADIGM FOR PSYCHOTHERAPY INTEGRATION

John D. W. Andrews

INTRODUCTION

A theoretical model that aims at being integrative must provide a consistent account of personality stability and change; it must be anchored in a scientifically valid body of data; it must take account of other therapy models; and it must enable us to assess client problems and intervene helpfully. In what follows, I will present the active self or self-confirmation account of personality and therapy, and will indicate how this model aspires to meet the criteria indicated above.

THE ACTIVE SELF

The Identity Image

Self-image is the touchstone of personal orientation, and from the concept of self each person generates a network of expectations, behaviors, perceptions of others, and interpretations of events that are consistent with it. By doing so, one forms

John D. W. Andrews • Psychological and Counseling Services, University of California, San Diego, La Jolla, California 92093.

Comprehensive Handbook of Psychotherapy Integration, edited by George Stricker and Jerold R. Gold. Plenum Press, New York, 1993.

a personal environment which, through its feedback, confirms one in a stable identity. Selectivity is at the heart of this process. Each choice or action implies a definition of self, the adding of one more piece to the mosaic of characteristics that conveys: "This is me." One is continually making choices for which one is responsible, and in each action one perceives oneself and is perceived by others as having followed a particular path and rejected alternatives. In this way, the individual puts his or her stamp on the action and expresses a distinctive personal style.

To convey anger, for example, may carry various self-defining overtones. It may imply that "I am a person capable of anger," "I am a person who will get angry in certain kinds of situations," or even "I am a dangerous person." Thus, any communication carries a metamessage concerning the person's underlying self-image.

The identity image is a creative construction, a synthesis of many experiences involving one's own activity as well as messages from others (Erikson, 1959). Each person strives to develop a configuration that will reconcile the complexities of experience and provide a central guiding orientation. Progressive reorganizations of problematic and conflicting information generate a sense of self that provides simplicity and pattern, giving the individual his or her characteristic style and "flavor" of personality. And it is these self-definitional messages that are of central concern to the therapist, because the client's self-image is both a focus of orientation and a major source of the problems for which therapy is sought.

By understanding identity patterning, the therapist can often conceptualize both the client's presenting problem and his or her main strengths within a single framework, bearing out the saying that "What gets us into the most trouble is not our weaknesses but rather the strengths that we carry too far." Therapeutic goals that deal with the alteration of identity style are the most challenging because they involve revising the core assumptions upon which expectations about self and others are built.

Self as Content and Self as Process

The sense of self is as much verb as noun, in that our habitual modes of engaging in self-confirmation are as much a part of our "selves" as the self-pictures they generate and sustain. The self as verb is the *active self* alluded to in the title of this chapter, which is similar to a self-schema, and must be distinguished from the individual's identity, which is the content of the self-concept. The distinction between the active self, on one hand, and the more "passive" *identity*, on the other, has been likened to the distinction between a computer program that processes data and the data processed by that program (Greenwald and Partkanis, 1984), or to the relationship between the *I* and the *me* as in the following statement by Mancuso and Sarbin (1983):

The first-order self, I, self-as-storyteller, is a construction that persons develop for use in understanding the creation of self-narratives. The protagonists in these self-narratives are selves-as-objects, that is, second-order selves. In explaining their own ongoing self-presentations, people act as if they held the belief that self-as-storyteller (the I) had authored a script to guide role enactment as heroes, villains, fools, or whatever. (p. 246)

In dealing with a client's active self processes, one comes to grips with the ways in which he or she maintains self-stability, which are also important leverage points for introducing change.

The Self-Confirmation Feedback Cycle

The view that self-concept is a key ingredient in the stability of personality has been central to several conceptualizations, including those of Lecky (1951), Rogers (1951), and Sullivan (1953); in addition, it has been proposed that people sustain continuity of self-concept through self-confirmatory interpersonal relationships (Leary, 1957; Secord & Backman, 1961).

Self-confirmation theory assumes, as well, that when faced with self-incongruent feedback the individual will find ways to counteract, avoid, or discount such disconcerting information and thus sustain the perception of a self-consistent environment. In other terms, the self-image serves as a homeostatic reference value (Andrews, 1977, 1991; Carver & Scheier, 1981). The individual endeavors to maintain self-consistency by arranging his or her interactions with the environment so that they form a negative feedback loop, that is, one in which information tends to return a system to a prior equilibrium.

This proposition is supported by a sizable body of experimental literature, reviewed by Andrews (1977, 1989, 1991), Burns (1979), Felker (1974), Rosenberg (1979), and Swann (1983, 1985, 1987). This research provides a solid evidential base from which to extrapolate a model of therapeutic intervention and client change. Some of this evidence also suggests that under favorable conditions, people will seek or accept experience that is moderately novel or self-dissonant (Andrews, 1990; Holloman & Hendrick, 1972; Poag, 1991). This readiness is a key factor in producing therapeutic change.

The self-confirmation feedback cycle, the processes of which constitute the active self, is diagrammed in Figure 1. At each stage in this loop, the individual channels action and experience in ways that are congruent with, and confirmatory of, the self-concept. These stages are described below and illustrated with sample findings from the research literature.

One begins with a self-concept (Stage I on the diagram), consisting of generalized self-perceptions concerning feelings, attitudes, capacities, styles of behavior, and so on—who one is on the whole and who one is not (Rogers, 1951). And the person attempts to maintain congruence among these self-perceptions. For example, Pyszczynski and Greenberg (1985) found that depressed subjects preferred self-focused attention (via a mirror) following task failure, whereas nondepressed individuals preferred self-focus following success; in this way, each type of person selec-

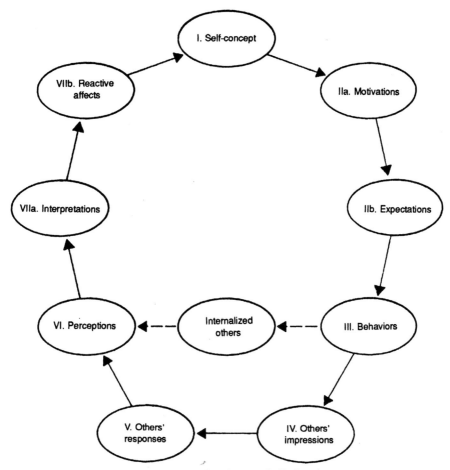

Figure 1. The self-confirmation feedback cycle.

tively directed attention to the aspect of self that was consistent with initial self-esteem level.

One's needs (Stage IIa) and expectations (Stage IIb) regarding specific people and situations tend to be consistent with, and to help sustain, one's generalized self-image. First, where needs are concerned, Dengerink and Myers (1977) found that after failure depressed men became less aggressive, whereas nondepressed subjects became more aggressive. They reasoned that failure would be self-confirming for the low self-esteem depressives, but that the nondepressives would need to react with anger in order to re-

affirm their self-confidence. With respect to expectations, McFarlin and Blascovich (1981) found that subjects' predictions of future performance following task success or failure were consistent with chronic self-esteem level. They also found that high self-esteem subjects in the failure condition predicted significantly higher levels of future performance than did high self-esteem subjects in the success condition. The authors suggest that this elevated expectation helped to restore self-esteem following the threat posed by the failure.

Behavior (Stage III), in turn, has a confirmatory relation to the self-image of the one who initiates an action and to the feelings and expectations which underlie that self-image. To test this connection, Swann and Hill (1982) provided subjects with self-confirming and self-discrepant feedback (supposedly from an experimental partner), and then arranged for half of each group to interact again with that partner. The discrepant-feedback subjects tried harder to change the partner's impression and also behaved more "in character" than subjects who were exposed to congruent feedback. Also, those subjects who had the opportunity to interact again with the partner (and hence to reconfirm their identities) changed their self-ratings less than those who lacked that opportunity.

In addition to meeting the needs of the initiator, behavior is an interpersonal message, a set of cues from which others form an image (Stage IV) of the person with whom they are dealing. This image will significantly overlap the person's own self-picture (Kiesler, 1983). Thus Swann and Ely (1984) studied interactions in which "perceivers" were induced to see "targets" in ways opposite to the latter's own self-perceptions. They found, as predicted, that in this conflict of expectations the targets "won" by bringing perceivers to treat them in a manner consistent with their (the targets') self-conceptions. As a result of such impressions, the responses of others (Stage V) will, on the whole, tend to confirm one's expectations about oneself (Leary, 1957).

This effect is further reinforced by the tendency to selectively associate with others who *do* provide self-confirmation and to avoid those who might challenge one's ideas about oneself. For example, Broxton (1963) found that among college roommates, friends usually held mutually confirming views of each other, and that when this congruence was not present there was a greater likelihood that one party would change roommates. This finding involves a combination of Stage III (selective interaction) and Stage V (self-confirming interpersonal response). How such friendship patterns can affect self-confirmation was shown by Swann and Predmore (1985); they found that following self-discrepant feedback, subjects who discussed the feedback with friends who saw them as they saw themselves manifested the least self-image change and were the most resistant to future disconfirming information.

Of course, the match between a person's self-image and the other's reaction is not perfect. The other person will have his or her own interactive patterns, and hence may present a disconfirming response. As is shown by the last sector of Figure 1, people have ways to deal with the dissonance and tension that can arise in such exchanges, in order to preserve their self-definitions intact. First, there is selective perception (Stage VI). One generally filters out social feedback that is not self-confirming, and pays particular attention to that which supports one's self-concept (Kiesler, 1982). Moreover, when people are unable to avoid perceiving such cues, it is still possible to reinterpret them, relabel them, or deny responsibility for them in some way (Stage VIIa). As Felker (1974) noted, the self-concept serves as an inner filter; as perceptions pass through the filter, they are given meanings which reflect the view the person has of himself or herself. Those meanings are the result of selective interpretation.

A study by Hamilton (1969) demonstrated a chaining among these perceptual and interpretive self-confirmation strategies. He provided subjects with self-discrepant feedback, supposedly based on a personality test. Some subjects underrecalled the dissonant items. Others reinterpreted the situation by either discrediting the test or disparaging the skills of the supposed test interpreter. Still others were "conformers": They changed their self-ratings in response to the feedback. And as in the Swann and Hill (1982) study, it was only when no self-reconfirmation strategy was used that such change occurred.

Finally, the affective impact (Stage VIIb) of an experience is often significantly determined by the person's self-image. Selective perception and interpretation shape the meaning of the event, and the individual's affective response generally reflects this meaning, thus further reinforcing his or her perception of self. For example, Conn and Crowne (1964) arranged for subjects to be confronted with hostile provocation by an experimental confederate. Individuals high in self-perceived need for approval (a characteristic which is incongruent with hostility) reacted with less anger and were more ingratiating than under non-provocation conditions, whereas other subjects showed the reverse pattern. Thus the approval-oriented subjects intensified their "agreeable" expressive styles when faced with a stimulus that might evoke self-inconsistently hostile emotions.

A further implication is shown by the interior dotted line of Figure 1. The person maintains continuity not only by engaging in "real-world" interactions, but also by engaging in intrapersonal or symbolic communications with *internalized others* (M. Horowitz, 1979; Stryker, 1985) that are the legacy of important early interactions such as parent–child relationships. The internalized other plays a role in an inner self-confirmation cycle that continues to operate even when the individual is alone or in a new environment. Thus, if one expresses one's self-concept through a certain action (Stage III), one can adopt an internalized-other stance toward one's own behavior and give oneself internal feedback; and one can even, in turn, reject or reinterpret (Stages VI and VIIa) that feedback as if it were an external stimulus.

Recent research has experimentally distinguished between internal and external self-presentation. Baumeister (1982) noted evidence for self-presentational factors in many studies of social behavior, and concluded that "the two main self-presentational motives are to please the audience and to construct (create, maintain, and modify) one's public self congruent to one's ideal" (p. 3). One type of evidence cited by Baumeister as demonstrating internal self-confirmation is the audience-transfer effect, in which an experience (usually involving self-image damage) leads the individual to counteractive behavior in the absence of the people who produced or witnessed the original event. Since influencing the original audience is not possible, the aim must be to reestablish one's generalized self-image, across audiences, as perceived by the only person present in both contexts: oneself.

A chain of causal influence is implicit in the self-confirmation feedback cycle. As the arrows in Figure 1 show, there is a continuous loop of time-sequenced stages[1] such that each stage leads to the next in order. Thus, the self-concept is generally expressed in behavior via the mediation of situation-specific needs and expectancies. Internal processes (self-perceptions, needs, expectancies) only influence other people via the medium

of overt (verbal and nonverbal) behavior. Cues from others' behavior and the nonsocial environment affect us by being perceived and by being interpreted in some fashion, however rudimentary. Finally, one's emotional response to a stimulus is dependent upon how that stimulus is perceived and interpreted. In this way, each stage is congruent with, and helps to reinforce the concept of self.

In sum, the appearance of fixity or stability in the self-concept is the product of an ongoing, though not usually conscious or deliberate, effort at self-confirmation involving self-fulfilling prophecies. By engaging in the processes described by the active-self model, the person maintains a complete negative feedback cycle, beginning and ending with the certainties of self; and in doing so defines much of his or her experience of the world as well. Such cycles, when too rigid or maladaptively selective, are a key ingredient in personal disturbance. Conversely, healthy functioning involves an appetite for novel experience so long as extreme self-dissonance is not generated. In this context, psychotherapy produces change by intervening at various stages of the cycle to help the client rechannel his or her self-confirmation system.

SELF-CONFIRMATION AND PSYCHOTHERAPY

Assessment of the Client

The therapist can assess a client's difficulties by characterizing his or her self-confirmation strategies at each stage in the feedback cycle. The stages set forth in Figure 1 can thus be used as a set of categories for defining how the client resists self-redefinition through the expression of needs, expectancies, interpersonal behavior, selective perception and interpretation, and reactive affect.

Targeting of Interventions

The self-confirmation cycle can also be used to characterize interventions, which are the means used by the therapist to help the client interrupt or rechannel the self-confirming feedback cycle. Each of the nine stages provides a leverage point for such intervention. Because each stage is dis-

[1]Exceptions to this sequencing may occur in certain areas. Exceptions (Stage IIb) may influence how strongly needs (IIa) are felt, and reactive feelings (VIIb) may affect the nature of selective interpretation (VIIa). It is for this reason that these processes are given an a/b designation in Figure 1.

tinctive, where and how one intervenes makes a difference, and various interventions may appear quite dissimilar because they take on the form of the stage toward which they are directed. At the same time, interventions that are very different on the surface may produce overlapping outcomes in the long run, because they have the common ultimate aim of redirecting the entire cycle of which each stage is a part. This commonality in diversity is the basis for the integrative model presented here. A significant benefit of this approach is that client characteristics and intervention styles are set forth in the same terms, thus enabling therapists to move clearly and directly from assessment to intervention.

In addition to being targeted toward particular stages of the self-confirmation cycle, interventions may be designed either to help the client gain awareness of his or her self-confirmation patterns, or to develop change experiments. With respect to the first of these goals, the therapist can show how problematic aspects of self-concept about which the client may feel helpless are actually generated by unnoticed or "unconscious" self-confirmatory activities. This helps to establish what Yalom (1980) calls *self-authorship*; the client is led to assume responsibility for his or her problematic view of self.

Secondly, therapist and client can build on this awareness by generating change-producing activities or assignments, using the stages of the cycle as leverage points. This can be used as a basis for conducting therapy collaboratively through homework assignments or in-therapy activities. These experiments involve reversing the client's habitual patterns at one or more of the stages of the self-confirmation process in order to introduce novelty into self-experience.

The distinction between awareness and change interventions, when combined with the nine cycle stages, produces a "menu" of eighteen types of interventions, which is portrayed in Table 1. This typology corresponds to, and thus helps to organize the rich repertoire of interventions available in current therapeutic practice.

To be fully effective therapeutically, the therapist needs interventions that deal with all aspects of the feedback cycle. By selecting an approach that addresses each self-confirmation strategy as it arises, one will have the best opportunity to carry the change process forward. And

using the confirmation cycle as a diagnostic template can help the therapist to scan for areas not addressed and to plan interventions.

Conversely, without this breadth of approach a change initiated at one point might encounter increasing resistance from novelty-reducing "filters" at other stages. When this happens, the change process is more likely to dissipate than to grow productively. For example, revision of self-perceptions (Stage I) may not be enduring if the client remains baffled about how to realign expectations (IIb) and behavior (III) accordingly, thus altering the messages received (IV) by other people. And even if these messages do change, significant others will often continue to respond (Stage V) on the basis of older images and expectations (IV). Change is apt to fade away unless the individual knows how to cope with this interpersonal resistance. Also, new behavior (Stage III) may be undercut if the client succeeds in selectively overlooking (VI) or distorting (VIIa) the reactions (V) this behavior is eliciting from others. Finally, insight into perceptual-cognitive filtering (Stages VI and VIIa) may not be implemented if one is not enabled to *see* what one has been overlooking and to assimilate its emotional meaning (VIIb) into a revised sense of self (I).

Effective psychotherapy can help the client to sustain the momentum of the change process by providing learning experiences that will foster the necessary self-revision skills at each stage of the confirmation cycle. And combinations of specific interventions add therapeutic power because they impact the feedback loop at multiple points. This gives the client the leverage needed to redefine his or her conception of self by initiating change experiments throughout the cycle.

Self-Confirmation within the Therapist–Client Relationship

Self-confirmation also enters directly into the therapeutic interaction, because the client will be endeavoring to sustain his or her self-concept within the therapeutic relationship as well as in outside life. (So, too, may the therapist!) In addition, the therapist–client interaction provides a context for the target-specific interventions discussed above, because each intervention has both form and content. When making an intervention, the therapist is talking about some aspect of the

Table 1. Intervention Styles Classified by Confirmation Cycle Categories

Cycle stage	Understanding/awareness	Change/experimentation
I. Self-concept	Empathically explore client's currently experienced self-image	Enable client to experience and assimilate new, dissonant self-perceptions
IIa. Motivations	Explore, reflect, interpret experienced wishes and motivations	Encourage client to experiment with unexpressed needs and to assimilate unrecognized wishes
IIb. Expectancies, plans	Clarify and reflect on client's expectancies and problem-solving modes	Provide training and modeling in problem solving and in reevaluating and revising expectancies
III. Behavior	Provide feedback on client's behavior patterns, including nonverbal style	Encourage client to experiment with new behavior; provide behavioral skill training
IV. Others' impressions	Provide feedback about own emotional reactions, impressions of client	Provide feedback about own reactions which offer client new images of self
V. Others' responses	Offer direct behavioral response which highlights client's characteristic evoking style	Act in ways which provide client with novel, self-image expanding feedback
VI. Selective perceptions	Point out ways in which client overlooks self-dissonant cues	Encourage client to focus on experiences which will provide novel self-perceptions
VIIa. Selective interpretations	Point out self-confirming interpretations, attributions, or ways of framing experience	Encourage client to experiment with alternative forms of interpretation or self-talk
VIIb. Reactive emotions	Elicit and support expressions of emotional response to experiences	Provide suggestions or skill training in alternative ways of coping with difficult emotions

Note. From *The Active Self in Psychotherapy: An Integration of Therapeutic Styles* by John D. W. Andrews, 1991. Boston: Allyn & Bacon. Copyright 1991 by Allyn & Bacon. Reprinted by permission.

client's life, and is also talking about it in a particular manner.

In self-confirmation theory, the form and content levels are linked by *their converging implications for self-definition*. Intervention content influences the client's self-confirmation tactics, and how these interventions are expressed conveys a definition of the relationship. This definition, in turn, implies a certain image of the client which is therapeutically important because it influences the client's own self-perceptions. The therapist, by engaging in *anticomplementary* behavior—that is, by declining to play a confirmatory role toward the client—introduces interpersonal novelty and thus stimulates self-concept change (Kiesler, 1983). The convergence between form and content is highlighted during *metacommunication*, that is, when the content of discussion refers to the interaction itself.

There is one additional component to therapeutic effectiveness. The accepting therapist–client relationship (Rogers, 1951) and the therapeutic working alliance (Bordin, 1979) provide an environment of psychological safety in which the

client can relax his or her urgent efforts at self-reconfirmation. In one of Aesop's fables, the sun and the storm compete to induce a man to remove his coat. As in the fable, the sun of positive regard is more effective in producing change than is the storm of unsupportive confrontation. The latter simply causes the individual to wrap himself or herself still more tightly in the cloak of self-consistency. Conversely, providing a safe environment for the client potentiates the effects of target-specific interventions and anticomplementary therapist–client interactions.

INTEGRATING THERAPEUTIC SCHOOLS

The foregoing analysis can be used as a tool for psychotherapy integration, in that various theories and principles of intervention can be "mapped" onto the 18-category array of intervention styles presented in Table 1. Many therapeutic models deal primarily with one or a few cycle stages, and hence the taxonomy can be used to locate them in relation to one another.

In previous research (Andrews, 1977, 1988), I have employed the self-confirmation model as a content analysis system for analyzing therapy transcripts. This work compared sessions conducted by five therapists who were either founders or spokespersons for major therapeutic schools: client-centered, psychoanalytic, gestalt, behavioral, and cognitive (rational-emotive). Table 2 gives my own placement of these therapies (as well as a number of others, which will be discussed at a later point).

In client-centered therapy (Rogers, 1951), the self-concept (Stage I) is crucial to personality and therapy, and the primary mode is understanding rather than change. Reactive feelings (VIIb) and needs (IIa) are also emphasized. Psychoanalysis (Wolberg, 1967) has traditionally focused on the understanding of motives or drives (Stage IIa) in personal functioning. Insight into transference-based emotional reactions (VIIb) is also important, and psychoanalysts are increasingly emphasizing work with the self (Stage I) as well (Kohut, 1984). Gestalt therapy is harder to place. On one hand, it minimizes interpretation and stresses awareness of needs and sensory experiences (Perls, 1969; Perls, Hefferline, & Goodman, 1951). Accordingly, we might portray it as understanding-oriented at Stages IIa and VI. However, gestaltists also stress the interactions between therapist and client (Simkin, 1979), and this involves change as well as awareness (at Stages III–V), via the gestalt experiment technique. Behaviorists use guided practice aimed at behavioral change (Stage III). This is especially characteristic of Wolpe's assertion method, the approach he used in the (1970) transcript studied. Wolpe assumes that expressing aggression will reciprocally inhibit fear, and hence changes in motivation (Stage IIa) are also involved. So, too, are the reinforcements provided by others' responses (V). Fi-

Table 2. Psychotherapeutic Schools: Primary Foci of Intervention

Cycle stage	Focus on awareness	Focus on change
I. Self-concept	Client-centered* Psychoanalytic*	Self-efficacy
IIa. Motivations	Client-centered* Psychoanalytic*	Behavioral* Multimodal
IIb. Expectations	Personal construct	Personal construct Learned helplessness
III. Behavior	Gestalt* Sensitivity training	Gestalt* Behavioral* Multimodal Rational-emotive*
IV. Others' impressions	Gestalt* Sensitivity training	Gestalt* Interpersonal
V. Others' responses	Gestalt* Sensitivity training	Gestalt* Behavioral* Multimodal
VI. Perceptions	Gestalt* Cognitive encoding	Cognitive encoding
VIIa. Interpretations	Rational-emotive* Cognitive	Rational-emotive* Multimodal Cognitive
VIIb. Reactive affect	Client-centered* Psychoanalytic	Behavioral* Multimodal

*Starred entries are therapeutic schools dealt with in the content analysis study.
Note. From *The Active Self in Psychotherapy: An Integration of Therapeutic Styles*, by John D. W. Andrews, 1991. Boston: Allyn & Bacon. Copyright 1991 by Allyn & Bacon. Reprinted by permission.

nally, rational-emotive therapy (Ellis, 1962) deals most directly with the information-processing segment of the feedback loop. Ellis's A-B-C (stimulus-cognition-emotion) model fits into the V–VIIb stage sequence, the therapeutic goal being to change cognitions (Stages VI and VIIa) and the emotions (VIIb) that follow from them. Ellis also has a strong secondary emphasis on practicing new behavior (Stage III). In the research studies mentioned above (Andrews, 1977, 1988), 95% of all interventions that were conceptualized as fitting a particular school were above the median in frequency of use in the interview representing that school. This finding leads credence to the typology presented in Tables 1 and 2.

In addition to these five schools, one can go further and look for other approaches to complete the cycle, as is also shown in Table 2. Just as the periodic table of elements provided a template whose unfilled categories guided scientists toward new discoveries, so might new psychotherapies be added until the entire cycle-stage system is completed. Thus, Bandura's (1978) approach to enhancing self-efficacy is a change technique directed toward Stage I, especially when it involves global self-efficacy beliefs (Goldfried & Robins, 1982). Also, none of the approaches discussed so far concentrates on expectations (Stage IIb), and George Kelly's (1955) psychology of personal constructs fills this gap. His fundamental postulate is that "a person's processes are psychologically channelized by the ways in which he anticipates events" (p. 46). Certain cognitive therapies have a similar emphasis; thus Hollon and Garber (1980) state that "negative expectations about the future produce much of the depressive symptomatology, and therefore . . . the major focus of the process and procedure of therapy should be on expectations" (p. 182).

The sensitivity training approach (Golombiewski & Blumberg, 1970) places a primary emphasis on learning about one's impact on other people, corresponding to Stages III to V of the cycle. And experimentation at Stage VI can also provide a therapeutic focus. Greenberg and Safran (1981) help clients to become aware of their perceptual selectivity; the clients are then asked to "intentionally change their perceptual behavior and focus on attributes hitherto ignored. These deliberate attempts at new microbehaviors . . . are explicitly designed to break old encoding patterns and lay the blueprint for new, more effective

patterns" (p. 166). Systematic desensitization (Wolpe, 1969) is an affective change intervention at Stage VIIb. Other therapeutic approaches could be located within the structure of Table 2 in a similar way.

Of course, these categories involve a certain unavoidable simplification; no therapy can be wholly effective by dealing exclusively with one process, or by failing to concern itself with a wide range of human experience. Yet the processes emphasized in various therapeutic models do represent distinctive choices of focus, and many theorists, while discussing a variety of processes, claim—like Bandura, Ellis, Freud, or Kelly—that "their" process should be the main therapeutic focus because it is the one that energizes all the others.

A SELF-CONFIRMATIONAL ANALYSIS OF DEPRESSION

The syndrome of depression provides a valuable realm for applying the self-confirmation model; in addition to being a prevalent complaint among clients, this syndrome has been studied and conceptualized from a wide variety of viewpoints. An examination of the complex literature on depression (Andrews, 1989) shows that most of the explanatory constructs used to account for this difficulty fit within the categories of the self-confirmation cycle. Moreover, when combined, they interlock and complement one another so as to "cover the map" of the cycle stages quite completely. This pattern will be examined in detail below. The discussion will begin with the depressive's self-concept and then move counterclockwise around the cycle. The reason for this ordering is related to the fact that in many formulations, the phenomena covered by a particular stage of the cycle are accounted for by the processes of the *preceding* stage. Thus, the counterclockwise approach highlights how the proposed causal connections are related to the assumptions of self-confirmation theory.

The Identity Prototype of the Depressive Person

Stage I: Self-Concept. In applying self-confirmation concepts to the depressive syndrome, we first ask: What is the identity image (Stage I) that characterizes the depressed person? This pattern corresponds to the *loss or lowering of self-esteem* stressed in psychoanalytic theories of depression. Freud (1959) writes that the depressed individual "reproaches himself, vilifies himself, and expects to be cast out and chastised. He abases himself before everyone and commiserates his own relatives for being connected with someone so unworthy" (p. 155). And Gaylin (1968), in summarizing the psychoanalytic literature on the syndrome, notes a trend that involves "an enlargement of the role of self-esteem and its movement from the periphery to [the view] that diminished self-esteem is the *cause* of depression" (p. 388). A similar idea is included in Blatt's (1974) account of introjective depression, which posits that punitive internal objects, derived from interaction with parents, generate self-perceptions of worthlessness, guilt, and failure.

Sociocognitive theories also stress the depressive self. Pyszczynski and Greenberg (1987) proposed that the depressed individual sustains his or her low self-esteem via a *negative self-focusing style* involving a tendency to become self-aware with respect to negative experiences; this tendency leads to other depressive features such as negative attributions, pessimism, and performance deficits. Kuiper and Olinger (1986) have proposed a *self-worth contingency* model of depression, according to which the clinically depressed individual has a strongly consolidated, negative self-schema that incorporates the "contractual contingency" that one's self-worth depends upon the approval of others. As a result, a cycle of depressogenic events often develops, in which the individual's negative view of self, and his or her perceived failure to meet self-esteem contingencies, leads to self-rejection. This produces a negativistic, self-critical presentation style that enhances the possibility that others will reject the vulnerable depressed individual.

Stage VIIb: Reactive Affect. As the defining characteristic of the "affective disorder" of depression, the reactive affects of sadness, disappointment, and self-hate are more typically looked upon as needing explanation than as sources of explanation in themselves. However, Rehm's (1977) *self-regulation* model is built around the variable of low self-reinforcement: the depressed individual's diminished capacity to provide positive emotional experiences for himself or herself. In this sense, self-reinforcement—which is a mixture of self-evaluation and self-reward—is viewed as causally producing depressive affect and low self-esteem.

Stage VIIa: Selective Interpretation. Beck's *cognitive* model (Beck, 1976; Beck, Rush, Shaw, & Emery, 1979) posits that depressives are characterized by a primary triad of negative cognitive patterns or schemata; depression is "primarily a result of the tendency to view the self, the future, and the world in an unrealistically negative manner" (Sacco & Beck, 1985, p. 4). The depressive person sustains these views through cognitive distortions such as selective abstraction, arbitrary inference, and overgeneralization.

The learned helplessness model (Seligman, 1975) is an expectancy theory, and is discussed under the heading below. However, the *revised learned helplessness model* (Abramson, Seligman, & Teasdale, 1978) includes attributions, and hence is relevant to Stage VIIa. According to this account, the depressive is one who makes internal, global, and stable attributions for negative outcomes, thereby reinforcing his or her sense of inadequacy, helplessness, and depression.

Stage VI: Selective Perception and Recall. The *information-processing* model of Kuiper, MacDonald, and Derry (1983) grew from the study of how self-schemata influence memory. These authors propose that information networks linked to the self provide the best memory access, and the depressives possess negatively toned networks that are associated with low self-esteem. Thus, they argue, the memory-processing system of the depressive person will retrieve predominantly negative experiences, thereby generating dysphoric affect.

Similarly, Ingram (1984) has proposed that the depressed person possesses an extensive cognitive network that incorporate negative affect nodes, and that as a result, negative information will be most elaborated and will occupy the greater proportion of cognitive capacity. He writes that "as activation cycles through the network, it is eventually fed back . . . to the depression node, causing it to remain activated. Phenomenologically, it may seem to the individual that negative memories keep coming back, again and again, thus maintaining depressive feelings" (p. 455).

Stages IV to V: Others' Impressions and Responses. A *cognitive prototype held by others* that shapes their impressions and responses (Stages IV–V) may contribute to maintaining the depressive pattern in still another way. Cane and Gotlib (1985) point out that many lay individuals hold a prototype of depression that includes such elements as withdrawal, self-blame, dependence, and sadness (see Horowitz, Wright, Lowenstein & Parad, 1981). Cane and Gotlib go on to suggest that when a person notices one or a few prototype features in a depressed other, he or she may apply the full prototype and hence assume the existence of additional features that are not necessarily present. This amounts to creating a stereotype of the depressed person that can function as a self-fulfilling prophecy. The depressed individual, finding himself or herself treated as more of a global depressive than is actually the case, may behave in accord with the expectation this response conveys, thereby intensifying the depressogenic cycle still further.

Stages III to V: Interpersonal Behavior and Response. According to *interpersonal* theories, what is distinctive about the depressive individual is the type of social environment he or she sets up in dealing with others. Leary (1957) identifies depression with the self-effacing personality type, and writes that "if a person acts in a glum, guilty, withdrawn, and weak manner, he will tend to train others to look down on him and to view him with varying amounts of contempt (p. 284).

Somewhat similarly, Coyne (1976) stresses the depressive's seeking of support from significant others, as well as the guilt and resentment generated by his or her attempts to shift the "interactive burden" to the other party. The resulting negative emotion, combined with growing impatience when reassurance seems to produce little effect, often leads to the very rejection the depressed person had been so anxious to avoid in the first place.

A related interpersonal portrayal is offered by Arieti and Bemporad (1978), who write from a psychodynamic perspective. They stress the depressive's lack of autonomy and self-direction and assert that this sort of individual typically looks to a *dominant other* or a *dominant goal* as the major source of gratification, self-direction, and self-esteem. Loss of the dominant other or dominant goal is often the event that precipitates a depressive episode.

Stage III: Social Behavior. Poor interpersonal functioning at Stage III—seen as lack of skill in eliciting positive social reinforcement (Stage V)—is a key ingredient in *behavioral* theories of depression (Costello, 1972; Ferster, 1966, 1973; Lazarus, 1968; Lewinsohn, 1974, 1976). Although the lack of positive reinforcement may initially be due to an external event (such as a failure or the loss of a relationship), it is the degree of interpersonal skill the person brings to the experience that determines how it will be handled and whether depression will develop. This account also assumes that as adjustive, reward-producing behaviors decrease, depressive behaviors become more prevalent and are often rewarded by social attention.

Stage IIb: Expectations. As noted earlier, the original *learned helplessness* model (Seligman, 1974, 1975) is built around an expectancy construct. The key expectation is that the probability of a particular consequence if one makes a response will equal the probability of the consequence if there is no response. In plain terms, no matter what you do it will not make any difference. Particularly when aversive consequences are involved, this results in learned helplessness—from which the depressive symptoms of passivity, negative cognitive set, lack of capacity for satisfaction, and dysphoria are assumed to follow. In addition, Beck's (1976) cognitive model of depression deals with expectancies in the sense that a negatively slanted view of the future is considered to be one component of the depressive pattern.

Stage IIa: Motivation. A *motivational* formulation that bridges the connection between expectancies and needs is offered by Layne (1980) and Layne, Merry, Christian, and Ginn (1982). These authors review a number of studies supporting the assumption that "depression is primarily a motivational deficit; motivation consists of the organism's expectancy of an outcome multiplied by the organism's valuation of that outcome. Therefore, depression is primarily a deficit in the person's expectancies and values" (Layne *et al.*, 1982,

p. 259). In this statement we see a close intertwining of Stages IIa and IIb.

Prototype Overview

It can be seen from the above account that a number of theories claim to hold the explanatory key to depressive functioning, arguing that phenomena made central in other theories are in fact secondary or noncausal processes. As various theorists pursue this reductionistic path, they often explain a given stage in the confirmation cycle by invoking another that is "upstream" from it in the feedback loop. Moreover, the very diversity of explanatory accounts, each supported by a body of evidence, calls into question the endeavor to derive all depressive characteristics from any one factor. This "dog-chasing-its-tail" circularity is a problem only if one is seeking "the" cause of depression; it is actually an asset from the perspective of self-confirmation theory, which is concerned with precisely this type of interactional phenomenon. Thus, it seems most useful to view the depressive syndrome as constituting a complex, multifeatured prototype, with features that correspond to the elements portrayed in Figure 2.

Implications for Psychotherapy of Depression

The self-confirmation cycle model helps the therapist to define leverage points for heightening self-awareness and stimulating change. One can introduce interventions that correspond to the depressogenic causal mechanisms reviewed above in order to target the corresponding aspects of the client's functioning, and combinations of interventions can be used to redirect the feedback cycle as a whole. In addition, the therapeutic relationship can serve as a new arena for identifying and revising the client's self-confirmation strategies.

The Effects of Interventions on Targeted Processes. At Stage I, many therapists redirect self-talk and self-reward to improve client self-esteem (e.g., Jackson, 1972; Mahoney, 1971). Mahoney provided positive self-statements for his client, who gradually learned to use them as rewards and to generate them for himself. The self-reward element in these cases is also pertinent to reactive

emotion (Stage VIIb), and some therapists focus on this stage by encouraging clients to expand their pleasant activities, especially as a means to counteract depressive ruminations (e.g., Anton, Dunbar, & Friedman, 1976; Tharp, Watson, & Kaya, 1974). Cognitive therapies are focused on Stages VIIa and VI, encouraging clients to replace their depressogenic attributional and attentional patterns with cognitions that are less globally negative and that imply more behavioral control and positive self-valuation (e.g., Rush, Khatami, & Beck, 1975; Schmickley, 1976).

Social reinforcement approaches deal partly with Stages IV and V, working to alter the interpersonal feedback given to the client. In this sphere, therapists often act to reward adaptive behavior and discourage depressive talk, and/or enlist the client's significant others for this purpose (e.g., Burgess, 1969; Johansson, Lewinsohn, & Flippo, 1969; Lewinsohn, 1976; Liberman & Raskin, 1971). The client's social behavior (Stage III) is also a focus of intervention. Typical programs involve practicing assertion and anger expression, as well as communication skills such as making eye contact and eliciting social reward (e.g., Lazarus, 1968; Shipley & Fazio, 1973; Wells, Hersen, Bellack, & Himmelhoch, 1977). The short-term interpersonal psychotherapy (IPT) method (Weisman, Klerman, Rounsaville, Chevron, & Neu, 1982) is focused on present interpersonal difficulties, such as role disputes and role transitions, and thus involves Stages III to V.

Cognitive therapists often work with helplessness expectancies (Stage IIb) in depression. For example, Glass (1978) helped clients to identify areas in which helplessness was experienced, and to generate alternative behaviors for anticipating and dealing with it. Problem-solving training works with the client's expectancies in a somewhat similar way (e.g., Caple & Blechman, 1976). Finally, motivation-oriented therapies help clients to reestablish the reward values (Stage IIa) that are often lacking in depression. Lazarus (1968) and Sammons (1974) used guided fantasy for this purpose, and Sammons incorporated the positive fantasy thus generated into an *in vivo* exercise, called "systematic resensitization," that leads to renewed seeking of reinforcement.

Combinations of Target-Specific Interventions. Each intervention principally affects the targeted process (Biglan & Dow, 1981), and therefore combinations of interventions will often be needed, especially for more complex depressive problems (Craighead, 1980; Lazarus, 1981; Liberman, 1981; McCullough, 1984; McLean, 1976; O'Brien, 1978). The combining of methods takes on additional importance when considered in the context of self-confirmation theory. Viewing various aspects of depressive functioning as causally related stages of an interactive cycle suggests that an intervention introduced at one stage may influence others as the individual strives to maintain consistency among different aspects of his or her experience; as a result, there can be a "ripple" of change that spreads throughout the client's self-confirmation system and facilitates the restructuring of that system. At the same time, a self-confirmation strategy associated with one stage of the cycle may be invoked by the client to counteract a change introduced at another stage. It is therefore important to select and sequence interventions in ways that strengthen the momentum of the change process.

The Therapeutic Relationship. As discussed previously, the depressive individual tends to establish dominant-submissive dyads with other people, and he or she will endeavor to draw the therapist into a similar pattern. The therapist, though he or she will be "pulled" to engage in this cycle, must gradually introduce anticomplementary responses that will change the client's self-confirmation patterns. Relationship issues of this sort are generally involved in the transferential interactions emphasized in psychoanalysis. Moreover, many psychodynamic writers (e.g., Arieti & Bemporad, 1978; Jacobson, 1968; Lorand, 1968) have recommended that the classical "blank screen" analytic technique be modified with depressives, in that the therapist should adopt an active, supportive, and visibly involved role. This provides positive mirroring of the sort emphasized by Kohut (1984), which helps to counteract the depressive's self-disparaging and self-effacing tendencies. For example, Lorand urges that therapists honor the client's inarticulate plea to "show me emotion, that I may know I make a difference to you" (1968, p. 336).

Arieti and Bemporad (1978) discuss how the therapist must initially reciprocate the depressive client's submissiveness, stating: "We have seen how often the difficulty of the depressed patient stems from his dependence on a dominant other. And now we would encourage him to substitute for the dominant other a dominant third (the therapist); in other words, we would not encourage him to assume an independent role" (p. 215). This is because initial rapport must be established within the client's accustomed interactive patterns, or else he or she will experience therapy as threatening and turn away from it.

Later, as the therapeutic alliance grows strong and trustworthy, the therapist can begin to enact the role of a *significant third*: "Whereas the dominant other was experienced as a rigid and static person, the significant third will change rapidly and will appear eventually as a person who shares life experiences without aiming to control and dominate. He may indicate alternative possibilities but he does not demand their implementation" (p. 216). The behavior of the significant third thus involves anticomplementarity; as discussed earlier, this therapeutic stance produces change by challenging the self-presentation and self-concept of the client.

A Multilevel Model of Psychotherapy for Depression

As noted at the start, therapeutic impact can be most fully understood by being viewed in terms of both intervention content and relationship form. With regard to depression, there is evidence for the efficacy of many content-focused (target-specific) therapeutic techniques, leading an increasing number of writers to propose that they be used in combination to deal with particular problem patterns and subtypes. The self-confirmation model provides a taxonomy of these methods and suggests ways of orchestrating them toward the goal of redirecting the depressive vicious cycle. And through the vehicle of the therapeutic relationship, the depressive client's tendency to confirm an identity of submissiveness and self-abnegation can be challenged as he or she is accepted unconditionally and encouraged to enact a more confident and assertive role. When target-specific methods are introduced in this interactive context, both the form and content of therapeutic intervention will facilitate the client's efforts to revise his or her self-confirming dealings with the world.

CASE EXAMPLE

Case Narrative

Neil came to me with recurrent episodes of depression and serious worries about his professional competence. Though he was doing very well at his job (his first), he was terrified to look at the performance evaluation he had received some months before. He was so sure it would be less than perfect that he even considered quitting and looking for a less demanding position.

Believing that selective avoidance of feedback is a legitimate therapeutic issue and as good a place as any to start, I gave Neil the initial assignment of reading his evaluation before our next session. I suggested that if he found doing so too hard, he could bring the report in and we would look at it together. This was intended to provide him with support and to offer a positive mirror that would help him correct his own selective interpretations. In fact, he did read the evaluation on his own. The few criticisms were far outweighed by its positive tone, and he felt elated.

As this progress was being made, I explored Neil's growing-up years. He was one of five siblings, and the children's performance had always been very important to his parents. They took the successful offspring for granted—giving them little real attention—but bragged about them to friends in a way that made Neil feel exploited. They also focused most of their concern and reassurance on the "problem" children. It seemed evident from these accounts that Neil had lacked positive, nonpossessive mirroring of his pleasure in accomplishment at the points when he had needed it most. As a result he felt obligated to provide material for his parents' pride, but was simultaneously tempted to reach for the only sustained attention that was available by becoming a depressive "problem child." His conviction that he would fail seemed to be a reflection of this need.

An opportunity to work on this issue arose when Neil discussed a project that had been highly praised by his supervisor. He called his success a "lucky accident." Being interested in the psychology of creativity, I soon saw that he had engaged in a typical creative sequence. Starting with one approach, he had become increasingly frustrated and had then stepped back to

restructure the situation. Subsequently he devised a new and original solution. I was able to convince Neil that his invention had not been a fluke but a product of his own prior efforts. In this way I helped him to engage in cognitive reattribution and also provided a positive mirror by acknowledging his imaginativeness. This was a corrective experience because such mirroring had been so lacking in his early family life.

To provide closure and practice at internalization, I then asked Neil to tell me about the project a second time while incorporating this new understanding. He did so very convincingly and with increasing pleasure. He also reported an interesting thought sequence: "At first I said to myself, 'Well I can do this (portray events more positively), but that's not really what *is*.' Then I began to feel that *was* what is!" He was beginning to absorb the reframing of this event. The purpose of my intervention was to establish an internalization step through a form of counterattitudinal role playing. I wanted Neil to identify actively with this new and more self-valuing attitude. Though it was I (and his boss) who had initially pointed out Neil's creative invention, he was now able to express greater ownership as he reworked it in his own terms. He then went on to talk animatedly about a new project, and I made a point of expressing my interest and pleasure: "It's nice to see you so full of enthusiasm now." My reaction was genuine, and was also intended to offer Neil, once again, a corrective mirroring experience.

This was not the end of the problem, of course; in subsequent sessions Neil often persisted in seeing the inadequate side of his accomplishments. On one occasion I said, "I'd like to get you curious about why you so often bounce back to the negative viewpoint." "Well," he insisted, "I just believe it." I pointed out how hard he worked at *proving* the negative view, even in spite of the previous counterattitudinal experiment—"Like a wily prosecutor bent on making his case." His strained efforts to convict himself were hardly deniable. In this way I hoped to show Neil that his depression-producing sense of inadequacy was not simply a fact about himself, but a self-definition he was repeatedly choosing to perpetuate.

I did succeed in making him curious, and together we sorted through various hunches. Neil suggested that "If I make myself look good, I'm vulnerable to being shot down." I turned his attention again to childhood memories, and he recalled how successes were taken for granted with "we expected that"; failures drew far more involvement from his parents. Then he recalled that when he did present a success, their first response was often to mention his brother: "And Jim did—" or "And won't it be nice if Jim can do the same?" Neil said, with a flash of anger, "Well, fuck Jim!" He was furious because his parents had been less interested in his positive achievements than in sympathizing with Jim's problems or trying to impress their friends. He added that his parents would call him "selfish" if they heard him express any of these thoughts.

I told Neil that this sort of parental response can make it very hard to approve of oneself; he had internalized their reflection—*absence* of a reflection, really—and turned it back on himself. I suggested that his wish for approval from his boss could be a way of compensating for this lack, but that eventually he could learn to provide it for himself and thereby counteract his depression. All he had to do, in fact, was to *stop withholding approval from himself*—to stop focusing on the negative side of his accomplishments and avoiding or disbelieving positive feedback.

To carry this idea a step further, we worked on desensitizing Neil's fear of feedback. We constructed a hierarchy of feedback opportunities, and he ranked them according to degree of threat. Then we make a contract that he would seek out feedback from his associates, beginning with the least disturbing situations and gradually moving up the hierarchy. As a result of doing this he became more comfortable and also learned to handle the criticisms he sometimes did receive. My first aim here was to help Neil desensitize himself. More basic was the aim of restructuring the confirmation cycles he had internalized from his parents. He could now begin to assimilate the new, positive feedback that was presently available to him as a young adult. In this way, cognitive restructuring served as the gateway to corrective internalization.

Soon afterward, Neil's boss took an extended business trip, an event that offered us the opportunity to deal with another aspect of this issue. Neil had been given a major project to work on, and following his supervisor's departure his efforts bogged down. He knew he needed to take a new approach to the problem, but kept becoming frustrated and distracting himself into busywork. I asked him what self-talk he used to distract himself, and he became aware of thinking, "But I'm just a kid. I can't do this!" Because his boss was away, Neil felt abandoned with no one to turn to for help. Without this external support (which Kohut, 1977, might view as a *selfobject*), he felt immobilized and demoralized. In response, I decided to try a two-chair exercise (Perls, 1969). I asked Neil to imagine that the second chair was occupied by himself 10 years hence, as a successful executive and supervisor. He was to ask this more confident self for advice. As his present self, he simply said, "I'm stuck. Now what?" But as "successful Neil" he proceeded to structure the situation thoughtfully, offering several concrete suggestions and indicating the steps needed to follow them through. I was increasingly impressed by the emergence of capacities that were not accessible to "kid Neil." By the end of the dialogue, this "team" had come up with an idea that was quite exciting and eventually led to the solution of the problem.

By imagining himself in this more mature role, Neil gained greater access to his own creative capabilities. Here, too, was progress in internalization. Formerly he would have needed to rely on his boss or me for positive feedback, but now he was able to take both roles himself. This was an important step in "owning" both sides of the supervisor–supervisee relationship; Neil thereby became, in effect, his own supervisor.

The role play exercise provided Neil with the opportunity to put into practice the guiding stance he had implicitly internalized from others. In doing this he invented a new self-regulatory role that was more than the sum of others' mirroring; it also included his own ideas, capabilities, and aspirations. What had made this hard to do previously was, of course, the lack of such mirroring in his childhood. In this sense the two-chair exercise was a corrective experience, a second chance at internalizing a positive perspective on himself. I pointed this out, and Neil found the idea especially convincing because of the new and pragmatically valuable ideas he had produced during the dialogue.

This success was followed by a flood of memories about how his attempts at independent problem solving had been undermined. One that Neil recalled with tears involved having been told, at about three, to "say good night to the (party) guests." He had gone around the room quite uncomfortably, saying goodnight to each one. At the end he had been admonished: "Why did you take so long? All you had to do was say goodnight to the group." He felt hurt and fooled. Having been given a task, he had solved it in his own way and then been told he was wrong. No wonder he was so reluctant to trust his own judgment!

Neil then associated to a puzzling contradiction in his behavior at work. In small informal brainstorming meetings, he was often hesitant and silent, fearing to say something stupid even though the norm in such sessions was to offer half-formed ideas and rework them as a group. By contrast, in formal meetings he liked to bring out "gems" of questions or critiques that impressed others and showed off his intelligence. I asked him, "How many gems would it take for you to believe in your own abilities?" He answered: "endless ones," and began to sob. This was an intense, moving moment in which we both realized the depth of the self-hate he was constantly trying to counteract by impressing others with his brilliance. "Maybe," he added, "if I work at it forever, I'll build up something around my ugly stupidity and be able to hide it for good."

Here Neil was expressing, in his own language, the notion of a *false self* (Winnicott, 1965) or a compensatory structure used to hide a *defective self* (Kohut, 1977). His struggles dealt with issues of self-acceptance and the conflicts generated by unassimilated (and punitive) internalized others. These internalized relationships were laden with double-bind messages. He had been pressured to perform well but was simultaneously treated with a subtle lack of respect. As a result, he had a deep-seated belief that his "stupid and bad" self-image was *the real Neil*. Because of this hopeless and depression-producing view of himself, he implicitly felt that his only alternative was to engage in coverup and compensation.

Accordingly, my first step in giving Neil hope was to challenge his unquestioned assumption of a "bad real me." This is where the idea of the active self—the ongoing, current self-confirmation system—is therapeutically valuable as contrasted with the view of the self as a passive

data structure. Instead of focusing on how the therapist can "repair" the client's self (Kohut, 1977), we begin by asking: How is the client, *right now*, maintaining this negative conception of self which he or she thinks is "just how I am"? And what positive self- perceptions might emerge if he or she could be helped to use self-confirmatory feedback in fresh ways? In implementing this notion I reminded Neil of the other times we had identified his negatively biased self-talk, perceptions, and expectancies, and I suggested that he was now *creating* his "stupid" self by the same sort of selectivity and by deflecting positive feedback away from his self-image. There was plenty of validation around, but he needed help in assimilating and internalizing it.

For this purpose I asked Neil to construct a new persona: the self he would be if he actually believed all the success experiences he had had and the good feedback he had received from others. I designated a chair for this confident Neil and asked him to leave aside his self-doubting, problem-child, stupid self. Neil said he felt very unnatural in the new role. I acknowledged that this would of course be the case, because he had so successfully blocked out the implications of his positive experiences, but asked him to persist in spite of the discomfort.

He did so, and I "interviewed" confident Neil for some time about his abilities and accomplishments. As I mirrored my enthusiasm back to him, adding my own impressions from previous interactions, he began to enjoy himself more and even became expansive. By the end, though not wholly convinced that this new self was "real," he had had quite a vivid and joyful experience. He acknowledged that he now found his positive qualities more believable and his depressogenic negative self-image somewhat less convincing.

Comments: The Case of Neil

Because of the mirroring deficits in Neil's childhood, his adulthood was shadowed by self-doubts. Despite many success experiences, he lived in fear of devaluation. His negative, depression-engendering self-image was sustained via his self-confirmation patterns. He selectively avoided positive feedback, negatively slanted the feedback he did receive, selectively presented an uncertain posture to others, and pictured himself as a helpless child. Even when he did make attempts to congratulate himself (as with his "gems"), this was not credible to him because he saw them as a coverup that did not dislodge his negative self-attributions.

I intervened to help Neil shift these patterns at several points, using target-specific interventions of various kinds. We gained understanding of the interpersonal system in which he grew up, and he reexperienced the hurt and anger he had felt at not being appreciated as a competent individual apart from his siblings. We worked to reverse his fear-driven avoidance of feedback and his tendency to attribute his accomplishments externally. I did this by offering him my own acceptance and positive mirroring, and also by encouraging reattribution activities such as "retelling" (reframing) his accomplishments and acting as his own supervisor. The two-chair conversation with his successful future self also grew into a planning and problem-solving activity. Desensitization and graded practice *in vivo* helped him to overcome his feedback avoidance. Finally, I encouraged him to challenge the underlying conviction that—despite much positive experience—his "stupid, ugly" self was his true identity, which could never be changed.

In my interventions I was active and reflective at different times, with the overall goal of orchestrating both styles in the service of Neil's autonomy and positive self-valuation. In this process, we helped him to rechannel the internal confirmation cycles by which he had been sustaining a depressogenic image of himself.

CONCLUSION

The self-confirmation model provides a template for understanding the dynamics of various therapeutic theories and for seeing them in relation to one another. The feedback loop schema portrays the individual's ways of perpetuating a stable sense of self in the midst of a variable environment. This is done largely by shunting aside experience that is too self-dissonant, although a moderate degree of novelty will be experienced as positive by most people and can be utilized as a force for therapeutic change.

Interventions of various kinds have primary impact on different stages of the feedback loop, thus differentiating them, and yet all interventions have the common effect of rechannelling the cycle as a whole. The latter characteristic provides a basis for integrating the methods emphasized by different schools. This has been exemplified above by comparing the general change principles espoused by different orientations, by coordinating various etiological-therapeutic accounts of depression, and in the closing case study. The self-confirmational model set forth in Table 1 also offers the possibility of devising new interventions to fill gaps in existing therapeutic methods.

REFERENCES

Abramson, L., Seligman, M., & Teasdale, J. (1978). Learned helplessness in humans: Critique and reformulation. *Journal of Abnormal Psychology, 87,* 49–74.

Andrews, J. (1977). Personal change and intervention style. *Journal of Humanistic Psychology, 17,* 41–63.

Andrews, J. (1988). Self-confirmation theory: A paradigm for psychotherapy integration. Part I. Content analysis of therapeutic styles. *Journal of Integrative and Eclectic Psychotherapy, 7,* 359–384.

Andrews, J. (1989). Psychotherapy of depression: A self-confirmation model. *Psychological Review, 96,* 576–607.

Andrews, J. (1990). Interpersonal self-confirmation and challenge in psychotherapy. *Psychotherapy, 27,* 485–504.

Andrews, J. (1981). *The active self in psychotherapy: An integration of therapeutic styles.* Boston: Allyn & Bacon.

Anton, J., Dunbar, J., & Friedman, L. (1976). Anticipation training in the treatment of depression. In J. Krumboltz and C. Thorensen (Eds.), *Counseling methods.* New York: Holt, Rinehart & Winston.

Arieti, S., & Bemporad J. (1978). *Severe and mild depression.* New York: Basic Books.

Bandura, A. (1978). Reflections on self-efficacy. *Advances in Behavior Research and Therapy, 1,* 237–269.

Baumeister, R. (1982). A self-presentational view of social phenomena. *Psychological Bulletin, 91,* 3–26.

Beck, A. (1976). *Cognitive therapy and the emotional disorders.* New York: International Universities Press.

Beck, A., Rush, A., Shaw, B., & Emery, G. (1979). *Cognitive therapy of depression.* New York: Guilford.

Biglan, A., & Dow, M. (1981). Toward a second-generation model: A problem-specific approach. In L. Rehm (Ed.), *Behavior therapy for depression: Present status and future directions.* New York: Academic.

Blatt, S. (1974). Levels of object representation in anaclitic and introjective depression. *Psychoanalytic Study of the Child, 29,* 107–157.

Bordin, E. (1979). The generalizability of the psychoanalytic concept of the working alliance. *Psychotherapy: Theory, Research, and Practice, 16,* 252–260.

Broxton, J. (1963). A rest of interpersonal attraction predictions derived from balance theory. *Journal of Abnormal and Social Psychology, 66,* 394–397.

Burgess, E. (1969). The modification of depressive behaviors. In R. Rubin and C. Franks (Eds.), *Advances in behavior therapy, 1968.* New York: Academic.

Burns, R. (1979). *The self-concept in theory, measurement, development, and behavior.* London: Longman.

Cane, D., & Gotlib, I. (1985). Implicit conceptualizations of depression: Implications for an interpersonal perspective. *Social Cognition, 3,* 341–368.

Caple, M., & Blechman, E. (1976). *Problem-solving and self-approval training with a depressed single mother.* Paper presented at the meeting of the Association for the Advancement of Behavior Therapy, New York.

Carver, C., & Scheier, M. (1981). *Attention and self-regulation.* New York: Springer-Verlag.

Conn, L., & Crowne, D. (1964). Instigation to aggression, emotional arousal and defensive emulation. *Journal of Personality, 32,* 163–179.

Costello, C. (1972). Depression: Loss of reinforcers or loss of reinforcer effectiveness? *Behavior Therapy, 3,* 240–247.

Coyne, J. (1976). Toward an interactional description of depression. *Psychiatry, 39,* 28–40.

Craighead, W. (1980). Away from a unitary model of depression. *Behavior Therapy, 11,* 122–128.

Dengerink, H., & Myers, J. (1977). The effects of failure and depression on subsequent aggression. *Journal of Personality and Social Psychology, 35,* 88–96.

Ellis, A. (1962). *Reason and emotion in psychotherapy.* New York: Lyle Stuart.

Erikson, E. (1959). *Identity and the life cycle.* New York: International Universities Press.

Felker, D. (1974). *Building positive self-concepts.* Minneapolis: Burgess.

Ferster, C. (1966). Animal behavior and mental illness. *Psychological Record, 16,* 345–356.

Ferster, C. (1973). A functional analysis of depression. *American Psychologist, 28,* 857–870.

Freud, S. (1959). Mourning and melancholia. In *Collected papers* (Vol. 3). New York: Basic Books.

Gaylin, W. (1968). *The meaning of despair: Psychoanalytic contributions to the understanding of depression.* New York: Science House.

Glass, D. (1978). An evaluation of a brief treatment for depression based on the learned helplessness model. *Dissertation Abstracts International, 39,* 2495B. (University Microfilms No. 78-20, 221).

Goldfried, M., & Robins, C. (1982). On the facilitation of self-efficacy. *Cognitive Therapy and Research, 6,* 361–379.

Golombiewski, R., & Blumberg, A. (1970). *Sensitivity training and the laboratory approach.* Itasca, IL: Peacock.

Greenberg, L., & Safran, J. (1981). Encoding and cognitive therapy: Changing what clients attend to. *Psychotherapy: Theory, Research, and Practice. 18,* 163–169.

Greenwald, A., & Pratkanis, A. (1984). The self. In R. Wyer & T. Srull (Eds.), *Handbook of social cognition* (Vol. 3). Hillsdale, NJ: Erlbaum.

Hamilton, D. (1969). Responses to cognitive inconsistencies: Personality, discrepancy level, and response stability. *Journal of Personality and Social Psychology, 11,* 351–362.

Holloman, C., & Hendrick, H. (1972). Effects of sensitivity training on tolerance for dissonance. *Journal of Applied Behavioral Science, 8,* 174–187.

Hollon, S., & Garber, J. (1980). A cognitive-expectancy theory of therapy for helplessness and depression. In J. Garber & M. Seligman (Eds.), *Human helplessness.* New York: Academic.

Horowitz, L., Wright, J., Lowenstein, E., & Parad, H. (1981). The prototype as a construct in abnormal psychology: I. A method for deriving prototypes. *Journal of Abnormal Psychology, 90,* 568–574.

Horowitz, M. (1979). *States of mind.* New York: Plenum Press.

Ingram, R. (1984). Toward an information-processing analysis of depression. *Cognitive Therapy and Research, 8,* 433–477.

Jackson, B. (1972). Treatment of depression by self-reinforcement. *Behavior Therapy, 3,* 298–307.

Jacobson, E. (1968). Transference problems in the psychoanalytic treatment of severely depressive patients. In W. Gaylin (Ed.), *The meaning of despair: Psychoanalytic contributions to the understanding of depression.* New York: Science House.

Johansson, S., Lewinsohn, P., & Flippo, J. (1969, November). *An application of the Premack principle to the verbal behavior of depressed subjects.* Paper presented at the meeting of the Association for the Advancement of Behavior Therapy. Washington, DC.

Kelly, G. (1955). *The psychology of personal constructs.* New York: Norton.

Kiesler, D. (1982). Interpersonal theory for personality and psychotherapy. In J. Anchin and D. Kiesler (Eds.), *Handbook of interpersonal psychotherapy.* New York: Pergamon.

Kiesler, D. (1983). The 1982 interpersonal circle: A taxonomy for complementarity in human transactions. *Psychological Review, 90,* 185–214.

Kohut, H. (1977). *The restoration of the self.* New York: International Universities Press.

Kohut, H. (1984). *How does analysis cure?* Chicago: University of Chicago Press.

Kuiper, N., MacDonald, M., & Derry, P. (1983). Parameters of a depressive self-schema. In J. Suls & A. Greenwald (Eds.), *Psychological perspectives on the self* (Vol. 2). Hillsdale, NJ: Erlbaum.

Kuiper, N., & Olinger, L. (1986). Dysfunctional attitudes and a self-worth contingency model of depression. In P. Kendall (Ed.), *Advances in cognitive-behavioral research and therapy* (Vol. 5). New York: Academic.

Layne, C. (1980). Motivational deficit in depression: People's expectations outcomes' impacts. *Journal of Clinical Psychology, 36,* 647–652.

Layne, C., Merry, J., Christian, J., & Ginn, P. (1982). Motivational deficit in depression. *Cognitive Therapy and Research, 6,* 259–274.

Lazarus, A. (1968). Learning theory and the treatment of depression. *Behavior Research and Therapy, 6,* 83–89.

Lazarus, A. (1981). *The practice of multimodal therapy.* New York: McGraw-Hill.

Leary, T. (1957). *Interpersonal diagnosis of personality.* New York: Ronald.

Lecky, P. (1951). *Self-consistency: A theory of personality* (2nd ed.). Long Island, NY: Island.

Lewinsohn, P. (1974). A behavioral approach to depression. In R. Friedman and M. Katz (Eds.), *The psychology of depression: Contemporary theory and research.* Washington, DC: Winston.

Lewinsohn, P. (1976). Behavioral treatment of depression. In P. Davidson (Ed.), *The behavioral management of anxiety, depression and pain.* New York: Brunner/Mazel.

Liberman, R. (1981). A model for individualizing treatment. In L. Rehm (Ed.), *Behavior therapy for depression: Present status and future directions.* New York: Academic.

Liberman, R., & Raskin, D. (1971). Depression: A behavioral formulation. *Archives of General Psychiatry, 24,* 515–523.

Lorand, S. (1968). Dynamics of therapy of depressive states. In W. Gaylin (Ed.), *The meaning of despair: Psycho-*

analytic contributions to the understanding of depression. New York: Science House.

Mahoney, M. (1971). The self-management of covert behavior: A case study. *Behavior Therapy, 2,* 575–578.

Mancuso, J., & Sarbin, T. (1983). The self-narrative in the enactment of roles. In T. Sarbin & K. Sheibe (Eds.), *Studies in social identity.* New York: Praeger.

McCullough, J. (1984). Cognitive-behavioral analysis system of psychotherapy: An interactional treatment approach for dysthymic disorder. *Psychiatry, 47,* 234–250.

McFarlin, D., & Blascovich, J. (1981). Effects of self-esteem and performance feedback on future affective preferences and cognitive expectations. *Journal of Personality and Social Psychology, 40,* 521–531.

McLean, P. (1976). Therapeutic decision-making in the behavioral treatment of depression. In P. Davison (Ed.), *The behavioral management of anxiety, depression, and pain.* New York: Brunner/Mazel.

O'Brien, J. (1978). The behavioral treatment of acute reactive depression involving psychotic manifestations. *Journal of Behavior Therapy and Experimental Psychiatry, 9,* 259–264.

Perls, F. (1969). *Gestalt therapy verbatim.* Lafayette, CA: Real People.

Perls, F., Hefferline, R., & Goodman, P. (1951). *Gestalt therapy.* New York: Julian.

Poag, J. (1991). *The effect of self-discrepancy feedback and the observation of therapist empathy on selective information seeking.* Unpublished doctoral dissertation, California School of Professional Psychology, San Diego, CA.

Pyszczynski, T., & Greenberg, J. (1985). Depression and preference for self-focusing stimuli after success and failure. *Journal of Personality and Social Psychology, 49,* 1066–1075.

Pyszczynski, T., & Greenberg, J. (1987). Self-regulatory perseveration and the depressive self-focusing style: A self-awareness theory of reactive depression. *Psychological Bulletin, 102,* 122–138.

Rehm, L. (1977). A self-control model of depression. *Behavior Therapy, 8,* 787–804.

Rogers, C. (1951). *Client-centered therapy.* Boston: Houghton Mifflin.

Rosenberg, M. (1979). *Conceiving the self.* New York: Basic Books.

Rush, A., Khatami, M., & Beck, A. (1975). Cognitive and behavior therapy in chronic depression. *Behavior Therapy, 6,* 398–404.

Sacco, W., and Beck, A. (1985). Cognitive therapy of depression. In E. Beckman & W. Leber (Eds.), *Handbook of depression: Treatment, assessment, and research.* Homewood, IL: Dorsey.

Sammons, R. (1974). *Systematic resensitization in the treatment of depression.* Paper presented at the meeting of the Association for the Advancement of Behavior Therapy, Chicago.

Schmickley, V. (1976). Effects of cognitive-behavior modification upon depressed outpatients. *Dissertation Abstracts International, 37,* 987–988B. (University Microfilms No. 76-18, 675).

Secord, P., & Backman, C. (1961). Personality theory and the problem of stability and change in individual behav-

ior: An interpersonal approach. *Psychological Review, 68,* 21–32.

Seligman, M. (1974). Depression and learned helplessness. In R. Friedman and M. Katz (Eds.), *The psychology of depression: Contemporary theory and research.* Washington, DC: Winston.

Seligman, M. (1975). *Helplessness: On depression, development, and death.* San Francisco: Freeman.

Shipley, C., & Fazio, A. (1973). Pilot study of a treatment for psychological depression. *Journal of Abnormal Psychology, 82,* 372–376.

Simkin, J. (1979). Gestalt therapy. In R. Corsini (Ed.), *Current psychotherapies* (2nd ed.). Itasca, IL: Peacock.

Stryker, S. (1985). Symbolic interaction and role theory. In G. Lindzey and E. Aronson (Eds.), *Handbook of social psychology* (3rd ed., Vol. I). New York: Random House.

Sullivan, H. (1953). *The interpersonal theory of psychiatry.* New York: Norton.

Swann, W. (1983). Self-verification: Bringing social reality into harmony with the self. In J. Suls & A. Greenwald (Eds.), *Psychological perspectives on the self* (Vol. 2). Hillsdale, NJ: Erlbaum.

Swann, W. (1985). The self as architect of social reality. In B. Schlenker (Ed.), *The self and social life.* New York: McGraw-Hill.

Swann, W. (1987). Identity negotiation: Where two roads meet. *Journal of Personality and Social Psychology, 53,* 1038–1051.

Swann, W., & Ely, R. (1984). A battle of wills: Self-verification versus behavioral confirmation. *Journal of Personality and Social Psychology, 46,* 1287–1302.

Swann, W., & Hill, C. (1982). When our identities are mistaken: Reaffirming self-conceptions through social interaction. *Journal of Personality and Social Psychology, 43,* 59–66.

Swann, W. & Predmore, S. (1985). Intimates as agents of social support: Sources of consolation or despair? *Journal of Personality and Social Psychology, 49,* 1609–1617.

Tharp, R., Watson, D., & Kaya, J. (1974). Self-modification of depression. *Journal of Consulting and Clinical Psychology, 42,* 624.

Weissman, M., Klerman, G., Rounsaville, B., Chevron, E., & Neu, C. (1982). Short-term interpersonal psychotherapy (IPT) for depression: Description and efficacy. In J. Anchin & D. Kiesler (Eds.), *Handbook of interpersonal psychotherapy.* New York: Pergamon.

Wells, K., Hersen, J., Bellack, A., & Himmelhoch, J. (1977). *Social skills training for unipolar depressive females.* Paper presented at the meeting of the Association for the Advancement of Behavior Therapy, Atlanta.

Winnicott, D. (1965). *The maturational processes and the facilitating environment.* New York: International Universities Press.

Wolberg, L. (1967). *The technique of psychotherapy* (2nd ed.). New York: Grune & Stratton.

Wolpe, J. (1969). *The practice of behavior therapy.* New York: Pergamon.

Wolpe, J. (1970). The instigation of assertive behavior: Transcripts from two cases. *Journal of Behavior Therapy and Experimental Psychiatry, 1,* 145–151.

Yalom, I. (1980). *Existential psychotherapy.* New York: Basic Books.

PART III

The Integration of Traditional and Nontraditional Approaches

A Hermeneutic Approach to Integration: Psychotherapy within the Circle of Practical Activity

Michael A. Westerman

INTRODUCTION

In many ways, psychotherapy appears to be characterized by circles. Patients want to change, but they approach their problems in a manner that reflects the very problems of concern. In particular, patients often engage in the therapeutic relationship in ways that replicate the interpersonal difficulties they hope to resolve. Therapists, for their part, try to help, but they bring their own feelings and conflicts to the therapeutic situation. Furthermore, insofar as therapy involves helping patients to accept more responsibility for their own lives, there is the circle or paradox of trying to influence another person so that he or she will become self-directed.

What if these observations are true in a fun-

Michael A. Westerman • Clinical Psychology Doctoral Program, New York University, New York, New York 10003.

Comprehensive Handbook of Psychotherapy Integration, edited by George Stricker and Jerold R. Gold. Plenum Press, New York, 1993.

damental sense? That is, what if psychotherapy *is* circular in nature? Beyond this, what if life in general is characterized by circles? These ideas actually reflect a particular philosophical perspective, which argues that we always approach things from within the context of our involvement with those things, never from the outside as an onlooker. We are always inside what is called the "hermeneutic circle."

In this chapter, I will try to show that it is useful for those interested in psychotherapy to turn to a consideration of basic philosophical issues. For one thing, this is true because current therapy models and, in good measure, actual clinical practice reflect the influence of basic ideas from the philosophical tradition. These ideas lead us to believe that we can explain away the circular nature of therapy in terms of some different picture of the therapeutic process. In what follows, I will suggest that these attempts to step outside of the circle have concrete implications for actual clinical work, limiting the effectiveness of therapists' efforts. I will also suggest that this is not an isolated "mistake." The view that we can step out of the circle as patients, therapists, therapy researchers, and philosophers is fundamental to the philosophical tradition. Moreover, I will suggest that the appearance of this "mistake" at the level of an individual person's approach to his or her life is central to the nature of psychopathology.

There is also a positive reason for engaging in basic philosophical considerations. Although the philosophical tradition suggests that we can step outside the circle, the hermeneutic philosophical perspective clearly points away from such an attempt. It provides a foundation for a different framework for psychotherapy. This framework includes useful ways to think about the nature of psychopathology, the roles of patient and therapist in the change process, the role played by the therapeutic relationship, and how to employ different intervention techniques.

With respect to interventions, the framework incorporates the major types of interventions with which we are familiar, including insight-oriented, behavioral, and strategic techniques. On the level of concepts, it reflects the influence of ideas from the psychodynamic, behavioral, and experiential traditions. What is different about the framework that will be presented here, first of all, is that it includes together these supposedly divergent and often warring sets of interventions and concepts. But it does not include them in an uncritical, "all are welcome" manner. The approach is an integrative framework that places these elements in a new light. It provides its own view of how to make best use of those elements, and it also helps us to avoid mistakes promoted by the other approaches.

I have discussed the hermeneutic therapy framework in several other places (Westerman, 1986, 1989). This chapter summarizes those presentations. It also includes several major additions to the earlier discussions.

THEORETICAL POSITION: THE PHILOSOPHICAL PERSPECTIVE

If we turn to a consideration of philosophical points of view, it becomes clear that the temptation to step outside the circle is strong. Our philosophical tradition is *based* on the notion of the uninvolved subject. As many scholars have pointed

out, the tradition includes two main currents, empiricism and rationalism. We typically view these two perspectives as very different from each other, but according to *both*, the basic question about how to understand the knowing relationship is the founding issue for philosophy. Furthermore, *both* assume that the knowing relationship involves a subject approaching an object, with subject and object conceptualized as separate, unrelated terms at the outset. This starting point leads to familiar conclusions: Either the subject or person is described as an active, free, autonomous agent *or* the person is taken to be a passive automaton with thoughts and behavior determined by the external world. Knowledge is said to reflect radical subjectivity *or* objective truth. The world of things and events is taken to reflect deep, abstract meanings *or* it is made up of many, many essentially dead or meaningless "building block" objects and behaviors.

The philosophical work of Wittgenstein (1958), Merleau-Ponty (1962), and Heidegger (1962) offers a very different perspective (cf. Dreyfus, 1979; Westerman, 1987) that takes the hermeneutic circle as fundamental. Prior to the knowing relationship, there is what Merleau-Ponty (1962) called "involved subjectivity." The subject or person is actively involved in practical activity in the world before he or she approaches any particular object of inquiry. First off, we are engaged in doing things as embodied and social beings. Our prior active involvement in the world provides a background against which we come to know any new thing. If we switch to this starting point instead of the one both wings of the philosophical tradition start from, we end up with practical activity as the bottom line when it comes to how to think about the nature of the person, meaning, knowledge, human behavior, and also psychotherapy. This bottom line is very different from the positions at *either* pole of the all too familiar antinomies.

Thinking and Self-Awareness

In order to clarify this perspective, I will need to point out a number of possible misinterpretations. First, the focus on practical activity does not lead to the conclusion that thinking and self-awareness, or what Merleau-Ponty (1962) referred to as "thematized understanding," do not exist. We can think about the world, ourselves, other people and events with ideas and beliefs, but when we reflect we always do this in terms of our prior familiarity with practical activities, which Merleau-Ponty (1962) called "prereflective understanding."

Does this mean that thematized understanding is merely epiphenomenal? No. The fact that we can think about things in a thematized way greatly changes our relationship to the world from what it would be if it were based on pre-reflective understanding alone. It makes a big difference that we can reflect on things, but thematized understanding is never complete and self-contained. It is always based on practical know-how and that is never completely transparent to us. Although at times it may seem otherwise, it is not possible to strike a third-person relationship to the world or to oneself. We always think about things from inside our active involvement in the world. Later, I will return to these remarks when I discuss the implications of the philosophical perspective for understanding the role played by insight in therapy.

The Nature of Practical Activity

Further clarification is called for because it may well seem that the insistence on the primacy of action indicates that, in the terms of traditional debates, the perspective is on the side of the world, not on the side of the subject. The key point concerns the question: What is practical know-how? According to the hermeneutic perspective, it is not made up of specific responses to stimuli in specific situations, no matter how complicated chains of behavior "simples" may be. Notwithstanding the emphasis on action, we are not turning to a behaviorist view or to any other empiricist position. The empiricist perspective assumes that the person is separate from the object (this is made explicit with the notion of the person as *tabula rasa*). The hermeneutic position, on the other hand, argues that the person always has a *starting point*. The object, or "stimulus," always has its significance with respect to the role it plays in a person's practical activities, which are characterized by purpose, goals, and meaning. Practices are not "just" a string of behaviors. We have not gone over to a dead, mechanical view of the world and life.

It is tempting to take recourse to other traditional notions in order to understand the starting point idea. The hermeneutic perspective emphasizes the role of interpretation (indeed, this is the most common association to the term *hermeneutic*), but this is not to say that there is an ideal realm of abstract meanings, templates, conventions, rules, or formal structures as the rationalists would have it. I am not saying, for example, that the thoughts we are aware of rest on pre-reflective understanding, which is out of awareness but still of the same basic nature as the processes described by rationalism. The abstract categories of rationalism provide one way of arguing that the object is always apprehended with respect to something the subject brings to the situation, not as a brute fact. But note that this reflects the idea of the removed knower. To begin with, subject and object are separate. The subject brings a set of categories, templates, and the like *to* the epistemic relationship. It is very different to suggest that the starting point is practical familiarity. First off, the person is involved in doing things in the world, not a knowing agent equipped with a theory or categories of understanding. Practical activity itself is meaningful. Meaning inheres in the activity, not in some realm of ideas that lies behind it. We view things from within them, from the viewpoint of a participant living life.

This is what Wittgenstein (1958) meant when he said the meaning of a word is its use, and when he said that what he called "our form of life," the "grammar" of our everyday lives, are bedrock. He pointed out that an activity can be orderly without being rule-governed. Practical activity is meaningful and *concrete* at the same time. We can never get beyond the need to point to *concrete* examples and say "this is an example of what I mean." If we take our involvement in the world as the starting point, we arrive at the view that there is meaning but it is what *cannot* be said. Instead, we can point to examples of meaningful things and we can engage in meaningful practices. Looking ahead, in the therapy framework based on this philosophical perspective the focus is on patterns of practical activity. These patterns are complex and meaningful, but they are also irreducibly concrete in nature, not ideal.

One more point should be made about practical activity. The emphasis on action is not meant to detract from the importance of emotions. The perspective is not about dispassionate behaviors. As noted above, intentions, purposes, goals—or what Heidegger (1962) called "concern" (how things matter to us)—are central to the nature of action patterns. Emotions are not left out of the picture. At the same time, the perspective offers its own view of emotion. According to the hermeneutic approach, emotions are not private, subjective experiences primarily. Rather, affective experiences *per se* play a part within patterns of action. Emotions themselves are organized action patterns. For example, anger refers to action patterns that are set in motion when a person is blocked in reaching a goal. I should note that this idea is entirely compatible with a recent view in the emotion literature that argues for a functionalist approach to emotion (Fischer, Shaver, & Carnochan, 1988, 1990; Greenberg & Safran, 1987; Safran & Greenberg, 1986; Westen, 1985, 1986). Hence, from the standpoint of the hermeneutic perspective, it is possible—indeed, it is absolutely necessary—to think about psychotherapy in a way in which emotion plays a central role.

View of the Person and an Ethics of Interdependence

The perspective is not on the "side of the world," but we did not get to this conclusion by placing the perspective on the "side of the subject." Rather, we arrived at the view that the person and life are more than mechanical and dead by sticking with the very commonsensical idea that from the outset we are engaged in the world *from our particular point within it* (our bodies, our community, general history, individual history, and particular location).

This leads to fundamental ideas about the person that are unsettling in some respects and also difficult to grasp as compared to the familiar ideas of the tradition (however extreme and noncommonsensical the notions of an unconditionally free, autonomous subject or a passive automaton may be). The hermeneutic perspective demotes the status of the person considerably as compared to how the person is viewed by rationalists. The person is not radically free nor fully autonomous. We always come to situations from our starting points. We can never see things "as they are" nor make choices *de novo*. As Sampson (1988)

argued in his recent discussion of "ensembled individualism," we can never be independent of the social world and our history. At the same time, with respect to autonomy, we are the ones leading our lives, and with respect to freedom, we can change—but always from our starting points.

Although this viewpoint demotes the status of the person in important respects, it is also empowering and constructive. It provides its own basis for respecting people. In contrast to the philosophical tradition, which argues that we should respect each other because as uninvolved subjects we share access to *the* point of view (the removed perspective of the knower), the hermeneutic perspective suggests that the basis for respect is the fact that each person lives his or her life from *a* point of view. The hermeneutic perspective provides the foundation for an *ethics of interdependence*. It provides a basis for sharing and helping, because we are all part of the shared world with similar bodies, a shared history as members of the species, and a largely shared history as members of the community. But by themselves these considerations point to an ethics of dependency—the notion that we are interchangeable bees in a bee hive. The hermeneutic perspective offers a different view from this because it clearly points out that there will be differences and conflict. Genuine respect, empathy, and compassion involve accepting and appreciating these fundamental differences—recognizing that one of the central things we "share" is the fact of being different, that we each lead our own lives. Looking ahead once again, these ideas about the person and an ethics of interdependence will provide a foundation for understanding the role of patient and therapist in therapy and the nature of the therapeutic relationship.

Stepping Outside the Circle

Why is it that these ideas are hard to grasp, while at the same time they represent very human, reasonable notions? Why are the traditional notions easier to understand although they lead to such longstanding conundrums as whether it is ever right for one person to try to influence another even if it is for the sake of offering help?

At the onset, I suggested that what is misguided about traditional philosophy does not simply reflect an isolated, albeit enormous, "mistake." Actually, it reflects a very basic phenomenon, one that occurs all the time, not just when it comes to philosophizing or thinking about therapy. Merleau-Ponty (1962) argued that by its nature perception "covers itself over." When we perceive something it is always against the background of our practical familiarity with things. But perception "covers over" this connection. We believe we see the object "out there" as it is "in itself." Merleau-Ponty (1962) referred to this as the "prejudice in favor of the world."

The idea here is similar to more recent work on cognitive development, such as Piaget's (e.g., 1983) well-known theory or Fischer's (1980) skill theory. The prejudice in favor of the world is a by-product of adaptation. Even though there is not a separate, dead world "out there," the world is not whatever we want it to be. It is real. By no means does it always conform to our wishes and expectations. Hence, we learn to modulate our behavior with respect to the things we encounter. We begin to shift away from an egocentric viewpoint during the early months of our lives (e.g., the development of the concept of the permanent object) and go on from there to develop increasingly adaptive ways of modulating our behavior.

Therefore, even in our most basic perceptions and actions there is the basis for the "mistake" of neglecting the connection to the object. For example, it becomes very tempting to neglect the fact that the cup over there has its place in a world of practical activity, namely, it is at the other end of my grasp, something to use for drinking (sustaining basic needs of the body), a tool that also plays a role in social practices about polite, hygienic eating and drinking, and so forth. The truth is that we learn to modulate our behavior with respect to the cup not for what it is "in itself" but rather in terms of what works with cups in the context of our practical activities given the purposes of those activities and the nature of our bodies. Nevertheless, learning to interact more and more successfully with the objects in our lives involves packing more of that connection into the background, organizing our behavior "as if" the things are out there in themselves.

This sets the stage at a very fundamental level for neglecting our connection to the things and events that make up our lives. It prepares the way for the philosophers who have advanced the notion of the uninvolved subject and makes that notion so appealing to the layman, notwithstanding the fact that it is extremely curious, even bizarre in many respects. But these are not the immediate consequences of the way perception and action "cover over" the person's connection to the world. Well before we get to the point of the philosopher's abstract theorizing, "covering over" processes can lead to problematic ways of relating to oneself and to the world at a very personal level. In what follows, I will suggest that this fundamental process not only sets the stage for misguided philosophizing and misguided theorizing when it comes to psychotherapy, but that it also plays a central role in psychopathology.

CLINICAL ANTECEDENTS

In what follows, I will present an approach to psychotherapy based on the hermeneutic philosophical perspective. The approach is an integrative framework that reflects the influence of the major established perspectives on therapy to a great extent. Specifically, the approach reflects the influence of behavior therapy in its use of active interventions, a psychodynamic orientation with its focus on defenses and transference phenomena, Sullivan's (1953) work because it emphasizes the role played by interpersonal processes in psychopathology and in the change process, and the experiential tradition by its insistence on recognizing and respecting what I refer to as the patient's starting point and his or her capacity to move beyond that starting point. But as noted at the outset, while the influence of these approaches on the present perspective is enormous when it comes to concepts and intervention techniques, the perspective places these influences in a new framework. The goal is to reinterpret and reinvigorate these influences by discovering and clarifying what is of value in them in terms of the new perspective, and also by identifying how clinical work is often limited when we employ those techniques in ways that reflect misguided features of the originating perspectives.

I should also note that this perspective is *not* similar to recent work along the lines of what has been called a hermeneutic approach to psychoanalysis (e.g., Spence, 1982), notwithstanding the common use of the label *hermeneutic*. The hermeneutic approach to psychoanalysis is actually based on a different philosophical perspective (e.g., Husserl, 1931) in which subjectivity is given preeminent status—and the subject is viewed as a bystander as in the philosophical tradition. The "circle" of interest to these philosophers and their exponents in the psychoanalytic camp has to do with how one's specific perceptions and beliefs cannot escape one's general viewpoint, which itself is conceptualized in ideal terms (how I think about things) rather than one's involvement in the shared world of practical activity. From this vantage point, we end up with radical subjectivity. Elsewhere, I have discussed the limitations of this approach as a basis for therapy (Westerman, 1984).

In this section on clinical antecedents, I should note that my approach reflects the influence of a number of contributors to the psychotherapy literature who also have endeavored to provide integrative frameworks that bring together valuable elements of traditional approaches—often with reference to general/philosophical considerations along lines similar to those offered here. My work draws on Wachtel's (1977, 1987a; Sollod & Wachtel, 1980) seminal contributions to therapy integration and important contributions by Safran and Greenberg (1986; Greenberg & Safran, 1987; Safran, 1989), Mahoney (1988), and Arkowitz (1989, Arkowitz & Hannah, 1989).

APPROACH TO PSYCHOTHERAPY

Conceptualization of Psychopathology

The hermeneutic philosophical perspective suggests an approach to psychotherapy aimed at helping patients make changes in the action patterns that make up how they live their lives. That is, the central focus is on patterns of action, not on how patients think about themselves and the world, nor on specific problematic behaviors— although cognitions and behaviors have a place within the general framework. This viewpoint follows directly from the idea that the person's involvement in the world of practical activities is the touchstone.

Several points should be made about the nature of problematic patterns. These are consistent with the basic perspective, although they are not necessarily implied by it. First, problems of concern in therapy are frequently interpersonal in nature. From the standpoint of the philosophical perspective, *all* human action is interpersonal in the sense that ultimately it must be understood in terms of the role it plays in the shared world of social practices. But what is meant here is a simpler idea. Most therapy issues concern interpersonal *relationships*—that is, the "social" comes into play in an intimate, personal sense. At times, this is obvious (e.g., a marital difficulty). At other times, it is not so obvious (e.g., a problem with schoolwork that reflects fears of becoming successful and independent from parents).

Another feature of problematic patterns is that typically they are very general, sometimes almost all-pervasive. They appear in many different domains of a person's life (relationships with spouse, parents, friends, in the realm of work, in the individual's relationship to self), and across different levels of analysis from the molar (e.g., choice of spouse) to the moment-to-moment (e.g., aspects of turn-taking in conversations). Note that these comments about the generality of problematic patterns are *not* meant to suggest that they are based on ideas, "internal" mental contents, or abstract structures that lie beneath them.

Another point is that patterns of concern usually have their origin in childhood. Interactions with caregivers and the family system at large lead to the internalization of what were initially patterns of interpersonal interaction, including patterns more or less general to the species or culture and patterns that are personal and idiosyncratic (cf. Kaye, 1984). It is important not to jump to conclusions about the therapeutic implications of this point. In particular, this claim (the childhood origins of *action patterns*) does not lead to suggestions about the value of archaeological reconstructions of early experience.

Defense. So far, I have suggested that the problems of interest are action patterns, that these patterns characterize a person's behavior quite generally, and that they often have their origin in childhood. But what is it about the patterns of concern in therapy that make them problematic? To be sure, these problems are quite diverse, but I believe that most are similar in one important sense. Furthermore, I believe the philosophical perspective provides the basis for understanding this key feature. At bottom, problematic patterns involve what is, in a sense, a breach in the connection of the person to the world. This connection is the founding term of the philosophical perspective, but with the notion of the prejudice in favor of the world, the perspective identifies a fundamental way in which we all step outside the circle of this connection in a sense. As I develop this point about how the prejudice in favor of the world provides a foundation for thinking about the nature of psychopathology, it will become clear that my remarks also reflect the influence of the Freudian notion of defense. Indeed, my viewpoint is similar enough to Freud's on this issue that I will use the term *defense*, notwithstanding the fact the term comes with a great deal of theoretical baggage I do not wish to import.

I explained above that patterns of interaction with objects, for example, a cup, have "packed" within them a rich background reflecting our connection to the object, for example, the characteristics of our hands, social practices about polite eating, and so forth. Paradoxically, precisely because we learn to modulate our behavior with respect to the object in a way that takes into account the background (goals, nature of our bodies, etc.)—to "pack" the background into what we do with the object—it is as if these things are what they are "in themselves." This makes for slippery footing. We can slip and find ourselves out of the circle. This is especially true when it comes to the personal realms of life. People also modulate what they do (including their actions, emotions, and views of others and themselves) to control what happens in their relationships with others. Powerful capacities of this sort are no doubt essential for participating in the complex social and personal activities basic to human life. But, to use Freudian concepts, our goals or *wishes* cannot always be realized. This leads to *fears* about how things will turn out. Frequently, we adapt our actions to take these fears into account in ways that work quite well (e.g., finding a polite way to request a raise from your boss even though you feel a raise is long overdue), but our rich and complex abilities for modulating our actions can also lead to pursuing a wish in a limited, distorted, overly protective, or defensive way. When that happens, we no longer fully embrace the wish. In fact, defensive action patterns actually

make it impossible to really have our wishes met, even though the patterns are safe in the sense that they make it less likely that feared consequences will occur.

To use Merleau-Ponty's phrase, our connection to the world gets "covered over." We have stepped out of the circle, not by adopting the philosopher's theoretical ideas about the "uninvolved subject," but by becoming less fully involved in our lives. I am suggesting that these two movements have a common basis. They are pitfalls created by the basic nature of our relationship to the world, which sets the stage for the prejudice in favor of the world.

Note that I have not said that the wish gets "covered over" because we deny or repress it, or that the fundamental problem in how a person deals with his or her fears is failing to be aware of them. These internal processes frequently occur but they are secondary to the basic process, which concerns organizing one's actions in a defensive way. It is not that we put the wish out of awareness and so we behave differently, but the other way around. Defense is primarily a matter of engaging in the world in ways that try to protect against feared consequences at the expense of pursuing our goals in action in a straightforward, direct manner. Internal processes play a role *within* these action patterns. This is the fundamental point of divergence between the view of defense offered here and the Freudian position. As will become clear below, this leads to important differences in terms of interventions.

Consider two examples of defensive action patterns. One example involved a male patient who was constantly striving—putting in long hours at his job as a manager, taking responsibility for many aspects of the care of his children, and devoting a great deal of time responding to his mother's requests for help running the small business she owned. This patient felt some sense of accomplishment and even enjoyment in these efforts, but there was also a great deal of resentment and strain. Nevertheless, he simply could not say "no." He had a deep longing to be noticed, that is, to be acknowledged as a person with feelings and needs. But he was also afraid that if noticed, he would be found to be incompetent, unintelligent, and unattractive. His pattern of living his life was a defensive attempt to avoid rejection by performing in response to others' requests. Another example involved a young woman who filled up sessions with almost nonstop, highly intellectualized talk, broken only occasionally by asking her therapist, "Does that make sense?" This patient had a powerful wish to be heard and understood, and a wish for guidance and direction. She was also extremely afraid that the others she turned to (including her therapist) would let her down by failing to be there for her or by taking a critical, harsh, demanding stance toward her. Her in-session behavior exemplified a defensive pattern in which she attempted to discover if others would be there for her in the sense of going along with her own very controlling way of doing things (e.g., attending to her long monologues and responding "on cue" to her requests for feedback).

These examples illustrate several key characteristics of defensive action patterns. First, they are characterized by what Freudians refer to as conflict. The issue is not the presence of an inappropriate behavior or a deficit of a desired behavior. This observation also does *not* mean that they are motivated by *internal* conflicts, or that there is strife between the person and others. Rather, the point is that the patterns are two-sided. For example, the patient in the second example sought concerned, attentive responsiveness from her therapist, but she pursued that wish in a way that greatly limited the therapist's opportunities to respond to her. Another characteristic is that people who live their lives defensively often experience themselves in binds. For example, it might well be very difficult for the patient who "fills up" sessions to figure out how to respond to a remark by her therapist that goes beyond the simple response, "Yes, that makes sense." Although such a remark may show interest and concern, the patient may well view it as an interruption or a "refusal" to respond in the expected manner. This example also illustrates another point about defensive patterns, which is that they create binds for the other people in a patient's life, including therapists. The therapist working with this patient might well believe that whichever way he goes, things will not go well. As just noted, a comment that goes beyond "Yes, that makes sense" might seem intrusive, but conforming to the patient's tight control of the session amounts to letting the patient down because the therapist is not making a contribution. All of these considera-

tions are related to one other characteristic of defensive patterns. As I mentioned above, these patterns actually work against fulfillment of patients' wishes. In the example we have been considering, it is clear that while the patient's approach to the session might avoid the type of therapist response she most fears, it also works against receiving the concerned, attentive response she hopes for—which really requires the therapist to be there in a concerned, nonintrusive way on his own initiative.

Although defense is primarily a matter of patterns of action, "inner" processes can also play a role because we modulate our views of ourselves and others as well as our behavior. Quite frequently, blaming, rejecting, or devaluing oneself are part of the picture. Some patients, on the other hand, take a blaming, critical stance toward others, but even in these cases, there is usually a devaluing/distorted view of self, for example, as a powerless victim. Grandiose self views also play a role in defensive patterns.

One example of how views of self can play a role in defensive action patterns involved a patient who ruminated in a self-critical way about whether she ended her work with a former therapist (who moved to another area of the country) the "right way," directing all of her energy along these lines rather than recognizing how she felt about the early termination of the treatment. Although it would be accurate to say that this critical approach to her own behavior represented a defense against experiencing anger and abandonment viewed as internal experiences, note that her view of herself played a part in a pattern in which she did not *act* in a straightforward way by expressing her feelings to either her first therapist or the new therapist. We will return to this example at a later point in the chapter.

Framework for Interventions

Based on the conceptualization of psychopathology offered above, the main questions about therapeutic interventions are: What can a therapist do to help a patient change problematic patterns in his or her life? and How do you intervene in a useful way when the patterns in question are defensive in nature?

I can introduce the response to these questions offered by the basic philosophical perspective by referring to Wittgenstein's (1958) thoughts about the role played by concrete examples, or what he called "perspicuous representations" in teaching a concept. Elsewhere, I have illustrated Wittgenstein's ideas about this with the example of teaching someone the concept "chair" (Westerman, 1986; also see Dreyfus, 1979):

The teacher could point to a number of examples: "There's one (pointing to a young man at a table having dinner). There's another (pointing to a woman sitting in an armchair and reading a book). That's not a chair (pointing to a sculpture in a museum that happens to have four "legs," "a seat," and "a back," which looks more like a chair than many real chairs). And that (a throne) is an unusual case of a chair." (p. 54)

Several things should be noted about this example. First, this illustration about teaching rests heavily on the use of examples. But Wittgenstein argued that the concept "chair," or any other concept, is not equivalent to the concrete instances pointed out. The term *example* captures the idea that what one is pointing out goes beyond the cases one actually points to. If the pupil in our example learns what "chair" means, he or she will come to understand what is really an incredibly complex set of relationships between certain objects (chairs) and the world of practical activity. In other words, the concept is *meaningful*, not just a laundry list of objects.

The next point is that the examples only succeed in teaching the concept because they build upon the pupil's prior practical familiarity with such human practices as sitting, reading books, creating artwork, political ceremonies, and so forth. It is because the pupil makes use of the examples with respect to this starting point that he or she ends up with a meaningful concept, not just a list of a few specific objects called "chair."

The final point is that according to Wittgenstein, even though the concept goes beyond the specific examples cited, it is not the case that the pupil learns some abstract, pure notion that is more real than and separate from the examples. The background knowledge about sitting and reading books the pupil brings to this learning situation is itself practical, concrete knowledge, not a filter of ideas. It is the pupil's familiarity with concrete practices that makes the examples useful. The concept chair is more than the examples pointed out, but it is not something other than concrete examples.

An intervention in therapy can also be viewed as an example, as a particular concrete event that points the way to a new pattern of activity. In one important respect, the discussion about chairs is misleading if we treat it literally as suggesting that a therapist should actually present examples of a new pattern for the patient to *look at*. Instead, therapy *examples*, or interventions, are most useful when they represent enactments of a new pattern. But otherwise, the remarks about the concept chair are very useful because they point out three key ideas about interventions.

The first point is that interventions should not aim at promoting change in specific behaviors, but in *meaningful* patterns of behavior. The teacher was not trying to help the pupil learn that this particular object was a chair, but rather the teacher tried to find examples that would help the student learn the concept.

The second point is that interventions help promote meaningful change when they build on a patient's *starting point*, or existing ways of doing things. A person is not a *tabula rasa* or blank slate. The process is a reflexive one. The impact of an intervention depends on how it relates to the patient's current approach to things. The therapist must take this into account. It is very tempting to mistakenly assume that the starting point idea refers to the importance of keeping in mind the ways patients think about things, not their current action patterns. Among other unfortunate outcomes, when the starting point idea is taken to refer to how the patient thinks about things, as in a psychodynamic approach, or for that matter, many types of cognitive-behavioral therapy, we are led to believe that fundamentally interventions should operate at the level of thinking (promoting insight or modifying beliefs).

The third point illustrated by the chair example concerns the essential role played by concrete examples. In order to help a patient change problematic action patterns, a therapist must provide concrete examples of new patterns. I refer to this point as the need for *prospective* interventions, interventions that concretely point the way to change. This point about prospective considerations diverges from the notion of unfolding in the experiential-humanistic tradition. Change is not a matter of providing nurturance so that a dormant potential can be realized, as when an acorn becomes an oak tree. Patients have to create new ways of living their lives that build upon, but are not implicit in, their starting point patterns. The psychodynamic tradition is also weak on this score. Supposedly, by making the unconscious conscious all will be set right by the ego faculties of rationality. (Some Freudians touch on helping patients develop new approaches to things with ideas about ego building through identification with the therapist, but these considerations are treated as secondary.) Unfortunately, many insight-oriented therapists frequently work with their patients on such things as how the patient feels about a recent event or why the patient is the way he or she is without ever wondering what this person would be like *concretely* if he or she were to change. Behavioral approaches to therapy are typically much stronger when it comes to prospective considerations. But what is often referred to as "skill learning" by behaviorally oriented clinicians proceeds as if the patient were a tabula rasa—as if the process involves simply inserting new building blocks into a patient's repertoire. Hence, these efforts fall short with respect to the starting point idea.

To summarize what has been said so far: Interventions can be viewed as examples that can help promote change in meaningful patterns of action if they take into consideration patients' current action patterns and insofar as they concretely exemplify new patterns. I will discuss how these points can be embodied in specific therapeutic interventions in later sections, which consider behavioral, strategic, and insight-oriented interventions from the point of view of this general framework.

Several additional points can be made based on the view that the problematic patterns under consideration are defensive in nature. To begin with, in order to help point the way to new meaningful action patterns, therapy must focus on patients' wishes. These wishes are a crucial aspect of the starting point. Therapists must build upon them. Typically, this involves helping patients acknowledge their wishes and then supporting and encouraging them to accept and trust their wishes. In a sense, everything that follows relates to how to accomplish this, but three components of the therapy process are directly relevant here. One is work directly aimed at helping patients identify their desires, hopes, longings. Relevant interventions here can be, but need not be, insight-oriented in nature. Arkowitz (1989) has shown how behavioral enactments can be employed to help patients recognize their wishes. Another component is helping patients find some satisfaction of those wishes in the context of the therapeutic relationship itself. For example, consider the case briefly described above involving the hard-working patient who attempted to do everything asked of him hoping to be recognized. This patient often talked in therapy about his efforts at work and at home. On some occasions, however, he expressed some wish or interest of his own. When he did, the therapist showed interest in learning about these parts of the patient's life. These simple expressions of interest played an important role in the treatment. The third component involves prospective efforts aimed at encouraging patients to embrace their wishes in the context of how they lead their day-to-day lives. I will return to this below.

The therapeutic process should also respond to patients' fears. Here again, helping patients acknowledge their fears typically is important. And again, therapeutic efforts can be insight-oriented in nature, but this is not necessarily the case (cf. Arkowitz, 1989). It is also important that the therapist relates to the patient in such a way that the patient feels safe in the therapeutic relationship. Talking about one's fears with a therapist is itself frightening, because it opens up the possibility of experiencing the feared outcomes in the context of the therapeutic relationship. For example, it was extremely difficult for the hard-working patient mentioned above to discuss his fears about being inadequate. By doing so, he opened the possibility that the therapist might find him lacking. That is, his fear itself might be viewed as a failing because he should be able to handle things, including his own anxieties about himself.

Making the therapeutic relationship a safe context is not a matter of helping patients find a way to stop being afraid. Rather, it involves helping patients act in the context of the relationship in ways that embrace their wishes while they are afraid. Therapists can help with this by not responding to patients in the extreme and hurtful ways their patients fear. But it would be impossible for a therapist to never respond in a way that reflects the patient's fears. Indeed, an important curative or healing aspect of the therapeutic relationship is that patients can encounter what they fear in ways that make for new learning, involving such things as discovering how to stay with a line of effort even though it did not lead to the hoped for result at first or discovering that one is strong enough to sustain a feared outcome that cannot be changed.

Another way in which therapy helps patients come to terms with their fears is by helping them develop an enhanced sense of personal strength and create supports for themselves. When patients recognize, acknowledge, and nurture their own capacities and emotional resources, and when they develop sources of support in their lives (including the therapeutic relationship itself but also including friendship networks, participating in community organizations, and the like), they become better able to face their fears.

Interventions aimed at encouraging patients to experiment with new alternatives in their day-to-day lives are perhaps especially important when it comes to work related to patients' fears and also their wishes. Often these interventions can be direct suggestions. For example, in the case involving the hardworking patient, the therapist might suggest to the patient the idea of setting some limits for his activities at work, at home, and at his mother's business in order to create some time for himself. There are risks is this way of proceeding related to how the intervention impacts the patient given his or her starting point. Among other things, change can become a matter of pleasing the therapist, which actually impedes progress (Messer, 1986). The suggestion may activate fears about outcomes in the extra-therapy events in question and in the therapeutic relationship itself. These concerns are important (and I will return to them below), but when properly employed such interventions can be used to point in very concrete ways to new ways of doing things.

So far, my comments have focused on wishes and fears, but what about defenses themselves? At times, it can be useful to help patients identify their defensive patterns and to challenge those patterns directly, but such efforts can be counterproductive. Many (not all) psychodynamically oriented therapists devote considerable energy trying to help patients recognize and understand their defenses in ways that amount to an attack on the patient that recreates examples of what the patient fears. For example, questions directed to

the patient we have been considering about his defensive pattern of straining to meet the demands of others might lead the patient to feel that he has fallen short. Therapeutic efforts of this type promote further activation of defenses, rather than a change for the better. The patient in the example might labor at explaining why his activities are really necessary even though they are so demanding, or he might explain that he realizes he needs to become more efficient. I believe that the most effective response to defenses involves the efforts described above aimed at wishes and fears. As patients begin to acknowledge and embrace their hopes and as they come to new terms with their fears, they shift away from defensive patterns to more straightforward ways of doing things.

It is useful to offer a general characterization of the result of the therapeutic change process when it is successful. A key element is that the patient becomes an active, open person. There is a healthy sense of agency, a readiness to explore and discover what the individual can do and what his or her life can be. There is also a sense of what one cannot do, a humility and an acceptance of losses and disappointments. Note that humility and acceptance are not bland rationalizations or a denial of hopes and longings. Rather, they involve deep feelings, which some patients describe as tenderness. Finally, as patients shift to nondefensive ways of living their lives they frequently become more compassionate. While an obligatory sense of doing for others may have been part of their defensive patterns, they often come to identify and embrace a more heartfelt giving stance to others in their lives. All of this is to say that they enter more fully into the circle of involvement in their own lives from the starting point of their wishes and fears and the possibilities that are there for them given who they are, with an enhanced sense of connection to other people.

Therapeutic Relationship

From the standpoint of the hermeneutic perspective, the therapeutic relationship is extremely important. Moreover, the perspective provides its own way of conceptualizing the nature of the therapeutic relationship and the role it plays in the change process.

No simple characterizations of how the therapeutic relationship is viewed in the established therapy approaches can do justice to the rich subtleties of clinical practice. Nevertheless, it is useful to point to two simple, misguided pictures that have been very influential. They reflect the major currents in the philosophical tradition, empiricism and rationalism, which in turn, reflect (albeit in different ways) the notion of the uninvolved subject. The therapeutic relationship is a circle, and the idea of uninvolved subjectivity does not provide an adequate basis for understanding how patient and therapist are involved together in this circle.

As noted above, the philosophical tradition suggests that we can think of a person (e.g., a patient) as a fully autonomous, independent agent, *or* as a passive, dependent automaton. These views of the person suggest that the therapeutic process involves essentially self-generated change *or* change that is other-generated. According to the first view, which characterizes insight-oriented therapy and, especially, analytically oriented therapy, a patient is an independent agent engaged in what is ultimately a removed third-person process of trying to understand oneself. Therapists participate in this process, but they should take a neutral stance in the therapeutic relationship. Their primary activity is offering interpretations, which is viewed as a neutral kind of "involvement."

This formulation denies the real nature of the therapeutic process, which is that although it is *about* the patient's life in general, it is itself a part of life, an activity patient and therapist are involved in together. In other words, it is a circle. Although it is true that analytically oriented therapy includes concern about transference and countertransference processes, these "circular" phenomena are viewed as taking place within the context of a third-person process. This can be seen most clearly in therapists' commitment to limit their efforts related to transference phenomena, as well as all other aspects of the process, to the supposedly neutral practices of the interpretive mode.

According to the second view, which is reflected in behavioral approaches, patients are passive and dependent. Therapists are viewed as removed experts who take an active, directive role to change patients' behavior. Here again, the nature of the therapy process as a circle is denied. Patient and therapist are not recognized as doing things with each other, actively involved in an activity as part of their lives as well as doing something *about* the other parts of the patient's life.[1]

The hermeneutic perspective points away from both positions described so far. The reason for this relates to the founding idea of the perspective, the belief that from the outset the person is involved in the world of practical activities. We can take a removed stance to particular objects, people, or ourselves in a sense, but this stance is always based on active involvement doing things. From this vantage point, the therapeutic relationship is first off viewed as an activity engaged in by two (or more) participants. The patient's objectives are to change his or her life, but in order to do that the patient engages in an activity, which is now part of the patient's life. The situation is not symmetrical for patient and therapist, but the therapist is also participating in an activity as part of his or her life. Once more, this process is *about* the patient's life, and it may well be very different from the other parts of the patient's life in many important respects, but it is not something fundamentally different in kind as it would be if it were an essentially removed process of reflection or a technical, expert process. It consists of people doing things together. This point is a more radical idea than the notions of transference and countertransference. The circular nature of the therapy process is irreducible; there is no outside vantage point.

Where does this viewpoint lead us? To begin with, it points away from the first position. According to the hermeneutic perspective, *everything* done by patient and therapist should be

[1]Although I believe this simple characterization serves to describe a good deal of actual behaviorally oriented work, some qualifications are in order. The first is that behavior therapists have begun to show some interest in the therapeutic relationship (e.g., Goldfried, 1982; Lazarus & Fay, 1982). Nevertheless, when they do so, they focus on ways to remove problematic relationship processes in order to make it possible to pursue therapeutic efforts in the manner described above (i.e., outside the circle). Another point is that when behavior therapists directly address ethical issues about their work they often take an extreme stance against therapists making any choices for their patients (cf. Kitchener, 1980; Woolfolk & Richardson, 1984). Curiously enough, with such comments, they actually flip over to the other side of the coin—and still remain outside the circle.

viewed as acts in the context of the therapy relationship. With respect to the patient's part, for example, I noted above how acknowledging a fear had significance as an interpersonal act for the overworked patient who was concerned that the therapist might view such feelings as a failure on his part. It is interesting to note that results from studies on relations between patient self-exploration and outcome have been inconsistent (cf. McDaniel, Stiles, & McGaughey, 1981). This may reflect the fact that most investigations in this area focus on whether patients disclose information rather than on the interpersonal role played by their disclosures. In my own process research, I have found that assessments related to defensiveness in patients' interpersonal behavior were very strongly related to improvement in insight- and action-oriented treatment contexts (Westerman, Foote, McCullough, & Winston, 1990; Westerman, Frankel, Tanaka, & Kahn, 1987; Westerman, Tanaka, Frankel, & Kahn 1986). I have also found evidence indicating that indices of the interpersonal significance of patients' in-session behavior play a more important role than measures of self-disclosure *per se* (Westerman & Foote, 1988).

Turning to the therapists' part, the foregoing remarks suggest therapists' contributions also have significance as interpersonal acts. This is true whether the contribution is a direct suggestion or a response to a disclosure. Recall the observation offered above about how an interpretation about the workaholic's defensive pattern could be taken as a criticism by that patient. Note that, as this example indicates, the therapist is not neutral even when his or her contributions are limited to the interpretive mode (cf. Wachtel, 1987b). It may well be that the repeated failures on the part of therapy researchers to identify intervention variables that make a difference in outcome (cf. Stiles, Shapiro, & Elliott, 1986) stem from the neglect of the interpersonal significance of what therapists do.

According to the hermeneutic perspective, the fact that therapist contributions have interpersonal significance, that they are not neutral, is not an unfortunate failing at all. Nor does this reinterpretation of the supposedly "neutral" practices of interpretive work simply point to a new way of looking at what patients and therapists do. The interpersonal significance of therapists' behaviors should be embraced in our efforts to help patients. (A simple example of this was offered above in connection with the case involving the overworked man, when it was noted that it was therapeutic for the therapist to show interest in the patient's wishes and interests.) Therapists should *cultivate* the interpersonal act dimension of what they do, not try to keep it to a bare minimum. One very useful tool for such efforts is Benjamin's (e.g., 1982) Structural Analysis of Social Behavior, which provides a model for characterizing the interpersonal significance of therapist and patient behaviors and includes theoretical propositions about what interpersonal stance on the therapist's part will be most helpful for a particular patient.[2]

The implications of cultivating the act dimension of what transpires in therapy are far reaching. Once one acknowledges that everything done by patients and therapists has interpersonal significance, the supposed boundary breaks down between the "neutral" practices of the interpretive mode and direct suggestions. As noted above, direct suggestions can play a valuable role in therapeutic work according to the hermeneutic perspective. The point here is that while direct interventions most definitely have interpersonal significance, this does not make them fundamentally different from interpretive efforts in the way others have suggested. It by no means leads to the conclusion that such interventions should not be employed.

The preceding comments present a view of the therapeutic relationship that contrasts markedly with the view held by dynamically oriented therapists. Does this mean that the hermeneutic perspective reflects the other side of the coin? In fact, it does not represent a view of the therapy process as an other-generated change process. The reason for this has to do with the starting point notion. The impact of an intervention always depends on the patient's starting point. The

[2]A point of clarification may be in order. Note that the present emphasis on the therapeutic relationship does not mean that all, or most, or, for that matter, *any* of the therapeutic process should be talk about the relationship. Nor does it imply that the interpersonal processes in the therapeutic relationship are the sole curative ingredients in therapy. The point is that therapeutic relationship processes are *always relevant*, although the therapeutic process includes many components in addition to the relationship.

patient is not a passive, blank slate. Patients change only when therapy helps them find ways to move from their starting points. Hence, the framework does not point to a controlling therapist as the counterpoint to a passive, dependent patient. My comments above about how interpreting defenses can augment them illustrate that therapists cannot "make" patients change and that such efforts often lead to results opposite from those intended. Similarly, when behavior therapists take a controlling stance, their efforts are often met by resistance or by compliance that is not therapeutic, as in Messer's (1986) example about a patient who complied with a behavioral suggestion in order to please the therapist.

The starting point idea does not only argue against taking a controlling stance because such efforts will not work. It involves a whole different viewpoint about the nature of the therapeutic relationship and relationships in general. Earlier in this chapter, I explained how the basic perspective leads to the idea of *interdependence* between people. We are not separate, independent agents. We are agents actively involved in the shared world of practical activities. This makes for a fundamental connection between people. But there is a distance or difference between people, because we each lead our lives from a different starting point. The basic reason why a therapist should not attempt to control a patient is not because such efforts will not work, but because therapists should *respect* the fact that the patient is another person who is involved in the world from the standpoint of his or her individual history, experience, interests, capacities, and so forth. In a very fundamental sense, personal change in one individual is not something that another person can accomplish. What this means for therapists is that their contributions to the process can only provide opportunities pointing to change. Interventions will only effectively promote change if they reflect appreciation of this fact, that is, reflect respect for the patient as a person with a starting point. What this means for patients is that therapy cannot change them. The process will only lead to change if the patient finds a way from his or her starting point to make use of the process to create new patterns in his or her life.

Note that these remarks offer a very different reason for rejecting a directive therapist/passive patient view of the therapeutic relationship than the traditional argument about patients being autonomous, independent agents. The view of the person as involved in the world from a starting point argues against the directive/passive view and *at the same time* it provides a basis for active involvement by patient and therapist. From the standpoint of the hermeneutic perspective, it is true in a fundamental sense that people are engaged in a shared world. They participate in the world from different starting points, but this provides the basis for empathy, another aspect of sharing. The hermeneutic perspective incorporates a view of respect for another person that argues against taking a controlling stance and *simultaneously* argues in favor of active involvement. As just noted above, for patients, this suggests that the therapeutic process involves the process of discovering ways to make use of the context so that it will help them move forward from their starting points. It suggests that therapists should actively join with their patients in ways that will help them move to change. These active efforts can run the gamut from recognizing and making good use of the interpersonal significance of what others might describe as the "neutral" activities of the interpretive mode to interventions that directly suggest new ways of doing things, so long as the therapist remains as faithful as he or she can to accepting the patient's starting point. Certainly, there are times when *certain* active interventions (e.g., a particular direct suggestion or a specific response to something the patient said, such as reaching out to take the patient's hand) are not indicated. But these contraindications have to do with specific features of the interpersonal significance of particular actions at specific points in a given case, rather than fundamental considerations about the nature of human beings as separate, removed, and fully autonomous.

It is worth noting that just as I described the patient who has shifted to nondefensive ways of living as *actively involved* and *accepting*, my remarks here offer a picture of the therapist as being *actively involved* (engaging in the circle as a participant, not as a removed observer) and *accepting* (recognizing and respecting the patient's starting point). This is not a coincidence. Both of these descriptions refer to central characteristics of participating fully in what you are doing when what you are doing is a circle, that is, an activity you are involved in from a particular starting point within the activity, rather than as an observer. Indeed, although this can only be mentioned here, in order for therapists to engage with patients in an active and accepting manner, they must find ways to incorporate their own personal starting point (wishes and fears) in their efforts so that they do not act defensively.

Reconsideration of Interventions: The "Direct Examples" of Behavior Therapy

According to the hermeneutic framework, interventions help promote change when they constitute concrete examples of new, meaningful action patterns. In order to function in this way, they must reflect appreciation of the patient's starting point and they must be prospective, that is, serve to concretely guide the patient to new patterns. They must also be responsive to the patient's wishes and fears in ways that point beyond defensive patterns. Finally, interventions should reflect respect for the patient. In what follows, I will show that the major types of interventions, behavioral, strategic, and insight-oriented, can all represent ways of meeting the requirements of this framework. Hence, the perspective offers an integrative approach that brings together the major kinds of techniques therapists employ to help their patients. But my remarks will not simply offer a reinterpretation of what therapists guided by the established approaches already do. When the major types of interventions are viewed in terms of the hermeneutic framework, they are not seen as mutually exclusive efforts. Also, it becomes possible to identify especially helpful ways of employing these interventions and to recognize how these interventions can be used in unhelpful ways, which unfortunately are suggested by the originating psychotherapy approaches. The following discussion will also serve to clarify and illustrate the basic perspective.

From the standpoint of the hermeneutic perspective, behavioral interventions can be viewed as "direct examples," because they directly point the patient to a concrete example of a new action pattern. As noted above, however, it frequently happens that behavioral interventions fail to serve as useful "direct examples" because they do not

build upon the patient's starting point. One of the clearest ways this occurs is when a behavior therapist responds to all cases with a given presenting problem, for example, test anxiety, with the same approach (e.g., systematic desensitization using a hierarchy of items about taking exams). Neglect of patients' starting points happens in other, less obvious, ways as well. For example, behavioral marriage therapists often direct uninvolved, withdrawn husbands to listen more attentively to their wives. In some cases, this can be useful. In other cases, it will not be useful or may well be counterproductive, because it represents an attack on the husband's defensive patterns for dealing with his fears about what he experiences as his wife's demandingness and his own disappointments about getting his wishes met in the marriage.

Behavioral interventions can be employed in ways that take the starting point into account and also conform to the other requirements of the framework presented above. For example, I have found that behavioral interventions can often be very useful in the kind of marital situation just described—but these interventions are quite different from those suggesting "better listening." Instead, they involve suggestions about how the husband might acknowledge his wishes about the relationship (that they are not simply "I wish she weren't so unhappy and that she would stop nagging me") and make requests of his wife based on those wishes. Such interventions can focus on in-session behavior (e.g., suggesting that the man ask his wife to stop interrupting him, or that he tell her that he likes it when she expresses concern about how he's feeling and that he would like it if she would do this more frequently) and new ways to interact with his wife at home (e.g., deciding what he would like to do the next time the two go out for the evening and asking his wife to join him). Typically, these interventions challenge the husband given his starting point, but they do not lead to a defensive response. The approach helps the man identify and acknowledge his wishes and helps point him concretely to discovering nondefensive ways of incorporating those wishes in his interactions with his wife. These interventions also can contribute to the identification of fears ("Well, yes, I would like her to do X, but I'm afraid she'll get really angry if I ask her") and lead to other therapeutic efforts designed to help the husband deal with real and anticipated feared responses from his wife—and, of course, efforts aimed at helping the wife with her side of the pattern. All of these efforts prepare things so that at a later point the therapist can turn to the husband's listening and help the couple make changes related to that problem too. This example illustrates the chief strengths of behavioral interventions: They exemplify new patterns in very concrete ways since they involve doing things; they prospectively point out what new action patterns might be like; and they provide effective ways to identify and support wishes, help patients recognize their fears, and try new nondefensive action patterns.

Again, behavioral interventions function in these ways only if they take the patient's starting point into account. The main problem here is that behavioral suggestions may be too frightening. Another concern is that patients may comply with the suggestion, but for the wrong reasons (e.g., as noted above, in order to please the therapist). Another problem is that the therapist's suggestion might be "wrong," that is, it may not point the way to a new pattern of interaction that is right for the patient given his or her starting point. The suggested action may be entirely off the mark or it may simply point to a particular way of doing things that differs in specifics from what is right for the patient (e.g., for a particular husband it may not fit to ask his wife to show concern for him, but giving his wife flowers when she's helped him cope with a difficult stretch at work may fit quite well).

I have found several techniques to be useful for dealing with these concerns. The first is to present the intervention as a suggestion, that is, in a way that makes it clear to the patient that he or she is free to say yes or no. Indeed, I frequently present suggestions in a way that downplays their implications for action (e.g., "What do you think would happen if you . . .", "Can you imagine yourself . . ."). This approach serves to put the suggestion on the table, while showing respect for the patient as the person who might or might not choose to pursue the idea. One positive feature of this approach is that for many patients responding to a suggestion with a direct and clear "no" is itself therapeutic. Another idea is to present the suggestion as an "experiment" (cf. Arkowitz, 1989). It is less frightening to try a new way

of doing things if the attempt has value whether or not it works out well because it will produce useful data. Another technique is to use suggestions for in-session behavior first or, instead of, suggestions about something the patient might try in the actual situation of concern. In-session suggestions can be role plays. For example, in a case involving a patient who finds it hard to believe that anyone really appreciates her or cares about her feelings, the therapist might suggest that she pretend that it is her birthday and somebody has just given her a present that she does not like. How would she feel about telling the person that she does not like the color or size of the present? Could she act out their response to such a comment imagining it to reflect genuine concern about whether or not she liked the gift? One other technique is what I call the *percolating* idea. At times, I bring up behavioral suggestions to patients but specifically state that the patient should not carry through the suggestion but simply think about it, perhaps when he or she encounters certain specific situations. Sometimes, this approach can be very useful in helping patients recognize what their wishes really are and/ or discover how scared they are about certain things. Not infrequently, patients will actually try some new way of doing things different from the specific suggestion they were "percolating" but similar in meaning.

Behavioral interventions can also be very useful for another line of therapeutic efforts. Here, I am referring to behavioral suggestions that do not relate directly to a patient's concerns, but instead focus on adding new positive aspects to the patient's life. Interventions of this type can include relaxation training or instruction in meditation, or encouraging patients to pursue hobbies, develop friendships, or to get involved in volunteer activities. As noted above, from the standpoint of the general framework, these interventions are valuable because they provide sources of pleasure, accomplishment, and support that strengthen the individual for moving ahead in the face of fear in the problematic domains of his or her life. They also cultivate more "self-directed" wishes. It is often important for patients to learn that they can find deep sources of satisfaction in their lives via activities they pursue separately from parents, spouses, children, or their boss or colleagues at work. Discoveries along these lines often impact fraught interpersonal areas and promote changes in problematic defensive patterns (e.g., when a patient discovers he or she not only wants caring and affection from the spouse, but also for the spouse to recognize and support his or her own independent pursuits).

One more point should be made about behavioral interventions. It is usually very important to help patients recognize that when they try new ways of doing things *two things* are going on, especially when interpersonal relationships are concerned. One thing concerns what they are doing. Another thing is the results of their efforts, including how other people in their lives respond. This is important because for many problematic interpersonal patterns, changes by one party often initially lead to an escalation of difficult responses by the other. Also, on a more fundamental level, in order to shift away from defensive patterns, there must be a "decoupling" of what one does from responses to one's actions. Acting in the face of one's fear (i.e., nondefensively) requires recognizing that things may not go well and developing personal resources to withstand experiences of disappointment and loss. Moreover, there can be a deep sense of satisfaction when a person acts in a manner that represents embracing wishes, hopes, and one's own sense about the best way to proceed, even when things do not work out well. It is helpful to point this out to patients so that they can discover this source of satisfaction.

Reconceptualizing Strategic Interventions

Strategic interventions were originally developed by the communications theorists (e.g., Haley, 1963; Watzlawick, Weakland, & Fisch, 1974). Paradoxical interventions, in which the therapist prescribes the symptom, are the most important example of this approach. For example, in a case involving a pessimist, Watzlawick *et al.* (1974) suggested that the therapist should point out to the patient that he failed to recognize how bad things were likely to get. Their rationale for this intervention was that the patient's pessimism was one pole of an interpersonal pattern that requires an optimistic stance at the other end. The intervention supposedly made it impossible for the patient to continue his end of the pattern.

I believe that this approach has a lot to offer. Indeed, in *certain* respects the theoretical framework upon which strategic interventions are based is similar to the hermeneutic perspective. Both focus on action patterns, place considerable emphasis on therapeutic relationship processes, and argue for active intervention strategies. Moreover, I believe that the communications theorists' interest in double-binding patterns overlaps closely with the present focus on defensive patterns. For example, I imagine the pessimist Watzlawick *et al.* spoke about was engaged in a defensive pattern in which fears about really getting what he needed from others were dealt with by always treating helpful responses by others as inadequate ("but that won't work because . . ."). Finally, the hermeneutic perspective incorporates the use of strategic interventions. These interventions can be quite useful, especially when working with highly defended, resistant patients (Horvath & Goheen, 1990; Kolko & Milan, 1983; Westerman *et al.*, 1987).

In spite of these similarities, the two perspectives are actually quite different. The hermeneutic framework includes use of strategic interventions, but it leads to different ways of employing them. In addition, it differs dramatically from communications theory with respect to how the two positions view the use of other interventions. The communications theorists see little value in behavioral interventions and no value in insight-oriented work.

One problem with strategic interventions as they are employed by the communications theorists is that they are insufficiently prospective. According to communications theory, an effective intervention can be viewed as a mathematical function that "operates on" the problematic pattern, which itself is viewed as an abstract formal structure, and flips it around all of a sudden. Supposedly, an intervention leads to change that is fully immediate and general, that is, a change in all instances of problematic interaction in the patient's life (Watzlawick *et al.*, 1974, pp. 1–28). This position is a fascinating and misguided example of rationalist philosophy (cf. Westerman, 1986). The hermeneutic perspective also focuses on action patterns, but these are not viewed as formal entities. They are meaningful and concrete at the same time. This theoretical difference has practical implications. As employed by the communications theorists, strategic interventions often fail to point the way to change because they do not reflect appreciation of the fact that patterns are not all of a piece. What strategic interventions actually accomplish is finding a way to get a resistant patient to change a particular behavior, not making a fully general change in a meaningful pattern. This change may lead to a more far-reaching change, but usually it does not by itself. This point has to do with the issue of the generalization of treatment effects. From the standpoint of the hermeneutic perspective, change can occur only through a process that involves many concrete steps because action patterns are concretely meaningful, not abstract (cf. Westerman, 1989).

Another problem with the communications theorists' approach is that it can be manipulative. Although the communications theorists are experts at taking a patient's starting point into account in an instrumental sense so that they can find ways to get even the most recalcitrant patient to change his or her behavior in certain respects, their approach does not reflect the respect called for by the starting point idea. They often get patients to change "in spite of themselves," and this actually has limitations of an instrumental nature. Patients can respond "positively" to paradoxical interventions for the wrong reasons (e.g., a husband and wife may stop arguing in a session when told by the therapist "your bickering shows how much you really love each other" in order to not be loving). When this happens, it is quite likely that the behavior change "induced" will not be part of a meaningful change in the action patterns of concern.

The hermeneutic perspective includes the use of strategic interventions, but it does so in a way that differs from communications theory in two crucial ways. First, strategic interventions are employed as part of a larger therapeutic process. A strategic intervention is not viewed as a mathematical "operator" that effects wholesale change by itself. There is no reason to expect that a single intervention (of any type) will be sufficient. For example, the paradoxical intervention "You don't recognize how bad things are likely to get" *might* lead the pessimist in the example above to shift to a more optimistic stance in his relationship with the therapist during that session, but this by no means guarantees that the patient will shift his outlook and behavior in all relationships and domains of his life. Also, the patient's response could be quite different. He might become very angry at the therapist. Hence, in the hermeneutic perspective, while it is recognized that a strategic intervention may make a very important contribution to therapeutic efforts in certain cases, such interventions are viewed as playing a role in a sequence of efforts. Moreover, behavioral and insight-oriented interventions will almost always play a crucial role in the overall process, notwithstanding the communications theorists' dismissive views of such efforts.

The second difference is the idea that therapists should use only strategic interventions when they can feel sincere about what they say to the patient. This follows from the emphasis on respecting, not "operating on," the patient. This can lead to differences in what one says. For example, in the case of the pessimist, the therapist might change Watzlawick *et al.*'s (1974) intervention so that it clearly reflects his or her appreciation of the fears that lie behind the pessimist's behavior as follows: "You've said that you think things are not going to go well, but I have a hunch that you actually feel that things in your life may go worse than what you've let on about so far. It's possible that you're right." Many therapists who might feel that it would be manipulative to employ the original version of the paradox, would find it quite acceptable to offer this revised statement. In fact, as this example suggests, the difference between even the most apparently outrageous paradoxical interventions and perfectly reasonable ways of responding to patients may not be all that great. One could say, for example, that an insight-oriented therapist is being "paradoxical" when he or she responds to a patient who is complaining about his boss at work by saying "I think you're angry at me too." This intervention "prescribes the symptom" in that it encourages the patient to express anger he was feeling toward the therapist. At bottom, there is a commonality between apparently outrageous paradoxical interventions and very reasonable, commonplace interventions, because both serve to recognize and validate patients' fears and/or their wishes in spite of the fact that the wishes and fears are being presented by the patient in a defensive manner.

The point here has two implications. The first is that not only is it possible to employ strategic interventions in perfectly reasonable ways that raise no concerns about sincerity, but that responses therapists make all the time can actually be viewed as examples of such interventions. Therapists should recognize this and cultivate their use of such reasonable, albeit paradoxical, responses. The other implication points in the opposite direction. Once a therapist realizes that paradoxical interventions, however outlandish they may appear to be, can often be rephrased in ways that seem quite acceptable, he or she may decide that the "outrageous" version itself can be presented with full sincerity. For example, a therapist might choose to use the original form of the intervention about the pessimist. One positive feature of the original version in comparison to the toned-down version is that it is more likely to lead to an angry response by the patient. This can be very therapeutic, so long as the therapist did not employ the intervention to "trick" the patient into being optimistic and cooperative, but rather as a sincere effort to respond to the fearful and defensive nature of the patient's stance in a way that might help him find new ways to integrate his hopes, his feelings of anger, and his fears in a nondefensive pattern.

Insight-Oriented Interventions: Thinking in the Service of Change

Insight-oriented interventions can also play a very important role in the therapeutic process according to the hermeneutic perspective, notwithstanding the use of action-oriented interventions in this approach and the fundamental role it ascribes to practical activity. But the perspective provides its own way of conceptualizing the role of insight. I should note that I am using the term *insight* broadly to refer to therapeutic work concerning cognitions, beliefs, and attitudes, as well as unconscious contents made conscious.

Insight-oriented efforts frequently reflect a very simple, misguided notion about the nature of thought and how it relates to action. This is the view, derived from rationalism, that thinking represents a removed third-person process of reflection, and that new thoughts, or insights, lead to change in behavior automatically. This model leads to a particular way of employing insight-oriented efforts. Following Wittgenstein's (1958) use of the term *grammar* to refer to the pattern describing an activity, we can say that this manner of pursuing insight-oriented work has the "grammar of understanding." I will elaborate on this point below, but the basic idea is that insight-oriented efforts frequently are employed as if the *point* of the work is increased self-understanding on the patient's part.

As I discussed at the outset, according to the hermeneutic perspective, thinking about things, other people, and oneself exists and it is very important, but our thoughts are never entirely reflective in nature. At bottom, they are always based on practical know-how. In order to clarify this point, consider some comments Wittgenstein (1958, pp. 39–40) made about how a signpost helps a traveler know which way to go. He offered these comments in a discussion about how rules guide behavior. He argued that the signpost does not guarantee that the traveler will know which way to go: "But where is it said which way I am to follow it; whether in the direction of its finger or (e.g.) in the opposite one?" The point is that rules are never sufficient in themselves, even though they can play a useful role. Fundamentally, our ability to make use of a rule is always based on practical know-how about what to do in concrete situations.

For Wittgenstein, this point applies not only to signposts and rules, but to all thoughts, beliefs, and ideas. I want to suggest that it applies to insight-oriented work in psychotherapy as well. This viewpoint *naturalizes* thinking. One implication of this naturalized view is that it demotes the status of insight from the lofty position ascribed to it by the top-down model. If the ideas that come up in therapy function as signposts, then there is no guarantee that they will lead to change. At the same time, recognizing that thinking is a reflective capacity rooted in practical activity, not an all-powerful, free-standing process, actually makes it possible to pursue insight-oriented efforts more effectively. It leads to employing them in a way that reflects appreciation of the need to link those efforts to action patterns.

In what follows, I will present three points about how to do this. Taken together these points map out an approach to insight-oriented work characterized by the grammar of "thinking in the service of change." I have presented the basic points elsewhere (Westerman, 1989), but the discussion that follows includes several important new ideas. Note that there is no suggestion here that efforts reflecting the grammar of understanding are never useful, nor that most insight-oriented therapists pursue their work in ways that never reflect the grammar of thinking in the service of change. My objective is to make several points about the characteristics of especially effective insight-oriented work, and to show that the hermeneutic perspective serves to direct us to these types of efforts and away from less useful approaches.[3]

Connecting Ideas to New Ways of Acting.
When insight-oriented work reflects the grammar of understanding, therapist and patient are likely to devote considerable attention to questions about why the patient is the way he or she is and what that way is like. One important limitation of such efforts is that they are not sufficiently prospective. Going back to Wittgenstein's example, these efforts do not serve to link the signpost to concrete examples of new action patterns. Consider a case involving a 30-year-old man who entered therapy because things were not going well in his relationship with a girlfriend. He reported that he had been in several relationships before which all ended because the women felt that he failed to be considerate and caring. In fact, he described his own behavior in those relationships as manipulative. Nevertheless, he was determined to behave in a different way in the present relationship, now that his current girlfriend was starting to move away from him just like the others before. Initial sessions, which were largely characterized by the grammar of understanding, focused on the very unhappy circumstances of his childhood. His parents died when he was young. He was raised by an uncle and his uncle's wife, who resented having him in her home. Although this patient was able to draw accurate and compelling connections between his history and his way of relating to women in his adult life,

[3]The interested reader is referred to the earlier article (Westerman, 1989) for a detailed discussion of how the naturalized view differs from cognitive-behavioral approaches. Although both call for efforts related to how patients think about things coupled with action-oriented interventions, the two are quite different. In particular, many cognitive-behavioral approaches reflect extreme examples of insight-oriented work characterized by the grammar of understanding (also see Greenberg & Safran, 1987; Mahoney, 1988; Safran & Greenberg, 1986; Schwartz, 1984; Sollod & Wachtel, 1980; Westen, 1985).

these insights left him with no idea at all about how he might change his behavior beyond very general thoughts, such as "I want to trust my girlfriend."

The first point about pursuing insight-oriented efforts so that they reflect the grammar of thinking in the service of change is that *insights can contribute to change if they are developed in ways that establish useful connections between ideas and new ways of acting in concrete situations.* In order to do this, it is necessary to pursue insight-oriented work in such a way that links are made between therapy talk and action. This does not necessarily involve prescriptions for action. Rather, it means that implications for action should be considered by means of such questions as "How would you like things to be (when you are in a particular situation)?" or "What do you think it would be like if you (acted in a certain way when a specific event happened)?" Note that these questions refer to specific situations. This is a crucial element of prospective efforts.

The point of drawing connections to action and doing so in a way that is tied to specific contexts is not to "get" the patient to act in a new way. Links must be forged between insight-oriented efforts and actions in concrete contexts because otherwise a patient may not understand what an insight *means*. This is a difficult idea to grasp. It is very tempting, for example, to think that the patient described above knew what it means to trust his girlfriend and that his problem was coming to believe that it would really be a good thing to trust her. But if insights function as Wittgenstein's signpost, the meaning of an insight or cognition is not at all transparent.

The case illustrates this point. The patient told me that his girlfriend was now seeing another man in addition to spending time with him, and that he was very upset because when he was out walking with her recently they didn't even hold hands. I asked him "What if you had asked her to hold hands, and if she said 'no' told her that her response made you very unhappy?" It was clear from the patient's reaction that he could not have imagined this way of relating to his girlfriend. He did not know that what "trusting" someone means includes letting them know what you want and sharing with them how much that matters to you. My question about a possible new way of acting in a particular concrete situation made our previous discussions meaningful. He could now begin to see where they pointed in terms of new ways of acting, recognize that the prospect of changing in these ways was very frightening for him, but also start to develop a real, concrete sense that this new kind of relationship was something he really wanted.

One other comment about prospective insight-oriented work: It follows directly from the basic framework that therapeutic efforts should help make connections from insights or new thoughts to a broad range of behaviors. A new action pattern goes well beyond a single, specific behavior. As noted above, the generalization of therapeutic effects is a crucial issue according to the hermeneutic perspective given its focus on concretely meaningful patterns, that is, patterns that go beyond individual behaviors but which do not have the nature of abstract entities that change all of a piece (cf. Westerman, 1989). The generalization of effects does not receive enough attention in most insight-oriented (broadly speaking) therapy approaches because the top-down model includes the idea that insights or cognitions are, by their nature, highly general. This is especially true in many cognitive-behavioral approaches, which reflect, as Braswell and Kendall (1988, p. 203) put it, a "pipe dream" about a "magical process" that leads directly to highly generalized effects (cf. Westerman, 1989).

The signpost analogy makes it clear that there is no automatic mapping from an idea to the whole range of relevant situations. It helps us to see that even when a patient "gets" an insight in connection with one context, there still remains the very real challenge of discovering whether and how that insight applies to a new situation. The connection is not automatic, and it is not simply a matter of choosing to act according to "the" insight in the new context. To point the way to new action patterns, insight-oriented efforts must move from consideration of one concrete situation to another, to another, and so on. Typically, the sequence of efforts includes many examples. It is often tempting to move from a specific example to insight-oriented discussion on a very general level. This can be useful, but such efforts can also take away from the concrete elaboration of the idea.

It is often extremely useful to include behavioral and, sometimes, strategic interventions. An insight is much more likely to function as a useful signpost once the patient has actually begun to use it as a guide in his or her life. Hence, it is often effective to move from insight-oriented work to a direct suggestion about trying a new behavior. Also, as Arkowitz (1989) has argued, behavioral interventions can lead to useful insight-oriented exploration of what it was like for the patient to act in the new way and the implications of the specific new experience for other domains of the patient's life.

Taking the Patient's Starting Point into Account. The preceding comments focused on ways to make forward-reaching connections between insight work and new action patterns, but Wittgenstein's analogy showed us that a signpost is only useful if it builds on a traveler's *prior* familiarity with practical activities. This idea leads to a second point about the grammar of thinking in the service of change. *In order for insight-oriented work to be effective, it must take the patient's starting point into account. The impact of an insight-oriented intervention depends very much on how it relates to the patient's current action patterns, including the very patterns one is trying to change, more so than on the "truth value" of the insight.* This point follows directly from the general framework's focus on starting points and the circular nature of the therapy process. I believe it helps to explain the often-occurring phenomenon in which a patient "gets" an insight but does not change, and that it provides a more useful explanation of this situation than discussions about "false insight."

The central idea here is that although thinking is rooted in action, the connections between the two can become very complicated. Thoughts can be tied to action in the very indirect sense of being part of defensive patterns. That is, there is a reflexive nature to how patients think about themselves. How they do this can itself reflect the problematic action patterns that are the targets of therapeutic efforts. Here, I will focus on two defensive approaches to insight work, an overly intellectualized approach and a self-critical approach in which patients view therapy as an opportunity to "make" themselves be the way they should be. These two approaches often overlap as in the case I briefly described earlier in the chapter involving a patient who recently transferred to a new therapist when her first therapist moved to a distant city. This patient explained that she "wanted to end my therapy with Dr. X the right way. I listened to what she (the therapist) said to figure out what I should do, but I didn't do a very good job." This statement was part of a much more long-winded analysis and critical assessment of how she ended her work with the first therapist. At no point did the patient express how she felt about having to stop her meetings with that therapist.

When patients think about themselves in a defensive manner in therapy, it is very likely that insight-oriented efforts will not function as signposts at all (cf. Safran, 1989). Those efforts are likely to get swallowed up by the way the patient engages in the work. This is especially true when insight-oriented efforts are guided by the grammar of understanding, although it may seem that many types of insight-oriented therapy are well-suited to "taking the patient's starting point into account" because they include exploration of the historical roots of the patient's difficulties and interpretation of defenses. But the starting point idea does not necessarily lead to work that focuses attention on the starting point as an object of inquiry. Rather, it raises the question of *how* to interact with the patient so that efforts will actually serve to help the patient move ahead.

One of the most useful answers to this question is to focus insight-oriented efforts on patients' wishes and fears, instead of on how the patient came to be the way he or she is or on an examination of what that way is like (i.e., the grammar of understanding). Often, insight-oriented work of this kind helps the intellectualizing patient and the patient bent on "self-improvement" engage their issues in a way that moves past defensive patterns. They become involved in a process of reflection that is in the service of change, not aimed primarily at understanding. This approach can help the intellectualizing patient identify and acknowledge feelings, and subsequently help the patient struggle with the challenge of embracing wishes and acting in the face of fear. For the "self-improvement" patient, it can help point to what the patient wants in contrast to what the patient feels obliged to do. It can help the patient identify fears that actually fuel the defensive stance, and it can do this in a way that does not make coming to terms with those fears another item on the patient's "to do" list. Note that these brief descriptions do not only point to different ways patients can *think* about their problems. When a patient acknowledges deep-felt wishes and fears to himself or herself and struggles in a first-person way with these feelings rather than a removed third-person manner, these efforts themselves are examples of engaging in nondefensive patterns.

It is often not easy to help a patient move to this different type of approach. In the example of the patient with a new therapist, useful questions to start with might include "How did you feel when she told you she was leaving?" "Were you angry (or sad or afraid)?" "Is there anything you thought about saying to her but didn't?" These questions may serve to shift the patient's manner of thinking about the event, but patients sometimes respond to questions aimed at their wishes and fears in ways that continue to reflect their defensive patterns. The patient in the example might acknowledge being scared, but only in the context of switching the issue to "Why was I scared when she told me that she was leaving?" (in the sense of "What caused me to have that type of reaction?" or "What is wrong with me so that I responded in that way?"). At such points, it may be sufficient to stay steadfast with the goal, for example, by simply saying to the patient in the example, "But tell me more about how you felt when you were scared." At other times, I have found it useful to explicitly stop the defensive response by labeling the patient's approach as getting in the way of exploring the patient's feelings. This last suggestion, however, can activate the circle, as I noted in the section on the general framework. An intellectualizing patient may well respond to a comment about his or her intellectualizing defensive pattern by turning to the issue of why he or she keeps avoiding feelings. By contrast, I believe that it is often useful to identify for patients how their self-critical views serve as a defense (e.g., "When you keep going back to evaluating whether you left therapy the right way, I hear how critical of yourself you can be. I also believe your view of yourself gives you a reason for not getting really angry"). This type of insight-oriented comment frequently helps patients acknowledge and share their wishes and fears, including those related to how they feel about themselves. It can help shift critical self-evaluations from the status of "facts" to an issue the patient can address.

The suggestion about focusing on wishes and fears does not preclude historical work or insight-oriented efforts examining patients' defenses, so long as these efforts are pursued in a way that takes the focus on wishes and fears as the goal. It is possible to consider childhood experiences in a way that provides central examples of wishes long since put aside and feared consequences the patient has tried to avoid for many years. Similarly, defenses can be discussed in order to illuminate what the patient wants and his or her fears, rather than for the sake of developing a removed understanding.

The remark above about patients' self-critical views is related to an idea about starting points that is as important as the suggestion about focusing on wishes and fears. Although only some patients are *especially* given to thinking about themselves in a self-critical way as part of their defensive action patterns, many patients are likely to take a self-critical stance when they encounter difficult situations in their lives and when they consider those issues in the course of insight-oriented work in therapy. When I describe effective insight work as "thinking in the service of change," this is not meant to suggest that patients should engage in the process in a way that reflects a constant *demand* on themselves to change. Such a stance constitutes self-rejection and it will contribute to, not promote, change in defensive patterns. In order for patients to move past their defensive action patterns, they must engage in a process of focusing on wishes they have not embraced and on their fears in a way that reflects *acceptance* of their starting points. Recognizing "Yes, I am afraid" leads to change more than thinking "I shouldn't be afraid" or "Why am I still afraid?"

Hence, it is important for therapists to help their patients accept themselves. The analyst, Merton Gill (1982), suggested one useful way to do this. Therapists can explain to their patients that during childhood they developed the best way of living their lives possible given the circumstances they encountered. This is a valuable suggestion, but it is also possible to directly suggest to patients that they acknowledge and accept their feelings, including negative ones (e.g., "I am very scared about changing").

This idea about helping patients move toward self-acceptance is the counterpart to what was said earlier about therapists accepting and respecting their patients' starting points. The two are closely tied together. In fact, it is probably true that the most effective way a therapist can help promote self-acceptance by a patient is by responding with empathy to the patient's difficulties, including difficulties experienced by the patient when it comes to changing.

Insight-Oriented Efforts as Interpersonal Acts. The previous point suggested that the process of insight-oriented work is circular in the sense that patients often think about themselves in ways that reflect defensive action patterns. This circularity includes interpersonal processes. When a patient engages in insight-oriented work in a way that reflects rather than helps change problematic patterns, one important aspect of what is going on concerns how the patient is relating to the therapist.

The third point about insight-oriented work characterized by thinking in the service of change concerns this aspect of the circularity of insight-oriented work. It follows directly from the idea that all contributions to the therapeutic process should be viewed as interpersonal acts, which was presented above as part of the general framework. It is perhaps especially important to keep this in mind when discussing insight (in contrast, say, to behavioral prescriptions) because it is tempting to think that when patient and therapist are engaged in insight-oriented work they are just talking *about* things, not doing things with each other. The third point is that *in order for insight-oriented work to be effective, it must reflect appreciation of the role played by therapists' insight-oriented interventions and patients' insight-related comments as acts in the therapeutic relationship.*

On the patient's side, it is important to recognize that insight-related comments by a patient are not just "viewpoints," nor even aspects of a defensive pattern in general, but a way of acting toward the therapist. For example, consider the patient who transferred to a new therapist. If that patient responded to the therapist's question "Were you afraid when you found out that your therapist was leaving?" by acknowledging being scared but switching immediately to a focus on "What is wrong with me that I responded in that way?" the response constitutes a refusal to trust the therapist. It probably reflects an unreadiness to believe that the therapist really cared about how she (the patient) feels, a sense that she would not be safe if she made herself vulnerable by sharing with the therapist how very scared she was (perhaps out of fear that this therapist would "leave" her by not showing interest in how she feels), and the belief that the therapist was going to judge her, that is, determine if she reacted in the "right" way. Conversely, if the patient responded to the question by moving away from her initial intellectualizing and self-critical stance to an open expression of how scared she felt, this would constitute an example of a new nondefensive, trusting pattern.

As this example suggests, it is crucial for therapists to recognize the interpersonal act significance of what patients say. By the same token, it is also crucial for therapists to appreciate the interpersonal significance of their own insight-oriented contributions. It is all too easy to say something to a patient that is true and even apparently useful but also counterproductive when understood in terms of its interpersonal significance. For example, I tentatively suggested above that a therapist might try to shift a patient away from an intellectualizing stance by labeling the stance as a defense. I went on to say that often such a bid actually serves to activate the defense. The reason this happens is not only because a therapist comment along these lines is easily linked to an intellectualized response by the patient in some impersonal sense. In large measure, the therapist's comment might activate the defensive response because it is likely to be experienced by the patient as a critical attack. It is all too often true that when insight-oriented work is conducted in a way that reflects the grammar of understanding, patients experience their therapists as critical and/or disinterested.

Indeed, this can even be true when a therapist is pursuing transference work. Such efforts may seem to reflect appreciation of the act significance of what patient and therapist say, but they may actually fall short. This is not to say that transference work cannot be useful. The point is that appreciating the interpersonal significance of insight work is not a matter of whether one *talks about* the relationship, but whether the therapist responds to the patient in a way that supports those aspects of the patient's attempts to change

how he or she is engaging with the therapist in the therapeutic process.

Indications for the Hermeneutic Approach

Although the preceding comments present the key features of the hermeneutic therapy framework, certain issues have not been addressed because they lie beyond the scope of this chapter. Most notably, there are specific questions about how to employ the approach, such as how to sequence insight-oriented efforts with behavioral interventions and exactly how to best use the interpersonal act dimension of therapist contributions (in particular types of cases, at specific moments in treatment).

Here, I would like to offer a few comments about the range of applicability of the approach. By its nature as a therapy approach founded on a general philosophical perspective, the hermeneutic framework promises to be relevant for a broad range of clinical problems. Nevertheless, it is no doubt true that the approach will prove to be useful only for certain types of cases. One important "boundary" regarding indications for the approach follows from its focus on defensive action patterns. Although I believe that such patterns play an important role in many psychotherapy cases, some cases do not involve defensive patterns. These are the less difficult situations therapists encounter, but they should not be ignored. They involve problems that can be described in terms of behavioral deficits or excesses, or a need for education about certain life issues, or situations in which patients simply need an opportunity to clarify and reflect upon their circumstances, goals, and so forth. Although these cases can be conceptualized in the terms of the framework (action patterns, starting points, prospective interventions), there may be little to recommend the hermeneutic approach over such alternatives as behavioral work or a client-centered approach.

Another boundary may exist at the other end of the difficulty continuum. I am not sure whether the framework provides a useful foundation for work with psychotic patients or patients with severe personality disorders (especially patients who would be described as distinctly "unrelated"). This is an extremely difficult issue that requires teasing apart what is probably the inherent intransigence of such problems from an evaluation of what can be gained by means of the hermeneutic approach in particular. One question here has to do with the role of medication. Although the hermeneutic framework is sufficiently far-reaching to incorporate this issue in some abstract sense (since it recognizes that people are embodied and all organismic factors are part of a patient's starting point), this is a purely theoretical point with no practical implications at this time. Another question concerns whether, in the terms of the model, there are certain requirements regarding a patient's starting point that must be met for the framework to be applicable (e.g., a minimal capacity for interpersonal relatedness). This issue remains open at the present time, but my experience suggests that the limits of applicability of the approach are broad enough to include some types of very difficult cases. The case example that follows illustrates this point.

CASE EXAMPLE

The following case presentation illustrates some of the main concepts of the hermeneutic approach and how they come together in the context of work with a patient. The case involved a patient I will call Sarah. The problems of concern included bulimia (Sarah was binging and purging daily at the outset of treatment, she was quite thin although still within normal limits), and depression (ongoing depressed mood accompanied by frequent bouts of uncontrollable crying, insomnia), and physical complaints (e.g., pressure in her ears). At the start of treatment, Sarah was 33 years old. She was married and had three young children. Her family of origin was of Eastern European Jewish descent. She had one brother and one sister. When she was 7 years old, her parents divorced. From that point on, she was raised by her mother and remained entirely estranged from her father, except for a brief time when she was a teenager. Sarah married a Syrian Jew. They lived close to her parents-in-law in a suburb of Los Angeles where many other Syrian Jews live. Sarah and her husband owned a restaurant in partnership with her mother- and father-in-law.

Sarah's behavior was characterized by a defensive action pattern. This pattern was longstanding (it began when she was a young girl) and it appeared in many areas of her adult life, including her relationship with her mother, her relationships with her husband and in-laws, and in her approach to the therapy context as well. In these areas and others, Sarah took a highly responsible, overly conscientious stance. She was intensely concerned about the well-being of significant others in her life and also keenly interested in how they viewed her. The pattern was defensive in nature because it represented an overly protective, indirect expression of a deep wish for nurturance and the hope that she would be respected and appreciated for who she is. Unhappily, for Sarah embracing these wishes seemed impossible because she also feared being rejected and abandoned.

At the outset of therapy, her defensive pattern appeared most prominently in her relationships with her husband and in-laws. This extended family was extremely enmeshed. In addition to shared ownership of the restaurant, family members were involved in almost all aspects of each others' lives. Sarah's overly responsible approach to things was reflected in long hours she put in at the restaurant. More importantly, it appeared as acting as a go-between mediating recurring disputes between her husband and his parents, primarily at the mother-in-law's request. In addition, it was reflected in the bulimia, because Sarah believed (accurately) that her husband and even more so his parents were extremely concerned about physical attractiveness and being thin.

The defensive pattern also characterized Sarah's relationship with her mother. Sarah felt that her mother was cold and distant. She believed that it would be threatening to her mother if she let her know that she wanted her to be more open and affectionate with her. Hence, she conformed to this unspoken request, but labored at securing her mother's approval by doing things she expected—this ranged from day-to-day issues such as buying clothes for herself based on her mother's preferences to deciding not to have any more children because her mother was opposed to large families. Shortly after Sarah entered therapy, her mother informed her that she was going to move to a retirement home in Arizona. Sarah realized that she was furious at her mother for making this decision, but when her mother visited her for a farewell get-together, Sarah left the room when she felt she could no longer control her emotions.

The defensive pattern also characterized Sarah's initial approach to therapy. It was very difficult for her to acknowledge any of her problems. In fact, at first she only mentioned the depression and her physical complaints, not the bulimia. She repeatedly returned to the idea that these problems might be caused by premenstrual syndrome. Even after she told me about her eating disorder (after about 6 weeks), she frequently brought up questions about how could therapy possibly help her. Her questions were based on her belief that the problem was her own failure at exerting sufficient self-control. Hence, only she could make things better. Sarah's stance reflected a difficulty asking for help. (Here it can be seen how harsh, critical views of self—"I should be able to control myself"—played a part in the defensive action pattern by contributing to her stance of taking care of things herself rather than asking for what she needed.)

The therapeutic approach was based on an appreciation of Sarah's starting point. To begin with, these considerations pointed away from efforts aimed directly at the eating disorder symptoms, because such efforts would amount to another demand for Sarah to comply with. Her own strained efforts along these lines had not worked and there was no reason to believe that direct interventions by a therapist would prove any more successful. More importantly, such efforts would not address Sarah's wishes or her fears.

I endeavored to help Sarah by focusing on her interpersonal relationships. We worked on her relationships with her in-laws first and went on to her relationships with her mother, father, husband, and children. Also, as I will explain later, one line of efforts focused on Sarah separate from involvements with others. The work included a combination of insight-oriented and behavioral interventions directed at helping Sarah to identify and acknowledge her wishes and her fears, and to develop ways of embracing the wishes and acting in the face of her fears in her day-to-day life. The treatment included antidepressant medication for a period of time.

The behavioral interventions were seldom direct suggestions. Sarah would have felt obliged to try to comply with them. Instead, I usually presented these suggestions in ways that downplayed their action implications or as ideas for "percolating." One important benefit derived from presenting these ideas about possible actions in specific situations was that it gave Sarah the opportunity to learn when suggestions seemed possible and appealing to her and when they did not, that is, to say "no" in a straightforward manner. It was extremely important for her to discover that another person would accept her even if she did not go along with them. Another thing accomplished by putting action suggestions on the table was that these concrete examples provided Sarah with opportunities to learn what it would *mean* to act in a new way. For example, I asked her what she thought it would be like to tell her mother-in-law that she was sorry about the problem she was having with Sarah's husband, but that she (the mother-in-law) should speak to him about it herself. It was clear that this suggestion served the prospective function of concretely pointing out a way of relating to others that was new to her—even though prior to this point Sarah had some general thoughts about wanting to be respected and recognized for her own sake.

Other examples of behavioral interventions focused on Sarah's relationship with her mother. For example, early in treatment I raised the possibility of buying clothes for herself that she liked whether or not her mother would like them. Other examples included telling her mother that she wished her mother would talk to her about her feelings, and letting her mother know how much she cared about her (Sarah had been very reserved in her expression of feelings toward her mother). These efforts proved to be very helpful. Sarah's relationship with her mother changed a good deal. Sarah reached out to her mother and her mother began to respond. A new issue came up in the therapy, however, when it was discovered that Sarah's mother had stomach cancer. There were setbacks when her mother began to deny her fears and temporarily became more reserved as in the past, but Sarah and her mother were able to recoup the gains they had made and build upon them right up until her mother died a year later. I made behavioral suggestions similar to those just mentioned throughout this period, but another important component of the work was helping Sarah "decouple" her actions from their consequences. She began to experience a certain kind of satisfaction when she acted in ways that were right for her even if her mother did not respond in the hoped for manner. Sarah was able to accept disappointments in an open, non-defended way, including the great sadness she experienced when her mother died.

Insight-oriented efforts were integrated with behavioral interventions throughout the course of therapy. While Sarah developed greater understanding of herself in terms of such issues as why she related to other people the way she did and what that way was like, such questions were seldom the focus of the work. Instead, my insight-oriented comments were aimed at helping her recognize and acknowledge her wishes and fears. We discussed her childhood at a number of points, but even at those times the focus was on her wishes and fears. For example, Sarah recalled that when she and her siblings were given their Chanukah presents, she would worry about whether her siblings got the presents they wanted. As she thought about this memory, Sarah realized how fearful she had been about letting her mother know what presents she wanted.

Insight-oriented efforts focused on wishes and fears also proved important when Sarah learned that her estranged father had cardiac myopathy and did not have long to live. She learned this shortly before her mother died. As we discussed her feelings about her father and whether she wanted to go see him, she realized she was afraid that he would turn his back on her again, especially if she were to let him know how angry she was at him because he abandoned the family. When Sarah was able to recognize this fear, she decided that she wanted to see him before he died. Sarah's relationship with her father was never transformed to the extent that had occurred in her relationship with her mother, but she made significant changes in that relationship too.

As noted above, one line of efforts focused on Sarah herself, separate from her relationships. At the beginning of therapy, Sarah's enmeshed involvements filled up virtually her whole life. Going to therapy was itself the first example of doing things for herself. Some of my behavioral interventions were suggestions about taking time to rest, read, take walks, and so forth. Sarah experimented with some of these suggestions.

About 2 years into the 3-year period of treatment, Sarah informed me that she had started to paint as a hobby.

A few comments about the role of the therapeutic relationship in the treatment process: One important component of the therapy was my consistent communication of concern about and interest in how Sarah was feeling, including both positive and negative emotions. I believe this gratified her wish for nurturance in a helpful way and that it led her to feel accepted. I also believe it was important that I avoided behavioral interventions aimed directly at the eating disorder symptoms, but I think it was even more important that I took an active stance in which I directed attention again and again to Sarah's wishes and fears by means of insight-oriented and behavioral interventions. Without this element, the therapy context would not have been a nurturing environment for her, because it would not have offered her opportunities to find new ways to incorporate these feelings in her life.

Although therapeutic relationship factors played a central role, the therapy included very little transference work. For example, when it seemed that Sarah was having trouble discussing something she was upset about, I usually (not always) directed attention to fears she had about the issue raised rather than to her difficulty talking to me about it. I have found transference work to be a helpful way to respond to therapeutic relationship concerns in other cases, but this case illustrates how attention to the therapeutic relationship can play a role even when transference work is minimal.

The treatment was successful. It helped Sarah make a broad range of changes in her life. These included changes in the eating disorder symptoms, even though these were never a direct focus of therapeutic efforts. About six months after the start of therapy, Sarah completely stopped binging and purging. She then gained a considerable amount of weight, but became less and less concerned about how others would view her. After about two years, she decided to go on a diet and got down to a healthy weight. In many ways, her relationships changed to reflect a nondefensive pattern. As noted above, this included creating a close, warm relationship with her mother. Her relationships with her in-laws, especially her mother-in-law, also changed for the better, but here her connections became less intense. She was able to free herself almost entirely from the old enmeshed pattern. She realized that her mother-in-law's apparent warmth and caring (which had always been contingent upon her playing the expected role) was not what she really wanted. Her relationship with her husband became stronger and more satisfying. Her relationships with her children deepened, but she also stopped being overinvolved in their lives. In general, she became more independent and at the same time closer to the people who were important to her. She stepped more fully into the circle of her life, more actively embracing her wishes and accepting pain and sorrow when that was part of her experience.

CONCLUDING COMMENTS

My objective in this chapter was to show that if we turn to a consideration of basic philosophical issues and adopt a perspective that represents fully stepping inside the circle (recognizing that we lead our lives as participants not removed onlookers), it is possible to discover the basis for an effective approach to psychotherapy. There is a need for additional work to explore and clarify the implications of the perspective, but I believe the framework is sufficiently promising to justify such efforts. These efforts should include additional clinical/theoretical investigation of the usefulness of the approach as well as systematic empirical research.

As I see it, empirical research efforts should not involve investigations pitting this approach against others—because the results of such "horse race" studies typically are uninformative—but rather attempts to examine specific phenomena from the viewpoint of the hermeneutic framework. For example, there is a need for research on defensive processes in psychopathology and psychotherapy. As I noted above, I have begun to investigate defensive patient interpersonal behavior in therapy (Westerman & Foote, 1988; Westerman et al., 1986, 1987, 1990). Recent research by Luborsky and Crits-Christoph (1990) on the Core Conflictual Relationship Theme and by Horowitz and his colleagues (Horowitz, Rosenberg, Ureno, Kalehzan, & O'Halloran, 1989) on the Consensual Response Method also suggest the value of focusing on defensive processes. The hermeneu-

tic framework offers guidelines for the direction of future efforts along these lines. In particular, it suggests that the primary focus should be on defensive action patterns rather than on internal processes of defense. The framework also points to the need for further research on the interpersonal significance of patient and therapist behavior, rather than work that reflects traditional notions about the value of adopting a reflective stance to oneself in treatment and coming to understand oneself better as an observer. The results of recent research challenging the old maxim about relations between psychological health and self-knowledge (Taylor & Brown, 1988) support the points made here about how the traditional perspective is misleading when it comes to conceptualizing the role played by insight or cognition. Indeed, the comments offered above about the differences between insight-oriented work that reflects the "grammar of understanding" versus the "grammar of thinking in the service of change" provide the basis for a very promising line of investigation about how insight-oriented work can be most helpful.

The thrust of this chapter has been to show that consideration of philosophical issues is worthwhile because it leads to useful ideas about therapeutic practice. In closing, I would like to suggest that it is also right and fitting for psychotherapists to be concerned about fundamental issues for their own sake. As we engage with our patients in the circle of the therapeutic process, we do this as participants in the larger circle of the world we share with others. Such starting point concerns as what it means to be a person inescapably play a role in our efforts.

REFERENCES

Arkowitz, H. (1989). From behavior change to insight. *Journal of Integrative and Eclectic Psychotherapy, 8,* 222–232.

Arkowitz, H., & Hannah, M. (1989). Cognitive, behavioral, and psychodynamic therapies: Converging or diverging pathways to change? In A. Freeman, K. Simon, L. Beutler, & H. Arkowitz (Eds.), *Comprehensive handbook of cognitive therapy* (pp. 144–167). New York: Plenum Press.

Benjamin, L. S. (1982). Use of Structural Analysis of Social Behavior (SASB) to guide intervention in psychotherapy. In J. Anchin & D. Kiesler (Eds.), *Handbook of interpersonal psychotherapy* (pp. 190–212). New York: Pergamon.

Braswell, L., & Kendall, P. C. (1988). Cognitive-behavioral methods with children. In K. S. Dobson (Ed.), *Handbook of cognitive-behavioral therapies* (pp. 167–213). New York: Guilford.

Dreyfus, H. L. (1979). *What computers can't do.* New York: Harper & Row.

Fischer, K. W. (1980). A theory of cognitive development: The control and construction of hierarchies of skills. *Psychological Review, 87,* 477–531.

Fischer, K. W., Shaver, P. R., & Carnochan, P. (1988). From basic- to subordinate-category emotions: A skill approach to emotional development. In W. Damon (Ed.), *Child development today and tomorrow,* New Directions for Child Development, No. 40. San Francisco: Jossey-Bass.

Fischer, K. W., Shaver, P. R., & Carnochan, P. (1990). How emotions develop and how they organise development. *Cognition and Emotion, 4,* 81–127.

Gill, M. M. (1982). Analysis of transference, Vol. 1: Theory and technique. *Psychological Issues,* Monograph 53.

Goldfried, M. R. (1982). Resistance and clinical behavior therapy. In P. L. Wachtel (Ed.), *Resistance: Psychodynamic and behavioral approaches* (pp. 95–113). New York: Plenum Press.

Greenberg, L. S., & Safran, J. D. (1987). *Emotion in psychotherapy: Affect, cognition and the process of change.* New York: Guilford.

Haley, J. (1963). *Strategies of psychotherapy.* New York: Grune & Stratton.

Heidegger, M. (1962). *Being and time* (M. Macquarrie & E. Robinson, Trans.). New York: Harper & Row.

Horowitz, L. M., Rosenberg, S. E., Ureno, G., Kalehzan, B. M., & O'Halloran, P. (1989). Psychodynamic formulations, consensual response method, and interpersonal problems. *Journal of Consulting and Clinical Psychology, 57,* 599–606.

Horvath, A. O., & Goheen, M. D. (1990). Factors mediating the success of defiance- and compliance-based interventions. *Journal of Counseling Psychology, 37,* 363–371.

Husserl, E. (1931). *Ideas: General introduction to pure phenomenology* (W.R.B. Gibson, Trans.). New York: Macmillan.

Kaye, K. (1984). Toward a developmental psychology of the family. In L. L'Abates (Ed.), *Handbook of family psychology and psychotherapy* (Vol.1, pp. 38–72). Homewood, IL: Dow Jones-Irwin.

Kitchener, R. F. (1980). Ethical relativism and behavior therapy. *Journal of Consulting and Clinical Psychology, 48,* 1–7.

Kolko, D. J., & Milan, M. A. (1983). Reframing and paradoxical instruction to overcome "resistance" in the treatment of delinquent youths: A multiple baseline analysis. *Journal of Consulting and Clinical Psychology, 51,* 655–660.

Lazarus, A. A., & Fay, A. (1982). Resistance or rationalization? A cognitive-behavioral perspective. In P. L. Wachtel (Ed.), *Resistance: Psychodynamic and behavioral approaches* (pp. 115–132). New York: Plenum Press.

Luborsky, L., & Crits-Christoph, P. (Eds.) (1990). *Understanding transference: The CCRT method.* New York: Basic Books.

Mahoney, M. J. (1988). The cognitive sciences and psychotherapy: Patterns in a developing relationship. In K. S. Dobson (Ed.), *Handbook of cognitive-behavioral therapies* (pp. 357–386). New York: Guilford.

McDaniel, S. H., Stiles, W. B., & McGaughey, K. J. (1981). Correlations of male college students' verbal response mode use in psychotherapy with measures of psychological disturbance and psychotherapy outcome. *Journal of Consulting and Clinical Psychology, 49,* 571–582.

Merleau-Ponty, M. (1962). *Phenomenology of perception* (C. Smith, Trans.). London: Routledge & Kegan Paul.

Messer, S. B. (1986). Behavioral and psychoanalytic perspectives at therapeutic choice points. *American Psychologist, 41,* 1261–1272.

Piaget, J. (1983). Piaget's theory. In W. Kessen (Ed.), *History, theory, and methods* (pp. 703–732), Vol. 1 in P. H. Mussen (Ed.), *Handbook of child psychology* (4th ed.). New York: Wiley.

Safran, J. D. (1989). Insight and action in psychotherapy. *Journal of Integrative and Eclectic Psychotherapy, 8,* 233–239.

Safran, J. D., & Greenberg, L. S. (1986). Hot cognition and psychotherapy process: An information processing/ecological approach. In P. C. Kendall (Ed.), *Advances in cognitive-behavioral research and therapy* (Vol. 5, pp. 143–177). New York: Academic Press.

Sampson, E. E. (1988). The debate on individualism: Indigenous psychologies of the individual and their role in personal and societal functioning. *American Psychologist, 43,* 15–22.

Schwartz, R. M. (1984). Is rational-emotive therapy a truly unified interactive approach? A reply to Ellis. *Clinical Psychology Review, 4,* 219–226.

Sollod, R. N., & Wachtel, P. L. (1980). A structural and transactional approach to cognition in clinical problems. In M. J. Mahoney (Ed.), *Psychotherapy process: Current issues and future directions* (pp. 1-27). New York: Plenum Press.

Spence, D. P. (1982). *Narrative truth and historical truth: Meaning and interpretation in psychoanalysis.* New York: Norton.

Stiles, W. B., Shapiro, D. A., & Elliott, R. (1986). "Are all psychotherapies equivalent?" *American Psychologist, 41,* 165–180.

Sullivan, H. S. (1953). *The interpersonal theory of psychiatry.* New York: Norton.

Taylor, S. E., & Brown, D. (1988). Illusion and well-being: A social psychological perspective on mental health. *Psychological Bulletin, 103,* 193–210.

Wachtel, P. L. (1977). *Psychoanalysis and behavior therapy: Toward an integration.* New York: Basic Books.

Wachtel, P. L. (1987a). *Action and insight.* New York: Guilford.

Wachtel, P. L. (1987b). The philosophic and the therapeutic: Considerations regarding the goals of psychoanalysis and other therapies. In P. L. Wachtel (Ed.), *Action and insight* (pp. 185–206). New York: Guilford.

Watzlawick, P., Weakland, J. H., & Fisch, R. (1974). *Change: Principles of problem formation and problem resolution.* New York: Norton.

Westen, D. (1985). *Self and society: Narcissism, collectivism, and the development of morals.* Cambridge: Cambridge University Press.

Westen, D. (1986). What changes in short-term psychodynamic psychotherapy? *Psychotherapy, 23,* 501–512.

Westerman, M. A. (1984). Standing outside the circle [Review of *Narrative truth and historical truth*]. *Contemporary Psychology, 29,* 277–279.

Westerman, M. A. (1986). Meaning and psychotherapy: A hermeneutic reconceptualization of insight-oriented, behavioral, and strategic approaches. *Journal of Integrative and Eclectic Psychotherapy, 5,* 47–68.

Westerman, M. A. (1987). Social interaction, goals, and cognition. *Journal of Mind and Behavior, 8,* 291–315.

Westerman, M. A. (1989). A naturalized view of the role

played by insight in psychotherapy. *Journal of Integrative and Eclectic Psychotherapy, 8,* 197–221.

Westerman, M. A., & Foote, J. P. (1988, June). *Revised scales for measuring coordinating style: Psychometric properties and relations with other patient interpersonal behavior variables.* Paper presented at the meetings of the Society for Psychotherapy Research, Santa Fe, NM.

Westerman, M. A., Tanaka, J. S., Frankel, A. S., & Kahn, J. (1986). The coordinating style construct: An approach to conceptualizing patient interpersonal behavior. *Psychotherapy, 23,* 540–547.

Westerman, M. A., Frankel, A. S., Tanaka, J. S., & Kahn, J. (1987). Client cooperative interview behavior and outcome in paradoxical and behavioral brief treatment approaches. *Journal of Counseling Psychology, 34,* 99–102.

Westerman, M. A., Foote, J. P., McCullough, L., & Winston, A. (1990, June). *Patient coordination in different phases of short-term therapy and process-outcome relations.* Paper presented at the meetings of the Society for Psychotherapy Research, Wintergreen, VA.

Wittgenstein, L. (1958). *Philosophical investigations* (3rd ed., G. E. M. Anscomb, Trans.). New York: Macmillan.

Woolfolk, R. L., & Richardson, F. C. (1984). Behavior therapy and the ideology of modernity. *American Psychologist, 39,* 777–786.

CHAPTER 15

A Feminist Framework for Integrative Psychotherapy

Iris G. Fodor

INTRODUCTION

Feminism: the doctrine of advocating social and political rights for women equal to men (Webster's New Collegiate Dictionary, 1979).

I have found that my own womanhood is a very important factor in my work as a therapist. With some women it adds an expectation of being understood in a way no man could understand them. This leads to a willingness to be open, to discuss things with me that they might "confess" to a man but they can tell me. It leads also, I believe to their become more confronting, less docile, less cowed by their therapist. Taking me on in an argument makes the odds seem a little more in their favor. . . . It gives me an advantage in working with women because there is a diminished likelihood that they can brush aside my disagreeable comments or observations as less relevant to them because I "don't really know how it is." I do know how it is, I have been there and I am still there. (Miriam Polster, 1974, p. 262)

For the past decade, one of the fastest growing therapies has been feminist therapy. The interest in women's issues and feminist therapy is evidenced in the appearance of dozens of books on feminist therapy, theory, or a feminist approach to particular clinical issues. The feminist approaches

to therapy stress the importance of paying attention to gender, sex role socialization, and expectations. In particular, they highlight the issues of inequality and the phenomenology of maleness and femaleness as central to the way clients and therapists construe the world and goals. Often the work in feminist therapy highlights the tension between changing the individual versus changing society. Feminist therapy ideally should be called nonsexist therapy, contextual therapy, or gender-based therapy since the approach is also applicable to men and their issues. In practice, however, feminist theory and therapy have been framed by women therapists working with women on women's issues, who prefer to call their approach feminist therapy.

In this chapter, I will review the history of feminism and feminist therapy, and outline the feminist framework for therapy. Next, I will present highlights from clinical cases to illustrate the integration of a feminist approach with two systems of therapy, cognitive behavioral therapy and gestalt therapy.

THE FEMINIST APPROACH TO THERAPY

Feminist therapy is more of an approach to therapy. It is a framework and way of analysis rather than a full system of therapy. There is not

Iris G. Fodor • Department of Applied Psychology, New York University, New York, New York 10003.

Comprehensive Handbook of Psychotherapy Integration, edited by George Stricker and Jerold R. Gold. Plenum Press, New York, 1993.

one feminist therapy but multiple feminist approaches to therapy. These approaches vary. The most radical approaches reject therapy training and traditional practice. In this chapter, I will try to highlight the most central features of feminist theory and practice commonly adapted by most feminist therapists (Brown & Brodsky, 1992, Sturdivant, 1980).

From their beginning, feminists in moving away from psychoanalytic theory and traditional therapeutic practice integrated feminist ways of thinking with the newer therapies, mainly humanistic and cognitive behavior therapy (CBT). I have had training and experience with three modalities of therapy: psychoanalysis, cognitive-behavioral therapy, and gestalt therapy and have practiced feminist therapy within each modality. Although feminist therapy originally rejected psychoanalysis, in recent years, many feminist psychoanalysts have built a case for a feminist approach to analysis (Alpert, 1987; Chodorow, 1989; Eichenbaum & Orbach, 1983; Miller, 1973; Mitchell, 1975). Recent work in integrating feminism and psychoanalysis has highlighted the gendered nature of self and reemphasized the important role of the mother in the psychological development of both male and female children (Chodorow, 1978, 1989; Dinnerstein, 1977; Jordan, Kaplan, Miller, Stiver, & Surrey, 1991; Kaplan & Yasinski, 1980). Most feminist therapists, including myself, utilize some psychoanalytic understanding and or methodology in their work, whatever their therapeutic orientation.

In this chapter, I will sketch out the main features of feminist therapy and will illustrate its integration with cognitive behavior therapy and gestalt therapy. The integration of feminist therapy and psychoanalysis will not be covered in this chapter. For a fuller discussion of this approach see (Alpert, 1987; Eichenbaum & Orbach, 1983; and Jordan et al., 1991).

Feminist therapy is very compatible with cognitive behavior therapy with its emphasis on social learning and the development of a systematic treatment. In fact, feminist cognitive behavior therapists have pioneered treatments for specific women's issues (e.g., battering, sexual abuse, eating disorders, phobias, lack of assertiveness) (Blechman, 1984; Fodor, 1988; Walker, 1984). However, feminist therapy in practice, is most similar to gestalt therapy. Both of these therapies stay close to the client's experience, highlight process, emphasize self-support, and espouse an equalitarian therapist–client relationship (Polster, 1974; Simkin & Yontef, 1984; Yontef, 1976).

FEMINIST THEORY/FEMINIST THERAPY

Feminist therapy, more than most other therapies, draws from anthropology, sociology, literary and art criticisms, philosophy, linguistics, and law as well as psychology. Thus, the basic theoretical framework is interdisciplinary. Most feminist therapists, expand their domain beyond psychology, drawing on and contributing to the intellectual richness of contemporary work in literary theory, the arts, history, sociolinguistics, and philosophy (Brown & Brodsky, 1992; Jagger & Rothenberg, 1984; Morgan, 1970; Snitow, Stansell, & Thomson, 1983).

Contemporary feminist theory highlights the patriarchal structure of society, the history of women's oppression, the special power inequities that exist between the sexes, particularly in the domain of sexuality and reproduction. Simone De Beavoir (1961) articulated the basic feminist philosophy with the publication of *The Second Sex*. She pointed out that throughout history, man has been cast as the central hero and his actions constitute the norm, while woman was the other, the object of his desires. Furthermore, she illustrated how most societies are organized around a patriarchal structure, which puts man in charge and delimits women's roles.

Contemporary feminist historians have stressed the fact that until recently women were invisible in history; history is *his story*. Feminist sociologists have highlighted the economic oppression of women, the appropriation of a woman's body and labor within the family, and the continued disadvantaged status of women today (Jagger & Rothenberg, 1984; Reiker & Carmen, 1984).

Literary critics focus on how most representations of women in literature are men's constructions. Kate Millet's (1969), *Sexual Politics* critically attacked Freud, Henry Miller, D. H. Lawrence, and Norman Mailer for their depictions of women. Her work led to a female constructed literary view of women and their sexuality. Discourse analysis and linguists have focused on the sexist aspects of language. They described how ordinary language often renders women invisible (e.g., they deplored the use of generic terms such as "mankind" to describe men and women). They argued that male dominant culture structures language and thought. Feminist philosophers have pointed out that enlightenment thinking is a male take on epistemology, while recent feminist work has focused on a woman's way of knowing (Belenkey, Clinchy, Goldberger, & Tarule, 1986). Many feminist thinkers have embraced deconstructionism, which emphasizes not one truth but multiple narratives and interpretations (Flax, 1990).

Within psychology, feminists provided an impetus for new research on sex role stereotyping, sex roles and bias, and gender development. Weinsstein's (1970) essay, entitled "Psychology Constructs the Female," first provided an impetus to look at the biased view of women in psychology. The psychology of women is now considered a legitimate field of study. Furthermore, this work has influenced understanding of the psychology of men and male roles. Attention has been also given to studying gender differences across various domains (e.g., morality, achievement, body image, etc. (Gilligan, 1982; Unger, 1979).

Another classic paper by Rich (1980) on compulsory heterosexuality challenged the view of heterosexuality as the norm for women. Women began to challenge psychology's take on female sexuality and began theory building and research toward a female defined sexuality, that included lesbian choice (Boston Lesbian Psychologies Collective, 1987; Brown, 1990; Snitow *et al.*, 1983; Vance, 1984).

CLINICAL AND THEORETICAL ANTECEDENTS OF FEMINIST THERAPY

Mainstream feminist therapy developed in the 1970s and grew out of the women's movement and the radical politics of the 1960s. More so than most psychotherapy writings, the feminist approach is political. Feminists adhere to a radical orientation, often Marxist, which looks beyond women's oppression to other oppressions (race, class) and posits a multicultural perspective (Brown, 1990).

In the 1960s, many traditions in our society were attacked and overturned. Within psychotherapy, there developed the antipsychiatry move-

ment led by Szasz (1961) and Laing (Boyers & Grill, 1971). Both Szasz and Laing were critical of the mental health establishment that labeled patients sick. Instead, they posited that the locus of mental illness lies in a sick society. About the same time, the humanistic psychology and the human potential movements began to espouse a different type of therapy emphasizing personal responsibility and self-actualization (Lerman, 1992). Additionally, they argued that therapy should not be limited to the emotionally disturbed, but available for everyone for personal growth.

As feminist ways of thinking emerged, women who were active in the antiwar and civil rights movements began to see that they were also an oppressed group. They argued for elimination of barriers that prevented their full participation in society. In 1970, the Boston Women's Health Book Collective published *Our Bodies Ourselves* (rev. ed., 1988) and women joined women's groups which focused on teaching about their bodies and sexuality.

Women therapists, like other women, formed consciousness-raising groups to share their stories and to question the traditional sex role programming. All aspects of their lives were examined. These included how they were raised, their sexual orientation, their relationships (e.g., with their parents, children, and mates). These therapists critically examined traditional therapy theory and practice (Kirsh, 1974; Kravetz, 1980). In 1972, Chessler, a feminist therapist, wrote *Women and Madness*. Her book was an angry attack on how a sick society had driven women mad. She was especially critical of psychotherapeutic treatments for women. Her causes were adapted by many feminist therapists.

Feminist therapists were particularly critical of mainstream psychoanalysis, the prevailing psychotherapy at that time, for assigning women to a second-class status. They rejected the psychoanalytic emphasis on the Oedipal complex, penis envy, and a limited view of femininity. In the beginning, feminist therapists worked to develop therapeutic practices that were distinctly different from the psychoanalytic way of working with clients. They formed feminist therapy collectives for support, training, and referral networks. They organized informal conferences and passed around unpublished manuscripts (Brodsky & Hare Mustin, 1980; Lerman, 1986).

Another major impetus to the development of feminist therapy practice was the grass roots women's movement. These grass roots feminists, often together in community collectives, were pioneers in setting up shelters and treatments for women. They developed crisis intervention and problem-solving treatments targeted to survivors of sexual abuse, rape, and battering, and helped put these issues on the national mental health agenda (Rosewater & Walker, 1985).

More than twenty years of feminist therapy has impacted psychotherapy practice and thinking in the mental health community. Contemporary feminist therapists have produced a large array of clinical books and publications. There is a national professional organization (Feminist Therapy Institute) and there are women's interests sections of major professional psychology and therapy organizations. In fact, feminist therapists are having increasing success in putting women's issues and shaping the agendas of national organizations and governmental funding agencies. (NIMH funded a conference to formulate a research agenda for women's mental health. The American Psychological Association put together a task force on sex bias in psychotherapy, and one on women and depression.) Other women's issues, for example, health, battering, and sexual abuse have also become national priorities (Dilling & Claster, 1985; McGrath, Puryear Keita, Strickland, & Russo, 1990).

FEMINIST THERAPY AS AN INTEGRATIONIST THERAPY

Feminist therapy does not posit one true therapy, nor do feminist therapists rally round one therapy guru. Although they do not represent any one specific therapeutic modality, feminist therapists tend to work together in their conferences and workshops, dialoguing with one another (Brodsky & Hare-Mustin, 1980; Brown, 1990; Rosewater & Walker, 1985). Most of the major writings in feminist therapy are by psychoanalysts, cognitive behavior therapists, and therapists who primarily identify themselves as feminist therapists (Brodsky & Hare-Mustin, 1980; Douglas & Walker, 1988; Rosewater & Walker, 1985). There is also a growing interest in the feminist approach to marital and family therapy (Bo-

grad, 1988; McGoldrick, Anderson, & Walsh, 1978). However, many eclectic and humanistic therapists, who have not fully articulated the feminist perspectives in writing also ascribe to the feminist approach (Polster, 1974). However, Lerman (1992) cautions that there is still bias and sexist thinking within the humanistic tradition.

On a theoretical basis, the approach is similar to the framing of radical psychiatry in that the client's problems can only be viewed in their social context. The therapy, however, integrates aspects of existential humanistic psychology (mostly Rogerian therapy). In feminist therapy, the therapist is equalitarian, and validates the clients' experience, while the clients are given the responsibility for their own choices and change process. The major goals derive from Maslow's theory of self-actualization (Lerman, 1992).

However, unlike existential and Rogerian therapy, feminist therapy emphasizes change. So feminists, to foster the goal of empowerment, utilize techniques from cognitive behavior therapy to teach new behaviors to clients. Feminist therapy is also constructivist and would fit a Kellian cognitive therapy model as well. In feminist therapy, the client is encouraged to examine her existing framing of experience and through therapy learns to construct a new way of thinking and behaving (Fodor, 1988).

Feminist therapists have also borrowed heavily from contemporary psychoanalytic theorizing from an object relations framework. Particularly germane to most feminist therapy is the highlighting of women's attachments, self development, individuation, and mother–daughter issues (Chodorow, 1989; Flax, 1990; Miller, 1976). How psychoanalysts who use feminist frameworks inform their work is beyond the scope of this chapter. Where possible, I will try to bring in some of the psychodynamic understanding into the case discussions.

BASIC PRINCIPLES OF FEMINIST THERAPY

The Centrality of Gender

Feminists believe gender is central to the way humans organize their lives and experience. Biologically, men and women are different, and this difference may influence temperament and emotional reactivity (Unger, 1979). Furthermore, women and men from birth onward have distinct psychological experiences and upbringing. Psychoanalysts posit that women stay more connected to their mothers, which inhibits individuation, while men achieve independence by separation (Chodorow, 1979). In addition, different key issues dominate the psychological life of men and women (e.g., reproductive options). Furthermore, as noted elsewhere, in our culture women and men are treated differentially by society.

Feminist Diagnosis

In general, feminist therapists are critical of traditional diagnostic categories. They will try not to label a patient as sick, but, instead, blame a sick society which delimits women's roles and possibilities as the problem. Rosewater (1988), a feminist critique of traditional labelings writes: "DSM-III (APA, 1980) and its proposed revision mirror the stereotyping and devaluing of feminine roles" (p. 139).

In looking at DSM-III diagnostic categories, we see that its classifications are consistent with male and female sex role stereotyping. Women predominate in depression, agoraphobia, sexual dysfunction, anxiety states, multiple personality, psychogenic pain disorder, bulimia, and anorexia. Among the personality disorders, women are more likely to be classified under histrionic, borderline, and dependent. Hence, we see women as more out of control emotionally and more hysterical and dependent. Men are more likely to be classified as alcoholics, drug abusers, or having an intermittent explosive, paranoid personality, antisocial, or compulsive personality disorder (Fodor & Rothblum, 1985). Feminists are protesting the new DSM-III-R (1987) categories (e.g., self-defeating personality disorder and premenstrual disorder) as perpetuating sexists ways of looking at women's mental problems.

Studies of mental health professionals suggest that they do use sex role stereotyping in differentially evaluating the mental health of males and females (American Psychological Association Task Force on Sex Bias and Sex-Role Stereotyping in Psychotherapeutic Practice, 1975; Broverman, Broverman, Clarkson, Rosenkrantz, &

Vogel, 1970; Sesan, 1988). However, when we examine feminist therapists' ratings of clients, they are found to present women as less mentally ill compared to other therapists (Gilbert, 1980).

Some theorists are moving beyond criticism and addressing diagnostic issues from a feminist perspective. Brown and Ballou (1992), have edited a book on feminism and psychopathology. They have highlighted key features of a feminist approach to many disorders (e.g., depression, PTSD, and agoraphobia). Their approach to diagnosis emphasizes socialization or the victimization process as the problem. They emphasize the interactive effect of person and environment.

IS FEMINIST THERAPY
FOR WOMEN ONLY?

Most feminist therapists, including myself, work with men, heterosexual and gay as well as couples. While there has been a beginning work on men's roles and male psychology, most of the research on gender issues in psychology has been done by women psychologists and therapists on women's issues.

The feminist approach to the study of male roles emphasizes that the way men are socialized and the pressure to conform to male sex role stereotypes creates barriers for males from developing their full potential. Male issues highlighted are: the pressure to achieve, the need for control, discomfort in being intimate and open about feelings, and an equation of sexuality with genital functioning (Pleck, 1976; Unger, 1979). Furthermore, these issues create problems for men and women in their relationships with one another. For example, Tannen (1990) in her popular book, *You Just Don't Understand*, illustrates how male and female differences relate to problems in communication for couples.

So a feminist approach similar to the one to be presented would work for both men and women and could be used by both male and female therapists. However, most men are not asking for training in feminist therapy. (This author found male students receptive to and appreciative of exposure to a feminist framework in her graduate courses.) Furthermore, while the basic feminist framework could be useful in working with men on male issues, it could also be adapted in work with diverse populations, highlighting class, race, or ethnicity.

THE THERAPEUTIC RELATIONSHIP

In feminist therapy, the therapist–client role is equalitarian as much as possible. However, in reality, the client is distressed and is seeking help from an expert. Feminist therapists try to be aware of this "temporary inequity" (Brown, 1985). They tend to view the client as the expert in that "they respect her perception of her world and credit her knowledge about herself and possible solutions to her problem" (Cammaert & Larsen, 1988, p. 18). They also encourage clients to shop around and interview potential therapists.

Feminist therapists see the validation of women's experience as a central feature of the therapy. Women come in berating themselves for being anxious, being in abusive relationships, not being able to handle being alone, and so forth. They worry about losing control of their lives and going mad. The feminist therapist will reframe the issue to help women make sense of what they are experiencing as normal or appropriate. For example, a woman who is battered may be unable or afraid to leave her husband. She worries about him and excuses his abuse. She berates herself for her weakness and continued attachment to her husband and for putting herself and her children in jeopardy. A feminist therapist helping the woman leave the abuse situation would gently sympathize with the woman's plight. She would let her know most women feel responsible for their relationships, often feel compassion for men who do not treat them well, and worry about how they are going to survive alone.

Since therapists are shaped by the culture as much as the clients, the therapist's own struggles as a woman are used as therapeutic tool. Modeling and self-disclosure are an important part of the therapy. "I know what you are going through." "Here's how I managed when I was divorced and had to care for small children." Feminist therapists believe that showing that you were able to cope with adverse situations is very important modeling for women clients.

THE THERAPY

A central tenet of feminist therapy is that *the personal is political*. Thus, in beginning feminist therapy, while the therapist listens to the presenting problem and the client's story, she frames the issues and personal narrative around the particular way the client was raised as a woman in our culture. She attends to the sex role messages the client received, the ways her parents modeled males and female behaviors, and the particular gendered experiences she had in her relationships and in society (Gilbert, 1980).

In working with a woman, we examine the wider social context. Thus, a woman may report feeling in despair, and berate herself for handling the depression badly or feel helpless to cope with her life situation. The feminist approach to interpretation would be not to blame her or suggest her response is sick or inappropriate. Instead, the therapist would link the helpless feelings to the way she as a woman was socialized in our society. They would point out the many realistic barriers that make life more difficult for a woman (e.g., being the primary caretaker for many young children, lack of economic or social supports, etc.).

Empowerment is the major therapeutic goal. The emphasis is on change, not adjustment. Self-knowledge, self-actualization, enhancing autonomy, and learning about choices and decision making are central for empowerment. A secondary not spelled out political goal is to enable women to become advocates for women's issues. Activity and action are encouraged, passivity and inaction are discouraged.

Feminist therapists support a continued focus on process and evaluation during the therapy. Therapist and client continuously evaluate the progress of therapy, goal setting, and choices. The client in consultation with the therapist will eventually decide when she has achieved her therapeutic goals.

THE CONTENT OF FEMINIST THERAPY

Feminist therapists address certain content domains. These include:

1. Socialization history. What does it mean to be a female? How was one raised? What are the client's societal and parental messages about gender roles?
2. Current life cycle issues. Where is the woman in her life cycle? How do life cycle issues influence current problems, expectancies, future goal setting?
3. Relationships. All important relationships are explored (parent, mother, wife, sister, mate, etc.) How is one in relationships? Is there a pattern of dependency or abuse? One goal of feminist therapy is learning how to be in charge of yourself, while still connected to others.
4. Work. In the work area, making choices, finding meaningful work, and juggling multiple roles are highlighted.
5. Dealing with anger and self-assertion. Are clients in touch with and able to express anger appropriately? Can they assert themselves? What are the barriers to self-assertion?
6. Sexuality. How much is the client in touch with her own sexual needs? Can she assert herself sexually? Is her sexuality defined by her partner?
7. Body image. How do clients feel about their bodies? What pressure are they putting on themselves to conform to a societal image of young, thin, as attractive?
8. Self-esteem. Does the client feel good about herself?
9. Key conflicts are also highlighted. These include the conflicts between caring for others versus caring for oneself, independence versus dependence, and conflicts over multiple roles (e.g., career versus family).

CASE EXAMPLES

Feminist therapy is an approach that can be integrated into any system of therapy. Some systems of therapy facilitate such an integrative process. For the case presentations, I will describe at length, a feminist framing of a cognitive behavior case. This presentation is similar to the case described in a chapter on cognitive-behavioral feminist therapy (Fodor, 1988). In this presentation, I will try to highlight the features of feminist therapy described above. I will also discuss some of the limitations of the piecemeal cognitive-behavioral approach. To address such limitations, I will then provide a short illustration of a gestalt feminist approach derived from ongoing work in integrating gestalt and cognitive therapy (Fodor, 1987).

Integration of Feminist Therapy and Cognitive Behavior Therapy: A Case Illustration

Feminists have been integrating their approach with cognitive behavior therapy since the mid 1970s. In many ways a feminist approach appears ideally suited for such an integration. What is common to both therapies is the following:

1. Problematic behavior is viewed in both systems as learned, shaped up by the environment.
2. Cognitive restructuring is the central focus of CBT. Learning new ways of thinking is central in feminist therapy. In both approaches, socialization messages, unproductive or outmoded ways of thinking, maladaptive schemata are identified and challenged to be replaced by newer, more adaptive ways of thinking.
3. CBT puts the client in change and so does feminist therapy. They both view therapy as a vehicle for teaching the client about herself, setting her own goals and learning techniques for change.
4. Both CBT and feminist therapy are optimistic about change. Neither therapy accepts the medical model. In CBT, the locus of change is on the individual. Any client with enough motivation could learn how to combat unproductive thinking, change their way of viewing the problem, and learn more productive coping strategies. Feminist therapy, while focusing on the individual and fostering change, additionally identifies societal barriers which limit a woman's potential.
5. Both treatments are programmatic. Clear goals are outlined. Techniques are speci-

fied. Many of the techniques of CBT (e.g., modeling, self-disclosure, cognitive restructuring, assertiveness training, teaching coping strategies) are congruent with feminist therapy and have been utilized in feminist treatments for the past twenty years.

6. In both approaches, the therapist is seen as a consultant/teacher to foster new learning, to help the clients understand their belief systems and be available to challenge maladaptive or obsolete belief systems.

The following case example presents an integrated feminist CBT approach for treating a recently separated depressed woman who needs to learn, at midlife, how to be single and cope with her new life situation. The case is a fictionalized composite of many clients, and it represents CBT as an ideal feminist therapy for helping a traditional woman, Mae, reshape her life. The case is an expanded version of a traditional woman's plight discussed previously by this author (Fodor, 1988).

MAE: A TRADITIONAL WOMAN IN CRISIS

Mae, aged 50, comes for therapy, depressed and unhappy. She has been separated from her husband, John, a prominent historian, for over a year. Now John is filing for divorce and she feels she cannot cope with her life. John left her to "find himself" and he is now living with his young research assistant. Before the separation, Mae's life has centered around her husband and family. As John's wife she had been not only the homemaker but his secretary, research assistant, traveling companion, social hostess, and so forth. All of her friends are from her husband's professional world. Mae has two children, a daughter aged 21, who is now living at home with her and a son, aged 26, who is in graduate school in Oregon.

Initial Interview: The Centrality of Gender

Mae's story is a woman's narrative. She is a small, thin, midwestern woman with straight, long, gray-blond hair. She looks tired and drained and speaks in a low voice. Mae reports she is lost without her husband. She has had little identity and life of her own and is clearly quite depressed. She admits to suicidal ideation, but she states that she has no wish to die. She just wishes her husband would come back and her life would fall back into place. Her daughter is planning to move out next fall to do graduate work in Boston, and Mae is worried about living alone.

The therapist asks Mae to talk about herself. Mae reports that she has moved frequently with her husband, and she still does not feel at home in New York after living there three years. Even though she loves her co-op, she still misses her big house and friends in Ohio. Her husband now wants to sell their co-op, claiming he needs the money to buy an apartment. Mae has not worked for wages since she moved to New York. She had started work on a Ph.D. in English, but never finished, citing the difficulty of caring for young children and the frequent moves. Mae had been teaching English, as an adjunct, at a community college in Ohio. For the year and a half before the separation, she had been helping her husband write and edit his latest book. She knows she has to look for a job, and is in despair about finding work at her age. Her husband John says he is not willing to give her support for more than two years. Mae's father died two years ago and her 80-year-old mother lives in Indiana and is not well. Mae is worried that she may have to live with her mother while she undergoes hip surgery. She does not feel she can cope with that problem now.

Diagnostic Framing: The Personal Is the Political

If, as feminists, we take seriously the centrality of gender, we see that Mae's plight is less likely to happen to a man. An educated man of her generation would probably not have interrupted his education to care for children. Nor would he have put his own aspirations on hold, moved around to follow a wife, or be expected to nurse an elderly parent. Her plight is not atypical for many late middle-age depressed women who seek therapy. They were raised to follow traditional role prescriptions, to be wives and mothers. However, more of these women find themselves at midlife and older divorced or widowed and seek help in finding new roles (Fodor, 1990; McGrath *et al.*, 1990).

Mae scores high for depression on the Beck Depression Inventory (BDI) and meets the criteria for a major depressive episode (Beck, Rush, Shaw, & Emery, 1979). Mae reports that she spends her time in the house alone during the day, sleeping a good deal. At night, if her daughter goes out, she sits in front of the TV waiting for her to come home. She has no appetite, and has lost ten pounds. She feels worthless, blames herself for her husband's leaving, and appears unable to do the most simple chores around the house. She reports despair for her future. Also, these symptoms have not subsided for almost a year.

Since, the primary diagnosis is depression, a cognitive feminist approach will first address the maladaptive beliefs assumed to be contributing to the depression. We assume that she is operating according to a schema that might have served her well in the traditional wife role, but is now contributing to her depression and despair. We identify those beliefs that are outmoded and need to be challenged. These beliefs are to be replaced by more adaptive beliefs to help her deal with her loss, to adapt to her changed life, and to serve as a new organizing schema for her current life (Ellis, 1984).

- *Loss of her husband and life without a man*: "Life has no meaning without a man. I cannot be happy without him. I will never find another husband like him."
- *Self-blame*: "It's my fault, I am responsible for his leaving. If only I was a better wife. I should have known he was unhappy. I should have catered to him more. I should be better able to cope."
- *Self-esteem*: "He was somebody, I'm a nobody, a nothing. I felt like I was worth something when I was married. Now, I feel worthless."
- *I can't cope with life right now*: "I can't handle my feelings. I am afraid of being alone. I hate myself for not coping better."
- *I'm too old*: "I will be alone in my old age. I'm too old to find someone else. I've lost my looks. I look old and dried up. I feel like a burden to my daughter."
- *I'm not going to be able to take care of myself*. "I don't have the energy to work, to fight for alimony. I'm not even sure I know what I want to do. I'm going to end up, a bag lady or living in a cardboard box on the street."

Given the way that Mae was socialized as a woman of her generation who followed the traditional script, we see that her beliefs are constructions based on the societal view of her role. The focus of a feminist cognitive behavior therapy will be to challenge these outmoded beliefs, help Mae construct an alternative belief system that reflects her current life. With a more realistic schema to guide her, she will build up her coping resources, move out of the depression, deal with her loss, and find new meaning in her life. We work on her beliefs as we deal with the specific problems that Mae brings to therapy.

The Therapeutic Relationship. Although feminist therapy espouses an equalitarian relationship, clearly the therapist and Mae are not in equally powerful places in their lives. Mae is seeking a consultant, the therapist is in the role of the expert.

In feminist therapy, we tell our stories, share our vulnerabilities and pain woman to woman as part of the therapeutic process. For a depressed woman like Mae, there may be a lot of pain involved in talking together about our lives. I am close to Mae's age and I have a career. Through self-disclosure, sensitively and appropriately timed, I can let her know how it feels to be divorced, sad, lose a husband, nurse a sick parent, experience a child leaving home, and so forth. However, the self-disclosures need to be short, in tune with where the client is at. They are used for empathetic bond and a building of hope. ("It's not easy, but look you too can make it.") We are sensitive to the impact of such sharing. Obviously, in an early session, when she is overwhelmed with her own depression and separation, I will not tell her about my own painful divorce. However, when she says later on, "Oh, you are so strong," or "You would know how to cope better," or "You wouldn't know what its like to fall apart" I might let her know the details of how hard it was, how I coped. We might also have a sharing session about being mothers, being raised in the 1940s and 1950s, talk about negative feelings about our own mothers, being academic wives, turning 50, dealing with the loss of a parent, and so forth.

Boundaries are not so rigidly drawn between therapist and client in feminist therapy. However, it is important for the feminist therapist to be aware of her own issues, what she is feeling, how she and the client are different, as well as any countertransference issues. The therapist needs to acknowledge these differences and how the two situations are not comparable. She also needs to be sensitive to the impact of self-disclosure on the client. Some clients do not want to hear about your history at all.

Goal Setting

Mae asks for help now for getting through this difficult period and accepting her loss. The therapist frames some additional goals which she shares with Mae. The therapy will proceed in stages. *Initial stage*: We will help Mae to cope with her losses and get her energy back. *Second stage*: We will work with the practical issues and stresses involved with the legal issues of the separation. Mae wants help in getting clear what she wants from the settlement. She needs to learn to assert herself with her husband and to understand the dynamics that contribute to her lack of assertion. *Third stage*: This stage will be the core work of the therapy. Work will be done on helping Mae learn more about herself and how to reach an independent life.

Stage 1. Dealing with the loss of the husband and her wife role. I typically begin work on loss with the client's story of the relationship and the meaning to her of the loss. As we go along, I try to understand her beliefs and the way she construes her past. As in any therapy, we also reveal the important family history and the patterns she carried over from her childhood.

What becomes clear, as we work in Stage 1, is that Mae had replicated her mother's marriage. Her father, who ran his own business, was the dominant one and the mother deferred and complied with his wishes. She describes her mother as dependent, weak, and helpless. She worries that she has now become her mother. In fact, her daughter is now also turning on her, disgusted with her crying and clinging, saying "She's just like grandma." In telling her story, we note that some of the self-blame relates to the shock of the divorce: "I did everything right, this was not sup-posed to happen, it's not fair" or "It happened because I was not a good enough wife."

Cognitive Restructuring. As Mae begins to get in touch with anger, she sees that she constructed her life according to her mother's plan and the social role for women laid out for women of her generation. This plan did not work well for her mother and she now is dealing with how it did not work for her either. Slowly, we begin to question the family values and the prescribed social role. Mae left home to start graduate school, began to be independent, and then like so many women of her generation she gave up her career for marriage. Very slowly, there is a shift from self-blame ("I wasn't a good enough wife"), to anger ("What a fool I was to have put all my eggs into his basket and now he's gone and knocked it over"). In mourning the loss of the husband, and her idealized view of her marriage, she is both very sad and angry.

Over six months, with many sessions devoted to crying about her husband, Mae begins to feel her anger. Slowly, she begins to let go of the desire to have her husband back and reports that she is willing to fight for a fair settlement.

Stage 2: Assertiveness Training. This phase may occur in overlapping phases with Stage 1. Mae has rarely stood up to her husband. In the marriage and in other relationships with her children and parents, she is accommodating the "nice" person, thinking of other peoples' feelings, putting her own needs last. Because of the economic crisis, she now has to fight for what she wants, to put her own needs first. We use assertiveness training for standing up to her husband (Fodor, 1985). (1) She needs to get clear on how she feels (Angry!). (2) Next, she needs to know what she wants (A fair settlement). (3) Next, she works on her rights. (She has worked without wages for 25 years; she has a right to her share of the family resources and some start-up money as well.)

As we work on assertiveness skills, Mae is able to be assertive in our role plays. However, she reports that when she meets her husband outside, she becomes a marshmallow. She reports feeling anxious when she has to confront her husband ("He sounds so right, he knows how to argue, he makes me feel ridiculous, like a child and I end up crying.")

Work on Overcoming Feelings of Intimidation and Lack of Self-Confidence. Mae reports that as she confronts her husband, she feels that she is weak and he is strong, and that he still has the power to intimidate her. We explore the history of the marriage. She reports that when she worked for him, he had a way of making her feel "dumb, insecure." She also felt this same lack of respect from her father. Mae handled these remarks by becoming childlike, crying which usually got them to stop criticizing her. She also reports how humiliated she felt when she cried.

In exploring these patterns, we talk about male–female relationships in general. (The therapist shares how she often felt intimated by her husband and father, too, and that it is a common problem for women.) To facilitate her ability to confront her husband without feeling anxious or weak, we try to pinpoint the specific triggers of the intimating feelings. (This boils down to "his look," "his self-confidence," "his knowing the facts," his ability to "argue"). We role play assertive behavior in the face of these triggers.

Letting Go—Reframing. As Mae becomes more assertive, John is still not willing to give her what she wants. Instead, she reports, he has become increasingly aggressive, putting her down, calling her a bitch. In addition, he presented her his past grievances, listing all the ways she displeased him in the marriage. Mae has a hard time in this phase of work. Her whole view of her marriage (which she saw as happy until he left) begins to crumble. She becomes depressed again. She is ready to sign away everything to avoid these encounters.

In this phase, we review her marriage and she begins to talk about John's way of criticizing her. When he did not get his way, he lost his temper, became abusive, throwing her faults in her face. She was stunned by his insisting now that he never loved her. Deep sobbing occurred during this phase, the therapist was there, often crying with her. Slowly, Mae's rage emerges. Earlier in the therapy, Mae in role play expressed some anger at John, while still excusing or protecting him. Now, she rages: "What right does he have to take away her memories?" "They were in love, most of the time, it was a good marriage." She also describes his infantile behaviors, how she had to mother him, how he needed her to be

there on his out-of-town trips. She calls him her "biggest spoiled baby." The rage energizes Mae enough to confront and stand up to John. She lets him know how unacceptable his behavior is. She lets him know, for the first time, how angry she was about how the marriage broke up. In this phase of therapy, she broke the mold of the accepting, understanding wife. She is also surprised to find her daughter supporting her growing assertion.

Finally, after three months of what she calls "a living hell," Mae was able to negotiate a reasonable settlement and felt up to compromising about the time frame for leaving the co-op. She reported upon signing the agreement: "I've just given birth to myself."

Stage 3: Building a Life of Her Own. This stage might be entitled. "I got my own life back and now what do I want?" Independence and empowerment are the themes of this phase of therapy (which takes about a year and a half).

By the time the divorce is over, Mae is in an urgency about making plans for her life. She has her energy back, is still angry at her husband, who is now getting married. She and her daughter are fighting more and she wants her daughter to leave, yet, doesn't think she can live alone. (Mae has never lived alone).

On the therapy agenda are: Coping with living alone. Figuring out what to do about work. Staying in New York or returning to Ohio. Building her own social network. Since Mae has few women friends in New York and is still intimidated by living there, I refer her to a women's group as an auxiliary to our individual work.

Independence—Living Alone. Mae is still having a hard time being independent and fears living alone. She is also encouraged to read about women's lives. We begin with Simone De Beauvoir's biography, *The Prime of Life.* Mae is intrigued with the descriptions of De Beauvoir's attempt to become the independent woman, going on trips by herself. Following the book, she tries eating alone in a restaurant, going to a movie alone. Her daughter takes a short trip and we plan a weekend alone, which we reframe as "being with yourself."

Working on Self-Nurturing. Mae was too dependent on her husband to provide all her nurturing and sexual needs. She often feels emotionally depleted and cut off from what she believed was her only source of nurturance. Furthermore, as we explore what she means by nurturance, she now reports that she mostly gave, and got very little back. Mae is next encouraged to learn how to use her own nurturing energies for herself, to self pleasure. For Mae, focusing on herself is quite novel. Often, she is not sure what she wants. Gestalt awareness is used to help Mae get more in touch with herself. (Nurturance training is used to counter the belief: I can only get what I need from a man; I can't learn how to nurture myself.) She is also encouraged to reach out to women and friends for friendship, intellectual stimulation, and fun. She takes a vacation with two women friends, the first woman's only vacation and has the "time of her life." They sat in a hot tub in a resort and compared stories about their marriages and sexual experiences. Mae has her first massage, ever, by a woman. Part of the self-nurturance also involves exploring her sexuality. Since Mae was married so early, she viewed sex in terms of the male framing of the main act—sexual intercourse. With her women's group, she attended a women's sexuality workshop and discovered her own sensuality.

Work. As we explore the issue of work, we take up the threads of her earlier interests. She takes a job teaching English at a private high school for about a quarter of her husband's salary. Mae is worried about being self-supporting. Since she loves teaching, she decides that she also would like to write to supplement her income. The first summer after therapy, she went to a women's writing workshop and came back full of excitement about a possible new supplemental career doing articles about women's lives. She has made friends with other writers and has decided that New York is an ideal place for a woman her age. While, previously, most of her life revolved around couples and her husband's friends, for the first time, she is selecting her own friends based on her own interests.

Relationship with Daughter. Over the course of the two years, her daughter left home, came back and finally moved to Boston. The therapist saw them together. Many of their issues were age-related separation individuation issues (La Sorsa & Fodor, 1990). They were encouraged to read some of the new literature on mother–daughter relationships.

Evaluation

Therapy lasted two years, once a week. By the end of therapy, Mae made a major cognitive shift from depressed, lost, abandoned wife to shaping her own life, making own choices. Her mother died and she handled that loss well. She began dating again, and seeking more equality in a relationship. Her friendships with women were now seen as central.

CBT AND FEMINIST THERAPY: SOME CRITICISM

The case history of Mae provides a positive example of the integration of CBT with feminist practice at its best, for a traditionally raised woman who needs to learn how to be in charge of her life. A woman therapist who has made similar shifts in her own life is an ideal teacher and role model for such a client. The situation for most women is more complex and certain issues need to be addressed about the efficacy of such an approach.

1. CBT, even though it is based on social learning theory, puts the onus of change on the client. It is up to you to change; we can help you undo poor parenting, bad prior conditioning, or sexist socialization practices. Such optimism, however, discounts both the difficult reality of women's lives as well as the sexist practices that exist in our society that make it hard for clients to change. For example, Mae's economic situation will probably be worse. Women earn less than men and divorced women's economic status worsens. Married couples and former friends often shun their friends when they divorce. There is discrimination against older women and a shortage of age eligible men to date. Much more work needs to be done to change social conditions directly and to prepare women in therapy to cope with reality, rather than put the onus of change on individual women seeking therapy (Fodor, 1988, 1990). There is very little discussion in the integrative therapy literature addressing ways of moving beyond individual work to change society.

2. While the therapist/client model for CBT is to have the therapist be a teacher/trainer, we are assuming that the therapist will not impose her values or agenda on the client. Yet, given the instructional nature of CBT, the therapist is certainly in a powerful position by using cognitive restructuring to impose her world view on the client. Where feminist cognitive behavior therapists may run into trouble is with clients who seek help for traditional goals that differ from feminist goals. What if Mae wanted to become an even more accommodating wife to hold on to her husband? Would we be willing to do such work uncritically? Therapists need to be aware and make clients aware of such value polarities. Since cognitive restructuring is a powerful tool in the hands of a therapist who is perceived by the clients as powerful as well, we must be careful that we also have respect for who the client is, what her life style preferences are, and where she is in her development. We also need to assess, as well, how much she is willing to risk being at odds with the culture.

3. CBT emphasizes rationality and teaches techniques to foster change. Cognitive therapists hold to the belief that thoughts control feelings and hence by changing thoughts, feelings are brought under control. Feminists have criticized this approach as a male rationalist model that may not fit a woman's way of being. Furthermore, feelings have a life of their own and too often cannot be controlled by thoughts or rational thinking (Fodor, 1988).

4. CBT does not address conflicts as central to the theory or practice. Typically, a feminist CBT may strengthen one side of a split (e.g., support independence over dependence) without fully exploring the dependent side.

5. CBT, even when conducted by a feminist therapist, is very task oriented. Close examination of the therapist–client interactions is not typically carried out or this aspect is minimized in the rush to follow a program. In particular, more work needs to be done in the CBT feminist integration to explore therapy process.

Hence, if we take the above into consideration, we see that a feminist integration with CBT has some serious limitations. This integration focuses mainly on content and beliefs, which I believe are only part of the picture. What I am proposing is to add a focus on process and affect

to the basic feminist cognitive formulation described above. Such an addition derives from ongoing work on integrating cognitive with a gestalt approach to therapy (Fodor, 1987).

A FEMINIST GESTALT APPROACH: A FOCUS ON PROCESS

Although feminist writing is almost absent in gestalt therapy, the approach is quite compatible with feminist therapy. In the first book published on women in therapy, Miriam Polster (1974) describes such an approach:

In gestalt therapy, a central focus of our work is the individual's responsibility for shaping his or her own existence. In spite of how her environment leans on her, a woman, nevertheless, has to know how to engage with it in ways that will be nourishing and zestful . . . she is creating her own life, bit by bit . . . to do this she has to be able to integrate her awareness of sensations, actions, wants and values, relationships and all the raw material of her life with her own personal willingness and skill in using this awareness as her basis for action. (pp. 249–250)

In gestalt therapy, the therapist is a facilitator for the development of self-awareness. She does this by sharing her own awareness with the client and underlining the recurrent patterns of behavior that are revealed in the therapeutic interaction (Simkin & Yontef, 1984). The following case description illustrates such an approach.

I have chosen a case of a modern young woman who has a career and is struggling with multiple roles and exhibits stress symptoms. I will not frame the case as fully as Mae's, but will use a few examples from the therapy to show how teaching awareness and attending to process enriches a feminist approach. In the integration of a feminist framework with a gestalt approach, cognitive therapy is used to underline the process, to help in conflict resolution, and to provide structure, meaning, and reframing (Fodor, 1987).

LIZ

Liz, a 32-year-old married corporate lawyer, comes for help for panic symptoms. She had a panic attack on the plane two months ago while on a business trip. Since then, she has become increasingly anxious on the subway and in crowded department stores. Several times in the past few weeks, she has had to leave a crowded train and take a taxi. She is very worried about her symptoms, stating they are "not like me." She reports feeling edgy and out of control.

As we go more into her story, Liz ties her anxiety symptoms to her feelings of being under constant stress, fatigue, and conflict in her personal life and at work. For the past year she has been trying to conceive; however, she reports she feels tired much of the time and has lost interest in sex. She and her husband have been fighting more; he wants to buy a house in the suburbs. Now, Liz is not sure whether she wants a baby or not, since she can hardly handle her life now. She worries that owning a house and commuting to the suburbs will lead to a full collapse.

The Personal Is the Political

Liz's history and her symptoms are not unusual in my New York practice. More and more I am seeing young professional women with anxiety, stress, or panic symptoms. They are juggling too many roles, have little time for themselves, and report conflicts about setting priorities. Liz is a member of a generation benefiting from the expansion of women's roles. She wants to "have it all."

Liz reports feeling under constant pressure. Her prestigious law firm expects her to work long hours and be available on weekends. She is very ambitious. She hopes to become a partner. Her husband Bill, a computer executive, wants to move out of the city. Liz reports he expects her to be available for weekday dinners with clients and to "play" and look for houses on the weekends. She reports that she loves him, and that she used to enjoy all their activities together. Bill is very athletic and on the weekends likes to jog with her. Vacations are spent hiking and skiing. Liz is very trim but also reports that she has been gaining weight lately. She says she is often too tired to run or care for her appearance and she worries that she is getting too fat. Lately, she has been depending on chocolate for extra energy boosts.

Setting the Therapeutic Goal. Linked to all of Liz's issues are out of control feelings. She reports anxiety, fatigue, feelings of emptiness, and cravings for chocolate. In combing a feminist framework with a gestalt approach, we begin with a focus on the stress symptoms. However, the approach differs from standard CBT, in that we will not initially directly treat the panic attacks associated with the stress symptoms, but instead, begin with awareness work, highlighting the therapeutic process.

Beginning Therapy: Becoming More Aware: Attending to Interruptions. As Liz tells her story, the therapist becomes aware of how she talks about her problems on an intellectual level. While Liz can frame her "story" in feminist terms, she seems disconnected from her feelings. In describing a recent argument with her husband about how she would hate to commute to the suburbs, Liz describes, in a detached way, how adamant her husband is about living in Connecticut, having a house, green space for the kids, and so forth.

THERAPIST: So, what do you want?

Liz: I don't know. I'm confused. I thought I wanted the house and children. But, I don't know.

THERAPIST: What are you feeling?

Liz: I don't know.

THERAPIST: I see tears, I feel a sadness as you speak.

Liz: (Begins to cry.) Sob . . . oh . . . there I go . . . out of control!

THERAPIST: If you feel sad . . . it's OK to cry. . . .

Liz: I feel overwhelmed with everything. (Begins to cry again and then stops herself.)

THERAPIST: What's happening? You look like you are choking.

Liz: Every time I try to focus on myself, I begin to cry. I can't stand crying. I feel like a baby, out of control, like my hysterical mother. (Begins to sob further.)

THERAPIST: Look, there's nothing wrong with crying. I don't experience you as hysterical right now. What's so wrong with crying?

Liz: If I let myself cry, I'll just end up being a puddle on the floor.

THERAPIST: So, be a puddle on the floor.

Liz: Here, I am, a big deal corporate lawyer bawling, in a therapist's office. I feel like a big crybaby. (Covers her face with her hands.) (Gently the therapist tells Liz that in her office "it's OK for even big deal corporate lawyers to cry." She moves closer and holds her hand. Liz begins to sob and the therapist quietly sits by her side.)

Liz: (Sighs, blows her nose, and says.) I feel better, I guess it's OK to cry.

THERAPIST: Yes, it's OK to cry. I've done it myself when I feel overwhelmed.

THERAPIST: So, what's happening now?

Liz: I feel so confused.

THERAPIST: Stay with the confusion.

LIZ: I don't like to be confused. I usually know where I am.
THERAPIST: How does that feel?
LIZ: I'm scared. I don't like being so fuzzy.
THERAPIST: Is it OK for you to be with me scared and fuzzy?
LIZ: I don't like it.
THERAPIST: Can you stay with being scared and fuzzy?
LIZ: I don't know what to do with my life. I feel pulled in all directions. *How do I know what I need and want?*

As Liz allows herself to feel her confusion and sadness about her lack of direction, we focus on helping her figure out what she wants. The gestalt therapy concept of self-support is central to helping Liz in understanding her needs and make choices. An intellectual like Liz has theories about what she needs (e.g., I need to be a good lawyer, work hard, be responsible, be a good wife, etc.). But, she has not learned how to sort out priorities among her needs and wishes. Too often she tries to work out her problems in her head and ignores what is happening in her body.

In the next phase of work we focus on utilizing her awareness of what is happening in her body to build self-support. The goal is to enable her to organize her experiences about what she really needs, as opposed to what she thinks she needs.

Central to self-support is the directed awareness. What do I really need at the moment? How do I keep myself from getting what I need? How can I organize my experience, my environment to give me what I need? How do I make choices? The therapist tracks Liz and points out what she is doing and how it is impacting her. (For example, one pattern might be how she looks for quick answers instead of staying in a confused state. At these times, the therapist might report to Liz that she then feels pressured to come up with solutions.)

We will illustrate the gestalt work by highlighting two conflicts: (1) Ambition versus an easier life. (Do I continue in a high-pressured career with long hours or do I find a less prestigeful job? Do I give up my goals of making partner to have more time for my personal life?) (2) Remaining in the city versus moving to the suburbs. (Do I do what I want as opposed to yielding to my husband's wishes?)

Ambition versus an Easier Life? First, we assess the nature of the work environment. By awareness exercises, the client is trained to pay more attention to what elements in her work setting contribute to her tension and fatigue.

As we continue this work, the client becomes aware of how tired she is from the pressure of handling too many cases, having to report to different partners, interruptions from clients, and late night writing of briefs with rush deadlines. Through the awareness work, Liz's thinking becomes less global. She shifts from the general view of requiring a less pressured job to specifying what is most tiring and stressful about the particulars of the current work situation.

As Liz becomes more in tune with her body, she notices that early in the day she is tired at work (noting aches in her shoulders and neck). As she learns to use the relaxation procedures and feels somewhat less fatigued, Liz begins to reassess whether the goal of making partner is worth the cost. We do gestalt two-chair work to have her talk to the split. She gets more in touch with the parts of the job that are energizing (working on specific projects, having contact with people rather than legal documents) and what aspects of the job that are deadening.

From this work, Liz is more in touch with a desire to find a different way of working as a lawyer. Liz acknowledges that she would like to have more free time, lunch hours, time for fun, to be with Bill and not have deadlines haunting her all weekends. The therapist and Liz have many long conversations about the realities of a modern woman's life. The therapist reveals her own struggles. She talks about how she left a desirable hospital position with fixed hours for a more flexible academic position. Gradually, Liz views her conflicts in terms of planning and choices. By knowing herself more fully, being clear that more time for herself at this phase of life is a priority, Liz envisions a different type of legal career.

Move to the City versus the Suburbs? Do I have to give him what he wants to keep the relationship? How can I still maintain my independence and still be in the relationship? Liz had an independent life for ten years before she married. She is used to making her own decisions about living, time allotment, when to eat in or out, how to spend her leisure time, and so forth. Being married for the past two years has been a major adjustment for her. While she loves Bill and his strong personality, they often fight over decisions, and she feels she either has to give in or lose him.

The decision about the move to the suburbs has now taken center stage and they are arguing daily. As we work on structuring a less stressful legal career, Liz is sure she does not want to leave the city. Bill is equally adamant about having a house out of the city. She worries that unless he has his way, she will lose him. We role play a recent fight. Liz reports that she cannot win with Bill and feels he does not hear her side of the story.

> LIZ: God, I'm so angry . . . he always seems to be so self-assured. He knows what's best for both of us, and when I cry, it's like he's vindicated. (She stops. As she begins to get angry, Liz stops herself almost to the point of swallowing the anger.)
> THERAPIST: What's happening?
> LIZ: What's the point of getting angry? (She becomes tense and stiff.) "He's impossible. It's impossible!"
> THERAPIST: I think I know how you feel. Sometimes when I talk to my husband, I feel he is so sure of his position, that he doesn't listen to me.
> LIZ: (Becomes more attentive.)—You know what I'm talking about.
> THERAPIST: What I've discovered, is that often I am so into feeling that he is overpowering me, that I refuse to budge and don't listen to him. At those times, we could be on opposite sides of a river.

We begin to explore this feeling of not being heard, feeling overpowered and holding back anger by studying our therapeutic interactions. (For a fuller description of this work, see Fodor, 1987.)

After a few sessions, Liz begins to see how quick she is to see any strong view, whether coming from the therapist or from Bill, as a possible compromise to her independence. We work together on her maintaining her independence and asserting what she wants, while listening to the other. We also explore her fear that unless she gives in, Bill will leave.

Next, we have a couples session. Bill and Liz discuss the move to the suburbs. As they listen to each other, Bill reveals that he does not like commuting daily either, while Liz admits she enjoys her time away with Bill out of the city.

After much discussion, they decide to get a country house not too far from the city for weekends. There is much relief in the compromise, Liz feels good that she was not wiped out and that getting away from work on the weekends fits her

desire to have more quality leisure time. Bill appreciates Liz's growing willingness to dialogue.

As Liz becomes more aware of her stressors and learns more about her patterns of handling stressful events and interpersonal conflict, she reports feeling under less pressure, more energetic, and less inclined to panic when she cannot come up with an immediate solution to a problem. The awareness work enabled Liz to feel more in charge of herself and less controlled by runaway emotions or external events.

CONCLUSION

In this chapter, I have presented a feminist framework for therapy highlighting women's issues. The feminist approach could be used with any therapy, but I feel that both gestalt and cognitive therapy, in combination, are ideal for achieving these goals. Gestalt therapy highlights awareness and process, the therapeutic work is facilitated by focusing on the therapeutic interaction and attention to what is happening in the moment. Furthermore, gestalt therapy is embedded in the theoretical framework of field theory, which highlights person–environmental interrelationships. Cognitive therapy, by accessing beliefs, helps clients access outdated core schemata and presents methods to help clients reframe their struggles and construct newer ways of being. This therapy enables women to come up with their own life scripts, their own understandings of how they got to be the way they are, where they are at, and where they want to go. In addition, the cognitive gestalt interface enables clients to understand their emotional system, how it works, how they use their evaluations and appraisals to distance themselves from charged issues and problematic feelings. A woman who understands herself is not afraid to look at patterns and behaviors she does not like. She can use her full awareness of who she is and what she needs to shape her goals.

In discussing this chapter with George Stricker, he asked if there was a difference between feminist therapy and good therapy. Ideally, there is no difference. The principles and techniques described in this chapter could inform any therapy.

However, the feminist approach and the integrations discussed in this chapter do raise issues for psychotherapy integration. Since clients and therapists are men and women who are influenced by the culture, gender issues need to be addressed in any attempt at developing an integrative psychotherapy.

I have not covered in this chapter recent attempts at integrating a feminist approach to psychoanalysis. The topic of gender in analytic theory has generated numerous controversies in the analytic literature. These include adapting traditional analytic procedures to consider feminist theory and practice. In particular, analysts have discussed gender and its relation to transference and countertransference and the Oedipus and Electra complexes. Many feminist analysts also emphasize the impact of the mother and consider attachment issues as primary. (See Alpert, 1987; Chodorow, 1989; Jordan *et al.*, 1991, for a fuller discussion of these issues.) The cases presented could have also been reframed from a psychoanalytic perspective which could have added another layer of depth and complexity to the work.

Moving away from analysis, one also needs to consider the "agenda" of feminist therapy. While all therapists claim to let the client set the agenda, feminist therapists do have specific goals for their clients. In choosing to integrate a feminist approach with other therapies, one needs to ask whether the feminist agenda is applicable to most clients. I would answer that for most women, wherever they are in their life cycle, being female is an essential part of their life and struggles. So a feminist approach ideally should be part of any good therapy for women.

Furthermore, although there is very little written about the feminist framing of male problems, clearly most males in therapy could benefit from a look at how being a man and socialized into the male role in our culture affects their life and struggles. Contemporary family therapists are beginning to consider gender as central in their work with couples and families (Bograd, 1988; Goodrich, Rampage, Ellman, & Halstead, 1988; Luepnitz, 1988; McGoldrick *et al.*, 1978).

In some sense, feminist therapy presents a challenge to the field of psychotherapy in general. In integrative psychotherapy, we are focused on the individual or the family. Yet, too many of our clients are suffering from the effects of societal inequity and discrimination. Integrative therapy may need to go beyond the individual to look at institutions and social structures that continue to adversely affect our potential clients, as well as the socialization process for the next generation.

Finally, as more and more of our clients are coming from diverse racial, class, and ethnic backgrounds, we may require a framing for integrative therapy that takes such diversity into account. The feminist framework could be broadened to address such differences.

REFERENCES

Alpert, J. (Ed.). (1987). *Women and psychoanalysis*. Hillsdale, NJ: Earlbaum.
American Psychiatric Association. (1980). *Diagnostic and statistical manual of mental disorders DSM-III* (3rd ed.). Washington, DC: Author.
American Psychiatric Association. (1987). *Diagnostic and statistical manual of mental disorders DSM-III-R*. (3rd edition revised). Washington, DC: Author.
American Psychological Association Task Force on Sex Bias and Sex-Role Stereotyping in Psychotherapeutic Practice. (1975). *Report of the task force*. Washington, DC: Author.
Beck, A. T., Rush, A. J., Shaw, B. F., & Emery, G. (1979). *Cognitive therapy of depression*. New York: Guilford Press.
Belenky, M., Clinchy, B., Goldberger, N., & Tarule, J. (1986). *Women's ways of knowing*. New York: Basic Books.
Blechman, E. (1984). Women's behavior in a man's world: Sex differences in competence. In E. Blechman (Ed.), *Behavior modification with women* (pp. 3–33). New York: Guilford.
Bograd, M. (1988). Power, gender and the family: Feminist perspectives on family systems theory. In M. A. Dutton-Douglas & L. E. Walker (Eds.), *Feminist psychotherapies: Integration of therapeutic and feminist systems* (pp. 118–133). Norwood, NJ: Ablex.
Boston Lesbian Psychologies Collective (Eds.). (1987). *Lesbian psychologies: Explorations and challenges*. Champaign, IL: University of Illinois Press.
Boston Women's Health Book Collective (Eds.). 1988. *Our bodies ourselves* (revised 3rd ed.). New York: Simon & Schuster.
Boyers, R., & Grill, R. (1971). *R. D. Laing and anti-psychiatry*. New York: Perennial Library.
Brodsky, A. M., & Hare-Mustin, R. (1980). *Women and psychotherapy: An assessment of research and practice*. New York: Guilford.
Broverman, I., Broverman, D., Clarkson, F., Rosenkrantz, P., & Vogel, S. (1970). Sex roles stereotypes and clinical judgments of mental health. *Journal of Counseling and Clinical Psychology 34*, 1–7.
Brown, L. (1985). Business practice in feminist therapy. In L. B. Rosewater, & L. E. Walker (Eds.), *Handbook of feminist therapy* (pp. 297–304). New York: Springer.
Brown, L. S. (1990). The meaning of a multicultural perspective for theory-building in feminist therapy. In L. S. Brown & M. P. Root (Eds.), *Diversity and complexity in feminist therapy* (pp. 1–22). New York: Haworth Press.
Brown, L., & Ballou, M. (Eds.). (1992). *Theories of personality*

and psychopathology. Feminist Appraisals. New York: Guilford.

Brown, L. S., & Brodsky, A. (1992). Feminist therapy: A look at the future. *Psychotherapy: Theory, research practice and training, 29,* 51–57.

Cammaert, L., & Larson, C. (1988). Feminist frameworks of psychotherapy. In M. A. Douglas & L. Walker (Eds.), *Feminist frameworks: Integration of therapeutic and feminist systems* (pp. 12–36). Norwood, NJ: Ablex.

Chessler, P. (1972). *Women and madness.* Garden City, NY: Doubleday.

Chodorow N. J. (1978). *The reproduction of mothering.* Berkeley: University of California Press.

Chodorow, N. J. (1989). *Feminism and psychoanalytic theory.* New Haven: Yale University Press.

De Beauvoir, S. (1961). *The second sex.* New York: Bantam.

Dinnerstein, D. (1977). *The Mermaid and minotaur: Sexual arrangements and human malaise.* New York: Harper.

Dilling, C., & Claster, B. (1985). *Female psychology: A partially annotated bibliography.* New York City Coalition for Women's Mental Health, %Joan Einwohner, 320 W. 86th St., N.Y., 10024.

Douglas, M. A., & Walker, L. (1988). *Feminist frameworks: Integration of therapeutic and feminist systems.* Norwood, NJ: Ablex.

Eichenbaum, L., & Orbach, S. (1983). *Understanding women: A feminist psychoanalytic view.* New York: Basic Books.

Ellis, A. (1984). Rational-emotive therapy. In R. J. Corsini (Ed.), *Current psychotherapies* (pp. 196–238). Itasca, IL: F. E. Peacock.

Flax, J. (1990). *Thinking fragments: Psychoanalysis, feminism, & post modernism in the contemporary west.* Berkeley: University of California Press.

Fodor, I. G. (1985). Assertiveness training in the 80's: Moving beyond the personal. In L. Rosewater & L. Walker (Eds.), *Handbook of feminist therapy* (pp. 257–265). New York: Springer.

Fodor, I. G. (1987). Moving beyond cognitive behavior therapy: Integrating gestalt therapy to facilitate personal and interpersonal awareness. In N. Jacobson (Ed.), *Psychotherapists in clinical practice: Cognitive and behavioral perspectives* (pp. 190–231). New York: Guilford.

Fodor, I. G. (1988). Cognitive behavior therapy: Evaluation of theory and practice for addressing women's issues. In M. A. Dutton-Douglas & L. E. Walker (Eds.), *Feminist Psychotherapies: Integration of therapeutic and feminist systems* (pp. 91–117). Norwood, NJ: Ablex.

Fodor, I. G. (1990). On turning 50: No longer young/not yet old: Shifting to a new paradigm. *Behavior Therapist, 13,* 2.

Fodor, I. G., & Rothblum, E. D. (1985). Strategies for dealing with sex role stereotypes. In C. Brody (Ed.), *Women therapists treating women* (pp. 86–95). New York: Springer.

Gilbert, L. A. (1980). Feminist therapy. In A. M. Brodsky & R. Hare-Mustin (Eds.), *Women and psychotherapy* (pp. 245–266). New York: Guilford.

Gilligan, C. (1982). *In a different voice.* Cambridge: Harvard University Press.

Goodrich, T. J., Rampage, C., Ellman, B., & Halstead, C. (1988). *Feminist family therapy.* New York: Norton.

Jagger, A. M., & Rothenberg, P. S. (1984). *Feminist frameworks: Alternative theoretical accounts of the relations between men and women* (2nd ed.), New York: McGraw-Hill.

Jordan, J., Kaplan, A., Miller, J., Stiver, I., & Surrey, J. (1991). *Women's growth in connection: Writings from the stone center.* New York: Guilford.

Kaplan, A. G., & Yasinski, L. (1980). Psychodynamic perspective. In A. M. Brodsky & R. Hare-Mustin (Eds.), *Women and psychotherapy* (pp. 191–211). New York: Guilford.

Kirsh, B. (1974). Consciousness raising groups as therapy for women. In V. Franks & V. Burtle (Eds.), *Women in therapy* (pp. 326–356). New York: Brunner/Mazel.

Kravetz, D. (1980). Consciousness-raising and self help. In A. M. Brodsky & R. Hare-Mustin (Eds.), *Women and psychotherapy* (pp. 267–281). New York: Guilford.

LaSorsa, V., & Fodor, I. (1990). The adolescent daughter/midlife mother dyad: A new look at separation and self definition. *Psychology of Women Quarterly, Vol. 14,* No. 4.

Lerman, H. (1986). *A mote in Freud's eye: From psychoanalysis to the psychology of women.* New York: Springer.

Lerman, H. (1992). The limits of phenomenology: A feminist critique of the humanistic personality theories. In L. Brown & M. Ballou (Eds.), *Theories of personality and psychopathology. Feminist appraisals* (pp. 8–19). New York: Guilford.

Luepnitz, D. A. (1988). *The family interpreted: Feminist theory in clinical practice.* New York: Basic Books.

McGoldrick, M., Anderson, C., & Walsh, F. (1978). *Women in families.* New York: Norton.

McGrath, E., Puryear Keita G., Strickland, B. R., & Russo, N. F. (1990). *Women and depression: Risk factors and treatment issues.* Washington, DC: American Psychological Association.

Miller, J. B. (1973). *Psychoanalysis and women.* New York: Brunner Mazel.

Millet, K. (1969). *Sexual politics.* New York: Avon.

Mitchell, J. (1975). *Psychoanalysis and Feminism: Freud, Rich, Laing, and women.* New York: Vintage.

Morgan, R. (Ed.). (1970). *Sisterhood is powerful.* New York: Random House.

Pleck, J. H. (1976). The male sex role: Definitions, problems, and sources of change. *Journal of Social Issues, 32,* 155–164.

Polster, M. (1974). Women in therapy—A Gestalt therapist's view. In V. Franks & V. Burtle (Eds.), *Women in therapy* (pp. 247–262). New York: Brunner/Mazel.

Rawlings, E., & Carter, D. (Eds.). (1977). *Psychotherapy for women: Treatment toward equality.* Springfield, IL: Charles C Thomas.

Reiker, P., & Carmen, E. (1984). *The gender gap in psychotherapy.* New York: Plenum Press.

Rich, A. (1980). Compulsory heterosexuality and lesbian existence. Reprinted in A. M. Jagger & P. S. Rothenberg (1984). *Feminist frameworks: Alternative theoretical accounts of the relations between men and women* (2nd ed., pp. 416–419). New York: McGraw-Hill.

Rosewater, L. (1988). Feminist therapies with women. In M. A. Douglas & L. Walker (Eds.), *Feminist frameworks: Integration of therapeutic and feminist systems* (pp. 135–155). Norwood, NJ: Ablex.

Rosewater, L., & Walker, L. (Eds.). 1985. *Handbook of feminist therapy.* New York: Springer.

Sesan, R. (1988). Sex bias and sex role stereotyping in psychotherapy with women: Survey results. *Psychotherapy, 25,* 107–116.

Simkin, J., & Yontef, G. (1984). Gestalt therapy. In R. J. Corsini (Ed.), *Current psychotherapies* (pp. 279–319). Itasca, IL: F. E. Peacock.

Snitow, A., Stansell, C., & Thomson, S. (1983). *Powers of desire: The politics of sexuality.* New York: Monthly Review Press.

Sturdivant, S. (1980). *Therapy with women: A feminist philosophy of treatment*. New York: Springer.

Szasz, T. (1961). *The myth of mental illness*. New York: Harper & Row.

Tannen, D. (1990). *You just don't understand*. New York: Ballantine Books.

Unger, R. K. (1979). *Female and male: Psychological perspectives*. New York: Harper & Row.

Vance, V. (Ed.). (1984). *Pleasure and danger: Exploring female sexuality*. Boston: Routledge & Kegan Paul.

Webster's New Collegiate Dictionary. (1979). Springfield, MA: Merriam-Webster.

Walker, L. E. (1984). *The battered woman syndrome*. New York: Springer.

Weisstein, N. (1970). "Kinde, Kuche, Kirche" as scientific law: Psychology constructs the female. In R. Morgan (Ed.), *Sisterhood is powerful* (pp. 205–219). New York: Random House.

Yontef, G. (1976). Gestalt therapy: Clinical phenomenology. I. V. Binder, A. Binder, & R. Rimland (Eds.), *Modern therapies*. New York: Prentice Hall.

CHAPTER 16

Integrating Spiritual Healing Approaches and Techniques into Psychotherapy

Robert N. Sollod

INTRODUCTION

The institution of verbal psychotherapy, as such, is a relatively recent historical development and one that first occurred in industrialized, Western societies. The precursor of contemporary verbal psychotherapy was a model that attributed the causes and cures of psychological problems to the levels of biology and physiology. Both models replaced millenia of traditional spiritual approaches to a variety of forms of malaise.

The term *successionism* refers to the negative attitude that religions have often evidenced toward their predecessors. For example, Judaism evidenced a negative view toward pagan religions. A type of successionism also may be found in the antagonism of the institutions of psychotherapy toward spiritual models of reality (Vitz, 1977) and toward associated healing traditions. Contemporary psychotherapy has thus lost sight

of important aspects of the human experience as well as of ways of helping people encumbered by life's difficulties.

Such a de-spiritualized psychotherapeutic endeavor overlooks the spiritual dimensions of life and of experience. A wide range of spiritual healing[1] traditions emphasizes the central importance of the connection of all life to spiritual or cosmic realities. In these views, healing is usually seen as restoring a condition of wholeness or harmony (Carlson & Shield, 1989). Contemporary psychology and many contemporary psychotherapeutic approaches express the perception of human beings as cut off and isolated, not only from nature and from other individuals, but more significantly from activities of cosmic purpose. Copernican, Newtonian and Freudian conceptual revolutions have led to the notion of human beings as purposeless, determined organisms acted upon by physical and biological laws. Even in

---

Robert N. Sollod • Department of Psychology, Cleveland State University, Cleveland, Ohio 44115.

Comprehensive Handbook of Psychotherapy Integration, edited by George Stricker and Jerold R. Gold. Plenum Press, New York, 1993.

[1]The term *spiritual healing* is not always clearly distinguishable from psychic healing or from shamanism. All three of these approaches share certain characteristics but may differ in major respects. Many healing traditions combine all three elements into a unitary form. In this chapter the term *spiritual healing* is used in a general way to refer to such traditions.

humanistic approaches, meaning is usually seen as a subjective and arbitrary creation (Tart, 1975). Beyond any specific techniques that may be derived from spiritual traditions, contemporary psychotherapy has much to gain from a worldview that reconnects human beings with one another and with universal and spiritual purposes (Bergin, 1980).

Frank (1973) has indicated that contemporary psychotherapies do have many features in common with traditional healing approaches. The underlying structure of psychotherapy itself, that is, of a person seeking help (healee) going to a specifically trained or qualified individual (healer) for the purpose of seeking some type of solace or remediation of a problem, appears to be derived either from healing traditions themselves or from aspects of human nature appreciated both by healing traditions and by contemporary practice.

Traditional spiritual forms of healing do consist, in part, of suggestion and placebo, but upon further examination it becomes apparent that active therapeutic ingredients[2] also must be present (Colijn & Sollod, 1990). Many such active ingredients which contribute to demonstrable changes in thinking, feeling, and behavior have been identified and utilized within various healing traditions during the millenia in which spiritual healing approaches have developed.

In addition, the significance of motives associated with the archetype of healer in the psychotherapist is an important factor that suggests the value of the integration of spiritual healing approaches and methods within psychotherapy. Many therapists appear to be motivated by an inner directionality similar to that experienced by healers in traditional societies (Guggenbuhl-Craig, 1971; Wilmer, 1987). Such an archetype involves service and the development of the power to change the lives of others as a result of specific training and experiences; privileged access to the often hidden experiential world of others and awareness of one's own problems (the "wounded healer") also are aspects of this archetypal pattern.

Some therapeutic training programs, most clearly psychoanalytic institutes, have already in-

[2]Pharmacologists have analogously discovered that traditional remedies are often potent cures and may consist of biologically active ingredients.

corporated elements of an initiatory school. From the standpoint of spiritual traditions, such programs represent pseudognostic initiations (Sollod, 1982); nonetheless, they engage the archetypal energies of would-be psychoanalysts. A more direct acknowledgment of the connection between the roles of psychotherapist and healer in the training of psychotherapists generally could foster their development.

The example of spiritual healing approaches also suggests that it is possible to work more sensitively and effectively with a variety of experiences that most contemporary psychotherapeutic approaches avoid or pathologize. Anomalous or paranormal experiences are often inexplicable in terms of current scientific views and are incompatible with normative perceptions and expectations about reality (Alcock, 1981; Braude, 1978; Tobacyk & Milford, 1983). Nonetheless, many reports indicate that such experiences are surprisingly prevalent. Greeley (1975, 1987) summarized his survey research to conclude that 29% of American adults reported visions, 67% reported ESP experiences, 67% indicated *déjà vu*, and 31% had experienced clairvoyance. According to a 1985 Gallup poll, 43% of American adults surveyed have reported an unusual spiritual experience and 15% have reported a near-death experience. Lukoff (1985) has written about the possibility of authentic mystical experiences and the frequent overlap of such experiences with psychotic disturbances. The spiritual healing traditions evidence a familiarity with and acceptance of a wide range of spiritual and anomalous experiences. This is, therefore, a domain in which contemporary psychotherapy could have much to gain by selectively incorporating aspects of spiritual healing approaches (Sollod, 1992).

THEORETICAL AND CONCEPTUAL POSITION

This chapter focuses upon the relevance of techniques, approaches, and concepts derived from spiritual healing traditions for the contemporary practice of psychotherapy. It also will present some guidelines and approaches to a possible psychotherapeutic integration of some insights and practices from spiritual healing traditions. As there are many different types of spiritual healing and a variety of viewpoints concerning them, there is no single available integration of such approaches within the practice of psychotherapy. The appraisal of frequent practices within spiritual healing approaches leads to the possibility of their integration within psychotherapeutic practice (Sollod, 1988). Some elements commonly found in spiritual healing may serve to reinforce or highlight aspects of current psychotherapeutic practice. Other elements may suggest that innovative techniques and approaches may be beneficial.

A sampling of current healing methods in a variety of traditions reveals major aspects of spiritual healing practices (Bloomfield, 1984; Carlson & Shield, 1989; Cooke, 1980; Goldsmith, 1959; Harner, 1980; LeShan, 1966; Markides, 1985, 1988). Principles and approaches considered important in many of these healing traditions include the following: (1) There is an alteration of the healer's state of consciousness. The healer has expertise in entering a variety of states of consciousness that differ from ordinary waking consciousness. These different states of consciousness are used to facilitate a variety of therapeutic processes. In such alternate states of consciousness, the healer relies on factors outside his or her ordinary ego to facilitate healing. The ego and its functions are kept in check during the process as they may interfere with the healing process. (2) The healer's view or manner of perceiving and conceptualizing the person seeking help is an important factor in spiritual healing. Seeing the person as deficient or impaired usually hinders the healing process, whereas seeing the person as freed of limitations is usually very therapeutic. The complementary client processes are disidentification and transcendence. (3) The healer accesses and uses intuitive understanding. (4) There is no clear separation between the processes of the healer and those of the person seeking healing. In some cases, a sense of fusion between the healer and the person seeking healing constitutes a basic element of the healing process. Healing may involve the healer successfully resolving certain personal issues. (5) There is considerable use of visualization by the therapist and by the healee. (6) Alteration of the healee's state of consciousness through trance induction is often used. (7) A spiritual or transpersonal model is used to explain illness and therapeutic recovery. (8) An implicit personality theory accompanying the spiritual tradition emphasizes the potential for change. Within Western monotheistic spiritual traditions, the individual is seen as a child of God and, as such, possessing rationality and free will. (9) Reestablishing a conscious relationship with spiritual life and developing an appreciation of divine or universal laws are often seen as resulting in the restoration of health. (10) Prayer or meditation are frequently viewed as therapeutic activities.

Although it is not feasible to illustrate the entire range of healing approaches here, space does allow a brief summary of the approaches of two healers—Joel Goldsmith and Stylianos Atteshlis. These examples illustrate some of the principles indicated above.

Joel Goldsmith (1958, 1959, 1983) was an American healer who led meditation, healing, and spiritual development circles throughout the world. Writing within a Judeo-Christian framework, Goldsmith emphasized the importance of the state of consciousness of the healer. He stressed that, in healing, it was important to enter a different state of consciousness in which one felt an inner wholeness or oneness with God. Goldsmith considered it unnecessary and even detrimental to focus on the type of illness or problem of the healee. The healing approach seemed to involve an effort to achieve "at-one-ment" and the healing thus was caused by spiritual forces beyond the activity of the ego. The healer's activity involved a suspension of normal ego functioning and an attempt to reach an inner stillness. The healing was said to take place within that stillness. Goldsmith did not do hands-on healing and indicated that healing could be done either in the presence of the healee or at a distance.

Stylianos Atteshlis[3] is a native of Cyprus who has engaged in spiritual healing and teaching for much of his life. He is commonly referred to as "Daskalos," which is the Greek word for *teacher*. His activities have been the subject of two books by the sociologist Kyriacos Markides (1985, 1988), and he has also contributed his own teachings and writings about spirituality and healing (Atteshlis, 1990a,b, 1991). Working within an esoteric Christian framework, Daskalos also emphasizes the importance of the state of consciousness

---

[3]Stylianos Atteshlis is referred to pseudonymously as Spyros Sathi in Markides' books.

of the healer. Unlike Goldsmith, he believes that the healer may try to affect the condition of the client through conscious control of the healer's own thoughts and feelings. He suggests that the energy of the healer can be intentionally directed, often through imagery, in such a way as to enhance the well-being of the healee on a variety of dimensions. He also states that the healer should be motivated by love and by a desire to be of service. He agrees with Goldsmith that healing is potentiated by spiritual forces beyond the ordinary ego functioning of the healer but teaches that such forces may be invoked and enhanced by the intention and directed consciousness of the healer. He also indicates that focusing on negative or limiting thoughts (either by the healer or the healee) limits and impairs the efficacy of healing but, unlike Goldsmith, does not think that the diagnostic process or recognition of the nature of a problem is inherently detrimental. Daskalos maintains that healing may be done in the presence of the healee or at a distance, and he also uses physical touch as one means of healing.

Daskalos has also devoted considerable attention to the art of psychotherapy (Atteshlis, personal communication, 1988, 1989, 1990a; Markides, 1985, 1988). He has stated that conventional psychotherapy does not get to the root causes of psychological problems. He often views such root causes as the thought–desire forms or patterns that a person has developed and energized over the years. He labels such patterns "elementals." Conventional approaches, through the process of catharsis, often prematurely bring to the surface some deeply hidden elementals with which a person may be unable to contend. Daskalos teaches that the process of psychotherapy, however, should instead include helping a person to develop more benign patterns of thought and feeling and to depotentiate destructive and negative patterns. This process may be aided, in Daskalos' view, through the creation of therapeutic elementals as well as by example and persuasion.

LeShan, who has developed conceptual models of alternate states of consciousness and meditation (1966, 1974), also presented a typology of healing approaches (Goodrich, 1978). In Type I healing, the healer enters an altered state of consciousness characterized by experiential fusion with the healee and a state of deep, caring love. Type I healing may be done in the presence of the

client or at a distance. In Type II healing, there is an attempt to direct the healing process. Therapeutic touch or the "laying on of hands" characterizes this approach. Applying this typology, it appears that the Type I approach best describes Goldsmith's approach to healing, whereas Daskalos' activities include both Type I and Type II processes as well as other aspects that do not fit into either pattern.

CLINICAL AND THEORETICAL ANTECEDENTS

The generally accepted assumption that psychotherapeutic approaches have been unequivocally derived from scientific roots has been challenged (Perrez, 1989; Sollod, 1982). The origins of psychotherapeutic forms are complex and consist, in part, of sociohistorical and biographical factors. Originators of psychotherapeutic approaches have drawn from a variety of extrascientific sources. Spiritual traditions and associated healing techniques have long been one major but largely hidden and poorly acknowledged source of psychotherapeutic innovation. A large portion of current psychotherapeutic practice appears either to have been derived from spiritual traditions and teachings or to consist of approaches and practices similar to those found in spiritual healing traditions.

From the development of psychotherapeutic uses for dreams to hypnosis, biofeedback, and relaxation techniques, Western psychotherapeutic innovators have been antedated by traditional sources and have drawn upon them. Rogers (1980) has indicated that Taoism was an influence on his development of client-centered therapy; secularized aspects of Protestantism also are present in his therapeutic approach (Sollod, 1978). Gnostic elements were prominent in aspects of Freudian psychotherapeutic techniques (Sollod, 1982). Freud traced his emphasis on the importance of dreams to Biblical writings; the idea of the subconscious mind was known to Cabalistic mystics (Bakan, 1958; Fodor, 1971).

Even when contemporary schools of thought may not have their origins in spiritual and healing traditions, surprising similarities are often present. For example, Adler's (1959) view of the individual as an active creator may be considered an exoteric version of Cabalistic thinking. Skinner's[4] model of individual behavior as completely conditioned and shaped by the environment was antedated by Uspenskii (1929), a Russian mystic and student of Gurdjieff. Albert Ellis (1970) has cited the insights of Epictetus, the ancient Greek spiritual master, to support the validity of his rational-emotive approach. A major tenet of rational-emotive therapy—that an individual's thought shapes experience—although presumably based upon empirical scientific considerations, is consistent with Stoicism as well as with some Christian, Buddhist, and Cabalistic teachings.

Another type of clinical antecedent is the fact that healers in a variety of traditions have not restricted themselves to physical illnesses but have also typically addressed problems and concerns that are commonly considered the exclusive province of psychotherapeutic intervention (Berthold, 1989; Edgerton, 1971). Traditional cultural and spiritual teachings have developed approaches to a variety of conditions that also could be described within the framework of psychiatric and psychological diagnosis (Buhrmann, 1984; Holdstock, 1979; Wilson, 1989). The integration of traditional healing approaches with more conventional practice has also been noted or suggested (Gordon, 1990; Rappaport & Rappaport, 1981).

Besides such considerations, several current forms of psychotherapy are based on specific spiritual or healing traditions. Such approaches may operate within the framework of a specific theology or spiritual tradition and consist of the application of principles and methods consistent with that worldview. Psychotherapies involving body work and therapeutic touch (Kepner, 1987; Krieger, 1975) also involve ideas and processes drawn from or similar to those found in spiritual healing traditions.

THE TECHNIQUE AND PROCESS OF PSYCHOTHERAPY

There is no one specific approach to psychotherapy that involves the integration of spiritual healing. Instead, there are some major types of

[4]Skinner (1976) indicates that he had read Uspenskii's *Tertium Organum* (1929) before beginning graduate school in psychology. Thus, there is a possibility that his thinking may have been influenced by Uspenskii's ideas.

emphases and a repertoire of techniques that may be adopted. In the spiritual traditions, the healer is the conduit of healing, and it is through the healer's inner activities that healing is enabled to take place. Such inner activities include the healer's state of consciousness and contents of consciousness.

Thus, a major emphasis in a psychotherapeutic approach incorporating the principles of spiritual healing is upon the inner activities of the therapist. The therapist in such an approach is ideally able to move into altered, often transcendent, states of consciousness that may be beneficial for the therapeutic process. Some such states may be similar though deeper than the empathic and the objective, almost meditative awareness of the therapist in various approaches of psychotherapy. Other states of receptivity, awareness, and nonordinary altered states of consciousness also may be accessed. Such states may involve a deep feeling of unselfish love, enhanced sensitivity to the other, contact with inner resources of compassion and understanding, and perception of the client as whole or potentially whole. Within Western monotheistic healing traditions, and in a psychotherapy incorporating these concepts, the therapist believes that the client is a loved and valued being—made in the image of God. He or she also can access states of consciousness in which the client's spiritual essence is perceived or directly experienced.

Conventional approaches to therapy also focus to a certain extent on the level of consciousness utilized by the therapist. Psychoanalysts, for example, are trained to develop a certain type of even-hovering attention. Therapists with a client-centered orientation evidence a special type of empathic awareness. Experiential psychotherapists access their embodied feeling states as an essential part of the therapeutic process (Mahrer, 1989). Conventional therapeutic approaches also emphasize the importance of therapists' specific thoughts and feelings, although in a different way for the most part than do spiritual traditions.

The therapist, as a result of training and experience, should be able to enter a variety of distinct states of consciousness. An ideal primary state is called self-observation, self-remembering (Tart, 1987), or witness-consciousness (Wilbur, 1977). In this state, the therapist is able both to attend to the communications of the client and to monitor reactions as they occur. This process goes beyond intellectual appreciation of one's own reactions and consists of a conscious, non-judgmental awareness of thoughts and emotions as they occur. This state may be accompanied by an associated emotional state that consists of access of deeply loving and compassionate feelings toward the client. For some therapists, self-remembering may be accessed only temporarily; for others, it can become a more pervasive or central state.

Besides this primary state, the psychotherapist should be able to shift to several additional states of consciousness. One is a state in which he or she accesses intuitive knowledge; another is a state of empathic fusion with the client. Additional states of consciousness also may branch off from the primary state of self-remembering. Some may represent a deepening of this state and a reduction of the influence of the therapist's own personality upon perception and thought. Others may combine benign intentions with the primary state of consciousness. Still other states may represent a deepening and transformation of the therapist's perceptions and experience of the client.

If possible, such states of consciousness may represent forms of split consciousness in which the therapist continues to interact on an ordinary level with the client. There is no need for the therapist who is trained and experienced in accessing such states of consciousness to go into a trance or to behave in any unusual fashion. The ability of therapists to enter such meditative states varies, and a therapist may find that he or she cannot reach one or more of the meditative states described. Participation in training programs as well as meditation and prayer may be of assistance.

The specific *contents* of the therapist's consciousness also are of particular relevance to a psychotherapeutic form integrating insights from healing traditions. Wilbur (1977, 1980, 1981) has written extensively about consciousness and has compared consciousness with a building. The levels of consciousness constitute a type of deep structure and are analogous to the different floors. Specific contents of consciousness are compared with the floor plans and the furniture. These contents of consciousness, although more superficial than the deep structure of levels of consciousness, are nonetheless significant.

Specifically, as in the healing traditions, seeing the client as deficient, defective, and diseased is viewed as detrimental, but seeing the client as potentially empowered, happy, healthy, and whole is beneficial. In such a psychotherapeutic approach, the diagnostic process is approached with caution. The therapist may utilize diagnostic constructs to assist in describing a case, but only if he or she realizes that the current pathological condition is not supported by the deepest level of reality of the client or of the cosmos. Such an insight should be conveyed to the client. As Daskalos (Atteshlis, personal communication, 1988) has said, "Help them [people seeking help] to see that their problems in time and space are just illusions." It is vital for the therapist not to become caught up in a sense of the client's limitations as it is precisely the therapist who is responsible for helping the client to relinquish views and activities that are causing difficulties.

Some techniques that emerge from these considerations emphasize pleasant, life-enhancing activities. For example, the client may be asked what activities he or she engages in or has engaged in that bring the most satisfaction and is encouraged to participate in one or more of those activities. This approach is very similar to that developed by LeShan (1990) for psychotherapy with cancer patients. He has indicated that another useful beginning point is to ask the client what he or she would most like to do with the gift of a year of life that could be shaped in any manner the client desired. LeShan has also indicated many additional techniques that can be used. The client also may be encouraged to undertake more helpful, altruistic activities in daily life. Such participation in new, life-enhancing activities should be deeply grounded in the therapist's belief that people have the power to change, that they are capable of rational choice, and that they are fundamentally responsible for the quality of their experiences and for the quality of their relationships with others.

Another technical consideration is the relative lack of emphasis on the problems, conflicts, and negative emotions of clients. The therapist is open to the expression of such concerns but does not want to potentiate them through undue attention or through repetition. Catharsis is not necessarily viewed as therapeutic—nor is trying to recover hidden, painful memories and concerns.

The effort is to help the client create areas of experience and associated thoughts and feelings that are satisfying and life-enhancing. Much of the therapeutic process is devoted to helping the client find out what would be most fulfilling and to encouraging inner and outer activities that correspond to selected goals.

Techniques that may be used to facilitate the building of new patterns of thought, feeling and behavior, in addition to those commonly used by cognitive therapists, are affirmations, prayers, and visualization techniques. These may be used by the therapist and by the client as well. In spiritual healing traditions, such techniques are thought to potentiate specific contents of thoughts and feelings. Thus, autosuggestion and suggestion are considered as potentially therapeutic processes. Both utilize the mind's ability to shape experience and even to affect physiological responses. Suggestion, in this approach, is not viewed as a placebo. It is an active ingredient of therapy (Barber, 1978). Hypnosis also may be used to enhance the impact of affirmations, visualization, suggestion, and autosuggestion.

An additional technique that may be incorporated into psychotherapy is that of hands-on healing. Therapeutic touch (Krieger, 1975) and a variety of other healing traditions employ a technique of touch or near-touch in which healing energy is assumed to pass from the healer to the healee (Brennan, 1987). Such an approach has been used for both physical and psychological problems. The psychotherapist incorporating techniques from healing traditions may develop expertise in hands-on healing and include such work as part of psychotherapy. This hands-on approach may be used to help a client become relaxed, to feel more energized, or even to resolve specific problems that might have a somatic representation. Empirical research has documented the impact of therapeutic touch and related approaches (Grad, 1965; Krieger, 1975; Krippner, 1980; Wirth, 1989). Therapists trained in therapeutic touch, reiki, or other related healing modalities can integrate such types of work with a variety of verbal psychotherapies. Kepner (1987) has presented a thorough integration of body work with gestalt therapy.

Meditation and prayer also may be used in a variety of ways to facilitate therapeutic change. Meditation, for example, has been found to result in greater relaxation, disidentification, alertness, awareness, empathy, sensitivity, and openness to change (Carrington, 1977; LeShan, 1974; Shafii, 1985). Both therapist and client may benefit from meditative practice. Meditation may be practiced both within and outside the therapist's office. Different types of prayer have been vital to many spiritual traditions (Bloom, 1980; Laubach, 1946). Prayer also may be part of spiritually oriented psychotherapy. The therapist may pray for and/or with the client as do a significant minority of therapists (Nix, 1978). The client's prayer life also may be supported in therapy.

Alongside the more conventional appreciation of the possible effects of such techniques, Jamesian parapsychic (Fuller, 1986) and transpersonal explanations also may be considered. A tenet of transpersonal psychology, consistent with spiritual healing traditions, is that the directed inner activities of a person may impact upon others. In addition to praying for the client, the therapist may direct visualizations or thoughts to facilitate beneficial changes in the client. Imagery that presumably results in changes in another person is termed *transpersonal imagery* (Braud & Schlitz, 1989; Samuels, 1990).

Some empirical support exists for the assertion of transpersonal influence. Over 35 studies have indicated that prayers and meditations can be beneficial for individuals at a distance (Byrd, 1988). The results of hundreds of studies have strongly suggested the possible influence of attention on electronic functioning as well as on living organisms. Changes in EEG patterns were recorded when persons tried to communicate with others at a distance (Orne-Johnson, Dilbeck, Wallace, & Landrith, 1982). Braud and Schlitz (1989) conducted a study in which transpersonal visualization was used to alter autonomic nervous system activities of others remotely. It appears that adequate methodological procedures were utilized in many of these studies.

Another characteristic of the therapeutic activity in a psychotherapeutic form that integrates spiritual healing techniques into psychotherapy is the reliance of the therapist on an intuitive process to guide therapeutic activities. Intuition, "listening with the third ear," involves the ability to access thoughts and feelings which reflect an inner knowing or understanding (Agor, 1984; Vaughan, 1979). Each person develops a particular means of contacting intuitive information. For many people, the ability to attain a relaxed, meditative state, to focus on a question for which an intuitive answer is desired, and to wait for relevant thoughts, feelings, or images to arise in answer constitute the intuitive process. Intuitive psychotherapists often experience ongoing access to a flow of intuitive information. Intuitively derived information should be examined rationally before being fully utilized.

In this psychotherapeutic approach, a close connection between the client and the therapist exists. At times, a sense of therapist/client experiential fusion is an important ingredient that facilitates therapeutic change. Also, the therapist seeks to find an underlying meaning for the therapeutic encounter and to understand what he or she is to learn through working with a specific client. Contact with a client may challenge the therapist to reexamine certain preconceptions, to learn to be more accepting of various aspects of experience, and to change his or her approach to life. Sometimes, this "work on oneself" is necessary for the therapist to be able to provide a truly therapeutic relationship.

Another feature of this approach is a collaborative, egalitarian relationship. There is a partnership between client and therapist. As in holistic approaches generally (Gordon, 1990), the client participates actively in recovery and can beneficially engage in a variety of activities. These might include instituting dietary changes, beginning an exercise program, engaging in meditation, visualization, relaxation exercises, self-analysis, or diary work. The specific content of exercises is usually developed collaboratively.

The process of therapy varies considerably from one client to another. Often, however, alleviation of symptoms occurs early in therapy. It is followed by the client learning to develop new patterns of living in order to "lock in" any symptomatic changes.

The utilization of such techniques drawn from spiritual healing approaches and their integration into psychotherapy depends upon both the readiness and openness of the client and upon the capacity of the therapist. Integration of these techniques occurs along a continuum ranging from a therapeutic approach virtually indistinguishable from the conventional (although affected by insights from spiritual healing traditions) to approaches consisting in large part of techniques derived from spiritual healing traditions. The therapist should be skilled and trained in the use of any such techniques, be familiar with their utilization, and be sure that clients are accepting of and comfortable with specific approaches that may be utilized. Prayer, for example, is usually inadvisable if the client is an atheist or agnostic or, for other reasons, does not believe in the efficacy of prayer. Visualization may not be suitable for clients who have a limited ability or disinclination to work with imagery. Specific visualizations and affirmations may be most suited to a given patient.

There are some potential pitfalls in the use of techniques drawn from spiritual approaches. It is important that such techniques and approaches be approached in a tactful and matter-of-fact way. Otherwise, the focus of therapy may center upon the apparent novelty of the techniques themselves and upon the effects that they may produce. More important than any specific techniques is the adherence to an underlying viewpoint based on an understanding and appreciation of spiritual principles. Emphasis on integrating spiritual healing techniques into psychotherapy does not invalidate the continuing application of other psychotherapeutic skills and methods or the importance of additional types of insights.

CASE EXAMPLES

It is not possible to present a single case that typifies all the principles indicated above. Each case is different, and practitioners vary in type and degree of training and expertise in this form of integration. Also, therapists may have different spiritual outlooks and have familiarity with a different range of associated techniques. Two cases will be summarized briefly to provide some sense of the broad range that is possible.

A 38-year-old man with a history of failed jobs and an unhappy marriage reported that he was feeling hopeless and depressed. He said that he had many conflicts with his wife and did not see much of a future in his job, at which he was failing. After initially forming a working therapeutic relationship, the therapist suggested that the client begin to engage in pleasant or fulfilling activities—no matter how unimportant they might seem. The client began gardening, taking long walks, and going sailing with some acquaintances. He objected at first, saying, "I have too many problems to enjoy myself." The therapist responded, "If your problems are so real, you don't have to worry about them all of the time. They will still be there after you spend the afternoon sailing on the lake."

The therapist began to limit the amount of time that the client could talk about his past and present problems to less than half of each session. Much of the rest of the time was focused on allowing him to explore what he wanted in his life and how he would like to be. The therapist encouraged the client to develop visualizations according to his stated goals. For example, one exercise was to visualize driving to work in a new car and looking forward to a pleasant and fulfilling workday. The therapist encouraged the client to plan and engage in specific behaviors that could lead to the fulfillment of his goals.

Dreams were also utilized and, when appropriate, were seen as indicating the potential for a more fulfilling life. As in healing traditions, the therapist encouraged the client to appreciate his dreams. For example he suggested that the client draw sketches of particularly significant dreams. Another possibility was to purchase small objects reminiscent of dream figures. Such measures were designed to help bring the feelings and thoughts expressed in dreams into the client's daily awareness.

Throughout the process of therapy, the therapist worked at maintaining a prayerful vision of the client as a being freed of limitations who could choose the direction of his life. He prayed that the client would have the wisdom to choose a good direction and the strength to carry out such a choice. Outside the therapy session, the therapist would meditate and visualize the client as happy, relaxed, and bathed in light.

The client seemed pleased and surprised at the direction of therapy. He had felt that something was deeply "wrong" with him and that psychotherapy should spend years getting to the root of his problems before change would be possible. Nonetheless, with the aid of this approach, he began to experience longer periods of positive moods and began making plans to move ahead in his career life. With an improvement in the client's mood, meditation training began. Meditation

gradually led to an increased awareness of the issues in his current relationship and, using a technique of self-analysis, he reviewed his responses to daily events in a meditative fashion upon falling asleep. Such efforts enabled him to develop more insight into his unfulfilling marital relationship. His frequent angry outbursts had distanced his wife. With more awareness, he was better able to apprehend the causes of his angry responses and to gain more self-control.

In a second case, an executive in his midforties reported a period of intense spiritual experiences. He was ecstatic and felt full of light, love, and forgiveness. The revelations he was experiencing were changing his life, but he was also frightened by the power and intensity of what he was experiencing. He also felt isolated and was somewhat confused about the meaning of his experiences. In addition, he stated that, at times, he sensed the presence of what he feared might be evil spirits. He was afraid of possession and of becoming or being considered insane. In addition, he reported becoming clairvoyant and was both frightened and intrigued by the possibility of the development of psychic abilities.

The approach used here was one of support and acceptance. Therapy provided a decentering context (Sollod & Wachtel, 1980) and support for the client to sort out aspects of his experience and to explore his spiritual opening (Sollod, 1992). The therapist addressed the sense of isolation and fear by discussing processes of spiritual opening (Greenwell, 1990) and describing experiences that people reported in altered states. Mystical states and psychotic experiences were compared and contrasted. The client was to engage in directed bibliotherapy involving reading descriptions of mystical states. He was encouraged to engage in visualizations and affirmations of protection according to his Christian beliefs. Grounding exercises were also suggested to help the client stay connected with his physical existence and daily life.

During the therapeutic process, the client moved from an apprehensive and fearful stance to one of more confident exploration of the new dimension of life that was opening for him. He indicated that he was learning to control or avoid the unpleasant and frightening aspects of such experiences. He continued to function effectively in his professional life. He became more committed to his religious tradition and began to participate in a study group to explore the dimensions of spiritual life.

CONCLUDING COMMENTS

It is possible that techniques and approaches indicated in this paper will be increasingly incorporated into psychotherapeutic practice during the coming years. Such a process would represent the continuation of a process that began with the earliest stages of verbal psychotherapy—the borrowing and integration of techniques and insights from traditional spiritual and healing approaches.

Many questions remain concerning how such an integration might occur. One area of concern is whether such methods would be subject to adequate empirical testing and outcome research before they become widely used. Are given techniques effective? If so, what are their strengths and limitations, their pros and cons? Some empirical research has already been conducted regarding the therapeutic impact of imagery (Sheikh, Kunzendorf & Sheikh, 1989), hypnosis (Bertrand & Spanos, 1989), and meditation (Shafii, 1985). The effects of prayer and hands-on healing, although studied outside of psychotherapy, have, as yet, been the focus of very little investigation within psychotherapeutic practice.

Another area of concern is the training of therapists in such techniques. Is it possible for therapists to learn such techniques through courses alone? Perhaps extensive workshops might be necessary to teach meditation or visualization skills. Or it might even be beneficial for therapists to participate in spiritual disciplines that involve extensive commitment to learning about such skills and approaches. Another question about the integration of such approaches and techniques into psychotherapy is to what extent the integration could occur on the level of technique, alone, and leave the underlying view of the model of personality and of psychopathology unaffected. The effect of techniques with origins in spiritual traditions might be explained by concepts derived from more conventional psychotherapeutic approaches. It is possible to use even such techniques as meditation, prayer, visualization, and therapeutic touch without equivalent consideration of the ethical, moral, and spiritual teachings of humanity's healing traditions. Ther-

apists might not be personally committed to a spiritual path and yet utilize these techniques. It is possible that some techniques could lose their effectiveness when separated from a spiritual tradition of which they were an integral part. Perhaps they would prove as effective even when practiced as part of a technically eclectic approach.

On the other hand, it is possible that the continuing integration of spiritually based healing techniques into psychotherapy will lead to a questioning and redefinition of the deepest levels of the psychotherapeutic enterprise. Such a modification of the psychotherapeutic enterprise would also bring along with it a series of additional questions and dilemmas. For which clients under which circumstances would it be ethically and professionally appropriate to utilize concepts and techniques drawn from spiritual traditions? Would it be possible to combine such approaches in a nonconfusing and effective way with elements of more conventional psychotherapies? Are not the views of reality implicit in spiritual approaches so divergent from those of prevalent psychodynamic, behavioral, and cognitive therapies as to prevent an adequate integration? Such considerations have been relevant in considering the integration of behavioral and psychodynamic psychotherapeutic approaches (Messer & Winokur, 1984). How would the role of the therapist change and how would the meaning of psychotherapy in a client's life become different? Could such an integration occur without radically changing the significance of psychotherapy? Or, if the meaning of psychotherapy did change radically, could the necessary accompanying shifts in the roles of therapist and client be feasible?

Depending on how these and related concerns are resolved, it is possible that empirically validated, spiritually oriented integrative psychotherapeutic forms will emerge within a contemporary, Western framework.

REFERENCES

Adler, A. (1959). *The practice and theory of individual psychology*. Totowa, NJ: Littlefield-Adams.
Agor, W. H. (1984). *The intuitive manager*. Englewood Cliffs, NJ: Prentice-Hall.
Alcock, J. (1981). *Parapsychology: Science or magic?* New York: Pergamon.

Atteshlis, S. (1990a). *Lectures*. Strovolos, Cyprus.

Atteshlis, S. (1990b). *Esoteric teachings* (R. Browning & A. Browning, Trans.). P.O. Box 4105, Nicosia, Cyprus: Imprinta, Ltd.

Atteshlis, S. (1991). *The parables and other stories*. P. O. Box 4105, Nicosia, Cyprus: Imprinta, Ltd.

Bakan, D. (1958). *Sigmund Freud and the Jewish mystical tradition*. Princeton, NJ: Van Nostrand.

Barber, T. X. (1978). "Hypnosis," suggestions, and psychosomatic phenomena: A new look from the standpoint of recent experimental studies. In J. L. Fosshage (Ed.), *Healing: implications for psychotherapy* (pp. 269–298). New York: Human Sciences Press.

Bergin, A. E. (1980). Psychotherapy and religious values. *Journal of Consulting and Clinical Psychology, 48*, 95–105.

Berthold, S. (1989). Spiritism as a form of psychotherapy: Implications for social work practice. *Social Casework, 70*(8), 502–509.

Bertrand, L. D. & Spanos, N. P. (1989). Hypnosis: Historical and social psychological aspects. In A. A. Sheikh, & K. S. Sheikh (Eds.), *Eastern and western approaches to healing: Ancient wisdom and modern knowledge*. New York: John Wiley & Sons.

Bloom, A. (1980). *School for prayer*. London: Darton, Longman & Todd. New York: Phoenix Press/Walker.

Bloomfield, R. (1984). *The mystique of healing*. Edinburgh, Scotland: Charles Skilton.

Braud, W., & Schlitz, M. (1989). A methodology for the objective study of transpersonal imagery. *Journal of Scientific Exploration, 3* 43–63.

Braude, S. (1978). On the meaning of paranormal. In J. Ludwig (Ed.), *Philosophy and parapsychology* (pp. 227–244). Buffalo, NY: Prometheus Books.

Brennan, B. A. (1987). *Hands of light: A guide to healing through the human energy field*. New York: Bantam.

Buhrmann, M. V. (1984). *Living in two worlds: Communication between a white healer and her black counterparts*. Cape Town: Human & Rousseau.

Byrd, R. C. (1988). Positive therapeutic effects of intercessory prayer in a coronary care unit population. *Southern Medical Journal, 81* (7), 826–829.

Carlson, R., & Shield, B. (1989). *Healers on healing*. Los Angeles: Tarcher.

Carrington, P. (1977). *Freedom in meditation*. Garden City, NY: Anchor Press/Doubleday.

Colijn, S., & Sollod, R. (April, 1991). *The relevance of traditional healing for psychotherapy: Content and/or context*. Paper presented to the 6th Annual Convention of the Society for the Exploration of Psychotherapy Integration, Philadelphia, Pa.

Cooke, I. (1980). *Healing by the spirit*. Hampshire, England: The White Eagle Publishing Trust.

Edgerton, R. B. (1971). A traditional African psychiatrist. *Southwestern Journal of Anthropology, 27*, 3–29.

Ellis, A. (1970). *Reason and emotion in psychotherapy*. New York: Lyle Stuart.

Fodor, N. (1971). *Freud, Jung and occultism*. New Hyde Park, NY: University Books.

Frank, J. D. (1973). *Persuasion and healing* (2nd ed.). Baltimore: Johns Hopkins University Press.

Fuller, R. C. (1986). *Americans and the unconscious*. New York: Oxford University Press.

Goldsmith, J. S. (1958). *Practicing the presence*. New York: Harper & Row.

Goldsmith, J. S. (1959). *The art of spiritual healing*. New York: Harper & Row.

Goldsmith, J. S. (1963). *Parenthesis in eternity*. New York: Harper & Row.

Goodrich, J. (1978). The psychic healing training and research project. In J. L. Fosshage (Ed.), *Healing: Implications for psychotherapy* (pp. 84–110). New York: Human Sciences Press.

Gordon, J. S. (1990). Holistic medicine and mental health practice: Toward a new synthesis. *American Journal of Orthopsychiatry, 60*(3), 357–370.

Grad, B. (1965). Some biological effects of "laying on of hands." *Journal of the American Society for Psychical Research, 59*(2), 95–127.

Greeley, A. M. (1975). *The sociology of the paranormal*. Beverly Hills, CA: Sage Press.

Greeley, A. M. (1987). Mysticism goes mainstream. *American Health*, January, pp. 47–49.

Greenwell, B. (1990). *Energies of transformation: A guide to the kundalini process*. Cupertino, CA: Shakti River Press.

Guggenbuhl-Craig, A. (1971). *Power in the helping profession*. New York: Spring.

Harner, M. (1980). *The way of the shaman: A guide to power and healing*. New York: Harper & Row.

Holdstock, T. L. (1979). Indigenous healing in South Africa: A neglected potential. *South African Journal of Psychology, 9*, 118–124.

Kepner, J. I. (1987). *Body process: A gestalt approach to working with the body in psychotherapy*. New York: Gardner Press.

Krieger, D. (1975). Therapeutic touch: The imprimatur of nursing. *American Journal of Nursing, 75*, 784–787.

Krippner, S. (1980). Psychic healing. In A. Hastings, J. Fadiman & J. S. Gordon (Eds.), *Health for the whole person* (pp. 169–177). Boulder, CO: Westview Press.

Laubach, F. (1946). *Prayer: The mightiest force in the world*. Westwood, NJ: Fleming Revell.

LeShan, L. (1966). *The medium, the mystic and the physicist: Toward a general theory of the paranormal*. New York: Viking Press.

LeShan, L. (1974). *How to meditate*. Boston: Little, Brown.

LeShan, L. (1990). *Cancer as a turning point: A handbook for people with cancer, their families, and health professionals*. New York: Flume.

Lukoff, D. (1985). The diagnosis of mystical experiences with psychotic features. *Journal of Transpersonal Psychology, 17*(2), 155–176.

Mahrer, A. R. (1989). *Experiential psychotherapy: basic practices*. Ottawa: University of Ottawa Press.

Markides, K. (1985). *The magus of Strovolos: The extraordinary world of a spiritual healer*. Boston: Routledge & Kegan Paul.

Markides, K. (1988). *Homage to the sun: The wisdom of the magus of Strovolos*. Boston: Routledge & Kegan Paul.

Messer, S., & Winokur, M. (1984). Ways of knowing and visions of reality in psychoanalytic therapy and behavior therapy. In H. Arkowitz, & S. Messer (Eds.), *Psychoanalytic therapy and behavior therapy: Is integration possible?* New York: Plenum Press.

Nix, V. (1978). *A study of the religious values of psychotherapists*. Unpublished doctoral dissertation, Department of Psychology, New York University.

Orne-Johnson, D., Dilbeck, M. C., Wallace, R. D., & Landrith III, G. S. (1982). Intersubject EEG coherence: Is consciousness a field? *International Journal of Neuroscience, 16*, 203–209.

Perrez, M. (1989). Psychotherapeutic methods: Between scientific foundation and everyday knowledge. *New Ideas in Psychology, 7*(2), 133–145.

Rappaport, H., & Rappaport, M. (1981). The integration of scientific and traditional medicine: A proposed model. *American Psychologist, 36,* 774–781.

Rogers, C. (1980). Personal correspondence. Sollod papers. *Archives of the History of American Psychology.* Akron, OH: University of Akron.

Samuels, N. (1990). *Healing with the mind's eye: A guide for using imagery and visions for personal growth and healing.* New York: Summit Books.

Shaffii, M. (1985). *Freedom from the self: Sufism, meditation and psychotherapy.* New York: Human Sciences Press.

Sheikh, A. A., Kunzendorf, R. G., & Sheikh, K. S. (1989). Healing images: From ancient wisdom to modern science. In A. A. Sheikh, & K. S. Sheikh, (Eds.), *Eastern and western approaches to healing: Ancient wisdom and modern knowledge.* New York: John Wiley & Sons.

Skinner, B. F. (1976). *Particulars of my life.* New York: Knopf.

Sollod, R. (1978). Carl Rogers and the origins of client-centered therapy. *Professional Psychology, 9,* 93–104.

Sollod, R. (1982). Non-scientific sources of psychotherapeutic approaches. In P. Sharkey (Ed.), *Philosophy, religion and psychotherapy* (pp. 41–56). Washington, DC: University Press of America.

Sollod, R. (August, 1988). *The relevance of healing techniques for the helping relationship.* Paper presented at the annual convention of the American Psychological Association, Atlanta, GA.

Sollod, R. (1992). Psychotherapy with anomalous experiences. In R. Laibow, R. Sollod, & J. Wilson (Eds.), *Current perspectives on anomalous experiences and trauma* (pp. 247–260). Dobbs Ferry, NY: Treat Publications.

Sollod, R., & Wachtel, P. (1980). A structural and transactional approach to cognition in clinical problems. In M. Mahoney (Ed.), *Psychotherapy process: current issues and future directions* (pp. 1–47). New York: Plenum Press.

Tart, C. (1975). *Transpersonal psychologies.* New York: Harper & Row.

Tart, C. (1987). *Waking up: Overcoming the obstacles to human potential.* Boston: Shambala.

Tobacyk, J., & Milford, G. (1983). Belief in paranormal phenomena: Assessment instrument development and implications for personality functioning. *Journal of Personality and Social Psychology, 44*(5), 1029–1037.

Uspenskii, P. D. (1929). *Tertium organum: The third organ of thought; a key to the enigmas of the world* (N. Bessaraboff & C. Bragdon, Trans., 2nd ed.). New York: Knopf.

Vaughan, F. E. (1979). *Awakening intuition.* New York: Anchor.

Vitz, P. C. (1977). *Psychology as religion: The cult of self-worship.* Grand Rapids, MI: Erdmans.

Wilbur, K. (1977). *The spectrum of consciousness.* Wheaton, IL: Theosophical Publishing House.

Wilbur, K. (1980). *The atman project: A transpersonal view of human development.* Wheaton, IL: Theosophical Publishing House.

Wilbur, K. (1981). *Up from Eden: A transpersonal view of human evolution.* New York: Doubleday.

Wilmer, H. A. (1987). *Practical Jung: Nuts and bolts of Jungian psychotherapy.* Wilmette, IL: Chiron.

Wilson, J. P. (1989). Culture and trauma: The sacred pipe revisited. In J. P. Wilson (Ed.), *Trauma, transformation and healing: An integrative approach to theory, research and post-traumatic therapy* (pp. 38–71). New York: Brunner/Mazel.

Wirth, D. P. (1989). Unorthodox healing: The effect of non-contact therapeutic touch on the healing rate of full-thickness dermal wounds. *Proceedings of Presented Papers: 32nd Annual Parapsychological Association Convention* (pp. 251–268). Durham, NC: Parapsychological Association.

CHAPTER 17

Psychoanalysis and Buddhism
TOWARD AN INTEGRATION

Jeffrey B. Rubin

INTRODUCTION

In recent years, there has been a burgeoning interest in the relationship between the Buddhist and the psychotherapeutic traditions among psychotherapists, researchers, and spiritual practitioners. The nascent dialogue between the Buddhist meditative and Western psychoanalytic traditions has been perhaps the most illuminating aspect of this historic encounter, yielding profound insights about human development, visions of selfhood, psychopathology, and cure (Engler, 1983; Rubin, 1989, 1991).

It is this encounter that I shall explore in this chapter. My focus on Asian psychology and psychoanalysis should not be construed as casting aspersions on, or discounting the value of, integrating other Western and non-Western psychologies.

In this chapter, I will compare and contrast psychoanalytic and Buddhist perspectives on subjectivity, pathology, and the process of change. This will serve as my template for an integrative

Jeffrey B. Rubin • Private Practice, New York, New York and Westchester, New York.

Comprehensive Handbook of Psychotherapy Integration, edited by George Stricker and Jerold R. Gold. Plenum Press, New York, 1993.

psychology. I shall be focusing on Theravadin Buddhism, a nontheistic ethical and psychological training system developed in India in the sixth century B.C. by Gotama Buddha which serves as a prototype for subsequent Buddhist schools such as Zen and Tibetan Buddhism (Goleman, 1977). This form of meditation has been well described in the classical and contemporary meditative literature and has been largely preserved in its original form in contemporary Southeast Asia, and since the 1970s, in the United States. There are three interconnected dimensions to this practice: the cultivation of (1) ethical purity, (2) mental clarity and (3) insight and wisdom. Training in ethics is usually the first stage of this practice. Classical Buddhist texts maintain that unethical behavior is motivated by and promotes mental states, such as greed, anger, and egotism which disrupt the mind and interfere with developing mental clarity and insight. Following ethical guidelines leads to mental "purification," in which counterproductive behaviors are gradually eroded and mental attentiveness and clarity are cultivated. Mental clarity facilitates the development of insight into the nature of selfhood and wisdom concerning oneself and the world.

There are two types of meditation practices: concentration and insight. Concentration meditation involves attending to the experience of one phenomena—such as the sensation of breathing—until the mind becomes focused and concentrated. In insight meditation, one attends, without judgment, to the experience of whatever mental or physical phenomena—thoughts, feelings, sensations or phantasies—are predominant in the field of awareness. This practice cultivates "mindfulness" or refined nonjudgmental awareness of whatever is occurring which leads to heightened perceptual acuity and attentiveness, increased control of voluntary processes, deepened insight into the nature of mental processes, selfhood and reality, the eradication of suffering, and the development of compassion and moral action.

THEORETICAL AND CONCEPTUAL POSITION

At first glance, psychoanalysis and Buddhism might seem to be too different to integrate. Several fundamental disparities between them are conspicuous. Buddhism is a spiritual system developed 2,500 years ago in India for attaining enlightenment; psychoanalysis is a psychotherapeutic system arising in Europe in the late nineteenth century addressing psychopathology and mental illness. To attain enlightenment, Buddhists recommend recognizing the illusory nature of selfhood—as we ordinarily understand it—as a unified, stable, unchanging, autonomous entity; whereas non-Lacanian psychoanalysts—of whatever theoretical orientation and consequent conception of subjectivity—encourage the discovery and development of a strong sense of self. Buddhism emphasizes the necessity of negating all desires and self-centeredness, while psychoanalysis—especially schools such as self psychology—maintain that ideals and goals play a crucial role in psychological well-being.

Certain crucial commonalities make a comparison between them intriguing. Both are concerned with the nature and alleviation of human suffering and each has both a diagnosis and "treatment plan" for alleviating human misery. The three other important things they share: (1) they are pursued within the crucible of an emotionally intimate relationship between either an analyst/analysand or a teacher/student; (2) they emphasize some similar experiential processes—evenly-hovering attention/free association and meditation; and (3) they recognize that obstacles

impede their attempts to facilitate change, for example, resistance/defensive processes in psychoanalysis and "hindrances"/"fetters"/"impediments" in Buddhism—make a comparison between them possible and potentially productive.

It will be the argument of this chapter that "there are more things in heaven and earth . . . than are dreamt of" in either psychoanalytic or Buddhist psychologies alone and that both psychoanalysis and Buddhism can enormously benefit from an egalitarian dialogue characterized by mutual respect, the absence of submission or deification, reciprocal communication, and a genuine interest in what they could teach each other. My stance of "bifocality" or "reciprocity of perspectives" (Fischer, 1986, p. 199) in which psychoanalysis and Buddhism are viewed in tandem so that they can mutually question and challenge each other, encourages a foregrounding of taken-for-granted assumptions, a relativizing of apparent eternal truths, a highlighting of theoretical blindspots, and an illuminating of unsuspected possibilities.

What I have discovered since approaching psychoanalysis and Buddhism in an egalitarian way is that both traditions have a great deal of merit but neither provides a complete picture of human nature, transformation, and liberation. Each offers a valuable and incomplete perspective—neglecting indispensable elements included in the other. For example, Buddhists could teach psychoanalysts about states of dereified, decommodified, and nonselfcentric subjectivity, while psychoanalysis could teach Buddhists about the recurrent, unconscious organizational patterns and self and object images and associated affects that shape and delimit human life and the psychological dangers of neglecting human agency.

Since neither tradition has the last word on these issues, both traditions could be enriched if their respective insights were integrated into a more inclusive and encompassing perspective—which currently does not exist—that takes into account their respective contributions and avoids their blindspots and limitations.

Beyond Self-Blindness: Psychoanalytic and Buddhist Visions of Subjectivity

The nature of the self is of central concern to psychoanalysis and Buddhism, which provide extremely sophisticated techniques for investigating and illuminating questions about its nature and status. "To study the Way [Zen] notes Zen master Dogen (1200–1253) "is to study the self." The self, according to psychoanalyst Heinz Kohut (1984) is the organizing center of the individual's psychological universe. Although differing significantly in theory and practice, both psychoanalysis and Buddhism share an assumption that optimal development involves a transformation of the self. But their differing viewpoints about how to investigate it and what it is lead in diametrically opposed theoretical and clinical directions.

Before presenting psychoanalytic and Buddhist conceptions of subjectivity, a brief excursus is necessary to put the following discussion in context. History (and I would add human subjectivity) can be studied, to borrow the French social historian Fernand Braudel's (1980) terminology, in terms of the immediate; the instant—"histoire événementielle"—or the long time span—"longée durée" (p. 27). Biologists distinguish between the "proximate" or the short-term causes of phenomena and the "ultimate" or long-term causes of phenomena (Modell, 1985, p. 85). Philosopher Richard Wollheim (1984) notes that there are three aspects to a person: the relationship between (1) conscious/preconscious/unconscious; (2) past/present/future; (3) transient and episodic "mental states"—such as thoughts, moments of interest, boredom, joy, lust, despair, and so forth—and recurrent "mental dispositions"—which do not occur and are not events—such as "knowledge and belief, emotions, desires, habits, virtues and vices, and skills" (pp. 33–34).

The consulting room is the laboratory in which psychoanalytic conceptions of subjectivity are formulated. The analyst listens with "evenly-hovering attention" to the patient's "free associations." What the analyst listens to is apprehended within a particular hermeneutical context, a genetic, linear perspective (Gold, 1992) in which it is assumed that the particular symptoms, traits, and conduct in the present—have been shaped in a linear way by formative experiences in the past. Psychoanalysts pay attention to the proximate aspects of the analysand's material but what Freud termed the attraction of the infantile prototypes may lead to a slight neglect of some of the "here-and-now" aspects of the person.

Through this kind of wide-angle attention to the patient's material the analyst "discovers" a substantial, enduring subject shaped by formative experiences and events from the long-term past.[1]

The typology of this substantial self varies depending on the school of psychoanalysis. In his synthetic overview of postclassical psychoanalytic views of the self, Mitchell (1991) demonstrates that each school of psychoanalysis construes selfhood differently. Mitchell distinguishes three views of the self: the Freudian view of the self as separate and integrated, the object relations and interpersonal view of it as multiple and discontinuous, and the self psychological view of it as integral and continuous.

The portrayal of self as multiple and continuous and the sense of self as separate, integral and continuous are referring to different aspects of self. The former refers to the multiple configurations of self patterned variably in different relational contexts. The latter refers to the subjective experience over time and across the different organizational schemes. The experience of patterning may be represented as having particular qualities or tones or content at different times; however, at every point, it is recognized as "mine," my particular way of processing and shaping experience. (Mitchell, 1991, p. 139)

But despite these differences there is a general agreement among psychoanalysts about two things: (1) the self exists; (2) strengthening and expanding the self is a fundamental goal of psychoanalysis. The outcome of psychoanalysis is an expanded and nuanced experience and understanding of "I-ness."

In a reflection late in his life on the nature of self-experience, Harry Stack Sullivan (1950) wondered if it were possible for there to be a completely different sort of self-system: "for all I know, there would not be evolved, in the course of becoming a person, anything like the sort of self-system that we always encounter" (p. 168). But Sullivan ultimately rejected his intriguing question, maintaining that a human being without a self-system is "beyond imagination" (p. 168). But it is not beyond a Buddhist imagination.

The experience of "I" is also of central concern in Buddhism. But in Buddhism it is no more than illusory. It is an epiphenomenon generated by our perceptual insensitivity.

The laboratory in which Buddhist views of subjectivity are formulated is the practice of meditation, which can occur either in a retreat context removed from the noise and sensory stimulation of daily life or in the midst of everyday life.

[1] This is not true of more interpersonally oriented analysts.

Meditation is the careful and detailed non-judgmental observation of the proximate dimensions of consciousness—mental states such as the feeling or thought or bodily sensation that just arose as you read this. Through this kind of microscopic "zoom lens" (Nozick, 1989) attention to consciousness, Buddhism "discovers" an ever-changing flux of thoughts, feelings, perceptions, memories, sensations which arise and pass away like clouds entering and exiting from the sky. The mind, in Buddhism, is like a movie screen: who we are is what is arising in the current moment on the surface of the screen. Each moment the screen, like the sky, is changing.

The consensually accepted belief—prevalent in most sectors of Western life—in the substantiality of this illusion is, according to Buddhism, problematic in several ways: (1) it presents a distorted view of how things really are; (2) it interferes with experiencing a deeper, more profound reality; (3) it generates suffering and interferes with our experiencing the greatest kind of contentment (cf. Nozick, 1989). Understanding the absence of an abiding self leads, according to Buddhism, to an absence of selfcentric preoccupations and a more engaged relationship to life. Competition and self-judgment decline as one accepts life more on its own terms. This leads to greater compassion and a sense of peace and openness. Rather than focusing on the development of the self, Buddhism recommends and attempts to facilitate seeing through the illusoriness of subjectivity.

Believing that the self is an illusion, a Buddhist would view one's quest in psychoanalysis to understand oneself or develop an identity or discover one's true self a misguided enterprise that would be a source of enormous psychological suffering. Buddhism would attempt to facilitate the radical transcendence of self-concern. In contrast, a psychoanalyst—depending on his or her theoretical orientation—would probably view the denial of selfhood as some kind of symptom of conflict or development arrest that needed to be understood and worked through psychoanalytically. Psychoanalytic and Buddhist views of the nature of subjectivity seem antithetical and irreconcilable.

There is no immaculate perception. There is no single, neutral, objective, ahistorical, transcendental viewpoint from which to view the self.

Our conception of subjectivity depends on how we look at it. What psychoanalysts and Buddhists "discover" about selfhood is often an artifact of the way they investigate it. A psychoanalyst approaching subjectivity with a wide-angle lens will "discover" different dimensions of subjectivity—the solidity and continuity of a unified subject shaped by a particular history of recurrent self and object images and mental dispositions—than a Buddhist who adopts a microscopic perspective and observes the proximate nature of subjectivity—the way we are shaped and created anew each moment by the arising of fluid and discontinuous mental states.

As a result of their different observation points in investigating subjectivity, psychoanalysis and Buddhism each illuminate and neglect different facets of it. Psychoanalysis highlights the substantial aspects of subjectivity, particularly the enduring patterns from the past that shape and delimit human experience, while Buddhism highlights the transitive dimensions of subjectivity particularly the fluid mental states arising and shaping subjectivity, moment-after-moment.

From my perspective, each view of subjectivity is illuminating and myopic. Neither is wrong; they are partial—valid under certain circumstances, false under others. They each eclipse some crucial aspect of subjectivity and thus offer a partial perspective on it which results in a fragmented portrait of its typology and fate.

Each conception fosters a complementary type of self-blindness. In exploring subjectivity meditatively, Buddhists are "near-sighted" and partially neglect the substantial, historical aspects of subjectivity. Questions of the subject's history and agency are eclipsed and the seeds of self-deception and self-blindness are planted. In examining subjectivity psychoanalytically, psychoanalysis is sometimes "far-sighted;" eclipsing several of the near-at-hand aspects of subjectivity.

Much Ado about Nothingness or Evading the Subject. Buddhism evades the subject and thus eclipses three of its important facets: (1) its embeddedness in history; (2) its idiosyncratic structure and design, and (3) the fact of human agency and moral responsibility.

The absence of a sense of history or personal continuity leaves one adrift without any anchor.

There would appear to be no basis for action because there is no reference point to evaluate phenomena, no previous experiences to learn from and no criteria to evaluate among various courses of action.

One consequence of this is that it helps people not to be critical of things they should be critical of. This can result in a self-induced historical "amnesia" in which amoral actions in spiritual communities, for example, can be rationalized as things in the past that are of no concern because they are not happening in, and do not pertain to, the present moment.

In addition, if there is no subject then there is no one who is exploited or alienated and no oppression to challenge or contest. There would appear to be no basis for morality or effective social criticism because there is no criteria for decisions or actions. Crucial questions about resistance to the existing order of society are eclipsed: Resistance in the name of what? For the sake of whom? To what end? (Walzer 1988, p. 191).

Evading the subject also leads to the "return of the repressed." Self-denial leads to self-centeredness. The result of denying the existence of a substantial self is a resurfacing of some of the disavowed aspects of psychic life. In recent years there has been an epidemic of scandals in American Buddhist communities involving Buddhist teachers illegally expropriating money from the community or sexually exploiting students (Boucher, 1988). The acting out of such self-centered behavior seems directly related to Buddhism's denial of self-existence. The return of the repressed emerges in this acting out on the part of Buddhist teachers. Thus, instead of a meditation teacher utilizing the feeling of sexual attraction to a student as feedback about important personal and perhaps interpersonal phenomena, these feelings may be denied or acted out. It is thus not incidental or accidental that there have been so many incidents of self-centered behavior in spiritual communities in the United States in recent years.

"Fixing" the Subject. But if Buddhism evades the subject, psychoanalysis tends to "fix it"; to cut off some of its life. The psychoanalytic approach to subjectivity leads to "far-sightedness"; particularly a neglect of certain near-at-hand aspects of subjectivity such as the (1) fluidity of episodic, transient mental states which arise moment-after-moment and may not neatly fit into or confirm our established, taken-for-granted view of ourselves and (2) the nonpathological, nonselfcentric aspects of subjectivity.

Self-reification is illustrated by classical psychoanalysis' conception of the mind, in which processes such as desiring/wishing, perceiving/adapting, and self-judging/self-punishing are made into tangible, thing-like, spatially localized entities—id, ego, and super-ego.

Neither the psychoanalytic nor the Buddhist view of subjectivity is wrong, but each falls victim to the *pars pro toto* fallacy, reducing subjectivity to the essentialistic core that derives from the unique vantage point they employ in investigating it. Buddhism takes the kaleidoscopic sense of subjectivity derived from its zoom lens approach and universalizes it as the essential constituent of subjectivity instead of as an aspect of subjectivity that inevitably emerges when selfhood is examined in the microscopic manner dictated by the Buddhist meditative approach. Psychoanalysis takes the substantive sense of self generated from its telescopic way of investigating subjectivity in the psychoanalytic consulting room and then universalizes that, instead of recognizing it as a facet of subjectivity that necessarily arises when selfhood is examined psychoanalytically. This eclipses other aspects of subjectivity that are invisible to the method currently being employed to investigate it. The universalization of the partial psychoanalytic and Buddhist viewpoints impedes the formulation of more encompassing views of subjectivity.

In my view, each view of subjectivity suggests important correctives to the blindspots of the other. Buddhism's dereifed conception of subjectivity can help psychoanalysis in several ways. Meditation could teach psychoanalysis that the apparently unified narrative that the analysand and the analyst have constructed about the patient's self is, in part, illusory. This homogeneous image of the self hides its heterogeneity; the discontinuities, fissures, and anomalous perceptions expressed in the transient and episodic mental states that arise moment-to-moment. Meditation facilitates, to borrow Foucault's (1977) terminology in a different but not incompatible context, an "'unrealization'" (p. 160) of our taken-for-granted, unified identity based teleologically on past experiences and conceptions of ourselves. An unreified and unconstricted sense of subjectivity would be facilitated.

Nonselfcentric moments of consciousness become more apparent when attention is paid to these proximate aspects of subjectivity. Moments of nonselfcentricity—whether surrendering, merging, yielding, letting go—seem part of most spiritual traditions. Autonomous, differentiated identity—which is a more selfcentric aspect of subjectivity—has been traditionally viewed as the apex of human development by most non-Kohutian psychoanalysts. Experiences of merger and nonselfcentric modes of being have been interpreted by most psychoanalysts, following Freud's unceremonious lead, as symptoms of psychopathology. In the self-psychology tradition, for example, fragmentation of self-boundaries and self-cohesion are viewed as symptoms of a vulnerable or besieged self.

But experiences of self-transcendence, in which there is a loss of self-differentiation and nonselfcentricity, may refer to nonpathological, expanded states of consciousness qualitatively different from more archaic states of undifferentiation. Because psychoanalysis lacks a psychology of transcendent states, these modes of being do not appear on its map of human development and are assumed to be pathological. Psychoanalysis is guilty of a "prestructural fallacy" (Wilber, 1984) in which these experiences are automatically correlated with archaic development and pathologized.[2]

Buddhism could teach psychoanalysts that such states of nonselfcentricity may represent not a pathological regression or a fragmentation-prone self-structure but spiritual experiences that can enhance self-experience by eroding restrictive identifications and facilitating greater freedom, flexibility, and inclusiveness of self-structures.

In detaching one from a hypertrophied, overly selfcentric sense of self, meditation opens subjects up to the possibility of greater intimacy; for rapport and love demand that we unconstrict and sometimes transcend our normally more restrictive sense of separateness from others and

the world. Loosening the grip of excessive self-preoccupation—whether one is deeply immersed in playing a musical instrument, watching an engrossing cultural event, or making love—often leads to a heightened sense of living.

In psychological and spiritual matters, like in real estate, practically no one voluntarily trades down. The vast majority of meditators would not meditate if they believed they would lose more than they would gain. Since practically no one—save the Huck Finn's of the world—enjoys his or her own funeral one wonders what are the unconscious attractions, what is the desire, underlying the Buddhist doctrine? Psychoanalytic understanding of self-protective strategies such as defensive processes can illuminate some aspects of this process and increase Buddhist understanding of some of the consequences and dangers of the self-deceptions endemic to Buddhism's stance of self-nullification.

In denying their own subjectivity, Buddhists unwittingly become its prisoner and reenact restrictive dramas of childhood such as deferentially submitting to idealized teachers or secretly condemning themselves and experiencing shame for actions that violate Buddhist ethical precepts.

They will also have greater difficulty, in certain ways, leading a full life in the present and creating an individualized array of goals and ideals than they would have if they did not deny their status as historical beings.

Disbelieving in the existence of selfhood is appealing to people who feel deep guilt, shame, or fear or wish to erase traumatic history. For example, one way of responding to an abusive childhood or coping with powerful guilt or shame is to deny one's existence and thus eliminate any responsibility.

One way of whitewashing the amorality of others—which in a given situation might include teachers in spiritual communities—is to deny the reality of subjectivity. If there is no subject than there is no impropriety or exploitation. It is all maya, illusion.

The nonexistence of the self might also be attractive to meditators with an apocalyptic sense of the future. For such a person, it might be less scary to imagine that one does not exist then to contemplate a nuclear winter in the near future.

Psychoanalysis and Buddhism alone provide an incomplete and inadequate rendering of

[2]My account has been enriched by Karen People's (1991) unpublished summary of a paper in progress entitled "The Paradox of Surrender: Constructing and Transcending the Self."

subjectivity. Both psychoanalytic and Buddhist conceptions of subjectivity would be enriched if the understandings obtained from their different ways of investigating subjectivity are integrated into a more encompassing and inclusive framework that values their unique insights into the different facets of subjectivity they each elucidate while avoiding their limitations—for example, the nearsightedness of Buddhism and the farsightedness of psychoanalysis.

A more encompassing model of subjectivity would investigate subjectivity "microscopically" and "telescopically" so that both its proximate and ultimate facets would emerge.

Subjectivity is composed of various dialectically related facets—selfcentricity and nonselfconsciousness; self-assertion and communion; substantiality and transiency/fluidity; history (embeddedness in time) and spirituality (the capacity for nonselfcentricity/dwelling in timelessness). Psychoanalysis and Buddhism each illuminate certain of these facets. Psychoanalysis highlights the selfcentricity, substantiality, and historicity of subjectivity, whereas Buddhism elucidates its fluidity, nonselfcentric and spiritual aspects. Typically psychoanalysts and Buddhists neglect, if not denigrate, those facets of subjectivity occluded by their conception of it. One facet of each of the five dialectical pairs is thus neglected by each theory. Buddhists neglect selfhood's substantiality and historicity, whereas psychoanalysts eclipse its nonsubstantiality and spirituality. To recognize only one of these aspects is to misperceive the multiplicity of subjectivity.

I do not view either facet as primary or superior. I disagree with Buddhism's insistence that emptiness is primary and psychoanalysis' belief that substantiality is primary. I find the popular transpersonal view that nonselfcenteredness is a higher state of being than selfcenteredness, illustrated in the oft repeated claim that "you have to be somebody before you are nobody," incomplete. Although it is true that you cannot disidentify from what you are not, both facets of subjectivity are interpenetrating aspects of human experience; alternating positions of being rather than hierarchically ordered stages.[3] The privileging of nonselfcenteredness and the consequent

devaluing and repression of selfcenteredness ultimately engender the egotistical behavior sometimes acted out in Buddhist communities. For as Jung frequently said: when one aspect of subjectivity is consciously overemphasized, its opposite takes on increased unconscious importance.

The expanded conception I am advocating involves thinking more dialectically; granting that both viewpoints have a range of applicability; recognizing that the two perspectives are alternative tools, useful for different purposes rather than contradictory claims.

It is impossible to address each of the facets of subjectivity within the scope of this chapter. I shall take one of the dialectical pairs and briefly discuss it in terms of the more inclusive perspective I am proposing.

Twentieth century physics teaches us that we may view phenomena in terms of particles (e.g., things and entities) or waves (e.g., movement and process).[4] When it comes to selfhood most analysts prereflectively adopt the "particulate" perspective—the self as a "fixed entity, separate particle" (Tart, 1990, p. 161). In Buddhist circles the "wave" perspective is valorized.

Life consists of both things and processes, entities and movement. In certain realms of life the "wave" paradigm is useful while the "particle" paradigm works better for others.

Sometimes when reflecting upon one's conduct or planning a course of action, we must fixate the self and view it as a concrete, substantial entity. Decisions and planning cannot occur without a human agent who envisions possibilities, weighs alternatives, and chooses specific courses of action. To deny this mode of being is to create chaos and undermine the basis for choice and action.

At other times, observing art, participating in athletics, or merging in love, unselfconsciousness—the view of subjectivity as a process—is valuable. The particle view of subjectivity interferes with participating in these activities and states of being in a complete way. For patients with an insufficiently consolidated self-structure a wave view of subjectivity would occasion terror and would be absolutely disastrous.

"Most people," as Young (Tart, 1990) observes, "are one-sided, always experiencing self

[3]My position is, in part, an outgrowth of Ogden's (1991) suggestive interpretation of the notion of "positions" in Melanie Klein.

[4]My view of subjectivity has greatly benefited from Shinzen Young's discussion in Tart (1990).

as particle, unfamiliar with self as wave" (p. 161). We often need to be able to oscillate between both modes of being during the course of a day.

Taken together psychoanalysis and Buddhism illuminate a more complete range of the multiplicity that is the self[5] than either pursued alone. A bifocal conception of subjectivity would help us be less myopic about selfhood's important features. Adopting such a complementary viewpoint would enable us to recognize that states of selfcentricity and unselfconsciousness are both part of living a full life. The former is necessary to assess situations, formulate plans and goals, and choose among potential courses of action. The latter is necessary in appreciating art, listening to patients, participating in athletics, and experiencing love. A complementary view of subjectivity would help us avoid Buddhism's far-sightedness and psychoanalysis's near-sightedness: neither eclipsing the view of self-fluidity, nonselfcentricity and self-transcendence suggested by Buddhism, nor the sense of self-substantiality, historicity and agency recognized by psychoanalysis.

Pathology: East and West

Asian and psychoanalytic perspectives on the etiology of pathology are quite different. Buddhist writings on attachment, greed, egoism, and desire (Kornfield, 1977) illuminate some of the "proximate" or immediate sources of pathology and suffering whereas psychoanalytic models of the causes of pathology, for example, unempathic parenting and consequent self-defects (Kohut, 1977), negative unconscious fantasies and introjects (Fairbairn, 1952), illuminate the "ultimate" aspects of why humans become ill and suffer.

Psychoanalytic perspectives on pathology suggest that the Buddhist view is naive about the tenacity of pathology and the possibilities of change. Buddhism neglects such aspects of mental life as unconscious commitments to restrictive relationships with self and others. Psychoanalysis could demonstrate to Buddhism that we may consciously desire change yet also maintain an allegiance to these past modes of being.

Buddhism is more skilled at working on

[5]My rendering of subjectivity is necessarily incomplete. Other investigators utilizing different approaches will undoubtedly detect and highlight other dimensions of selfhood.

pathology than diagnosing it. This is not surprising given its lack of a fully delineated developmental framework, its neglect of the impact of the long-term past on personality, and its underemphasis on types of character. Because of its developmental viewpoint, its sensitivity to the influence of the past on the present and its more extensive cartography of types of pathology, psychoanalysis is more able to diagnose pathology.

CLINICAL AND THEORETICAL ANTECEDENTS

There are few antecedents in the literature for integrating psychoanalysis and Buddhism. Traditionally non-Western psychologies in general, and Asian psychology in particular, have rarely been discussed in Western psychology. Asian psychology has been virtually ignored in the psychoanalytic literature. The few exceptions, for example, Alexander (1931) and Masson & Masson (1978), present distorted and reductionistic accounts of it: falsely equating it with mysticism (Masson & Masson, 1978), regression and pathology (Alexander, 1931). In his blanket dismissal of Buddhism as a training in an artificial catatonia, psychoanalyst Franz Alexander (1931) illustrates the Eurocentrism that has plagued psychoanalysis.

The more sympathetic non-Eurocentric work of Horney (1945; 1987), Jung (1958), Kelman (1960), Fromm, Suzuki, & DeMartino (1960), Roland (1988), Suler (1991) and myself (Rubin, 1985; 1989; 1991) are the exceptions that demonstrate the rule. Although they have pointed to various aspects of Buddhism's salutary dimensions including its ability to sensitize us to the inner life (Jung, 1958), enrich psychoanalytic listening (Rubin, 1985), promote "well-being"—being fully awake and alive (Fromm, Suzuki, & DeMartino, 1960), and expand psychoanalytic conceptions of subjectivity (Roland, 1988), they tend, with the exception of the work of Roland (1988) and Rubin (1989; 1991) to neglect both clinical issues and clinical material.

The most compelling effort to integrate Asian and Western psychology is transpersonal theorist Ken Wilber's "spectrum psychology" which attempts to create a marriage between Western and Asian psychological perspectives on human development, psychopathology, and cure.

The central underlying assumption of Wilber's model is that consciousness, like light, is composed of various bands or spectrums which develop through a series of stages. In a recent article, Wilber (1986) proposes ten levels to the spectrum. In ascending order,. they are: sensoriphysical, phantasmic-emotional, representational mind, rule/role mind, formal-reflexive mind, vision-logic, psychic, subtle, causal, and ultimate. It would distract from the central argument to define Wilber's terms. For our purposes it is sufficient to note that each stage of development has it own particular type of self experience, cognitive development, moral sensibilities, potential distortions, and pathologies. Each level is characterized by a different sense of personal identity ranging from the sensoriphysical level in which one identifies only with the realms of matter, sensation, and perception to the ultimate level in which one is identified with the totality of the universe. Each higher stage is less "selfcentric" than its predecessors (Wilber, 1986).

Wilber maintains that different psychotherapeutic and spiritual traditions address and are best suited for different levels of the spectrum. Western psychotherapies, for example, psychoanalysis, gestalt therapy, and transactional analysis, address pathology on lower levels of the spectrum while contemplative disciplines such as Buddhism are recommended for higher stages of the spectrum and the deepest kinds of transformation and liberation. For Wilber, psychoanalysis and Buddhism are complementary.

Wilber's model does not achieve genuine integration. The apparent marriage of psychological and spiritual perspectives is an asymmetrical affair with psychoanalysis relegated to an inferior status. While psychoanalysis and Buddhism are said to be complementary, Buddhism is actually viewed as superior: offering a privileged and true description of how humans really are. A tacit inequality is hidden underneath the nominal complementarity. Whereas psychoanalysis usually pathologizes non-Western thought, transpersonal theorists tend to deify it.

Within the transpersonal ranks what I would term "Orientocentrism" not Eurocentrism tends to predominate. By Orientocentrism I mean not the "Orientalism" literary and culture critic Edward Said (1978) refers to when he describes the tendency among Western commentators on the Orient to utilize an imperialistic discourse about Asia which presents a distorted and reductionistic picture of "the East" in order to intellectually colonialize Asia and psychologically fortify itself, but rather the mirror opposite danger to Eurocentrism: the valorizing and privileging of Asian thought and the neglect if not dismissal of Western psychological perspectives. The Zen master who told the student of Zen who indicated that psychotherapy and Zen had similar effects in overcoming suffering that the psychotherapist is just another patient (Matthiessen, 1985, p. 160) and the revealing and never cited fact that none of the articles in the preeminent, extant anthologies in the field of east/west studies (e.g., Welwood's *Meetings of the Ways*, 1979; Tart's *Transpersonal Psychologies*, 1975; Boorstein's *Transpersonal Psychotherapy*, 1980; Walsh & Vaughan's *Beyond Ego*, 1980) explore what value Western psychotherapies might have for Asian thought illustrates Orientocentrism.

The Eurocentrism of traditional Western psychology and the "Orientocentrism" of transpersonal psychology both inhibit the creation of an integrative psychology because they establish an intellectual embargo on commerce between Asian and Western psychology: traditional Western psychology does not import Asian perspectives while transpersonal psychology does not import Western perspectives.

An alternative perspective is necessary if the genuine insights of both traditions are to emerge. In contrast to the Eurocentrism of psychoanalysis and the "Orientocentrism" of transpersonal psychology, I will be recommending a more egalitarian relationship in which both differences and similarities and strengths and limitations of each are acknowledged.

THE TECHNIQUE AND PROCESS OF PSYCHOTHERAPY

Two major difficulties arise when one attempts to discuss the actual integration of psychoanalysis and Buddhism. Because some of the qualities cultivated by each discipline which might play a significant role in integration—such as the spirit cultivated by long immersion in eastern disciplines or years of exposure to the "analytic attitude" (Schafer, 1983)—may not be completely amenable to verbal delineation although they profoundly affect the person; an integration of psychoanalysis and Buddhism does not always lend itself to concrete specifications.

Second, because certain features that each tradition emphasizes—such as psychopathology in psychoanalysis and meditation in Buddhism—may not be viewed as essential ingredients of the process of change by the other tradition, the very template one employs in attempting to integrate them cannot avoid being ethnocentric. The clinician interested in integration must strive to be aware of and open to the various ways in which intellectual xenophobia and colonialism implicitly or explicitly operates in his or her theoretical framework. For example, the very attempt to integrate psychoanalytic and Buddhist views of pathology may be an act of intellectual colonialism toward Buddhism because the notion of pathology may be more endemic to Western modes of thinking than to Buddhist ones. Ways of thinking and being that are somewhat foreign to one's own preferred approach need to be respected.

In the following section, I shall attempt to highlight some of the ways I currently think about integrating psychoanalysis and Buddhism. Believing with Wittgenstein that we cannot avoid creating models which simplify a more complex reality, my recommendations are offered in the spirit of provisional suggestions rather than conclusive pronouncements.

Buddhist and Psychoanalytic Paths

The Buddhist and psychoanalytic paths to transformation—the Buddhist "eightfold path" and "factors of enlightenment"—and psychoanalytic writings on transference, resistance, and the therapeutic action of psychoanalysis may be synergistic in that combining certain aspects of each could make them both more effective than if pursued alone. Thus, studying them together could be mutually enriching. Both follow a similar process which includes (1) presenting the problem of human suffering; (2) diagnosing its causes; (3) offering a remedy. In this section, I will suggest that each tradition's remedy has elements that could be usefully applied by the other.

The Seven Factors of Enlightenment, a classical Buddhist delineation of the seven factors leading to awakening, provides a possible template for integrating the psychoanalytic and Buddhist paths of transformation. The seven factors are (1) mindfulness, or awareness without judgment, attachment or aversion to what is happening in the present moment; (2) investigation, or actively probing, exploring and analyzing the nature of things and the various dimensions of experience; (3) energy, that is, the focus on being attentive and awake and seeing clearly; (4) rapture, or the curiosity about and delight in, each moment of experience; (5) calm, that is "quietness of mind" (Kornfield, 1977, p. 17); (6) concentration, that is a state in which the mind is deeply immersed with lazerlike "one-pointedness" in whatever it experiences; (7) equanimity, or a balance and evenness of mind in which one is receptive and impartial toward whatever is occurring.

There are two possible ways the factors of enlightenment could serve as a template to integrate or at least critically compare the psychoanalytic and Buddhist path. To illuminate the first, I must provide a gloss on mindfulness, the first and most important factor of enlightenment. As the Russian mystic Gurdjieff aptly noted, most humans are "asleep"—unaware of the actual texture of their experience. They are like the president of a pluralistic democracy—they hopefully have a general sense of what is going on but lack an understanding of certain crucial specifics that shape daily lived life. All authentic, noncultish psychological and spiritual systems attempt to cultivate wakefulness—the attentiveness and awareness of the actual texture of experience.

In the Satipatthana Sutra (Thera, 1962), perhaps the locus classicus for Buddhist views on training mindfulness, Buddha said that mindfulness—awareness without judgment, attachment or aversion to what is happening in the present moment—was the important factor in diminishing unwholesome states of mind and cultivating wholesome ones. The sole route to freedom, according to Buddha, is the development of mindfulness in four areas: (1) bodily phenomena, for example, physical sensations, breathing, body postures such as sitting, standing, lying, and walking; (2) "feelings," which refer not to what Westerners ordinarily mean by "emotions" but rather to the reactions of "pleasantness," "unpleasantness," and "neutrality" which accompany every moment of consciousness—every experience of seeing, hearing, smelling, tasting, touching, and thinking; (3) consciousness or mental phenomena, for example, all mental states: anger, love, joy, lust, fear, compassion, and so forth; and (4) "dharma"—the universal laws underlying life: for example, the four noble truths, the Eightfold path, the Seven Factors of Enlightenment, and the five hindrances to enlightenment.

Since all aspects of human experience are arguably contained within these four dimensions of mindfulness broadly construed, psychoanalysis and Buddhism can be viewed in terms of which of these four areas each cultivates and neglects. Psychoanalysis, for example, attends to mental phenomena to the relative neglect of "feeling," while Buddhism highlights "feeling" to the relative neglect of certain aspects of consciousness, for example, emotions related to interpersonal relationships and intimacy.

Various aspects of mental content, such as the dynamics of interpersonal relationships, intimacy, and sexuality are often suppressed or dealt with abstractly in Buddhism. These topics are often not addressed directly by meditation teachers. Clear guidelines about how to deal with them are rarely offered. Given the rash of sexual scandals emanating from Buddhist communities in America in recent years Buddhism would be enriched by psychoanalysis' illumination of mental content, particularly its understanding of unconscious resistance, transference, and countertransference. This is not to say that psychoanalysis offers a comprehensive or even balanced account of certain facets of mental content such as intimacy, which it does not, because its understanding of intimacy is also incomplete and reductionistic.

Human liberation, as I perceive it, involves the balanced development of two different but mutually enhancing types of forces—receptive, tranquilizing, and stabilizing energies, and active arousing and energizing factors (Goldstein, 1976; Kornfield, Dass, & Miyuki, 1979). This relates to the second possible way the factors of enlightment can be employed to integrate the Buddhist and psychoanalytic path. Various psychological and spiritual paths can be considered in terms of which of these factors are developed and neglected (Kornfield, Dass, & Miyuki, 1979). Some traditions cultivate active qualities while others

strengthen tranquilizing qualities. For example, in psychoanalysis there is a predominant emphasis on active, energetic factors, such as investigation into various aspects of internal and interpersonal life and a relative neglect of the value of the tranquilizing factors such as concentration (and equanimity). Buddhism is enormously effective in developing "receptive" factors such as concentration, calm, tranquility, and equanimity, but has tended to neglect the cultivation of active factors such as investigation. The balanced development of both kinds of factors is necessary to promote human liberation. One needs to concentrate the mind and then investigate from the place of heightened clarity which it engenders.

To give one specific example: listening to ourselves and our patients is the cornerstone of psychoanalytic inquiry and technique. Freud suggested what analysts need to do in this area— listen with "evenly-hovering attention"—but he did not prescribe *how* to do this. He presented a "negative" account—what to avoid, namely censorship and prior expectations—not what to do, that is, how to cultivate "evenly-hovering attention." No systematic procedure and no specific positive recommendations have ever been offered to cultivate this capacity by subsequent analysts. This omission has hampered the optimal development of psychoanalytic listening. Since meditation trains exactly this state of mind, it could enrich psychoanalytic listening (cf. Rubin, 1985, for a more detailed demonstration).

Psychoanalysis' skill in "investigation"— which I just alluded to in the previous section— emerges in its understanding of how and why we become ill—questions related to psychopathology. Because psychoanalysis is underwritten by a "tragic" worldview (Schafer, 1976), with its recognition of the inescapable mysteries, dilemmas, and afflictions pervading human existence, and is thus essentially a psychology of illness, and Buddhism offers a "romantic" psychology of wellness in which it is assumed that psychological conditioning can be transcended and ultimate meaning on a grand design can be achieved, the relative emphasis on pathology seems to differ in each tradition.

Psychoanalysis seems more interested in and offers a more extensive cartography of pathology. And yet, understanding Buddhist and psychoanalytic conceptions of pathology—particularly the former's focus on the "proximate" or immediate causes of pathology and the latter's relative emphasis on the "ultimate" or long-term sources of pathology, such as the effects of unempathetic parenting on self-development (Kohut, 1984) and the unconscious commitments to old and restrictive interpersonal ways of being (Fairbairn, 1952), allows the analyst to have a wider latitude in conceptualizing the nature of the patient's difficulty than either viewpoint adopted alone.

Buddhist explanations of pathology—unconscious attachments based on greed, hatred and delusion—can be reductionistic. Why greed, hatred and delusion? What is the unconscious meaning and purpose of living in this way? What unconscious self and object images are being recreated? There is more to pathology than "attachment" to illusory views of subjectivity or greed, hatred, and delusion. Why do we cling to self-damaging ways of being? In the service of what? For whom? Who gets protected? What gets warded off or avoided when we do this? Adopting the Buddhist view alone eclipses these and other important questions about the nature and cause of pathology. Psychoanalytic perspectives on the earlier, unconscious sources of pathology can temper Buddhism's tendency to neglect some of the unconscious self issues that cause greed, hatred, and delusion whereas Buddhist sensitivity to the proximate causes of pathology—the "here and now"—reveals certain problems in the analytic perspective. The analyst who attends to the proximate causes of pathology as well as the ultimate sources of pathology has less chance of neglecting either facet of pathology.

The analyst who attends to the facets of subjectivity uniquely illuminated by psychoanalysis and Buddhism will also approach the patient's problems in living more completely. The integrative analyst recognizes the value of all of the dialectically related facets of subjectivity. When only one aspect of subjectivity predominates or when one is excluded, illness is not far behind. An understanding of both conceptions of subjectivity can help the integrative therapist comprehend in a more nuanced way where the patient is struggling. The integrative therapist would also point out and help the patient work through barriers to either type of self-experience.

The therapeutic relationship plays a crucial role in my model of integration. Psychoanalysis is a testament to the human capacity for self-deception. Most people believe that they are acting in a rational, intelligent manner. It is nearly impossible to see our own blindnesses. The therapist can point out blindspots that the analysand cannot see and thus open up formerly unconscious sectors of the person's life.

The therapeutic relationship has other crucial benefits. Since Freud, psychoanalysts have recognized that the patients typical, formative ways of approaching self and others usually manifest in analysis and in the analytic relationship in the form of transference. The Eastern literature has anecdotes of teachers and masters interacting with students and disciples in ways that are designed to help them recognize characterological patterns. But the use of transference is sporadic and unsystematic. Psychoanalysis can enrich Buddhist understandings because in the psychoanalytic situation transference can be systematically analyzed. Psychoanalytic examination of transference can illuminate ways of being that may either go unnoticed or be submerged in Buddhism—such as the idealization of the teacher and the concomitant submission of the student (Tart & Deikman, 1991). In Buddhism this dynamic may remain unexamined and the student's self-devaluation and deferentiality may never get resolved and may play itself out in various other relationships.

The psychoanalytic relationship has other values for Buddhists. It can be the crucible for the reemergence of archaic transferences and can aid in the process of aborted development being recognized, reinstated, and worked through.

The practice of meditation and therapy in tandem is not for everybody. Most of my patients do not meditate and as a rule I do not introduce it. Introducing it could interfere with the treatment process by unconsciously compromising the impartiality of the analytic environment. Since the field of Buddhist-psychoanalytic integration is in its relative infancy and there is scant data on the question of indications and contraindications for working in this way I do not yet feel comfortable commenting on it. The available studies tend to link questions of indications and contraindications with diagnosis. Since I have come across schizophrenics who meditate without reporting negative side effects and neurotics who do, suitability, in my experience, depends on many more factors than diagnosis. This certainly is a question that future research needs to address.

CASE EXAMPLE

Clinical case studies of religion in general and Buddhism in particular are rare in psychoanalysis (Rubin, 1989). There is thus a dearth of clinical data regarding Buddhism in psychoanalysis. In this section, I shall present a clinical case of a Buddhist in psychoanalytic treatment. This is the only clinical data about this topic I have seen in the psychoanalytic or Buddhist literature.[6]

Steven, a man in his late-twenties, sought psychoanalytic treatment because of periodic bouts of mild frustration about his career, self-esteem issues, and as part of a more extensive quest for self-development and perfection. When he began analysis, he was attending graduate school and pursuing an advanced degree in the social sciences. In graduate school, Steven became very interested in Asian thought. He read widely in Asian philosophy and psychology and practiced insight meditation on a regular basis.

Steven was the oldest of two brothers in a middle-class family. His parents were atheists. Steven was raised as a secular humanist. As a child, Steven and his mother were quite close. Initially, he described her as a kind, sensitive and curious woman who valued him very much. He had fond memories of the time they spent together in his childhood.

In the course of analysis, Steven's impression of his mother altered. He came to feel that she was an anxious, overly protective woman who was deeply concerned about the opinions of others and avoided conflict at any cost. He recovered childhood memories of her "controlling" and infantilizing behavior. He felt that she viewed him as if he were an extension of herself and demanded that he conform to her vision of what he should be. He expended a great deal of effort molding himself into the sort of person that would make her feel proud and successful as a parent.

Their relationship changed for the worse

6This is a greatly revised and expanded version of a case discussed in two papers (Rubin, 1989, 1991).

when Steven was an adolescent. At that time family life began revolving around the plight of his troubled and enigmatic younger brother. His brother was constantly involved in some sort of trouble usually involving stealing or lying. When Steven was twelve, his brother stole his coin collection and bought candy with the proceeds. Steven remembered that his parents did not force his brother to make any sort of restitution.

Steven felt that his mother recruited him to assist her in handling his brother. Steven became the family "moderator," adjudicating between his brother's garbled explanations of his transgressions and his angry and baffled parents.

For his mother, he became a kind of a surrogate husband, providing advice and support about how to handle her youngest son and ministering to her emotional needs. As treatment progressed, Steven became aware of resenting that he had been cast in the role of family "redeemer." His parents and especially his mother had expected him to become accomplished and provide vicarious glory for her and the family so as to compensate for her sense of herself as a parental failure.

Steven felt he had a distant and unfulfilling relationship with his father whom he described as a competent, critical, emotionally constrained, and perfectionistic man with a bad temper. Steven and his father seemed to share very little.

Steven feared that any affectively charged situation might ignite his father's temper. He described his father as susceptible to severe periodic emotional outbursts accompanied by loss of temper, yelling, and screaming. His father tended to become angry or panic when things did not conform to his rigid expectations. In one particularly traumatic incident when Steven was in elementary school, his father whipped him with a belt after learning that Steven had gotten in trouble in school. Afterward Steven made a secret vow to himself that he would never lose his temper and become an "animal" like his father.

His father placed a great premium on performance. Steven presented various memories of his father criticizing and correcting his school work or athletic performance. Steven felt that he could never please his father and believed that if he was not perfect, then his father viewed him as a failure.

Steven felt that he had subordinated himself

to his parents' demands to such an extent that he had sacrificed and lost touch with his own needs and goals. He described this process of neglecting his own needs and life and subordinating himself to what others wanted as "Stevelessness." It involved both deferring to the needs of others and "straitjacketing" himself. He was afraid that self-assertion would result in his being shunned and "orphaned." In later stages of analysis he described this as being "buried alive."

He strove to be supersuccessful so as to compensate for his brother's difficulties and his parent's sense of failure and win his father's approval. But his childhood and adolescence were pervaded by the sense that he had failed his entire family: he had not cured his troubled brother, redeemed his mother, or pleased his father. He never felt admired for his own accomplishments, which he kept essentially hidden so as not to threaten his brother's precarious self-esteem. He felt he would never live up to his father's ambitions for him.

In relation to me, Steven was at first somewhat guarded and compliant. Although he seemed to speak with a minimum of self-censorship and inhibition, he was fearful that I would be judgmental, controlling, and intrusive; tacitly or covertly imposing my own agenda on him like his mother.

As his fantasies about these dangers were explored within the transference, his need for me to be an idealizable person whose insight and wisdom he could utilize and incorporate emerged. He also expressed an intense need for me to be perfectly attuned to the subtlety of his thoughts and feelings.

As the analysis proceeded, material about Buddhism periodically emerged. Buddhism was introduced in terms of Steven's experiences at a recent meditation retreat. He described the way in which meditation practice cultivated increased attentiveness and self-awareness and decreased self-contempt. At first Steven treated Buddhism like a historic building in a changing neighborhood, and accorded it a kind of "landmark status" in which it was exempt from critical examination and the threat of demolition and preserved in its original form. Gradually, curiosity about Buddhism replaced veneration.

I did not challenge Buddhism's protected status. I proceeded slowly, alert to Steven's sensitivity to intrusion. For several years, references to Buddhism were sparse and uniformedly positive. He continued to report that on-going meditation practice increased self-knowledge, insight, and acceptance.

My own stance, which was never stated explicitly, but was probably implicit, was to approach his involvement in Buddhism with neither unbridled reverence nor defensive renunciation. I attempted to avoid the twin dangers of *a priori* pathologizing which would reject Buddhism automatically, or uncritical acceptance, which would accept it without critical examination. Clinically we treated Buddhism like a dream—examining his associations to it—rather than assigning it a standardized meaning.

Buddhism's skill in addressing pathology was illustrated by the ways meditation increased his self-awareness, reduced self-criticism, and facilitated greater freedom. Since meditation cultivates increased attentiveness, exactly the state of mind that is essential for psychoanalytic listening, it can enrich psychoanalytic listening. Steven demonstrated a tremendous ability to access and describe nuances of his thoughts, feelings, and fantasies. Meditation practice seemed to cultivate this unusual degree of self-awareness. Since successful analysis also does this, it seems impossible to ascertain the relative influence of each discipline in promoting it. As I stated earlier, at the beginning of analysis Steven evidenced a great deal of self-awareness and an unusual ability to access his inner world. One factor that suggested to me that meditation practice seemed to greatly promote this was that several times he returned from meditation retreats the day of our session and seemed unusually attentive in our sessions to nuances of his thoughts, feelings, and fantasies. This awareness seemed more related to meditation than psychoanalysis.

This increased awareness facilitated greater access to formerly unconscious material. To cite one example among many: on several occasions while meditating, Steven became aware of the formerly unconscious hurt and rage he felt about the way his parents made him feel responsible for family difficulties and the extent to which they encouraged him to fulfill their own needs and goals.

His stance toward himself and negative, affect-laden feelings also changed. Nonjudgmental attentiveness—the ability to experience thoughts and feelings impartially—replaced his perfectionistic father's criticalness. His tendency to use imperfections as ammunition for self-prosecution subsided. This was illustrated by his growing capacity to examine imperfections during and outside sessions without lapsing into self-attacks. As he gradually experienced decreased self-criticalness, he came to feel more compassion.

In his studies of mystical practices and psychotherapy, Arthur Deikman (1982) emphasizes the centrality of "de-automatization"—an undoing of automatized, habitual thought and action. In cultivating perceptual acuity and attentiveness, meditation fostered awareness of, and de-automatization from, previously habitual patterns. This led Steven to feel an increased freedom of action while also lessening the potential for the emergence of unconscious negative affects associated with danger to himself and his family. Being de-automatized minimized the chances of his being out of control like his punitive father. Thus there was less chance of him acting like an "animal" or anyone getting "whipped."

Psychoanalytic understanding of pathology helped me recognize some of the unconscious limitations of Steven's involvement in Buddhism. It gradually became evident that Buddhism's emphasis on cultivating "cool" rather than "hot" emotions—equanimity rather than *passion* (Kramer & Alstad, 1989)—actually inhibited Steven in certain ways, reinforcing his defensive passivity. In attempting to develop such qualities as equanimity and compassion, Steven focused on detaching from negative affects rather than experiencing them. This blocked the emergence of normal outrage against his parents for neglecting his needs and allowing his disturbed brother to dominate family life. The possibility of Steven being appropriately assertive or angry was thus unfortunately stifled.

Psychoanalytic views of pathology also helped me understand the attraction of Buddhist views of health. Inquiry into the origins and functions of his ambitions revealed that he was haunted by his failure to receive his critical father's approval, save his damaged brother, and redeem his mother. He had a deep fear that to abandon these strivings as compulsive necessities would be to lose forever any possibility of his being important and exciting to his parents (or anyone else).

Because of his father's remoteness and vol-atility, he never provided Steven with an image of "idealized strength and calmness" (Kohut, 1984, p. 52) which Steven could utilize as a model for cultivating his own goals, ideals, and values. Consequently, this aspect of himself was underdeveloped. He became what Kohut (1971) termed an "ideal hungry personality" seeking to identify with exemplary figures and exalted theories in the external world. In offering an image of, and a vehicle for, self-perfection, Buddhism afforded him a substitute set of missing ideals and values thus strengthening a dimension of himself that he needed to fortify to feel good about himself.

Psychoanalytic investigation revealed that these ideals were restitutive and restrictive. Buddhist emphasis on self-purification and transformation had a dual unconscious function: it provided a means of attempting to win his perfectionistic father's approval and atone for his unconscious guilt over his imagined crime of not saving, and sometimes wishing to destroy, his damaged brother. Perhaps if he was perfect then his father would accept him. Buddhism offered an opportunity to offset his sense of badness and repair the damage he felt he had committed. Buddhism thus became what Melanie Klein (Klein & Riviere, 1964), in another context, termed a vehicle for "reparation."

Psychoanalytic views of pathology aided me in recognizing that Buddhist ideals also became an agent of self-condemnation and self-inhibition. The quest for purity of action—like his father's demand for perfection—became one more ideal that he could never attain and thus one more occasion for self-condemnation. He periodically spoke of the guilt he felt when he was not meditating on a regular basis or not completely living up to Buddhism's ethical ideals.

Psychoanalytic perspectives on subjectivity elucidated another aspect of his interest in Buddhism. Asceticism—having little—also protected him from reliving the trauma of being robbed by his brother and unprotected and undefended by his parents. If he had scant possessions—only some "spare change"—then less could be taken from him than if he was wealthy and had a "large coin collection."

Psychoanalytic perspectives on subjectivity helped me realize the way Buddhism unconsciously contributed to "Stevelessness." Analytic investigation revealed that Steven's attraction to the no-self doctrine of Buddhism had at least three possible meanings. (1) The problem of self-assertion—being orphaned—was avoided by embracing this doctrine. If there was no-*self* then there was no self-*assertion*. If there was no self-assertion then there was no threat of being abandoned and orphaned. (2) The doctrine of no-self had an important emotional resonance for Steven because it captured his experience of "Steveless-ness." It embodied the subjective sense of self-lessness he felt about his eviscerated life. (3) The doctrine of no-self also relieved the emotional pain of not being who he could have become: being "Stevefull." If we follow Christopher Bollas (1989) in *Forces of Destiny*, all humans share a desire to discover and actualize their "destiny"—their unique, personal idiom. Embracing the no-self doctrine of Buddhism anaesthetized Steven's excruciatingly painful sense of having missed out on his potential. But in his associations, Steven described our work as "a crane pulling the buried coffin out of the earth."

A bifocal view of subjectivity helped me be more attentive to a different aspect of it—the way the dereified Buddhist view was also *liberating* for Steven. Meditation offered Steven an alternative way of experiencing subjectivity—the view of the self as "a fluid process" (Tart, 1990, p. 161).

Buddhism's sensitivity to the dangers of self-reification helped me recognize and avoid the subtle self-commodification that occurred in his family, his relationship to himself, and periodically in his previous analysis and our analysis. In these four situations he was made into a thing; a means rather than an end; an *it* rather than a *Thou*. Self-commodification happened in his family when he was narcissistically viewed as an extension of them. His parents were more concerned with making him into the sort of person they needed him to be for them to feel better about themselves than to facilitate his own differentiated development.

In our analysis, a pattern emerged that had apparently shadowed his previous analysis in which he would almost instantaneously bury negative feelings—for example, the feeling that I had not fully appreciated a particular accomplishment—and shift the analytic focus onto understanding what he had done wrong. His self-bashing was sometimes quite subtle and not easy

to detect both because it was so automatic and because the concomitant shift in focus had some plausibility; in other words, he would direct us toward areas that seemed to be troublesome for him. For example, after one session in which he had discussed what he had learned from both Buddhism and psychoanalysis he suggested that we examine the way in which he sometimes undermines himself and hides his intellectual potential. He suggested that his convoluted and complex presentation of his ideas during the previous session could provide a clue to what he needs help with in this area. He suggested that his presentation was symptomatic of a difficulty he sometimes has in his intellectual work. My experience of the previous session was that he had made some subtle and important points about both psychoanalysis and Buddhism but that some of his ideas were still inchoate. I also felt that I had not offered him much assistance in further clarifying the material. After I commented in the current session about one of his ideas that I believed was quite interesting he realized that the last session had been disappointing for him. Further exploration revealed that he was disappointed that I had not been more effusive about his ideas. He realized that when he suggested at the beginning of the current session that we examine the negative way he thinks that he was both obscuring his disappointment in me for not being more enthusiastic about his intellectual work and making himself into a "commodity" to be worked on and improved. He indicated that he felt that this kind of process pervaded his previous analysis and occurred periodically in our work. The Buddhist dereified view of subjectivity—particularly recognition of the fluidity of consciousness and the importance of the transient, episodic mental states arising moment-after-moment—helped both of us be sensitive to the way self-commodification occurred in our work and in his life outside analysis which led to a more unconstricted view of himself, as evidenced by increased participation in non-instrumental activities. For example, he became more involved in athletic and nature-related activities.

In terms of an integrated view of the psychoanalytic and Buddhist path, the combination of meditation's capacity to quiet and focus the mind and facilitate lapidary receptivity to unconscious material and psychoanalysis' capacity to investigate and interpret pathology and utilize the psychoanalytic relationship as a crucible for the past to reemerge and be resolved, provided Steven and I with a more comprehensive way of approaching his life than either pursued alone.

REFERENCES

Alexander, F. (1931). Buddhistic training as an artificial catatonia: The biological meaning of psychological occurrences. *Psychoanalytic Review*, *18*, 129–145.

Bollas, C. (1989). *Forces of destiny: Psychoanalysis and human idiom*. London: Free Association Books.

Boorstein, S. (Ed.). (1980). *Transpersonal psychotherapy*. Palo Alto: Science and Behavior Books.

Boucher, S. (1988). *Turning the wheel: American women creating the new Buddhism*. San Francisco: Harper & Row.

Braudel, F. (1980). *On history* (S. Matthews, Trans.). Chicago: University of Chicago Press.

Deikman, A. (1982). *The observing self: Mysticism and psychotherapy*. Boston: Beacon Press.

Engler, J. (1983). Vicissitudes of the self according to psychoanalysis and Buddhism: A spectrum model of object relations development. *Psychoanalysis and Contemporary Thought*, *6*, 29–72.

Fairbairn, R. (1952). *Psychoanalytic studies of the personality*. London: Routledge & Kegan Paul.

Fischer, M. (1986). Ethnicity and the post-modern arts of memory. In J. Clifford & G. E. Marcus (Eds.), *Writing culture, the poetics and politics of ethnography* (pp. 194–233). Berkeley: University of California Press.

Foucault, M. (1977). Nietzsche, genealogy, history. In D. F. Bouchard (Ed.), *Language, counter-memory, practice* (pp. 139–164). Ithaca: Cornell University Press.

Fromm, E., Suzuki, D. T., & DeMartino, R. (1960). *Zen Buddhism and psychoanalysis*. New York: Harper & Row.

Gold, J. (1992). An Integrative-Systemic Treatment Approach to Severe Psychopathology of Children and Adolescents. *Journal of Integrative and Eclectic Psychotherapy*, *11*, 55–70.

Goldstein, J. (1976). *The experience of insight: A natural unfolding*. Santa Cruz: Unity Press.

Goleman, D. (1977). *The varieties of the meditative experience*. New York: E. P. Dutton.

Gordon, J. S. (1987). *The golden guru: The strange journey of Bhagwan Shree Rajneesh*. Lexington: The Stephen Greene Press.

Horney, K. (1945). *Our inner conflicts*. New York: Norton.

Horney, K. (1987). *Final lectures*. New York: Norton.

Jung, C. (1958). *Psychology and religion: West and East*. Princeton: Princeton University Press.

Kelman, H. (1960). Psychoanalytic thought and eastern wisdom. In J. Ehrenwald (Ed.), *The history of psychotherapy* (pp. 328–333). New York: Jason Aronson.

Klein, M., & Riviere, J. (1964). *Love, hate and reparation*. New York: Norton.

Kohut, H. (1971). *The analysis of the self*. New York: International Universities Press.

Kohut, H. (1977). *The restoration of the self*. New York: International Universities Press.

Kohut, H. (1984). *How does analysis cure?* Chicago: University of Chicago Press.

Kornfield, J. (1977). *Living Buddhist masters*. Santa Cruz: Unity Press.

Kornfield, J., Dass, R., & Miyuki, M. (1979). Psychological adjustment is not liberation: A symposium. In *Zero: Contemporary Buddhist Life and Thought* (pp. 72–87). Los Angeles: Zero Press.

Kramer, J., & Alstad, D. (1989). *The guru papers*. Unpublished manuscript.

Matthiessen, P. (1985). *Nine-headed dragon: Zen journals 1969–1982*. Boston: Shambhala.

Mitchell, S. A. (1991). Contemporary perspectives on self: Toward an Integration. *Psychoanalytic Dialogues: A Journal of Relational Perspectives*, *1*(2), 121–172.

Masson, J. M., & Masson, T. C. (1978). Buried memories on the Acropolis: Freud's response to mysticism and anti-semitism. *International Journal of Psychoanalysis*, *59*, 199–208.

Modell, A. H. (1985). The two contexts of the self. *Contemporary Psychoanalysis*, *21*(1), 70–90.

Nozick, R. (1989). *The examined life: Philosophical meditations*. New York: Simon & Schuster.

Ogden, T. H. (1991). An interview with Thomas Ogden. *Psychoanalytic Dialogues: A Journal of Relational Perspectives*, *1*(3), 361–376.

Peoples, K. (1991). *The paradox of surrender: Constructing and transcending the self*. Unpublished manuscript.

Roland, A. (1988). *In search of self in India and Japan: Toward a cross-cultural psychology*. Princeton: Princeton University Press.

Rubin, J. B. (1985). Meditation and psychoanalytic listening. *Psychoanalytic Review*, *2*(4), 599–612.

Rubin, J. B. (1989). Psychoanalytic treatment with a Buddhist meditator. In M. Finn & J. Gartner (Eds.), *Object relations and Religion: Clinical Applications* (pp. 87–107). New York: Praeger.

Rubin, J. B. (1991). The clinical integration of Buddhist meditation and psychoanalysis. *Journal of Integrative and Eclectic Psychotherapy*, *10*(2): 173–181.

Rubin, J. B., & Suler, J. (Eds.). (1991). *Self Psychology and Religion*. Unpublished manuscript.

Said, E. (1978). *Orientalism*. New York: Vintage Books.

Schafer, R. (1976). *A new language for psychoanalysis*. New Haven: Yale University Press.

Schafer, R. (1983). *The analytic attitude*. New York: Basic Books.

Stolorow, R. D., & Atwood, G. E. (1979). *Faces in a cloud: Subjectivity in personality theory*. New York: Jason Aronson.

Suler, J. (1991). Self psychology and Zen. In J. Rubin & J. Suler (Eds.), *Self psychology and religion*. Unpublished manuscript.

Sullivan, H. S. (1950). The illusion of personal individuality. In *The fusion of psychiatry and social science*. New York: Norton.

Tart, C. (Ed.). (1975). *Transpersonal psychologies*. New York: Harper & Row.

Tart, C. (1990). Adapting Eastern spiritual teachings to Western culture: A discussion with Shinzen Young. *Journal of Transpersonal Psychology*, *22*(2), 149–165.

Tart, C., & Deikman, A. (1991). Mindfulness, spiritual

seeking and psychotherapy. *Journal of Transpersonal Psychology, 23*(1), 29–52.

Thera, S. (1962). *The Way of mindfulness: The Satipatthana Sutra and commentary.* Kandy, Sri Lanka: Buddhist Publication Society.

Walsh, R. N., & Vaughan, F. (Ed.). (1980). *Beyond ego: Transpersonal dimensions in psychology.* Los Angeles: J. P. Tarcher.

Walzer, M. (1988). *The company of critics: Social criticism and political commitment in the twentieth century.* New York: Basic Books.

Welwood, J. (Ed.). (1979). *The meeting of the ways.* New York: Schocken Books.

Wilber, K. (1984). The developmental spectrum and psychopathology. Part I. Stages and types of pathology. *Journal of Transpersonal Psychology, 16*(1), 75–118.

Wilber K. (1986). The spectrum of development. In K. Wilber, J. Engler, & D. P. Brown (Eds.), *Transformations of consciousness: Conventional and contemplative perspectives on development* (pp. 65–105). Boston: Shambhala.

Wollheim, R. (1984). *The thread of life.* Cambridge: Harvard University Press.

CHAPTER 18

Psychotherapy and Religious Experience

INTEGRATING PSYCHOANALYTIC PSYCHOTHERAPY WITH CHRISTIAN RELIGIOUS EXPERIENCE

Bede J. Healey

INTRODUCTION

In some respects, consideration of the integration of psychotherapy and religious experience has come full circle. In the earliest societies, the responsibility for all types of healing resided with the religious leaders of the community (Pattison, 1990). There was a gradual separation of religious and psychological issues, and, for a while there was considerable antipathy between the two groups. It is only in the past few decades that there has been a rapprochement, with an increasing interest in the ways in which religious experience and psychotherapy interact. The antipathy was perhaps nowhere more apparent than in psychoanalytic circles; interestingly enough, it is in this area that some of the most exciting work is being done to integrate these areas.

Pruyser (1968) quotes Even Ferm's comment regarding the definition of religion: "The term

religion belongs to that large class of popular words which seems acceptable as common coin of communicative exchange but which on closer examination fails to carry the imprint of exact meaning" (p. 329). Indeed, many authors write about it without defining it. Among the many definitions, a few have special relevance for this discussion. Rizzuto (1979), in her book on the psychoanalytic study of religious experience, uses Spiro's definition of religion as "an institution consisting of culturally patterned interactions with culturally postulated superhuman beings" (p. 3). Haule (1990) states that "religion is any complex of interlocking beliefs, explanations, symbols, and behaviors to which an individual, community, or society appeals, for the most part unconsciously, in order to understand itself ultimately" (p. 1056). Pruyser (1968) thinks of religion as "perspectival," having "a perspective on things, a certain way of looking at the world and all reality, including ourselves" (p. 329). Homans sees religion as a cultural symbol, a component of common culture (Homans, 1989). In addition to these definitions, religion is often considered by believers to be the vehicle for development of a faith-based spiritual life, including a relation with God or the Tran-

Bede J. Healey • The Menninger Clinic, Topeka, Kansas 66601-0829.

Comprehensive Handbook of Psychotherapy Integration, edited by George Stricker and Jerold R. Gold. Plenum Press, New York, 1993.

scendent. From all of these definitions three key elements surface: religion (1) as a cultural component, (2) as a vehicle for the development of spiritual experiences, and (3) as a particular perspective from which to understand reality. Any effort to integrate psychology and religious experience will need to keep these elements in mind.

There is a long and relatively unexplored history of the living out of psychological reality in the Christian tradition. Long before the dualism that separated religious from psychological experiences entered the scene, early Christians grappled with the totality of the human experience, and did not parcel out certain aspects of an individual's life for exploration by specialists. Here, religion as culture and as experience were completely intermingled. The writings and sayings of the Desert Fathers and Mothers (Ward, 1975) give testimony to their efforts to work with the combined religious/psychological issues. Men and women of the fourth and fifth centuries, dedicated to a more complete and intense religious experience, would go out into the wilderness to devote themselves totally to seeking God. They would not do this alone, but under the direction of a spiritual master. Ward (1975) states that this relationship was a vital, life-giving one, not solely a theological teaching relationship nor a counseling experience, but a full, complete relationship that addressed all aspects of life. For example, one of the most frequent admonitions given by a master to a disciple was to reveal not only one's actions, but all of one's most inmost thoughts. Thus, everything was open to examination.

Religion and psychotherapy are distinct fields now. However, as knowledge of psychotherapy increased, knowledge about religious experience by therapists did not keep pace. Even today there still exists a lack of understanding about religious experience. There are those who hold that certain kinds of involvement in religious experience, such as heavy involvement in mysticism or a belief in a personal god, should preclude an individual from becoming a psychoanalyst (Burke, 1991). This line of thinking may reflect only a superficial understanding of religious experience. Burke goes on to indicate that religious solace and comfort come at the cost of giving up rationality, which is the basis for psychoanalysis. Even if this were true, it reflects a limited understanding of the extensive cultural and spiritual impact of reli-gion that goes far beyond solace and comfort. With these beliefs, it would be difficult indeed to approach the religious experience of patients in an open and objective manner, and to be open to understanding the particular individual meaning religion may have for a given patient.

Religious experience is a complex phenomenon, and is too often oversimplified. Bergin (1983) argues for a nuanced approach to understanding the complexity of religious experience. Examples of recent research that appreciate the complexity of religious experience and take a nuanced approach include the work of MacPhillamy (1986), who studied the personality effects of long-term Zen monasticism, and Dudley and Hillery (1979), who explored the complex nature of freedom as lived out in a cloistered Christian monastic community of men.

In an earlier article, Bergin (1980) argues forcefully for the integration of psychotherapy and values, including specifically religious values, stating there is a growing dissatisfaction with a purely secular approach to therapy. Sevensky (1984) provides an exceptionally clear presentation of critical issues salient to any discussion of integration of psychotherapy and religious experience. Regarding the disparity in belief systems that exists between the mental health professionals in general and the general public, he makes the following points:

> many people hold beliefs which most doctors and scientists deem false; they claim as possible actual experiences which most doctors and scientists . . . regard as impossible; they organize and make sense of their lives around meanings and goals which a majority of the scientific-medical establishment considers mistaken. (Sevensky, 1984, p. 75)

He then points out the real likelihood for misinterpretation or error if these differences are not considered. Recently, Shafranske and Malony (1990) reported on the religiosity of a group of clinical psychologists. A majority of these psychologists address religious issues in their personal and professional lives. Thus, in practice, there is a movement toward integrating these areas, but the authors point out that there has been very little training in addressing religious issues in the therapeutic process. Other writers echo this point (Sansone, Khatain, & Rodenhauser, 1990). This chapter will speak to some of the ways religious experience and psychotherapy can be integrated.

THEORETICAL AND
CONCEPTUAL POSITION

In thinking about points of common ground between psychotherapy and religious experience, the relational character of both stands out. Object relations theory emphasizes both the relational role as well as the internal processes that affect interpersonal relations.

Broadly speaking, psychoanalytic object relations theory places emphasis on the relational nature of human existence and development. Unlike other strands of psychoanalytic thinking, psychoanalytic object relations theory regards relationships as central, the ground from which all development proceeds. A complete description of this field is beyond the scope of this chapter, but Greenberg and Mitchell's book (1983) provides a comprehensive discussion of this, as well as other varieties of psychoanalytic theory.

The role of the earliest relationships, how they worked well, and how they went awry, are critical to understanding an individual, and crucial in any therapeutic endeavor. This is not only a theoretical position, but is supported by empirical research in developmental psychology (Mahler, Pine, & Bergman, 1975; Stern, 1985). The human infant is object seeking from birth, and development takes place in the context of interactions with significant others. This, in turn, contributes to the build-up of the individual's internal object world, those unconscious internal schemata through which we build up and filter our experiences of ourselves and others. When informed by this theory, the therapeutic relationship provides the ground for the reworking of past problems. Although this is hardly new, inasmuch as work on the transferential relationship forms the basis for much psychoanalytic work, the primacy of relatedness and the role of the internal object world separates psychoanalytic object relations theory from classical and ego psychology.

Object relations theory, although concerned with the inner world of internal objects, is also of necessity concerned, as is religious experience, with the interpersonal milieu in which an individual exists. Although Christian religious experience can be intensely personal, it is grounded in the communal dimension, and has been from its earliest descriptions. This is perhaps best exemplified in the writings about the earliest Christians in the Acts of the Apostles of the New Testament of the Bible. It is clear from these writings that the church is more properly understood not as the building in which worshippers gather, but as a gathering of people, come together for a shared religious experience. More recently, the communal dimension has been neglected, or, at best, improperly understood. Perhaps one of the greatest fallacies in the Christian spiritual tradition is that religious experience is primarily a personal, individual experience, somehow almost unknowable by others, and ultimately unshareable. Although there certainly is that element, religious experience in general proceeds out of a communal experience. Even hermits, those who choose to live apart in their search for God, have their spiritual grounding in a faith community before moving to a life in solitude (Fry, 1981). The communal nature is deeply embedded, is part of the deep structure of the Christian experience, and is unconsciously present in all aspects of religious experience.

Homans' (1989) recent book provides a fresh understanding on the origins of psychoanalysis. He makes the point that psychoanalysis is deeply social in nature and arose out of the loss of important cultural symbols and values of the past. According to Homans,

the origins of psychoanalysis lie deep in the cultural traditions of the West and in its relationship to the religious symbols and values which inform these traditions. There are, in other words, complex "internal relations" between psychoanalysis and the Western cultural and religious traditions. (p. 3)

In general terms, he discusses the process whereby the role of religion and religious ideas has declined in power over the centuries, and that there has been a gradual mourning of this loss, particularly the loss of important symbols and the wholeness that religion provided. He goes on to point out that through the process of individuation, which he defines as "the ways the self can remain integrated and psychological while also appropriating meanings from the past in the form of cultural symbols which infuse it" (p. 9), an individual can become involved in the creation of meaning, in which "the self both appropriates from the past what has been lost and at the same time actually creates for itself in a fresh way" (p. 9) new meanings. This involves both common culture and the analytic process.

This cursory presentation of Homans' ideas does not do justice to the rich development of these ideas, nor is it in any way a complete synopsis of his ideas. But it provides another useful way to think about the integration of religious ideas with the psychotherapeutic process. Homans makes the point that the early analysts were all alienated from their own religious traditions, and too quickly "deidealized" religion and other cultural values. This may still be somewhat true as regards current therapists (Sevensky, 1984; Shafranske & Malony, 1990). However, the denial of the importance of religion in the personal life of the therapist does not negate the role it plays in the patient's life specifically, nor in the culture at large. As Homans points out, it is through an analytic process in the context of a common culture that meaning is created. Surely, the finding and creating of meaning is an integral component of a therapeutic process, and understanding the cultural impact of religion, as well as the spiritual element, can be complementary to the therapeutic process. Even though, as Homans argues, the impact of religion on culture has diminished, it is not gone, and for some individuals religion can still be a central element in their lives, either as a cultural influence or as an important spiritual dimension.

These elements then, form the framework for this particular approach. Object relations theory expands the psychological dimension to include an emphasis on the exploration of real and fantasied relationships, and relationships are at the root of Christian religious experience. In addition, the role of religion as a key component in culture is emphasized.

Others have wondered about whether psychotherapy is the new religion of our day. Without being disrespectful to either field, it seems that psychoanalytic psychotherapy could be considered a religious system in its own right. As Homans (1989) points out, psychoanalysis developed in the void caused by the diminishment of the cultural impact of religion, and it is certainly perspectival, just as Pruyser (1968) points out religion is perspectival. Although there is no belief in a transcendent being, there are fundamental shared beliefs held by those who practice this form of therapy. All of this is to point out that religion and psychotherapy are, in some ways at

least, more alike than different, and that integration need not be antithetical to either field.

CLINICAL AND THEORETICAL ANTECEDENTS

There are many and varied approaches to integrating psychotherapy and religious experience. It is possible to think of a continuum, with one end where religious experience is totally understood and explained by standard psychoanalytic principles; most simply stated, religion could be seen as a neurotic defense, similar to Freud's early writings on the subject. Another point along the continuum would recognize the relative autonomy of both psychological and religious experience. Here some might look at religious experience from a psychological perspective, not denying its own existence, but not denying the psychological component as well. Alternately, one could view these fields as separate and perhaps at odds with each other. And finally, the other end point would be to see all experience as primarily religious, with psychological principles used in an overall Christian theological framework. Strong's (1980) Christian counseling would be an example of this.

The approach discussed here lies more in the middle area. That is, religious experience is acknowledged as real and important in its own right, but can be understood and utilized as it emerges in the psychotherapy process.

John McDargh has written extensively (1984, 1985, 1986) on issues of integration of psychology and religion. His writings reflect a subtle, general shift in the literature toward the increasing autonomy of religion, and more assurance of its value in its own right. Rather than psychology explaining away religion, scholars of religious experience are using psychology to help explain, in part, the complex field of religious experience. Religion is no longer the universal obsessional neurosis (Freud, 1907), and no longer needs to be looked at reductionistically as a regressive experience. Object relations theory in particular can provide a nonreductive psychological lens through which to view religious experience. From this viewpoint, "the human person is born with a primary and irreducible need for the confirmation and affirmation of relationship" (McDargh, 1986, p. 255). An individual's relationship with God and with a religious community can be examined in this light and this information can be used in the overall understanding of the whole person.

There are various ways in which clinicians have integrated religious issues in the psychotherapy process. Sevensky (1984) explores the ways in which religion can be distorted in the psychiatric situation. His approach is broadly psychodynamic. He mentions two important facts: religious concerns are no more or less an issue for psychiatric patients, and that religion can be distorted. Religious experience should not be considered in a vacuum. Sevensky then lists a number of religious distortions and points out the psychological components associated with them. Work on these issues not only frees the individual psychologically, it also allows for fuller and freer religious experiences. He identifies eight syndromes or ways in which religion can be distorted and suggests treatment interventions designed to respectfully address the distortion. These include such problems as demands for a therapist of the same faith, what he calls the "Witch of Endor syndrome" (p. 79) (which refers to the belief that therapy is magical and contrary to religious belief), mistaken identity, demonic possession, the inability to feel forgiven, the feeling of being abandoned by God, and the "weak faith" (p. 78) syndrome. Sevensky points out that in this last syndrome it can be helpful to separate spiritual beliefs from psychological disturbance. He indicates that at times this work may challenge certain faith positions. Throughout his presentation, Sevensky frequently suggests that it may be necessary to consult with or simultaneously refer to a pastoral counselor to work through some of these problems, or to learn more about a patient's particular denomination. Although not specifically stated, there is a continual reference to the role and function of the religious community in understanding and working through the distortions.

Fitzgibbons (1987) takes a slightly different approach. He focuses on the development of religious maturity and then discusses pathology in religious development resulting from arrest or fixation in that development. Fitzgibbons integrates the ideas of Meissner (1984) and Fowler (1981), and utilizes a primarily ego psychological approach. His discussion of one case highlights the importance of the communal dimension in working with religious experience in the psychotherapeutic setting. Although the patient had used religious practices to ward off and avoid conflict at first, he later was able to use the religious community of which he was a part to both broaden his religious experience and to also work through his interpersonal difficulties. Here, effective exploration of the religious experience of this patient helped him grow both spiritually and psychologically. Fitzgibbons comments that a knowledge of the normal pathway to religious maturity can lead to wiser psychotherapy.

Rosenberger (1990) approaches the integration process from a self-psychology perspective. She details her work with a Roman Catholic priest who left his religious order. In discussing her approach, she points out that a powerful self-object bond exists in any highly valued relationship, including one's relationship with God, and that disturbances in this relationship can have an impact on other relationships. She believes that "self-psychology can offer the religious patient a means of being understood in terms in which he already knows himself" (p. 122). She also points out the challenge to the therapist:

Seeing potential cohesion between aspects of the secular self and aspects of religious and spiritual self-experience may require the analyst to reach for an understanding that surpasses his or her familiar explanations. Empathic attunement as a clinical guide demands an abandonment of a priori postulations about religious experience and practice, and instead defines a developmental process to be shared by patient and analyst alike. (p. 122)

Roland's (1988) seminal work on applying psychoanalytic principles to other cultures includes one contribution helpful to this discussion: that of the difference between the "I-ness" of Western cultures and the "we-self regard" of the cultures of India and Japan. There is also a fundamental familial or communal self that is a part of every Christian's experience, and this is more or less developed. Although it is common to speak of Eastern and Western traditions in religious experience, this is often erroneously used to separate Christianity from Buddhism, Taoism, and other non-Christian religions. Christianity has its roots in the east as well, and although

Christianity has become Westernized, the early Eastern roots still undergird Christianity.

The "I-ness" Roland discusses is related to the considerable autonomy granted to individuals in Western society. The "we-self regard," whereby an individual's self-esteem comes from a strong identification with other groups, is related to the "familial self" of Eastern cultures, which is the "basic inner psychological organization that enables women and men to function well within the hierarchical intimacy relationships of the extended family community or other groups" (p. 7). This distinction between the individual self and the familial self provides an interesting way of understanding Christian religious experience, one that closely mirrors object relations views. Knowing the historical roots of the communal dimension of Christian religious experience can keep one alert to a heretofore relatively neglected aspect of Christian experience, and allow therapists to consider this dimension in their work, as well as the more personal relationship between the individual and God.

Roland's views, described above, provide an additional way to understand religious experience in the psychotherapeutic situation, but his ideas are not completely new. The notion of a communal self existing in Western culture has been defined, although not in so many words, by Smucker (1986) in his research on religious community and individualism in a group of Mennonites. He describes the adaptations this group has made to urban living and the adaptations they made in their definition of community, a central component to their religious experience and identity.

This section touches on only a few of the many ways psychotherapy and religious experience have been integrated. What comes through clearly is the richness and complexity of religion and its use in psychotherapy.

THE TECHNIQUE AND PROCESS

The approach presented here reflects more of an attitude or listening perspective to religious themes in psychotherapy. It is a first step in integrating these areas. As such, there are few specifics about how one must concretely act in order to integrate religious experience with psycho-

therapy. Again, the central theme presented here is that the religious dimension can and should be included in the overall psychotherapeutic process. Religious experience has had a profound impact on the common culture in general, and is also an important spiritual dimension in the lives of many people. However, there are some general guidelines that may be helpful to follow.

Addressing religious issues begins in the assessment process. As Rizzuto (1979) points out, routine inquiry should be made with all patients as to their religious experience and development, just as one would do for other areas of development, including sexuality and family history. Questions such as the role of religion or spirituality in their life now, as well as when they were growing up, how their religious or spiritual sense has changed, the nature of the religious life of the parents, their thoughts and feelings about religion, and so forth, will prove helpful. Questions about the individual's internalized sense of God are also important, as parallels or discontinuities with other primary introjects can provide valuable information regarding salient issues that may need to be addressed in therapy. In keeping with the relational nature of the orientation espoused here, the role of religious experience in the context of relationships bears special study. In addition, it is crucial to pay attention to the communal elements of religious experience and to inquire about this as well. This serves two purposes. First, to gather information about the extent of their communal involvement, and second to set the stage for further work in this arena.

It is not necessary to disclose one's own religious preference or practices, although this may be considered (please refer to *Self Disclosure in the Therapeutic Relationship*, edited by Stricker and Fisher (1990), for a fuller discussion about this). For those patients for whom religious experience is a central part of their lives, questions about it and references to it from time to time may signal to the patient the therapist's willingness to explore and address these issues. Even for those for whom it is not, some exploration as to why this may be, and their reaction to the religious experiences of others may be helpful, given the impact of religion on the common culture.

Religious experience does not assume paramount or exclusive role in the psychotherapeutic process. Rather it is one among many aspects of the patient's experience that is addressed. It would be inappropriate to force patients to explore religious issues if they do not wish to; a fine balance needs to be maintained between active interest and a too directive attitude. Nevertheless, there may be times when an arousal of commitment to spirituality may be a goal of treatment. For example, some people move away from religious experience because they have changed in some areas of their lives, but not in the religious dimension. It would not be out of order to consider this discrepancy in therapy.

It is important not to avoid religious issues in therapy. Wallerstein (1991) points out in his discussion of a failed therapy case that one of the reasons for the failure may have been the therapist's treading too lightly and failing to analyze the patient's religious beliefs. There is a common fear that to analyze religious beliefs will take away a person's religious faith. That may be true if religion is viewed totally as a defensive compensation. However, if Homans' (1989) views about religion, culture, and psychoanalysis are kept in mind, the task can be to create new meanings, and this can be in the religious realm as well.

The reworking of the internal object world, characteristic of an object relations approach, can lead to a reworking of religious experience as well. Recalling Homans' ideas, the analysis of the religious beliefs can lead to the creation of a new meaning as regards religion and spirituality for the patient. This may involve mourning the loss of beliefs and old systems of meaning, but a thorough exploration of religious issues in treatment can lead to new, more personally meaningful religious experiences. The faith of the patient grows and develops in tandem with the growth and development of the self. In a less spiritual sense, the cultural component of religious experience can be reworked, giving the individual a new and creative connection with the cultural past.

As the patient discusses religious issues, the role of the communal dimension needs to be assessed. The communal dimension provides a special arena for growth and understanding. Specifically, the presence, quality, and intensity of I-ness versus we-self regard can be explored. We-self regard is not a slavish adherence to hierarchical authority qua authority, but can be understood in this context as a genuine commitment to a group, based on a desire and need to move beyond one-

self, in order to truly find oneself and one's relation to God through relations with others.

In many ways, the application of this technique depends heavily on the personal preparation of the therapist. In general, an openness to the possibility that by exploring religious issues in therapy, an individual can create new, different, and more personally satisfying meanings in his or her life, seems to be a minimal requirement. It means being open to the creative power in the patient to chart his or her course. Predetermined views need to be held in abeyance. A personal belief in the importance of religious experience does not necessarily make one an expert in exploring religious issues, however, for there is the potential for seeing the patient's experience only through one's own eyes, and denying the patient the opportunity to develop his or her own meanings.

CASE EXAMPLE

The patient, an unmarried male in his 30s, was in weekly psychotherapy. He had been sexually abused by a father figure from early childhood to early adolescence, and had many difficulties in developing and sustaining relationships. Now, as an adult, he lived alone in an apartment, had perennial difficulties at work, was transferred often, and frequently was on the verge of being fired. His more intimate interpersonal relationships were also stormy, as he frequently tested those close to him, placing unreasonable demands on them, and then feeling confirmed in both his and their badness when they could not meet his impossible demands. However, the one area where he experienced relative calm in the midst of his interpersonal turmoil was his involvement with his church and in his prayer life. Religion was an important, organizing force in his life. He was a member of a number of church groups, and would spend a number of evenings, and much of the weekend involved with church activities. Here, and in prayer, he was able at times to experience the acceptance and affirmation he so very much wanted. Many, though not all, of the church members knew of his past history.

He would talk frequently in his therapy hours about the positive experiences he had at church, as well as the conflicts and problems he experienced there. He struggled with his relationship with God, repeatedly stating he had no trouble identifying with God as Lord or Savior, but, not surprisingly, real problems in relating to God as Father. This conflict echoed his traumatic past. The abuser was a father figure to him, and his own father was apparently unaware of the abuse and so did not intervene. Although his involvement with the church community was not completely free from the pervasive interpersonal difficulties he experienced in all other areas of life, it was considerably less.

Therapeutically, the patient's involvement with the church was actively supported and encouraged. From a religious perspective, the patient experienced some fulfillment of the "primary and irreducible need for the confirmation and affirmation of relationship" (McDargh, 1986, p. 255). From a psychotherapeutic perspective, the church provided some measure of reparenting for him. For this patient, who was organized at a lower borderline level and was subject to psychotic lapses, the therapy was more supportive in nature. The therapist accepted the importance of the patient's religious beliefs and practice, and the patient felt free to explore the ramifications of his involvement, to find new ways to utilize religious experience in his life. The patient's sense of familial self was strengthened by his involvement with the church community, and the repeated involvement with the church community provided another and very important arena for the patient to rework his distorted object relations, and build up more benign and loving images, including that of God. It is worth noting that the evolving image of God changed more slowly than did his internal representations of others, but change it did.

In this example, little interpretive work was done to directly point this out to the patient. Rather, an active choice by the therapist to encourage and foster the patient's involvement with the church, and to explore the effects of this in therapy helped this patient grow and develop. This patient was initially more developed in his church relationships, and this then later spread to his other relationships. Changes in his level of functioning in the church setting would then be echoed in the workplace. Work became less chaotic and he developed an increased capacity to maintain sustained interpersonal relationships, with a marked decrease in the testing that so frequently marked his previous attempts at forming relationships. Clearly, the patient was able, through this work, to transform his understanding of himself and others, and create new meanings in his life.

CONCLUDING COMMENTS

There are many ways in which religious issues and psychotherapy mingle. This discussion highlights only a few ideas. As a first start to the effort to integrate these two areas, an openness to the broad, rich, and complex cultural and spiritual elements of religious experience is required. A too shallow understanding of religious experience can hamper both patient and therapist.

The work of Leavy (1988) lends itself to this closing section. An Episcopalian and an analyst, he points out that the analytic task can be considered a task of "unconcealing." Becoming aware of hidden motives and ways of relating allows for the possibility for something new to develop. This creative work parallels an age old religious theme first articulated in the Hebrew scripture and echoed through the centuries in religious writings. This theme is that humanity is created in the image of God, and to know oneself more fully and more clearly, and to see others in the same way, is to acknowledge the presence of God or the transcendent in everyone. Therapy, then, can enrich the creative potential of religious experience, and religious experience can reclaim its place in psychological theory, not as a neurotic compensation, but as one of the many salient components of human growth and development, a rich and complex and life-giving aspect of both humanity and the culture at large.

REFERENCES

Bergin, A. E. (1980). Psychotherapy and religious values. *Journal of Consulting and Clinical Psychology, 48*, 95–105.
Bergin, A. E. (1983). Religion and mental health: A critical reevaluation and meta-analysis. *Professional Psychology: Theory and Practice, 14*, 170–184.
Burke, M. O. (1991). A philosophy of psychoanalytic training. *Psychologist Psychoanalyst, 11*, 28–31.
Dudley, C. J., & Hillery, G. A. (1979). Freedom and monas-

tery life. *Journal for the Scientific Study of Religion, 18*, 18–28.

Fitzgibbons, J. (1987). Developmental approaches to the psychology of religion. *Psychoanalytic Review, 74*, 125–134.

Fowler, J. (1981). *Stages of faith: The psychology of human development and the quest for meaning*. San Francisco: Harper & Row.

Freud, S. (1907). Obsessive actions and religious practices. In J. Strachey (Ed. and Trans.) *The standard edition of the complete psychological works of Sigmund Freud* (Vol. 9). London: Hogarth Press.

Fry, T. (Ed.). (1981). *RB 1980: The rule of St. Benedict*. Collegeville, MN: Liturgical Press.

Greenberg, J., & Mitchell, S. (1983). *Object relations in psychoanalytic theory*. Cambridge: Harvard University Press.

Haule, J. (1990). Religion and psychotherapy. In R. J. Hunter (Ed.), *Dictionary of pastoral care and counseling* (pp. 1056–1058). Nashville: Abington Press.

Homans, P. (1989). *The ability to mourn: Disillusionment and the social origins of psychoanalysis*. Chicago: University of Chicago Press.

Leavy, S. A. (1988). *In the image of God: A psychoanalyst's view*. New Haven: Yale University Press.

MacPhillamy, D. J. (1986). The personality effects of long-term Zen monasticism and religious understanding. *Journal for the Scientific Study of Religion, 25*, 304–319.

Mahler, M., Pine, F., & Bergman, A. (1975). *The psychological birth of the human infant*. New York: Basic Books.

McDargh, J. (1984). The life of the self in Christian spirituality and contemporary psychoanalysis. *Horizons, 11*, 344–360.

McDargh, J. (1985). Theological uses of psychology: Retrospective and prospective. *Horizons, 12*, 247–264.

McDargh, J. (1986). God, mother and me: An object relational perspective on religious material. *Pastoral Psychology, 34*, 251–263.

Meissner, W. W. (1984). *Psychoanalysis and religious experience*. New Haven: Yale University Press.

Pattison, E. M. (1990). Psychiatry and pastoral care. In R. J. Hunter (Ed.), *Dictionary of pastoral care and counseling* (p. 972). Nashville: Abington Press.

Pruyser, P. (1968). *A dynamic psychology of religion*. New York: Harper & Row.

Rizzuto, A.-M. (1979). *The birth of the living God: A psychoanalytic study*. Chicago: University of Chicago Press.

Roland, A. (1988). *In search of self in India and Japan: Toward a cross-cultural psychology*. Princeton: Princeton University Press.

Rosenberger, J. (1990). Religious self and secular self: Clinical transitions. *Journal of Religion and Health, 29*, 113–123.

Sansone, R., Khatain, K., & Rodenhauser, P. (1990). The role of religion in psychiatric study: A national survey. *Academic Psychiatry, 14*, 34–38.

Sevensky, R. (1984). Religion, psychology, and mental health. *American Journal of Psychotherapy, 38*, 73–86.

Shafranske, E. P., & Malony, H. H. (1990). California psychologists' religiosity and psychotherapy. *Journal of Religion and Health, 29*, 219–231.

Smucker, J. (1986). Religious community and individualism: Conceptual adaptations by one group of Mennonites. *Journal for the Scientific Study of Religion, 25*, 273–291.

Stern, D. (1985). *The interpersonal world of the infant*. New York: Basic Books.

Stricker, G., & Fisher, M. (Eds.). (1990). *Self disclosure in the therapeutic relationship*. New York: Plenum Press.

Strong, S. R. (1980). Christian counseling: A synthesis of psychological and Christian concepts. *The Personnel and Guidance Journal, 58*, 589–597.

Wallerstein, R. (1991). Assessment of structural change in psychoanalytic therapy and research. In T. Shapiro, (Ed.), *The concept of structure in psychoanalysis* (pp. 263–282). New York: International Universities Press.

Ward, B. (1975). *The sayings of the desert fathers*. Kalamazoo, MI: Cistercian Publications.

CHAPTER 19

A "Social" Clinical Theory of Therapy
INTEGRATING SOCIAL AND CLINICAL PSYCHOLOGY

Rebecca Curtis

Of the best leaders
The people do not know they exist. . . .
But (of the best) when their task is accomplished, Their work done,
The people all remark, "We have done it ourselves."

Lao Tzu, *The Way of Life*

INTRODUCTION

Why yet another theory of therapy? With at least 250 such theories, we certainly do not need another one. Yet another theory appears to have emerged, needed or not. From a speciality within philosophy, psychology has grown into at least three subdisciplines. One, modeling itself after the natural sciences, includes behaviorism and behavior therapies. A second, social psychology, attempts to understand people and their relationships and uses the tools of social science. The third, situating itself with the humanities, draws upon the wisdom of poets and the arts of charismatic leaders and healers. Psychoanalysis and several other therapies are in this third subdiscipline. A "social" clinical psychology tries to integrate these three psychologies.

THEORETICAL INFLUENCES

The major theoretical influences in social psychology have come from Kurt Lewin and his field theory and from gestalt psychology. When one attempts to integrate these theories with the cognitive-behavioral and psychodynamic theories of clinical psychology, one is integrating the major theories of the art and science of psychology. This task seems as enormous as deriving a "unified field theory" (Brehm & Smith, 1986).

Rebecca Curtis • Derner Institute of Advanced Psychological Studies, Adelphi University, Garden City, New York 11530.

Comprehensive Handbook of Psychotherapy Integration, edited by George Stricker and Jerold R. Gold. Plenum Press, New York, 1993.

Social psychologists are trained to think about the processes occurring simultaneously at several different levels—the intrapsychic, the interpersonal, the group-as-a-whole, and between groups. The heritage of research on attitude change leads one to think about the cognitive, affective, and behavioral components of dispositions, to think about how to lead to change in all three, and the best order in which to proceed. Both situational and dispositional factors, and their interactions, are always considered. The heritage of Lewin is also to study interpersonal processes both objectively through research and subjectively through the experience of one's own thoughts and feelings. Neither alone is sufficient. The group dynamics and human relations training which Lewin spawned led to training in social skills not unlike that of cognitive-behavioral approaches, but with a different philosophical underpinning.

During World War II, Lewin (1943) had been interested in how to change the eating patterns of Americans in order to export larger quantities of desirable, nutritional foods to American soldiers abroad. American housewives would agree to serve horsemeat to their families, but when they returned to their own neighborhoods would refrain from doing so. Lewin, realizing the power of group dynamics, decided to assemble the women of particular neighborhoods together and obtain a public agreement. When the women knew that their neighbors were committed to the same objective, they then served horsemeat to their own families. The power of a commitment to an action made in the presence of a group is recognized in the marriage and religious ceremonies of many communities in many cultures. With knowledge of the enormous power of influence in groups, of the pressure in groups toward conformity, and of expectancy-confirmation effects, no one knowledgeable about social psychology would attempt to aid the person to make serious changes in her or his life by using only a relationship of at most several hours a week with one person from outside the client's community, that is, only the influence of the therapist. Why make things so difficult when we can also utilize the group process?

With strong influences upon social-clinical research coming from field and gestalt theories, and less so from behavioral and psychodynamic orientations, social-clinical theory emphasizes the meanings people make of their existence and their social environments or "fields," to use the Lewinian term. Embedded in a context of twentieth century physics, the mutuality of influence of the person and the situation, and the observer and the observed, is kept in mind. From a social science perspective, the conditions under which a phenomenon is more likely to occur are predicted. The social world is a world in the process of becoming, of possibility and potentiality, of "indeterminacy" (Lewin, 1936), not of certain cause and effect.

The first training groups designed to educate leaders in the Lewinian tradition met in New Britain, Connecticut, in 1946 and in Bethel, Maine, in 1947 (Benne, 1964). Consistent with Lewin's belief in the value of both subjective and objective knowledge, the participants who met to study group process, including Kurt Lewin, Morton Deutsch, Murray Horwitz, Martin Seeman, Kenneth Beenne, Leland Bradford, and Ron Lippitt, were expected to alternate their roles as experiential group members and as researchers/observers. Having conducted research upon the effects of authoritarian and democratic styles of leadership, this group stated explicitly the value of democratic leadership in a situation designed to foster self-awareness. All group members have important contributions to make; each member is the expert about what he or she is feeling in response to any other person's behavior. Consistent with the notion of the interaction of the person and the situation, the "t-group" promoted the value of "learning-how-to-learn." The learner is not a passive receiver of information dispensed by others or by an authority, but an active participant who can gain knowledge in a situation by attempting to make sense of the events transpiring and actively seeking the desired information. The questions are as important as the answers. Knowledge must have a scientific (research) basis.

Group goals emerge as the group attempts to fulfill individual needs. The norms developed in the group will greatly affect the attainment of goals and must be monitored and changed, if necessary. Information about the feelings of others will be the primary source of learning about the consequences of one's style of interaction, and will provide the stimulus for learning about the anxious feelings within oneself that have been warded off by particular behaviors and ways of coping that may be inappropriately generalized to the current situation. A good leader in this type of situation is one who facilitates learning in an atmosphere of trust and one who helps people to attain a realistic assessment of their strengths and weaknesses and a sense of confidence in contributing to the well-being of self and others—a leader who meets the standards of Lao Tzu.

A "social" clinical theory of therapy has not been articulated previously, to my knowledge, in the sense that there is a "cognitive-behavioral" or "multimodal" theory, for example. I shall attempt to articulate some major assumptions and hypotheses of such a theory in the sections which follow.

CONCEPTUAL FRAMEWORK OF A SOCIAL CLINICAL THEORY OF PERSONALITY, BEHAVIOR, AND CHANGE

Major Assumptions

1. Behavior is a function of the person and the situation. Both external realities and people's perceptions of them have profound effects upon people's behavior.

2. People formulate goals, both consciously and unconsciously, which guide their behaviors.

3. Goals are organized hierarchically, with self-preservation (physical or symbolic), arousal regulation, positive affect, and the avoidance of negative affect as primary goals. Emotions are felt as a function of goal attainment or the lack thereof, and of assessments, both conscious and unconscious, of progress toward goal attainment.

4. People formulate theories of themselves, others, and causality. That is, people make meanings derived from individual and cultural experiences of their existence, and these meanings influence their future behaviors. Preservation of the self-theory and world-theory are high-order goals.

5. Conflicts arise, intrapsychically, interpersonally, and between groups, to the extent to which attaining one goal is incompatible with the attainment of another goal.

6. Change occurs by altering the means of attaining a goal, changing the person's goal, the group's goal, the interrelationships among goals,

external realities, or psychic realities, that is, the meaning made of an experience.

7. Change occurs in a system (a person or a group) through a process of assimilation and accommodation. Sometimes the whole system changes to such an extent that one system disintegrates and another system emerges. The integration of warded-off affect can lead to such changes. Changes may be physical or symbolic.

View of Human Nature, of Personality, and of the Self

People are capable of making decisions of creating their "selves" within the context of their past histories and current goals. Given the complexity of the social world, it is almost impossible to determine the relevance of many past "reinforcements" to any current situation, that is the meaning of such reinforcements. Drives, themselves, of course, cannot be measured, but social-clinical psychologists have adeptly created situations to vary the degree of frustration of goal attainment and examine the effects upon behavior. Although people are capable of being aggressive, the twentieth century social science view of aggression is that there are conditions which make people more or less likely to act upon their aggressive impulses. Frustration, neglect, and harm are among such conditions.

Goals can be conscious or unconscious. Social-clinical psychologists have demonstrated the effects of unconscious motivation (McClelland, Koestner, & Weinberger, 1989) upon the achievement of goals. The major goals of an individual self-system are to preserve its theory of itself, its theory of the world, its theory of causation, and self-esteem (Epstein, 1973, 1980). When individuals fail to achieve their goals, they may adjust their strategies and increase their effort to achieve the goals, or they may begin a process of rumination (or obsession) over the goal (Martin & Tesser, 1989), failing to abandon appropriately important goals they are likely unable ever to attain. Curtis (1989, 1991) has argued this occurs to the extent that failure to attain a goal results in pain and anxiety that the self-system senses as unbearable. Pyszczynski and Greenberg (1987) proposed that depression results when people fail to abandon an unattainable goal, not when people experience a loss of a goal, as might be implied from clinical theories alone. When people are unable to attain a goal in reality or have not yet done so, they are more likely to engage in behaviors symbolic of the goal attainment. Wicklund and Gollwitzer (1982) have shown in a variety of studies that people who have not yet attained a goal to which they aspire are more likely to display visible signs of the goal, such as on clothing, refuse to admit shortcomings, and attempt to influence others.

Personality is a term which refers to all of the aspects of the person. The "self" has come to be used most frequently to mean "self-awareness," what Allport (1968) described as its second or more limited meaning. Because of the limitations of space, and the preponderance of recent research and theory on the self, the present chapter will focus upon some major aspects of recent social/clinical theory of the self, and not attempt to present a summary of a social/clinical theory of personality.

The theories of the self in social-cognitive and psychoanalytic psychology have been reviewed recently by Westen (1992) and criticized by Sampson (1981, 1985), Cushman (1991), Curtis (1992), and others as placing too much emphasis on a sense of agency and mastery, in keeping with the values of contemporary Western culture. Curtis (1992a) has also criticized these models for excluding the alogical, nonverbal, spiritual self important to the self-representations of many non-Western people and others who are rejecting of the rational-materialistic self of contemporary Western culture. This non-verbal self will be discussed further in the section below.

The Role of Self-Knowledge (and Insight)

Although much research has been conducted regarding people's beliefs about themselves, particularly the beliefs of normally happy people (Taylor, 1989; Taylor & Brown, 1988), depressed people (Alloy, 1988), and more recently anxious people (Greenberg, Vazquez, & Alloy, 1988), the cognitions about oneself which are not verbally mediated have been understandably slower to receive the attention of social/clinical researchers. The self which is known as the self-concept, or more recently the self-schema, is the self as the object of its own consciousness, the self as has been studied by Western science. The subjective self which focuses its attention upon the activities and stimuli with which it is involved at the moment, akin to James's spiritual self, has come under scrutiny again by psychologists who are aware of the incomplete vision of a verbal self. The nonverbal self is also the subject of study of infant researchers, who have been able to document the expectations of preverbal infants in interpersonal interactions (Beebee, 1986; Stern, 1985). Epstein (1980, 1991) has described this type of cognition as the experiential conceptual system. Neisser (1967) has called it secondary process thinking (using this term somewhat differently from Freud). It has also been called free association (Bollas, 1991), associational or vertical thinking (Noy, 1969, 1973), and alogical thinking (Bucci, 1985; Paivio, 1971, 1986).

As people become more aware of their inner states and feelings, that is, as they ward off less from their experience out of a sense of threat to their self-system, they also become more aware of the feelings of others, about what hurts others, and how their own failings cause suffering in others (Curtis & Zaslow, 1991). Research regarding empathy has shown that empathy is related to greater altruism (Eisenberg & Miller, 1987; Feshbach, 1979, 1982; Iannotti, 1978; Leiman, 1978; Staub, 1971) and less aggression (Feshbach & Feshbach, 1969, 1982; Feshbach, 1984; Miller & Eisenberg, 1988). Pennebaker (1989a,b) has also demonstrated that people who are physiologically responsive to the distress of others at the time that distress is occurring exhibit fewer symptoms of physical illness later. People who let themselves feel and know of their distress are healthier than the people who attempt to block awareness of such distress (Shedler, Mayman, & Manis, 1991).

The goal of social clinical therapy is to increase awareness. The therapist may help a person become aware of a particular behavior, its consequences, affect, or the meaning of events, depending upon the client's goals.

Self-Esteem Maintenance

In addition to self-preservation, and preservation of the self- and world views, the self-system is motivated to obtain pleasure and avoid pain. Pleasure is felt when one values oneself, or has self-esteem. According to the terror-management theory of self-esteem and social behavior (Greenberg, Pyszczynski, & Solomon, 1986; Solomon, Greenberg, & Pyszczynski, 1991a; Solomon, Greenberg, & Pyszczynski, 1991b), "self-esteem consists of the perception that one is a valuable part of a meaningful universe, and that self-esteem serves the essentially defensive purpose of buffering anxiety" (Solomon *et al.*, 1991a, p. 23). Children learn to behave in ways that are rewarded by their parents, reducing among other anxieties the anxiety of being abandoned. The vague fear of annihilation via abandonment is replaced by the existential fear of death as the child becomes aware of the mortality of all living creatures. The cultural worldview provides a basis for minimizing anxiety by imbuing the universe with order, stability, and permanence. The knowledge of the continuity of the culture after one's personal death provides a symbolic sense of immortality, as described by Becker (1962, 1973, 1975). Conformity to parental and cultural dictates provides self-esteem. Self-esteem thus has two components: (1) a meaningful world view and (2) a perception that one is meeting the standards for value within the culturally constructed view of reality.

Considerable research by these theorists demonstrates that positive feedback about one's personality buffers a person against the anxiety reported by experimental participants given only neutral information about their personality when the fear of death and other threats are made salient (Greenberg, Solomon, Pyszczynski, Rosenblatt, Burling, Lyon, & Simon, 1991). Studies have also found that when mortality is made salient, people are especially punitive toward people who violate their own cultural values and especially favorable toward people who validate their world view (Greenberg, Pyszczynski, Solomon, Rosenblatt, Veeder, Kirkland, & Lyon, 1990; Rosenblatt, Greenberg, Solomon, Pyszczynski, Kirkland, & Lyon, 1989).

Terror-management theory, like social/clinical theory in general, suggests that self-worth must be based internally, not upon external standards. It must be validated externally, however, as it is inherently a cultural construction. One's theory of oneself and of the world must be negotiated with reality (Higgins & Snyder, 1991).

Terror-management theory as articulated thus far has focused upon the avoidance of pain and anxiety. It has not included a motivation simply to achieve pleasure, or a motivation to recreate past pleasures, what might be akin to Freud's life force, or sex drive. Recent work by Hazan and Shaver (1990) has demonstrated that people who recall secure attachments with their parents are more likely to feel secure in current relationships and maintain them longer than people who recall less secure attachments. Franz, McClelland, and Weinberger (1991) have found that people who recall warm relationships with their father or mother were more likely to have long, happy marriages, children, and close friends at midlife, greater work accomplishment, and feel better about themselves. If a positive motivation is added to the avoidance of negative affect posited by terror-management theory, then a more complete theory of human motivation is conceptualized.

The maintenance of self-evaluations has been demonstrated to be a consequence of basking in the reflected glory of similar others when they have been successful at tasks not essential to one's own self-evaluation and feeling superior to others on dimensions central to one's own self-evaluations (Tesser, 1988). Similar processes of reflection and mirroring in order to have a positive sense of self-worth have been described by Kohut (1971, 1977). The basking process is probably more likely to occur in cooperative situations and the superiority-seeking is probably more likely in competitive situations (Manion, 1991). Downward social comparisons are particularly desirable in a contemporary Western culture devoid of sources of self-worth other than material possessions distributed inequitably and accomplishments measured against those of others (Solomon *et al.*, 1991a).

The motive to maintain a consistent theory about oneself can sometimes clash with the motive to have positive feelings about oneself. Considerable research has been conducted by Swann and his colleagues regarding such at times conflicting self-verifying and self-enhancing behaviors. People who are certain of particular negative qualities prefer negative feedback about such qualities over positive feedback, regardless of whether their overall self-view is positive or negative (Swann, Pelham, & Krull, 1989).

Discrepancies between various aspects of the self, such as the actual self, the ideal self, the "ought" self, the future self, the can self (cf. Higgins, Tykocinski, & Vookles, 1990), the undesirable self (Ogilvie, 1987) produce different affects and emotions. The ability to cope with the anxiety of unmet goals determines the strength of the self-system [cf. Bandura's (1977) concept of self-efficacy and McClelland's view of anxiety in achievement motivation theory]. The more complex a person's self-view, the better able the person is at coping with failures within any specific area (Linville, 1987).

Views of Other People and Assumptions about the World

Research on social cognition over the past two decades has provided us with considerable knowledge regarding the development and maintenance of person schemata. Recently, the similarities between the representations of self and others as described by social psychologists and as described by psychoanalytically oriented object relations theorists have been noted (Horowitz, 1991; Singer & Salovey, 1991; Westen, 1992). Research regarding the perseverance of erroneous beliefs has demonstrated that beliefs are especially likely to persist in the face of contradictory evidence when people have used their beliefs to explain other events (Slusher & Anderson, 1989) and when people have focused upon their feelings in relation to such beliefs.

An extensive theory regarding the perception of causality and the consequences of such perceptions has been developed by attribution theorists (Heider, 1958; Jones, Kanouse, Kelley, Nisbett, Valins, & Weiner, 1971; Kelley, 1967). People who achieve their goals are more likely to attribute their successes to ability and effort and their failures to a lack of effort, the difficulty of the task, or luck. People who are low achievers are more likely to attribute their successes to luck or the ease of the task and their failures to a lack of ability. The value of redirecting attributions in therapy has been discussed by Brehm (1976). In the therapy process, clients must come to attribute positive gains they are making to internal qualities about themselves, not simply to following the therapist's good suggestions. In Lao Tzu's phrase, their experience will hopefully be "We did it ourselves." In most therapies it is hoped that the client will gain a sense of responsibility, personal freedom, and sense of control over exter-

nal forces. Attributional changes in the other direction—toward external causes—may also be useful. Clients can be helped to understand that their choices were limited in many situations, especially as children, and that the self-defeating patterns they have developed may have been quite functional in the situation in which they began. Thus, self-blaming attributions to internal causes can be changed as the therapist focuses upon the external or situational constraints upon behavior. By learning that most people would have reacted similarly in the original situation ("consensus," in attribution theory terminology), the person can come to feel less pathological. People make many attributions of causality on the basis of heuristics which are not rational, such as availability or salience of particular causes, their vividness, their representativeness, and illusory correlations of two kinds of stimuli appearing infrequently.

Theory of Motivation and Emotion

Although social-cognitive theories of the self (Greenwald & Pratkanis, 1984; Markus, 1977) have invoked the metaphor of a computer and regard the self-system as an information-processor, social-clinical theorists (Curtis, 1989, 1991; Westen, 1985) have considered affect as motivating self-regulation, assuming that people are motivated to achieve pleasure and to avoid pain. People are motivated to maintain an optimum level of arousal. This requires an optimum level of familiar and consistent information and novel or inconsistent information. In some individuals, much familiar information is provided by an overarching confidence in an ability to tolerate pain and anxiety, even when such confidence seems unwarranted, what Fromm (1947) called faith, and Kierkegaard (1955) called a "leap of faith."

Emotions are experienced in relation to progress toward goal attainment. Depression occurs when people fail to make adequate progress toward goal attainment and do not relinquish the goal. Higgins and his colleagues have collected considerable data from both depressed students and clinical samples showing that people with large discrepancies between their actual and ideal self-views become depressed when these discrepancies are made salient. Research regarding the revised theory of learned helplessness has provided considerable evidence that people most at risk for depression after uncontrollable outcomes are those who attribute their loss to enduring, difficult-to-change personality characteristics. Optimism, as measured by scores on scales of explanatory styles and life orientation, makes people less vulnerable to depression after loss (Seligman, 1991), less vulnerable to physical illness (Scheier & Carver, 1985; Seligman, 1991), and more resilient after illness (Strack, Carver, & Blaney, 1987). Although there is an enormous social clinical literature on depression (Alloy, 1988; Brehm & Smith, 1986; Curtis, 1990), research from the social-clinical interface is just beginning on anxiety (Greenberg et al., 1988). Most of this work is limited to a social cognition perspective. Social clinical theorists have conducted large amounts of research on anger (Averill, 1982; Zillman, 1979) and also on positive emotions (Argyle, 1987; Freedman, 1978). Space in the present chapter precludes further discussion of the various particular emotions.

Theory of Change and Therapy

When people fail in their attempts to make greater progress toward their goals, they abandon the goal unless failure to attain the goal is believed to result in intolerable pain and anxiety. Change agents are useful in that they provide (1) a sense of hope for an alternative perspective—either new strategies for achieving unmet goals or the capability of relinquishing unrealistic goals and formulating new ones; (2) a refocusing of attention on neglected aspects of the situation; and (3) the perception that people can cope with the failure to achieve a current goal. Change involving goals central to the self-theory of a system occurs only when the affect associated with the failure to achieve highly valued goals is assimilated into the self-system. New goals, appropriate to current realities, then emerge. Because coping with failure to attain one's goals is so essential to this model of change, the modeling of admission of failure by the therapists when such failure is veridical, as when the therapist is not being of help to the client, is appropriate. The therapist must model an openness to change.

Change requires risking a disconfirmation of one's theories of self, others, and the world when beliefs, behaviors, or affect central to the self-

organizing process are involved (Curtis, 1992b). The risk may require not warding off a feeling or engaging in a new behavior to disconfirm one's self-view or one's believed inability to cope with the consequences of such a behavior. Dissonance theory research has demonstrated the value of making behavioral changes first, in order to then obtain desired changes in beliefs and affect.

Major Similarities with and Differences between the Social/Clinical Model and Other Models

The values of a social clinical theory of therapy are derived primarily from those of gestalt and field theory in their American context. The content of the theory is similar to that derived from a common-factors approach to the extent that each is founded upon research. Status is achieved more from what one knows and what one can do than from ascribed characteristics, such as social position or birth. The differentiation in status of therapist and client beyond that appropriate to the differing roles and abilities to accomplish the goals in the therapy situation is only helpful in facilitating an adjustment to a hierarchical status system in postindustrial society, one of questionable value in fostering a sense of self-worth in most of its people (Solomon et al., 1991a). Change is a process of reorganization, not simply a change in structures. In contrast to the heritage of cognitive-behavioral theory, the meanings people make of their behaviors and their perceptions of themselves and their situations play a central role in the change of any behaviors related to goals in the higher levels of the goal hierarchy, that is, those related to the preservation of the self and world representations. Affect organizes the self-system, thus being an end in itself, and not subsidiary to behaviors and cognitions in the change process. In contrast to many adherents of psychoanalytic theory, those with a social clinical theory value the data of nomothetic research as much as the narratives of the in-depth case study. "Knowing" requires confirmation from the objective data of experience as well as consensual validation.

With the role of meaning central to any understanding of people, the attributions of causality made by clients is central to the process of change. This emphasis upon implicit theories of causality, while not ignored by therapists of other orientations, has not been articulated forcefully.

The person and the situation create one another. As acknowledged by systems theorists, to attempt to change the individual without changing the system is an extremely difficult tact to take.

The social clinical model emphasizes the functional aspects of the social group—the community and the culture—as well as the dysfunctional aspects of generalizing adaptations made to previous groups, such as the family and school, to new groups and cultures in which other behaviors would enable a person better to achieve her or his goals. In other words, a social clinical model emphasizes both normal behaviors and the conditions under which they occur (formerly studied primarily by social and personality psychologists), and abnormal behaviors and the conditions under which they occur (formerly studied primarily by clinicians). The consequences of the norms prevalent in any group must also be taken into consideration. A person may decide to attempt to change these norms, rather than herself or himself.

TECHNIQUE AND PROCESS OF PSYCHOTHERAPY

A social clinical therapy has not evolved to the extent that it can be considered to have "a technique." Those practicing a social/clinical therapy in the past have largely included cognitive behaviorists knowledgeable about social psychology and psychoanalysts trained before the specializations in psychology became so separate. Recently, however, a view of normal behavior and dysfunctional behavior has emerged which is cognizant of social and psychoanalytic theory, as well as other approaches to therapy and personality.

Conceptualization of Psychopathology

Stemming from a perceptual model rather than a medical model, behaviors are considered dysfunctional or self-defeating, rather than pathological. Obviously, people have biological conditions which may predispose them to some types of behaviors more than others. Given a person's biological heritage, self-defeating behaviors are learned just as self-enhancing and others behaviors are learned, principally through reinforcement, punishment, and imitation. Specifically, self-defeating behaviors have been learned through positive reinforcement for self-defeating behaviors, negative reinforcement for self-defeating behaviors (by providing escape to a less anxiety-producing situation), lack of positive reinforcement for self-enhancing behaviors, contingent punishment for failure to engage in self-enhancing behaviors, contingent punishment for self-enhancing behaviors, noncontingent punishment of behaviors, and noncontingent reinforcement for behaviors. To the extent that people have experienced punishment, negative, and/or noncontingent reinforcement—or in the language of other theories, to the extent that they have experienced difficulty coping with anxiety—they will be more likely to fear engaging in the behaviors which were punished and continue to engage in a vicious circle of expectancy-confirming behaviors. This view of pathology has been expressed in more detail elsewhere (Curtis, 1989). Anxiety-provoking situations lead to a greater rigidity in the self-system, a greater recall of self-consistent as compared to inconsistent information (Curtis, Pacell, & Garczynski, 1991) and more information about others, both positive and negative, which is consistent with prior beliefs (Curtis & Hillman, 1992). In brief, people engage in self-defeating behaviors in order to avoid situations which they expect will lead to greater intolerable anxiety. This view of self-defeating behaviors is derived from Adler, as well as from experiential, cognitive-behavioral, and psychoanalytic theories.

Social clinical theory leads to an assessment of a person's strengths and weaknesses, view of self, others, and the world, and views of contingencies. Such views are both self-reported and implicit. Use of formal means of assessment can be used at the therapist's discretion.

Therapeutic Relationship. The therapeutic relationship is one of mutual respect, a process in which the self-systems of both therapist and client are open to change to the extent that they feel safe and open to new experiences. Frustration of the client can lead to an iatragenic aggression. The therapists will at all times be aware that the client may bring expectations from previous relationships into the present relationship and will bring to the client's awareness such data if it is occurring. Although what is going on in the "here and now" will be used extensively, the analysis of such phenomena will only take place to the extent it is relevant to the client's goals in seeking therapy. Because feelings in the "here and now" can be very anxiety-provoking, they will not be discussed when doing so will lead to greater resistance to change.

The therapist must always keep the client's goals in mind, but must state as clearly as possible what will be required to attain these goals, to the extent the therapist can say. This means an explicit cost/benefit analysis in some cases. It is the task of the therapist to help the client attain a goal, or for the therapist to state her or his unwillingness to help work toward that goal and why.

Timing of Interventions. Based upon Lewin's idea that when there are barriers (or defenses) to goal attainment, that is, forces against change, increasing forces for change will only create greater tension, conflict, and rigidity, the therapist attempts to avoid creating more resistance or reactance. Thus, empathic responses, the modern psychoanalytic technique of "joining the resistance" (Spotnitz, 1985) and paradoxical interventions may be required (cf. Shoham-Solomon & Rosenthal, 1987; Shoham-Solomon, Avner, & Neeman, 1989; Tennen & Affleck, 1991). The ways in which a person is keeping material out of awareness will be focused upon when the client feels safe enough to do so.

Interventions which would have the greatest impact upon all of the factors affecting an individual are given the greatest priority. The social support system is considered primary. Therefore impulses to withdraw from situations of social support helpful to the client's goals will be explored fully. The research regarding the value of social support for psychological functioning is reviewed by Brehm and Smith (1986) and for physical health is reported by Berkman and Syme (1979). Friends are known to aid the psychological and physical well-being of all people, not simply those, according to psychoanalytic theory, who have achieved a capacity for object relations commensurate with reaching an Oedipal level of development. Therefore, ways of tolerating feelings

of anxiety and rage without acting upon dysfunctional flight-and-fight impulses while remaining in anxiety-provoking situations will be explored. Although the therapist may wish to have as positive and as influential role as possible, such influence should accrue naturally to the extent the therapist is able to help the client attain his or her goals. Unlike psychoanalytic therapists who may wish to avoid "diluting the transference," the social clinical therapist will want the client to participate in as many groups as possible which will facilitate goal attainment.

Use of Fantasies and Dreams. Fantasies and dreams represent not only wishes and fears, but plans for the future and varying aspects of self. With an emphasis on the experience of consciousness in the here and now and the organizational process of the self-system, the gestalt technique of becoming each aspect of the dream is a useful one.

CASE EXAMPLE

Ms. C. was a 29-year-old woman hospitalized for major depression. She had made three prior suicide attempts and had spent a year and a half in a treatment facility for borderline patients. She had been physically abused by her paternal grandmother who had taken care of her during her preschool years and was subsequently abused by her father. Her mother and father had separated when she was 7 years old. She had lived with her mother, sister, and two brothers since that time. Her mother reported that her daughter had never had any friends, but always did very well in school. The mother had immigrated to this country and worked as a practical nurse. The family had lived in dire poverty and was ridiculed by the neighbors for their quiet, hard-working life-style and for not participating in the normative life-style of contemporary urban ghettos. Ms. C. was very intelligent. As a college student she had been working in a university biology lab and was hoping to attend medical school. She became severely depressed when her local pharmacist, to whom she had become attracted, explicitly rejected her romantic overtures. She was under the care of a pharmacological psychologist when she was hospitalized. Both the psychologist and Ms.

C. agreed that she appeared to be suffering from a "biological depression." The therapist considered the hospitalization necessary for a readjustment in the medications. Our overall goal was a decrease in Ms. C.'s depression.

Ms. C. would not get out of bed when I first went to see her. For several days she did not speak to me. I would simply go to her room and sit by her and tell her I was there to help her in whatever way might be useful. She eventually told me she had a "biological depression" and that I could be of no use to her. Getting her out of bed and attending the required activities on the unit was the first behavioral objective in our treatment plan. I told her she was required to participate in the activities on the unit and that normal daily activities were required to get her body out of its biological depression. She complained that the light bothered her eyes so much she could not leave her room. I told her the nurse would bring her sunglasses. She complained she could not attend group therapy because people would stare at her. Refusing to discuss anything psychological, I suggested she place a bag over her head. She did. After two group sessions with the bag, she came without it. By this time she clearly liked me a lot, probably because she found me quite different from the therapists of a very rigid psychoanalytic orientation on the borderline treatment unit. The first requirement for a relationship was accomplished. We had established an alliance positive enough to begin work.

By this time Ms. C. was ready to talk with me. I explained that I was a psychologist, that we were required to meet three times a week for forty-five minutes, and questioned her about anything in her life with which I might be of assistance. After several sessions of resistance, she told me that I could help her with her social skills, that she was afraid to go into the school cafeteria and speak to people, and that she was afraid to speak to other patients on the ward. I told her that I had another patient with similar problems who was hoping someone would speak to her because she was afraid to speak to someone first. This patient was someone with quite good social skills. Ms. C. wrote down several questions and agreed to approach the other patient, if she could tell the new patient that her therapist required her to speak to other people, and to ask several questions. Ms. C. took her brief questionnaire with

her, and like the excellent student that she was, continued to ask questions after she finished the three she had read from her list. The two patients became quite friendly and soon asked to be placed in the same room. Ms. C.'s belief that she could never make friends was beginning to change. The goal of the social skills treatment was not at this point to help Ms. C. make friends at college, although that outcome would have been welcomed gladly, but to give her some hope that she, too, could have friends to decrease her suicidal thinking.

One of Ms. C.'s major goals was to return to college the following semester (she would lose her scholarship if she did not). Although this did not necessarily seem to me to be the best plan for someone so impulsive and self-destructive, I also thought she might kill herself if she did not have another attempt at it again soon. In order to attain this goal and also the goal of not attempting suicide, the next objective was for Ms. C. to be able to tolerate her feelings of anger and terror without acting upon them. Being able to stay throughout group and community meetings was a good way to practice such affective tolerance. Leaving a group is a flight response, with impulsive leaving of relationships and jobs, and suicide as more extreme examples of the flight response. When patients leave groups, they are frequently afraid of psychologically decompensating, hurting others, or both. Ms. C. left because she was afraid she would hurt someone else. Exploration of this belief revealed that she feared she was like her father, although she did not *think* she was like her father. I suggested that she remind herself that she was not like her father when she was feeling like leaving the group. She began to stay in the groups, although she did not speak in them. The next behavioral goal was to get her to speak in the groups. Very afraid of being ridiculed and rejected, Ms. C. knew she was talented artistically. She did not expect the other patients to ridicule her art work, and quite realistically, expected to be admired for it. The art therapist encouraged her to talk about her drawings in the art group, and again, the good student complied. She received the admiration we all expected. With admiration in the art group and the encouragement of her roommates, Ms. C. began to take care of her personal appearance. Her appearance changed from that of a psychotic to that of a very attractive woman. I then assured her that if people stared at her when she spoke, it was because she was beautiful. She believed me. Her roommates and the whole staff were quite complimentary about her appearance.

It was now time to speak in the therapy group. Ms. C., of course, still considered her depression to be a totally biological one, but was invested in improving her social skills. She knew that I taught group courses to college students, and was able to work on her interpersonal skills as any good student would, not as a part of "therapy" *per se*, but as a college subject. She knew that I and the other staff watched the group therapy sessions and was looking forward to being admired if she spoke in the group. Our goal was one comment or question in the group. She started speaking. Once she was able to speak comfortably in the small group therapy session, we set a goal of speaking in the community meeting. She was so bright, perceptive, and experienced in therapy that her comments were very well received and the staff soon told her that she sounded like another staff member. She frequently did. Sometimes, she would jokingly predict what the staff would say, and I do not remember the staff thinking she was wrong. Through her behavioral participation in therapy and the benefits she received from participating in it, Ms. C. came to believe that therapy was very useful. The individual therapy had become so rewarding for Ms. C. that it could be used as a reinforcement for other behaviors.

This, of course, was just the initial phase of treatment of Ms. C. The power of the whole inpatient unit as a community was used to reinforce appropriate behaviors. Transferentially, the patient, the staff, and I saw me as the good mother, taking care of the patient and her roommate "sister" in whatever ways were most needed. Although there were initially objections to my suggestion that my patient practice social skills with another of my patients, and there was certainly some "sibling rivalry" at times, both patients stated eventually that they were convinced that I could take care of both of them, and would not treat either preferentially.

Ms. C. met her goal of returning to school the following semester. When I phoned her to ask permission to describe her treatment, I had not seen her for more than three years. She had found a good psychiatrist who accepted medicaid, spent some time in a day treatment program, both full- and part-time, had only been hospitalized once during the three years (again after a romantic rejection), and was in college and hoping to graduate soon.

CONCLUSIONS

Although "social" clinical therapy is re-emerging, testable hypotheses regarding the effectiveness of such therapy is awaiting the time when social psychological researchers begin to study in earnest the interpersonal processes occurring in the therapy situation. As social psychologists become less devoted to the experimental laboratory and are willing to investigate experimental variables in other settings, such research will hopefully burgeon. If research psychologists begin to emphasize the study of meaningful variables in real life situations, as some critics of contemporary psychology have encouraged (Bevan, 1991), the psychotherapy situation is a rich and valuable one in which they can examine interpersonal influence processes of clear importance. If psychotherapists of all perspectives value an objective way of knowing, as well as a subjective one, they will support such efforts in their practice. Both conditions are required if we are to know how best to integrate our theories of psychotherapy and our major modes of intervention. The above presentation, while extremely limited, provides many testable hypotheses.

ACKNOWLEDGMENTS. I wish to thank Jeff Greenberg and Ruth Mechanic for their helpful comments on an earlier version of this chapter.

REFERENCES

Alloy, L. B. (Ed.). (1988). *Cognitive processes in depression.* New York: Guilford.
Allport, G. W. (1968). The historical background of modern psychology. In G. Lindzey & E. Aronson (Eds.), *The handbook of social psychology* (Vol. 1, 2nd ed., pp. 1–80). Reading, MA: Addison-Wesley.
Argyle, M. (1987). *The pursuit of happiness.* London: Methuen.
Averill, J. R. (1982). *Anger and aggression: An essay on emotion.* New York: Springer-Verlag.
Bandura, A. (1977). Toward a unifying theory of behavioral change. *Psychological Review, 84,* 191–215.

Becker, E. (1962). *The birth and death of meaning*. New York: Free Press.

Becker, E. (1973). *The denial of death*. New York: Free Press.

Becker, E. (1975). *Escape from evil*. New York: Free Press.

Beebee, B. (1986). Mother-infant mutual influence and precursors of self and object representation. In J. Masling (Ed.), *Empirical studies of psychoanalytic theories 2* (pp. 27–48). Hillsdale, NJ: Analytic Press.

Benne, K. D. (1964). History of the T-group in the laboratory setting. In L. P. Bradford, T. R. Gibb, & K. D. Benne (Eds.), *T-group theory and the laboratory method* (pp. 80–135). New York: Wiley.

Berkman, L., & Syme, S. L. (1979). Social networks, host resistance, and mortality: A nine-year follow-up study of Alameda County residents. *American Journal of Epidemiology, 109*, 186–204.

Bevan, W. (1991). Contemporary psychology: A tour inside the onion. *American Psychologist, 46*, 475–483.

Bollas, (1991, March). *The psychoanalyst's use of free association*. Paper presented at the Ethical Cultural Society, New York.

Brehm, S. S. (1976). *The application of social psychology to clinical practice*. New York: Wiley.

Brehm, S., & Smith, T. (1986). Social psychological approaches to psychotherapy and behavior change. In S. L. Garfield & A. E. Bergin (Eds.), *Handbook of psychotherapy and behavior change* (3rd ed., pp. 69–115). New York: Wiley.

Bucci, W. (1985). Dual coding: A cognitive model for psychoanalytic research. *Journal of the American Psychoanalytic Association, 33*, 571–608.

Curtis, R. C. (1989). Integration: Conditions under which self-defeating and self-enhancing behaviors develop. In R. C. Curtis (Ed.), *Self-defeating behaviors: Experimental research, clinical impressions, and practical implications* (pp. 343–361). New York: Plenum Press.

Curtis, R. C. (1990). Mood disorders and self-defeating behaviors. In B. B. Wolman & G. Stricker (Eds.), *Depressive disorders: Facts, theories, and treatment methods*. New York: Wiley.

Curtis, R. C. (1991). Toward an integrative theory of psychological change in individuals and organizations: A cognitive-affective regulation model. In R. C. Curtis & G. Stricker (Eds.), *How people change: Inside and outside therapy* (pp. 191–210). New York: Plenum Press.

Curtis, R. C. (1992a). A process model of the self and consciousness integrating our rational and experiential selves. *Psychological Inquiry, 3*, 29–32.

Curtis, R. C. (1992b). Self-organizing processes, anxiety, and change. *Journal of Psychotherapy Integration, 4*, 295–319.

Curtis, R. C., & Hillman, J. (1992). Do negative moods lead to unfavorable views of others or more rigid stereotypes? Manuscript submitted for publication.

Curtis, R. C., & Zaslow, G. (1991). Seeing with the third eye: Cognitive-affective regulation and the acquisition of self-knowledge. In R. C. Curtis (Ed.), *The relational self: Theoretical convergences in psychoanalysis and social psychology* (pp. 138–159). New York: Guilford.

Curtis, R., Pacell, D., & Garczynski, J. (1991, April). *Anxiety and self-confirming behavior*. Paper presented at the annual meeting of the Eastern Psychological Association, New York.

Cushman, P. (1991). Ideology obscured: Political uses of the self in Daniel Stern's infant. *American Psychologist, 46*, 206–219.

Eisenberg, N., & Miller, P. (1987). The relation of empathy to prosocial and related behaviors. *Psychological Bulletin, 101*, 91–119.

Epstein, S. (1973). The self-concept revisited, or a theory of a theory. *American Psychologist, 28*, 404–416.

Epstein, S. (1980). The self-concept. A review and a proposal of an integrated theory of personality. In E. Staub (Ed.), *Personality: Basic issues and current research*. Englewood Cliffs, NJ: Prentice-Hall.

Epstein, S. (1991). Cognitive-experiential self theory: An integrated theory of personality. In R. C. Curtis (Ed.), *The relational self: Theoretical convergences in psychoanalysis and social psychology*. NY: Guilford.

Feshbach, N. D. (1984). Empathy, empathy training, and the regulation of aggression in elementary school children. In B. M. Kaplan, V. J. Konecni, R. W. Novaco (Eds.), *Aggression in children and youth* (pp. 192–208). Boston: Martinus Nijhoff.

Feshbach, N. D., & Feshbach, S. (1969). The relationship between empathy and aggression in two age groups. *Developmental Psychology, 1*, 102–107.

Feshbach, N. D., & Feshbach, S. (1982). Empathy training and the regulation of aggression potentialities and limitations. *Academic Psychological Bulletins, 4*, 399–412.

Franz, C. E., McClelland, D. C., & Weinberger, J. (1991). Childhood antecedents of conventional social accomplishments in midlife adults: A 36-year prospective study. *Journal of Personality and Social Psychology, 60*, 586–595.

Freedman, J. L. (1978). *Happy people: What happiness is, who has it, and why*. New York: Harcourt Brace Jovanovich.

Fromm, E. (1947). *Man for himself: An inquiry into the psychology of ethics*. New York: Holt, Rinehart, & Winston.

Greenberg, J., Pyszczynski, T., & Solomon, S. (1986). The causes and consequences of the need for self-esteem: A terror management theory. In R. Baumeister (Ed.), *Public self and private self* (pp. 189–207). New York: Springer-Verlag.

Greenberg, J., Pyszczynski, T., Solomon, S., Rosenblatt, A., Veeder, M., Kirkland, S., & Lyon, D. (1990). Evidence for terror management theory: II. The effects of mortality salience on reactions to those who threaten or bolster the cultural worldview. *Journal of Personality and Social Psychology, 58*, 308–318.

Greenberg, M. S., Vazquez, C. V., & Alloy, L. B. (1988). Depression versus anxiety: Differences in self- and other-schemata. In L. B. Alloy (Ed.), *Cognitive processes in depression* (pp. 109–142). New York: Guilford.

Greenwald, A., & Pratkanis, H. K. (1984). The self. In R. S. Wyer & T. K. Srull (Eds.), *Handbook of social cognition* (Vol. 3, pp. 129–178). Hillsdale, NJ: Lawrence Erlbaum.

Hazan, C., & Shaver, P. R. (1990). Love and work: An attachment-theoretical perspective. *Journal of Personality and Social Psychology, 59*, 270–280.

Heider, F. (1958). *The psychology of interpersonal relations*. New York: Wiley.

Higgins, E. T. (1987). Self-discrepancy: A theory relating self and affect. *Psychological Review, 94*, 319–340.

Higgins, E. T., Tykocinski, O., & Vookles, J. (1990). The psychological significance of relations among the actual, ideal, ought, can, and future selves. In J. M. Olson & M. P. Zanna (Eds.), *Self-inference processes: The Ontario Symposium* (Vol. 6, pp. 153–190). Hillsdale, NJ: Lawrence Erlbaum.

Higgins, R. L., & Snyder, C. R. (1991). Reality negotiation and excuse-making. In C. R. Snyder & D. R. Forsyth

(Eds.), Handbook of social and clinical psychology (pp. 79–95). New York: Pergamon Press.

Horowitz, M. (1991). Person schemas and maladaptive behaviors. Chicago: University of Chicago Press.

Iannotti, R. J. (1978). Effect of role-taking experience on role taking, empathy, altruism, and aggression. Developmental Psychology, 14, 119–124.

Jones, E. E., Kanouse, D. E., Kelley, H. H., Nisbett, R. E., Valins, S., & Weiner, B. (Eds.). (1971/1972). Attribution: Perceiving the causes of behavior. Morristown, NJ: General Learning Press.

Kelley, H. H. (1967). Attribution theory in social psychology. In D. Levine (Ed.), Nebraska symposium on motivation (pp. 192–238). Lincoln: University of Nebraska Press.

Kelley, H. H. (1971/1972). Attribution in social interaction. In E. E. Jones, D. E. Kanouse, H. H. Kelley, R. E. Nisbett, S. Valins, & B. Weiner (Eds.), Attribution: Perceiving the causes of behavior (pp. 1–26). Morristown, NJ: General Learning Press.

Kierkegaard, S. (1955). Fear and trembling and the sickness unto death (W. Lourie, Trans.). Garden City, NY: Doubleday. (Original work published 1849).

Kohut, H. (1971). The analysis of the self. New York: International Universities Press.

Kohut, H. (1977). The restoration of the self. New York: International Universities Press.

Lao Tzu (1955). The way of life. (R. B. Blakney, Tr.). New York: New American Library.

Leiman, B. (1978, August). Affective empathy and subsequent altruism in kindergartners and first graders. Paper presented at the annual meeting of the American Psychological Association, Toronto.

Lewin, K. (1936). Principles of topological psychology. New York: McGraw-Hill.

Lewin, K. (1943). Forces behind food habits and methods of change. Bulletin of the National Research Council, 108, 35–65.

Lewin, K. (1951). Field theory in social science. New York: Harper & Row.

Linville, P. W. (1987). Self-complexity as a cognitive buffer against stress-related depression and illness. Journal of Personality and Social Psychology, 52, 663–676.

Manion, A. (1991). Self-evaluation maintenance in cooperative and competitive situations. Unpublished doctoral dissertation, Adelphi University.

Markus, H. (1977). Self-schemata and processing information about the self. Journal of Personality and Social Psychology, 35, 63–78.

Martin, L. L., & Tesser, A. (1989). Toward a motivational and structural theory of ruminative thought. In J. Uleman & J. Bargh (Eds.), Unintended thought (pp. 306–326). New York: Guilford.

McClelland, D. C., Atkinson, J. W., Clark, R. A., & Lowell, E. L. (1953). The achievement motive. New York: Irvington.

McClelland, D. C., Koestner, R., & Weinberger, J. (1989). How do self-attributed and implicit motives differ? Psychological Review, 96, 690–702.

Miller, P., & Eisenberg, N. (1988). The relation of empathy to aggressive and externalizing/antisocial behavior. Psychological Bulletin, 103, 324–344.

Neisser, U. (1967). Cognitive psychology. Englewood Cliffs, NJ: Prentice-Hall.

Noy, P. (1969). A revision of the psychoanalytic theory of the primary process. International Journal of Psychoanalysis, 56, 155–178.

Noy, P. (1973). Symbolism and mental representation. The Annual of Psychoanalysis (Vol. 1, pp. 125–158). New York: Quadrangle.

Ogilvie, D. M. (1987). The undesired self: A neglected variable in personality research. Journal of Personality and Social Psychology, 52, 379–385.

Paivio, A. (1971). Imagery and verbal processes. New York: Holt, Rinehart & Winston.

Paivio, A. (1986). Mental representations: A dual coding approach. New York: Oxford University Press.

Pennebaker, J. W. (1989a). Confession, inhibition and disease. In L. Berkowitz (Ed.), Advances in experimental social psychology (Vol. 22, pp. 211–244). New York: Academic Press.

Pennebaker, J. W. (1989b, October). Confronting vs. confronted by upsetting experience: Health risks of providing social support. Paper presented at the meeting of the Society for Experimental Social Psychology, Santa Monica, California.

Pyszczynski, T., & Greenberg, J. (1987). Self-regulating perseveration and the depressive self-focusing style: A self-awareness theory of reactive depression. Psychological Bulletin, 102, 122–138.

Sampson, E. E. (1981). Cognitive psychology as ideology. American Psychologist, 36, 730–743.

Sampson, E. E. (1985). The decentralization of identity: Toward a revised concept of personal and social order. American Psychologist, 40, 1203–1211.

Scheier, M. F., & Carver, C. S. (1985). Optimism, coping, and health: Assessment and implications of generalized outcome expectancies. Health Psychology, 4, 219–247.

Scheier, M. F., Weintraub, J. K., & Carver, C. S. (1986). Coping with stress: Divergent strategies of optimists and pessimists. Journal of Personality and Social Psychology, 51, 1257–1264.

Seligman, M. E. P. (1991). Learned optimism: The skill to conquer life's obstacles, large and small. New York: Random House.

Shedler, J., Mayman, M., & Manis, M. (in press). The illusion of mental health. American Psychologist.

Shoham-Salomon, V., & Rosenthal, R. (1987). Paradoxical interventions: A meta-analysis. Journal of Consulting and Clinical Psychology, 55, 22–28.

Shoham-Salomon, V., Avner, R., & Neeman, R. (1989). You're changed if you do and changed if you don't: Mechanisms underlying paradoxical interventions. Journal of Consulting and Clinical Psychology, 57, 590–598.

Singer, J. L., & Salovey, P. (1991). Organized knowledge structures and personality: Person schemas, self-schemas, prototypes and scripts. In M. Horowitz (Ed.), Person schemas and maladaptive interpersonal behavior patterns (pp. 33–79). Chicago: University of Chicago Press.

Slusher, M. P., & Anderson, C. A. (1989). Belief perseverance and self-defeating behavior. In R. C. Curtis (Ed.). Self-defeating behaviors: Experimental research, clinical impressions, and practical implications (pp. 11–40). New York: Plenum Press.

Solomon, S., Greenberg, J., & Pyszcznski, T. (1991a). Terror-management theory of self-esteem. In C. R. Snyder & D. R. Forsyth (Eds.), Handbook of social and clinical psychology (pp. 21–40). New York: Pergamon Press.

Solomon, S., Greenberg, J., & Pyszczynski, T. (1991b). A terror-management theory of social behavior: The psychological functions of self-esteem and the cultural worldview. In M. P. Zanna (Ed.), Advances in experimental *social psychology* (Vol. 24, pp. 93–159). New York: Academic Press.

Spotnitz, H. (1985). *Modern psychoanalysis of the schizophrenic patient: Theory of the technique.* New York, Human Sciences Press.

Staub, E. (1971). The use of role-playing and reduction in children's learning of helping and sharing behavior. *Child Development, 42,* 805–816.

Stern, D. N. (1985). *The interpersonal world of the infant.* New York: Basic Books.

Strack, S., Carver, C. S., & Blaney, P. H. (1987). Predicting successful completion of an aftercare program following treatment for alcoholism: The role of dispositional optimism. *Journal of Personality and Social Psychology, 53,* 579–584.

Swann, W. B., Jr., Pelham, B. W., & Krull, D. S. (1989). Agreeable fancy or disagreeable truth? How people reconcile their self-enhancement and self-verification needs. *Journal of Personality and Social Psychology, 57,* 672–680.

Taylor, S. E. (1989). *Positive illusions: Creative self-deception and the healthy mind.* New York: Basic Books.

Taylor, S. E., & Brown, J. (1988). Illusion and well-being. A social psychological perspective on mental health. *Psychological Bulletin, 103,* 193–210.

Tennen, H., & Affleck, G. (1991). Paradox-based treatments. In C. R. Snyder & D. R. Forsyth, *Handbook of social and clinical psychology* (pp. 624–639). New York: Pergamon Press.

Tesser, A. (1988). Toward a self-evaluation maintenance model of social behavior. In L. Berkowitz (Ed.), *Advances in experimental social psychology* (Vol. 21, pp. 181–227). New York: Academic Press.

Westen, D. (1985). *Self and society: Narcissism, collectivism, and the development of morals.* Cambridge, England: Cambridge University Press.

Westen, D. (1992). Integrating the cognitive and psychoanalytic selves: Can we put our "selves" together? *Psychological Inquiry, 3,* 1–13.

Wicklund, R. A., & Gollwitzer, P. M. (1982). *Symbolic self-completion.* Hillsdale, NJ: Lawrence Erlbaum.

Zillman, D. (1979). *Hostility and aggression.* Hillsdale, NJ: Lawrence Erlbaum.

PART IV

Psychotherapy Integration with Specific Disorders

CHAPTER 20

An Integrated Approach to the Treatment of Anxiety Disorders and Phobias

Jerold R. Gold

Anxiety is a human experience which many assume is universal. Excessive or inappropriate "amounts" or overly frequent occurrences of this state, in its biopsychologically pure form or in the form of anxiety-based symptoms, have been the concern of all schools of psychotherapy since the field was born. Phobias and anxiety disorders often have been at the center of fierce disputes, controversies, and battles between therapists of one sectarian approach or another. Such acrimonious debates go back as far as the "Little Hans" and "Little Albert" discussions (Freud, 1909; Watson & Reyner, 1920), in which the psychoanalytic and behavioral theories of phobic etiology first were described as mutually exclusive. As behavior therapy developed as a viable alternative to analytic and humanistic therapies, the disorders which were taken as its testing ground were phobias and anxiety. Even today, the treatment of these problems is discussed with anger

and with much insistence upon the exclusive superiority or correctness of one position or another (Lazarus, 1991).

In this chapter, I will present a theoretical and technical approach to anxiety disorders and phobias which integrates valuable concepts and methods from behavioral, dynamic, cognitive, and humanistic therapies. The central theoretical constructs which are used to explain the etiology and phenomenology of anxiety disorders are drawn from attachment theory and from its applications to psychopathology and psychotherapy (Bowlby, 1980; Guidano, 1987). Attachment theory provides a developmental and explanatory model in which the discrete phenomena described and emphasized by the competing schools of psychopathology can be related to each other in an integrative manner which is not reductionistic and which avoids the problem of unidirectional causality. In other words, behavior, cognition, affect, self-experience, and motivation do not have to be seen strictly in cause and effect relations with each other, nor do one or several of these variables have to be identified as singularly important or unimportant. Instead, each variable and its role in the etiology and maintenance of

Jerold R. Gold • Doctoral Program in Clinical Psychology, Long Island University, Brooklyn, New York 11201.

Comprehensive Handbook of Psychotherapy Integration, edited by George Stricker and Jerold R. Gold. Plenum Press, New York, 1993.

the anxiety disorder or phobia can be placed within a larger context and can be understood to have developed out of the matrix of the individual's early and ongoing attachment relationships.

AN INTEGRATED, ATTACHMENT-BASED APPROACH

The phenomenology of anxiety disorders and phobias is marked by fear, the occurrence of which is judged subjectively by the individual and or by others to be inappropriate to the situation in which it occurs, or is construed as excessive in its frequency of occurrence or in its intensity. The similarities and differences between normal fear and pathological anxiety have been the subject of extensive scrutiny by clinicians and theorists for many years (cf. Freud, 1926; Dollard & Miller, 1950; Sullivan, 1953; among many others). Regardless of the specific vocabulary and constructs used, most students of anxiety agree that its occurrence is based upon the conscious or unconscious perception of danger or threat, at times and in situations which to others seem benign or unthreatening. Such perceptions of danger are based upon, and constitute, an entrenched and pervasive world view which reflects and is a consequence of the person's developmental history. Attachment theorists (Bowlby, 1980; Guidano, 1987) have established that anxiety is the felt component of a perceived threat to an attachment bond. Such threats may be external and situational, or they may be internal states, such as ideas, wishes, or needs, which the individual construes as threatening or unacceptable to attachment figures. Anxiety disorders and phobias have been traced to certain maladaptive patterns of relatedness around attachment and its counterpart, exploratory behavior (Bowlby, 1980; Guidano, 1987; Guidano & Liotti, 1983). An adult with clinically significant phobias or anxiety symptoms is considered to have had unstable, unreliable, conflictual, or rejecting attachment figures. In these relationships attachment was perceived by the child to be conditional, exclusive, or impossible, and exploration and separation were demonstrated to be awful and dangerous, or to be the cause of a breach in attachment bonds. Guidano and Liotti (1983) note that when such pathology of attachment and exploration exists,

the child's most basic and important representations of the self, of other people, and of the environment are shaped and structured into forms which predispose him or her to pathological anxiety in later life.

These skewed representations of experience, the self, and of others are identical to the "object" of psychoanalytic theory, and to the "schemata" of cognitive theory and therapy. Anxiety-provoking representations are concerned with the identification of threat and danger. Connection to others is depicted as unlikely or impossible without significant cost or compromise in autonomy and the ability to explore the world. Attachment figures and their equivalents are represented as fickle, weak, unreliable, or consuming, and the self is represented as unworthy, incompetent, and always in danger of loss or abandonment.

Such structural derivations of attachment experiences largely are unconscious and are unformulated at a verbal, cognitive level. But these structures shape and color all other levels and types of experience and behavior, making any or all a stimulus for anxiety. In this way motives, thoughts, behavior, affects, or situations may be perceived as a symbol or equivalent of an earlier threat, and thus become the immediate cause of anxiety. The sectarian schools of thought about anxiety disorders each have identified one sector of experience as the key component of these disorders. From the perspective just described it is apparent that wishes, thoughts, feelings, behaviors, and perceptions all share a deeper and more unconscious structure which is the foundation of their ability to elicit symptoms and distress.

The specific organization of each anxiety disorder will vary from individual to individual. For some, the behavioral and cognitive components will be most evident in the form of conscious preoccupations about or hypervigilant scanning for threat and danger, that are linked to and that cause avoidance of certain situations or actions. Such patients fit the cognitive pattern of hypervigilant alarming described by Beck (1976) in which certain events and experiences automatically elicit predictions of danger or harm to the person despite the availability of signs of safety. Other patients will report nonspecific or generalized anxieties which on examination do not have specific cognitive sets or situations attached. This latter group seems to become anxious when certain motives, fantasies or wishes are activated. In fact, it is likely that all patients with these disorders are beset by cognitive-perceptual and dynamic stimuli, with the phenomenology of the disorder differing from person to person. These differences may be traced individually to the person's history and to the way he or she construed and interpreted the fear and uncertainty in attachment relationships. Each child who is faced with unstable and threatening attachment bonding will in some way attempt to find an explanation for such experiences. The locus of blame may be attached to the child's sexual, aggressive, or loving wishes and feelings, or his or her needs for autonomy, achievement, dependency, or separation, or to certain conscious ideas or perceptions, or to particular ways of behaving and interacting. Most likely, the more serious and pervasive the clinical disorder, the broader and more inclusive was the construal of the reasons for failures in attachment by the child. Conversely, simple phobias and circumscribed anxiety symptoms most likely are based upon attachment and exploration experiences which were more largely adequate but which contained certain themes and situations of danger. These experiences led to the identification by the child of one or a few internal states or external events as the source of the anxiety. In all cases of attachment difficulties, the organization of attachment representations and attachment and exploratory behavior are effected by the developmental level of the child, by the ideology, myths, attitudes, and rationales for behavior offered by parents and other important persons, and by the operation of defenses, such as repression, displacement, denial, and dissociation. In particular, parents who approach the anxiety prone child in a hypocritical, mystifying, and condescending way are more likely to intensify and reinforce the child's self-blaming explanations, and therefore raise the probability of that child developing an anxiety disorder in later life (Laing, 1960; Levenson, 1983; Sullivan, 1956).

Once attachments or exploration are structuralized in negative and dangerous terms, a considerable portion of the person's activity is organized around identifying threats to the tenuous ties to safety which exist in his or her own experiences, thoughts, wishes, and behavior, and in the actions of others. As even the possibility of such a threat can be the stimulus for tremendous anxiety, a hypervigilant and protective perceptual set is established, along with an overemphasized need for control or protection in those areas of life which represent, actually or symbolically, the person's subjective point of vulnerability to loss, abandonment, irrevocable separation, or to the surrender of autonomy and independence. Because anxiety is intensely uncomfortable, its removability is highly desirable. Therefore, any intrapsychic action, thought, or behavior which lessens or banishes anxiety will be highly reinforced by the pleasure and comfort which such avoidances, defenses, distorting cognitions, or behavior patterns yield.

This pattern of reinforcement inhibits new learning and testing of novel modes of experience which might serve to correct the anxiogenic representations and more peripheral sources of the anxiety. New learning also is prevented by the fact that high levels of anxiety tend to interfere with the clarity of thought and with the ability to accurately process information (Sullivan, 1953), thus forcing the person to interpret situations and experiences through the anxiogenic concepts and ideas which were previously established.

The interpersonal world in which the anxious person lives often is a major obstacle to change and to the remediation of his or her attachment/exploration concerns. Skewed developmental experiences tend to be repeated and recreated unconsciously as the person chooses people who are unreliable or are threatened by the patient's need for individuation and autonomy, or, as Wachtel (1977; Gold & Wachtel, Chapter 5, this volume) points out, the nature of the anxious patient's fearful interactions evokes complementary responses in others, who become unwitting but reinforcing accomplices in the person's avoidances and anxious modes of representing experience.

The avoidant and restrictive way of life in which the anxious patient is trapped has serious and poignant effects on his or her sense of self-worth, authenticity, and upon the perception of the meaningfulness of his or her actions. With continued reinforcement of anxiety and of self-protective ways of life, the person finds himself or herself giving up some measure of what is meaningful, real, and important in terms of self-actualization, in favor of security and safety. Often, such choices are accompanied by shame, guilt, self-hatred, embarrassment, and by a sense of self-estrangement, phoniness, hopelessness, and emptiness. Such experiences are more likely and extensive in more severe and pervasive cases of anxiety disorder, but most patients seem to have some combination of these feelings. As the avoidance or reduction of anxiety becomes a predominant motive in the person's life, his or her sense of freedom and purpose, and ability to attain goals and to reach ideals is compromised and perverted. What emerges instead is a mechanical need for control and a personality which is hamstrung, superficial, and out of touch with the interpersonal environment and with what is most vital and enriching in the person's inner life. Such issues have been described most completely in the literature on humanistic, existential, and experiential psychotherapy (cf. Fromm, 1941; Rogers, 1961; Bugenthal, 1965; Perls, 1973) as well as by psychoanalysts such as Winnicott (1971), and Kohut (1971).

CLINICAL AND THEORETICAL ANTECEDANTS

The two most important sources for the ideas and methods described in this chapter are the works of Bowlby (1971, 1980), and the cognitive-developmental theories of Guidano (Guidano & Liotti, 1983; Guidano, 1987), who expanded Bowlby's attachment theory and applied those ideas most specifically to the etiology and treatment of several types of psychopathology, including anxiety disorders. Bowlby's (1971, 1980) descriptions of the reverberation of attachment and exploration throughout life, and of the consequences of pathology within the parent–child bond for secure growth and on the representation of experience are critical foundations upon which this work is built. Guidano's (Guidano & Liotti, 1983; Guidano, 1987) application of these concepts was important in so far as he was able to link specific syndromes to particular types of interpersonal deviations around attachment.

The understanding that anxiety is an interpersonal and developmental phenomenon which is self-reinforcing and which creates secondary experiential problems, particularly in the area of self-actualization, is a major tenet of interpersonal psychoanalysis (Fromm, 1941; Levenson, 1983;

Sullivan, 1953, 1956), and of humanistic theory and therapy (Perls, 1973; Rogers, 1961). That anxiety can cause a loss of self-integrity and of authenticity, particularly as it is connected to shame and to familial patterns of hypocrisy, is an idea learned from such authors as Sullivan (1956), Laing (1960), and Bugenthal (1965).

Among integrative therapists and theorists this work is closest to, and has been most influenced by Wachtel's (1977; Gold & Wachtel, Chapter 5, this volume) theory of cyclical psychodynamics, which opened a way toward understanding motivation, cognition, behavior, and character as being mutually influenced by each other and as arising out of common developmental and current experiences. In such a view, no one aspect of experience or behavior takes precedence over any other. As a result, the complex interrelationships between components of the person's psychological makeup, and the interactions of intrapsychic life with the environment may be studied and targeted for intervention. Other integrative therapists whose work has been influential include Beier (1966), who demonstrated how interpersonal events may serve as operant reinforcers for dynamic issues and for defenses, and the work on integrative implosion therapy of Stampfl & Levis (1967), which points to the efficacy of integrative work with anxiety disorders.

THE TECHNIQUE AND PROCESS OF PSYCHOTHERAPY

An integrated psychotherapy of anxiety disorders unfolds in three phases, each of the first two becoming the anchor of the last phase. The first part of the therapy is an extensive evaluation and assessment, in which the immediate intrapsychic, interpersonal, and situational causes of the patient's symptoms are identified. Along with this task, an attempt is made to begin an assessment and formulation of the deviant and skewed representations of the self, attachment figures, and of exploratory behavior and experience, which are the central structure of the pathology. The second phase of the therapy is identified by efforts aimed at symptom relief, behavioral and cognitive restructuring, and interpersonal and psychodynamic exploration. This work often will lead to major additions to, or revisions in, the

formulation of the person's unconscious representations. Major effects toward the establishment of
a safe, warm, and collaborative therapeutic relationship typify this part of the therapy as well.
The third and last phase of the therapy is dedicated to the reconstruction and understanding of
the patient's early experiences of attachment and
exploration. The specific goals of this phase include the modification of pathogenic representations, the creation and internalization of new and
beneficial representations of the self and of others,
and assisting the patient to experience himself or
herself in an authentic, congruent, and actualized
way. This last phase is dependent to a large degree upon both insight and the provision of new
experiences within and outside of the therapeutic
relationship. I will now discuss each phase of the
therapy in a more extensive way.

Assessment

The integrative assessment of anxiety disorders is conducted during the first several contacts
with the patient. Technically, it involves a semi-
structured interview in which the patient's phobic
symptoms and experiences of anxiety are placed
within a contemporary and historical context. Of
particular interest to the therapist are the immediate interpersonal and situational antecedents to
the onset of a symptom, and the cognitions,
meanings, affects, feelings, fantasies, and motives which are consciously and unconsciously
evoked by those transactions and events. Some of
the meanings and thoughts which elicit anxiety
will be readily accessible through direct inquiry,
while others will become apparent only through
indirect means and through interpretative work
(dreams, daydreams and fantasies, slips, etc.).
The ways that the patient relates to the therapist
come under careful study as well, though at this
point in the treatment they may become the focus
of overt discussion only rarely, and then when
they seem to pose a problem for continuity and
cooperation. The therapist will take note of avoidances, defenses, cognitive and memory lapses,
and most importantly, the appearance of anxiety
or phobic responses to the treatment situation,
interventions, and in relation to the therapist.

The assessment of current functioning has as
one crucial aim the identification of those aspects
of experience which early in life were identified

as threatening and as destructive to secure attachment. As noted earlier, each patient will bring a
unique blend of dynamics, beliefs, affects, and
actions, some number and combination of which
will be anxiety-producing. The therapist will attempt to label and discuss just which thoughts,
meanings, actions, feelings, and personal traits
were threatening to others and to the patient. The
hypervigilant perceptual style and ready cognitive tendencies to interpret unknown, unfamiliar,
or ambiguous stimuli as dangerous also come
under scrutiny and often are the first issues addressed in the intervention phases of the treatment. This process will further the introduction of
specific dynamic, cognitive-behavioral, or experiential interventions according to each patient's
idiosyncratic needs.

As data about the patient's current life is compiled and understood, information about his or
her attachment and exploratory experiences in the
earlier period of life is obtained. This information often will be spotty, inconsistent, and subject
to the distorting effects of memory, shame, guilt,
and defense mechanisms. While much of the relevant developmental data may only be accessible
after behavioral change has occurred (Alexander
& French, 1946; Wachtel, 1977; Gold & Wachtel,
Chapter 5, this volume), it is sought out in order
to construct an initial and tentative formulation of
the patient's basic experiential representations.
Such a formulation, with the ongoing revisions
occasioned by new data obtained at later points in
the therapy, becomes a blueprint for work in the
next phases of therapy. As the therapy progresses,
the therapist is increasingly able to understand
how, and in what specific ways the person construes attachment as unreliable or unavailable, or
exploration as impossible, dangerous, or disloyal.
The consequences for the self-representation of
these constructs guide the therapist in the selection of interventions which will offer corrective
emotional experiences in these spheres (Alexander & French, 1946).

Graded Exposure and
the Resolution of Fears

The main purpose of the careful assessment
described above is the pinpointing of the specific
interventions to be suggested to the patient. The
reduction of anxiety is dependent upon the pa-

tient's becoming able to face and experience the specific immediate sources. Exposure may be made possible through the use of behavioral techniques and homework assignments, such as relaxation, systematic or *in vivo* desensitization, or social skills training. It is also assisted by employing cognitive restructuring exercises when irrational or distorted beliefs are a main source of anxiety or are an important impediment toward behavioral change. The interpretive and experiential tools of dynamic psychotherapy and humanistic psychotherapy also are powerful vehicles for exposure when the patient's anxiety occurs as a response to unconscious wishes and motives or to unacknowledged and unintegrated affects and self-perceptions. The choice of intervention must be tailored to the unique and idiosyncratic balance of dynamic, affective, cognitive, and behavioral sources of anxiety, and will be most effective when two principles are followed.

First, the level of exposure must be gradual and tolerable for the patient (Wachtel, 1977). Sudden, severe jumps in the patient's anxiety will make new learning impossible (Sullivan, 1953), can cause severe strains in the therapeutic relationship which may contribute to resistances, and will add to the reinforcement value of the patient's avoidances and defenses. Exposure, through any technical procedure, must be graded to maximize the chance of success and to reinforce the development of tolerance of anxiety to a degree that exposure becomes reinforcing of the willingness to experience slightly greater levels of discomfort.

It is useful during this period of the therapy, and is congruent with the notion of graded exposure, to focus upon the automatic thoughts and hypervigilant perceptual set which cause the patient to find danger and threat where it does not exist. Such ideas often cause great resistance to *in vivo* exposure, imagery exposure, or interpretation, and often yield only when addressed through cognitive restructuring.

The second foundation of successful exposure is the formulation by the therapist of modes and experiences in which the meaning of the source of the anxiety can be identified and changed. As noted above, thoughts, behaviors, wishes, and emotions are anxiety provoking to the extent that such variables were considered to be symbolic or actual threats to attachment or autonomy by the patient. It is highly important therefore to help the patient to learn that his or her thoughts, feelings, desires, or behaviors did not and do not have the toxic and destructive potential with which they were associated. This is done in two ways. Much work will be carried out within the context of the patient's ongoing significant relationships, with gradual exposure to anxiety provoking stimuli being the aim. Patients will be encouraged to try out new ways of behavior with those individuals who have become conscious or unwitting reinforcers or accomplices to the patient's continuing anxiety and attachment difficulties. For example, patients who fear voicing certain opinions or expressing certain affects if they differ from that of a spouse may benefit from assertiveness training to add new behaviors but also to change their construal of, and relationship to, those intrapsychic issues. This work in modifying the interpersonal context of the patient's life will also go on in the therapeutic interaction. Patients often will bring their avoidances, anxieties, and ways of covertly obtaining reinforcement into the therapeutic situation. Such enactments will become the focus of intensive historical scrutiny and interpretation, as well as the data of cognitive and behavioral interventions aimed at modifying old beliefs and establishing new, anxiety-free ways of thinking and acting.

As the patient is successful in exposing himself or herself to the dynamic, cognitive, and behavioral sources of the anxiety, the symptoms will diminish. Additionally, as his or her symptoms come to make more sense historically and in the context of current relationships, the anxiety will decrease also, and the need for control and distance will lessen. Usually, such progress intensifies and deepens the patients' feelings for the therapist, and a more open, warm, and trusting interaction ensues. This interactional climate is the linchpin upon which the third and last phase of the therapy is built.

Therapeutic Enactment and Correction of Dysfunctional Attachment

The heightened emotional relationship between patient and therapist becomes a fertile field for transference reactions in which the patient's deepest and most unconscious representations of the self and significant others are exposed and enacted. The therapist will be perceived, and will often be induced to behave, as the parents and others who instilled a sense of doubt and fear about attachment or exploration. The therapist will encourage such enactments by relating induced feelings, attitudes, and ideas to the patient's significant object images, and as understanding the dyad as immersed in a "transitional" (Winnicott, 1971) interaction which is made up of experience from past and present encounters.

Such enactments require subtle and exhaustive interpretive work, historical reconstruction, and empathic and authentic warmth and resonance by the therapist. The therapist must help the patient to grapple with the conflicts and ambivalence, sadness, rage, guilt, and loss which inevitably are connected to the discovery and exploration of parental failures, abandonment, or hypocrisy. The therapist must work carefully also with the frustrated love and divided loyalties which will prompt defensive activity and resistances, as will the other emotions just mentioned.

As insight develops and the patient's self awareness expands and deepens, opportunities for considering people, the self, attachment, and exploration in new and positive ways emerge. Often, new self and object images are internalized within the therapeutic interaction and within the positive encounters which mark the patient's ongoing relationships. However, such experiences often need to be advanced or supplemented by *in vivo* exercises, or imagery, in which the self and others are consciously experienced and thought about in new and constructive ways (Gold, 1991).

With the discovery and understanding of the familial legacy of the patient's anxiety often comes a period of depression. This depression seems to be a necessary and belated state of mourning and grief, centered around the loss of past opportunities for successful attachment with the parents. This depression also is an expression of sorrow about the ongoing restrictions on experience and on the person's loss of a sense of authenticity and genuineness because of these restrictions. The therapy may turn to an exploration of these issues, as the patient attempts to construct a new, postanxiety identity which may contain old and unrealized abilities and potentials, or which may be permanently shrunken in some aspects. This phase of the treatment often is the final

one, and the work moves toward the experiential and existential, and away from symptoms or dynamics. Instead, the patient is assisted and accompanied on a path of self-discovery by the therapist's empathy, warmth, concern, and ability to reflect the patient's experiences (Rogers, 1961) and to provide a holding environment in which a genuine self can form (Winnicott, 1971). Such an encounter aids the patient in establishing useful and productive attachment and exploration representations, but as importantly, the patient's longstanding sense of guilt and shame may be explored and lessened. Such feelings often are the result of a life led inauthentically, where the goal of avoidance has taken precedence over self-actualization. As the patient finds new hope and courage, and examines what potentials have been retained and lost, shame and guilt may be replaced by determination, pride, ambition or regret and sorrow. Whether the affective transformation is completely positive or is largely mixed, it is a blend of more genuine experience which will advance new ways of relating to others. In turn these new relationships may reinforce the representational changes made within the therapy.

Pitfalls, Concerns, and Contraindications

I believe that this therapy is among the most comprehensive and flexible available for sufferers of anxiety and phobias. There is great potential for relatively rapid and complete symptom resolution, and its insistence on deep structural change offers the patient an opportunity for personal growth which makes relapse or new symptoms less likely than would be the case in a strictly symptom-oriented therapy. In these ways this integrative approach contains the greatest advantages of the competing cognitive-behavioral, dynamic, and humanistic systems, while avoiding the potential superficiality of the former, and the exclusive depth emphases of the latter two approaches. The sectarian schools of psychotherapy all address significant areas of anxiogenic functioning directly, and ameliorate some of the others indirectly through the benign aspects of the therapeutic relationship. However, all of these therapies miss some aspects of the immediate causes of the anxiety and of the underlying representational structures.

This therapy probably is most appropriate for those anxiety disorders or phobic conditions in which the person's life is moderately to severely compromised, and in which the disorder is more chronic, entrenched, and supported by a combination of dynamic factors, distorted cognitions, affective and experiential dissonances, and by pervasive representational problems. As Lazarus (1971) discovered, often symptom reduction is followed by rapid relapse or by the discovery of more basic and severe problems in other areas of the patient's psychology and interpersonal life. It would be something of an overkill experience for a patient with a discrete simple phobia or circumscribed anxiety symptom which appear in an otherwise healthy and productive life and history. Such delimited pathology might be best served by a short-term cognitive or behavioral intervention. Conversely, often multiple phobias, pervasive and unexplained anxiety and widespread panic are indicative of severe character pathology (Kernberg, 1975) which may indicate an extensive and prolonged reconstructive therapy based on a more formal psychoanalytic or humanistic approach, or a different approach to psychotherapy integration (see Gold & Stricker, Chapter 5, this volume) than that described in this chapter.

CASE EXAMPLE

Judy was a pediatrician in her early thirties who sought therapy because of frequent and intense bouts of panic and anxiety. While describing herself as having "always been tense and nervous," Judy dated the onset of symptoms to the time of having completed her residency in pediatrics. She immediately had begun a job as a half-time clinical physician in an outpatient setting, which was combined with another part-time position as a researcher in an affiliated medical school. Judy reported that her panic and anxiety were worst in the morning and then decreased throughout the day, although she experienced a resurgence of symptoms each time she saw a new patient or had a consultation with a new parent. Her time at her research job was relatively anxiety free, as were her weekends, though as the time approached to return to her clinical duties she would become preoccupied and frightened.

Inquiry into the conscious cognitive and ex-

periential components of Judy's symptoms revealed that she doubted her competence as a diagnostician and clinician, and that she continually thought she would miss something and that a child patient would sicken or die. She also considered herself to be unlikable to children and parents, and was deeply concerned with potential rejections. On an affective level Judy was dimly aware of feelings of anger and resentment about having to care for and minister to sick children, and of the need to put her own concerns aside while at the clinic. She alluded to other more unconscious affective trends such as envy and jealousy about the bonds she observed between mothers and children, and to a sense of isolation from intimate contacts with other people. These emotions were highly painful to Judy, causing her anxiety, guilt, and shame, and were a second (along with the cognitive components mentioned above) source of her panic and anxiety.

The initial interventions which were suggested on a trial, exploratory basis were cognitive monitoring and restructuring (testing out the validity of her doubts and self-criticism) and relaxation. These interventions were useful in assisting Judy in the task of exposure to the anxiety-provoking situations and to the cognitive and dynamic underpinnings of the symptoms.

As these interventions were attempted and applied *in vivo*, assessment and historical exploration continued apace. Judy's early life and attachment experiences were predictably implicated in her current difficulties. The second child of a physician father and nurse mother, Judy's life was marked irrevocably by the death of her brother when he was 7 years old and Judy herself was 18 months old. Her parents were inconsolable, and the mother particularly became depressed and withdrawn. Judy soon became an "adult" or "parentified" child who was able to be involved with her parents only as long as she cared for them and made her own needs secondary to theirs. This pattern of relatedness has been described by Bowlby (1980) as "compulsive caregiving," a variant of anxious attachment in which Judy's hopes for true attachment and positive exploration were replaced by an inauthentic and precocious maturity in which she became the attachment figure for her parents.

Intrapsychically, Judy's representational world included no significant figures who could protect or care for her. She unconsciously considered herself to be the only adult in a sea of needy and dependent children. Most powerfully, she believed that it was her responsibility to keep all of these children alive. However, she also portrayed herself as toxically destructive, incompetent, and a failure, since she has failed to win her parents, love and care, and had understood this to be a reflection of having had a role in her brother's death.

As these issues were brought to light, Judy understood that she had been on a mission for most of her life, which had dictated her career choices and had caused her to warp herself and to give up on interests and relationships which were more connected to her authentic self. Her anxieties about clinical work diminished significantly through this combination of exploration and the initial active techniques.

As Judy gained in self-awareness and confidence, she was able to examine her relationships with her patients and their families, and understood that this interaction often increased her anxiety by reinforcing her conscious doubts, and her deeper self-representations. Judy saw that her hesitant, subtly resentful and envious manner caused parents and children to be more formal, distant, and cold with her, thus confirming her beliefs and images of herself, and reinforcing her anxieties. As she explored these interactions, she spontaneously tried out newer and more open ways of behaving and also worked on these issues through a combination of modeling and behavior rehearsal. As her interactions with her patients changed, her clinical work became more personally rewarding to her. She was more frequently asked for by the parents who used the clinic, and developed several mutually satisfying social relationships with parents and staff members in which she was able to lessen or give up her role as the exclusive caregiver.

As Judy's symptoms diminished, the therapy moved toward the deeper and earlier levels of her attachment difficulties. Immense feelings of sorrow and loss, coupled with intense rage, guilt, and a sense of herself as unlovable, destructive, and unworthy dominated her experience and her interactions with the therapist. The therapist came to be for Judy her unattainable and needy parents, and in some ways this interaction was unwittingly reestablished as the therapist would

at times become preoccupied and insensitive to Judy's needs, and Judy would respond through caretaking activities which stimulated comparable rageful and sad feelings to those which typified her earliest parental interactions. As these issues were explored and understood, a deeper and more authentic interaction emerged, in which Judy was more free to make her needs known, to make demands on the therapist, and to be angry openly if he were inattentive or self-absorbed.

These interactions were accompanied by an expansion of Judy's affective involvement with the therapist, and with peers and friends who liked her and who did not want her or need her to care for them most of the time. Her awareness of real affection and concern for her, in and out of therapy, led to major revisions in her self-representation and in her images of others.

The last part of the therapy centered around the losses of potential and authentic experience which Judy's life had included. Although she had grown more comfortable with her clinical tasks, and took some satisfaction from her research, she now saw both of those aspects of her professional life as belonging to her past and to a mission of salvation which she had ended. She also felt sorrowfully the gaps in her intellectual, cultural, and social activities which her attachment to her parents and to caregiving had caused. Such exploration did not lead to specific changes but to a more active and openly adventurous style of interaction with the world which seemed likely to continue well after the therapy ended.

REFERENCES

Alexander, F., & French, T. (1946). *Psychoanalytic therapy*. New York: Ronald Press.

Beck, A. T. (1976). *Cognitive therapy and the emotional disorders*. New York: International Universities Press.

Beier, E. G. (1966). *The silent language of psychotherapy*. Chicago: Aldine.

Bowlby, J. (1971). *Attachment and loss, Vol. 1: Attachment*. London: Penguin.

Bowlby, J. (1980). *Attachment and loss, Vol. 3: Loss*. London: Penguin.

Bugenthal, J. F. T. (1965). *The search for authenticity*. New York: Holt, Rinehart, and Winston.

Dollard, J., & Miller, N. E. (1950). *Personality and psychotherapy*. New York: McGraw-Hill.

Freud, S. (1909). Analysis of a phobia in a five year old boy. In J. Strachey (Ed. and Trans.), *The standard edition of the complete psychological works of Sigmund Freud*, Vol. 10. London: Hogarth Press.

Freud, S. (1926). Inhibitions, symptoms, and anxiety. In J. Strachey (Ed. and Trans.), *The standard edition of the complete psychological works of Sigmund Freud*, Vol. 20. London: Hogarth Press.

Fromm, E. (1941). *Escape from freedom*. New York: Rinehart.

Gold, J. R. (1991). Repairing narcissistic deficits through the use of imagery. In R. Kunzendorf (Ed.), *Mental imagery*. New York: Plenum Press.

Guidano, V. (1987). *The development of the self*. New York: Guilford.

Guidano, V., & Liotti, G. (1983). *Cognitive processes and the emotional disorders*. New York: Guilford.

Kernberg, O. (1975). *Borderline conditions and pathological narcissism*. New York: Jason Aronson.

Kohut, H. (1971). *The analysis of the self*. New York: International Universities Press.

Laing, R. D. (1960). *The divided self*. Baltimore: Penguin.

Lazarus, A. A. (1971). *Behavior therapy and beyond*. New York: McGraw-Hill.

Lazarus, A. A. (1991). A plague on Little Hans and Little Albert. *Psychotherapy: Theory, Research, Practice, Training*, 28, 444–447.

Levenson, E. A. (1983). *The ambiguity of change*. New York: Basic Books.

Perls, F. (1973). *The gestalt approach: An eye witness to therapy*. Palo Alto: Science and Behavior Books.

Rogers, C. R. (1961). *On becoming a person*. Boston: Houghton Mifflin.

Stampfl, T. G., & Levis, D. L. (1967). The essentials of implosive therapy: A learning theory based psychodynamic behavior therapy. *Journal of Abnormal Psychology*, 72, 496–503.

Sullivan, H. S. (1953). *The interpersonal theory of psychiatry*. New York: W. W. Norton.

Sullivan, H. S. (1956). *Clinical studies in psychiatry*. New York: W. W. Norton.

Wachtel, P. L. (1977). *Psychoanalysis and behavior therapy: Towards an integration*. New York: Basic Books.

Watson, J. B., & Reyner, M. (1920). Conditioned emotional reactions. *Journal of Experimental Psychology*, 3, 1–14.

Winnicott, D. W. (1971). *Maturational processes and the facilitating environment*. New York: International Universities Press.

CHAPTER 21

Depression

AN INTEGRATIVE PERSPECTIVE

Adele M. Hayes and Cory F. Newman

Unipolar depression is one of the most prevalent of the major psychiatric disorders. Epidemiological studies estimate that one in five people in the United States will experience an episode of depression sufficient to warrant treatment (Weissman & Myers, 1978) and 3% to 5% of the general population will require hospitalization (Craighead, Kennedy, Raczynski, & Dow, 1984). Depression is a serious and recurrent disorder that can cause immense suffering and carries with it a suicide risk that is 30 times greater than that of the general population (Guze & Robins, 1970). The challenge in the treatment of depression is not only to relieve the client's/patient's suffering, but also to prevent its recurrence.

Depression is complex in its manifestations and has numerous sequelae that affect almost every aspect of the client's/patient's functioning.

In addition to the affective component, depression includes behavioral (e.g., psychomotor retardation, decreased activity, social withdrawal), cognitive (e.g., hopelessness, helplessness, low self-esteem), and somatic (e.g., decreased sleep, weight loss) symptoms. This ubiquitous disorder often coexists with a variety of other psychiatric disorders, as well as with an assortment of physical and medical problems, especially those that involve a reduction in autonomy (e.g., chronic pain, loss of limb).

Given the complexity of this disorder, we believe that depression demands a broad-based, integrative approach to treat not only the symptoms of depression, but also the psychosocial sequelae. Our approach does not represent a single integrative treatment for depression, as we believe that the spirit of integrationism is to move toward more idiographic approaches. Rather, we outline a framework with which to conceptualize the depression for a given individual and provide guidelines for selecting interventions to meet the needs of that person. The framework is based on an understanding of the intrapersonal, interpersonal, and environmental factors that have been identified in the research as influencing the course of depression. We will review this literature briefly.

Adele M. Hayes • Affective Disorders Program, Duke University Medical Center, Durham, North Carolina 27710. Cory F. Newman • Center for Cognitive Therapy, University of Pennsylvania, Philadelphia, Pennsylvania 19104-3246.

Comprehensive Handbook of Psychotherapy Integration, edited by George Stricker and Jerold R. Gold. Plenum Press, New York, 1993.

PSYCHOSOCIAL FACTORS ASSOCIATED WITH THE COURSE OF DEPRESSION

Intrapersonal Factors

Cognitions. In a recent review of the cognitive theory of depression, Haaga, Dyck, and Ernst (1991) conclude that depressed people tend to think negatively about themselves, their future, and their aptitude for coping with the world. There is little support for causal hypotheses regarding the role of cognitions in depression, but these authors contend that the verdict is not in until studies are conducted that prime latent cognitions. Nonetheless, it is clear that negative cognitions are an integral part of the constellation of symptoms and problems that characterize depression. There is some evidence that attributional style, dysfunctional attitudes, and hopelessness may play a role in the recovery and relapse processes.

There is general agreement that depressed clients/patients are more likely than nondepressed individuals to attribute the cause of negative events to internal (rather than external), global (rather than specific), and stable (rather than unstable) causes (see Robins & Hayes, in press, for a recent review). This attributional style is hypothesized to play a central role in depression, according to the most recent revision of the learned helplessness model, the hopelessness theory (Abramson, Metalsky, & Alloy, 1989). Although there is little support for attributional style as a predictor of the onset of depression, there is some evidence that it may be associated with recovery and relapse. For example, in a study of the process of change in cognitive therapy, pharmacotherapy, and a combination group, DeRubeis, Evans, Hollon, Garvey, Grove, and Tuason (1990) found that change in attributional style was related to improvement in depressive symptoms, especially in the groups that received cognitive therapy. Furthermore, the attributional styles of the responders at the end of treatment predicted the likelihood of relapse over a 2-year follow-up period (Evans, Hollon, & DeRubeis, 1989).

Beck (e.g., 1976) also maintains that negative cognitions play a central role in depression. This negative thinking involves the cognitive triad (negative view of self, world, and future) and schemata (or core beliefs) that develop during early life experiences. These schemata are presumed to be latent until activated by life events. The most likely activating events are those that are perceived to be similar to the past experiences involved in the development of the schemata. For example, a client/patient who was neglected during childhood may have formulated the schema that he is "unlovable." When in a satisfying relationship with his girlfriend, this schema may lie dormant, but it may be triggered when she suggests that they postpone their plans to marry.

As with attributional style, depressed individuals report a greater number of dysfunctional attitudes than do nondepressed people (Haaga et al., 1991). Whisman, Miller, Norman, and Keitner (1991) suggested that cognitive therapy may change dysfunctional attitudes. They found that depressed in-patients who received cognitive therapy in addition to the standard pharmacological treatment, reported fewer dysfunctional attitudes 1 year after discharge than did patients who did not receive cognitive therapy. Dysfunctional attitudes among remitted depressed clients/patients also have predicted increased depressive symptoms 6 months (Rush, Weissenburger, & Eaves, 1986) and 1 year (Simons, Murphy, Levine, & Wetzel, 1986) after treatment.

Another class of cognitions that plays an important role in depression is hopelessness. Hopelessness depression has recently been proposed as a subtype of depression, which the attributional model specifically addressed (Abramson et al., 1989). There is some evidence that hopelessness is involved in the recovery process because cognitive therapy is associated with lower levels of hopelessness at the end of therapy (Rush, Beck, Kovacs, Weissenburger, & Hollon, 1982). Additionally, depressed in-patients receiving cognitive therapy reported less hopelessness 6 and 12 months after treatment than patients receiving only pharmacotherapy (Whisman et al., 1991). Prospective studies have supported the relationship between hopelessness and suicide, independent of the severity of the depression (Beck, Brown, & Steer, 1989). Beck and Steer (1990) report that outpatients in their study who had high levels of hopelessness were 11 times as likely as those with lower levels of hopelessness to commit suicide. Taken together, these findings suggest that hopelessness may be important in the recovery and relapse processes.

Personality. In a review of the literature on interpersonal factors in depression, Barnett and Gotlib (1988) conclude that interpersonal dependency and introversion are enduring traits of remitted depressives that differ from never-depressed controls. Dependency is hypothesized to develop in those who experienced difficulties in establishing secure relationships early in life. Theoretically, a dependent person becomes preoccupied with interpersonal security and cannot maintain a positive sense of self without external support. Introversion refers to a generalized tendency to avoid social interactions. This tendency restricts the individual's range of social interactions, thus decreasing the potential sources of emotional support. Introversion has an inverse relationship with marital satisfaction (Renne, 1970), another very important variable in depression (Beach, Sandeen, & O'Leary, 1990). Although prospective studies have not been conducted yet, interpersonal dependency and introversion show promise as variables that may be related to relapse.

Coping Skills. Barnett and Gotlib (1988) conceptualize coping skills as internal and external resources used to regulate emotion and behaviors as a way to remove or decrease stress. Their review of the coping literature indicates that depressed people use more *emotion*-focused coping strategies (e.g., emotional release and seeking emotional support) than the nondepressed controls. They also use fewer *active* strategies (e.g., problem-solving, assertiveness) and engage in more avoidance than controls. There is some evidence that having better problem-solving skills may serve as a buffer against the effects of negative events, even though the individual has a self-deprecating style of attributing the cause of the events to internal, stable, and global factors (Nezu, Kalmar, Ronan, & Clarijo, 1986). Furthermore, *perceptions* of one's ability to cope are important in that individuals who view themselves as ineffective problem-solvers have been found to be more depressed than those who view themselves as effective problem-solvers (Heppner, Baumgardner, & Jackson, 1985). It is likely that individuals with low coping expectancies will develop

"hopeless expectancies" when encountering negative events.

Interpersonal and Environmental Factors

Social Skills. Coyne's (1990) recent review of the literature on interpersonal processes in depression concludes that when compared to nondepressed controls, depressed individuals have poorer social skills and they quickly evoke negative affect and tension in interactions with their spouses and with strangers. These deficits persist even when the symptoms of depression have remitted, thus increasing the likelihood of marital and family disturbances, as well as general social difficulties. These negative effects on others may reinforce depressed persons' negative views of themselves and reduce their social support.

Significant Relationships. Compared to nondepressed women, depressed women report more impairment in marital and parental adjustment, as well as problems with work, social interactions, and leisure (Weissman & Paykel, 1974). Recent reviews (e.g., Barnett & Gotlib, 1988; Coyne, 1990) conclude that marital discord appears to have an impact on the onset and course of depression, and that continued problems may impede the recovery process. Depressed persons appear to be at continued risk for interpersonal problems beyond the acute episode and these problems predict the persistence or recurrence of depression. Coyne (1990) proposes that marital distress may be an interpersonal diathesis in that it chronically erodes self-esteem and general coping resources. Moreover, when spouses agree with a person's negative self-view, they may insulate that person from positive experiences that might otherwise challenge this depressive view (Swann & Predmore, 1985).

Current family pathology also plays a major role in the course of depression, and even in suicidal behavior (Keitner & Miller, 1990). There is a substantial body of literature documenting the relationship between high levels of critical communication (a factor of a construct called "expressed emotion") in the families of depressives and higher rates of relapse (Hooley, 1990). Critical communication is also associated with marital distress (Hooley & Teasdale, 1989).

Another important interpersonal variable is level of social integration. Social integration is a term that describes the extent of a patients' extramarital support, as measured by social participation and the number of important relationships. Level of social integration predicts the onset of depression, its course, and relapse, and does not automatically improve after the symptoms of depression have remitted (Barnett & Gotlib, 1988). Low social integration is related to low ratings of marital satisfaction, as is introversion (Barry, 1970; Renne, 1970). Coyne and his colleagues (Coyne, Kahn, & Gotlib, 1987) have hypothesized a process whereby depressed people alienate those closest to them by escalating their demands for support and other depressive behaviors. Prospective research suggests that this alienation within the individual's interpersonal system may precede and possibly precipitate the onset of depressive symptoms (Gotlib & Hooley, 1988). The intractable interpersonal difficulties of depressed persons deserves greater attention as a target for treatment, especially in chronic and recurrent depression (Coyne, 1990).

General Life Events. There is a relationship between depression and a higher frequency of recent negative life events (Brown & Harris, 1978; Paykel, 1979), but causality is difficult to demonstrate because reports of recent life events are generally retrospective and open to the negatively biased recall associated with depression. It is also difficult to separate the occurrence of life events from the symptoms of the illness. Although the etiological status of life events is controversial, Brown and Harris found that 89% of new cases of depression in a community sample reported a severe event or chronic difficulty in the previous 9 months, whereas only 30% of noncases reported this. In chronic depression, a decrease in ongoing difficulties and in the occurrence of "fresh starts" seems to engender hope and to facilitate the recovery process (Brown, Adler, & Bifulco, 1988).

Additionally, there are data to suggest that life events can interact with the personality characteristics of sociotropy (interpersonal dependency) and autonomy (vulnerability to failure, lack of control, and lack of mobility) described by Beck (1983) and Blatt, D'Afflitti, and Quinlan (1976). For instance, Hammen, Ellicott, Gitlin, & Jamison (1989) found that clients/patients who experienced more negative events congruent with their personality mode than events that were not congruent, were more depressed 6 months after remission. In other words, a person with a sociotropic personality style was more likely to have a recurrence of depressive symptoms following an interpersonal rejection, while an autonomous person was more likely to become depressed in conjunction with a business setback.

In summary, the psychosocial factors that are important for the clinician to consider when treating depressed clients/patients include: attributional style, dysfunctional attitudes, hopelessness, interpersonal dependency, introversion, coping skills, social skills, marital, family, and social dysfunction, level of social integration, and life events. These findings challenge the notion that depression is a homogeneous disorder with discrete episodes that are resolved with few residual difficulties. Instead, depression is a complex syndrome with multiple points of intervention for symptom relief and relapse prevention.

THERAPIES FOR DEPRESSION

The following are brief summaries of a number of well-known treatment modalities that have been developed specifically for depression and that have been evaluated empirically. They do not represent an exhaustive list—indeed, the proliferation of psychotherapies makes such a review impractical, and has served as one of the motivating forces behind the movement toward the exploration of psychotherapy integration. In addition, we do not mean to imply that the following therapies are completely separate and distinct entities. Many theoretically and therapeutically significant points of commonality have been discovered across different psychotherapeutic approaches as they currently exist (cf. Arkowitz & Hannah, 1989; Goldfried, 1980; Goldfried & Newman, 1986; Hayes, 1990). Such areas of convergence will be most evident in the following summaries. Our intention is to highlight treatment approaches from which an integrative therapy may be derived.

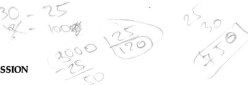

Cognitive Therapy

In the cognitive model (Beck, 1976), dysfunctional cognitions and maladaptive information processing are viewed as central to depression. Thus, cognitive therapy (Beck, Rush, Shaw, & Emery, 1979) emphasizes changing depressogenic attitudes and engrained thinking patterns by evaluating them logically and constructively. Patients are taught systematically to review available evidence for their beliefs and to conduct hypothesis-testing exercises between sessions. Beck's cognitive therapy has been demonstrated to be effective in alleviating the symptoms of depression and preventing relapse (see Hollon, Shelton, & Loosen, 1991 for a review).

Behavioral Therapy

In the behavioral models (Hoberman, 1990; Lewinsohn, Antonuccio, Steinmetz, & Teri, 1984), low rates of response-contingent positive reinforcement and high rates of aversive experiences are viewed as the central mediating factors in the onset of depression. These conditions arise for several reasons: (1) the immediate environment has too few positives and too many punishing aspects, (2) the individual's capacity to enjoy positives is reduced and/or sensitivity to aversive events heightened, and (3) the person lacks the skills necessary to obtain the available positives and/or to cope with aversive events. The first step in behavior therapy is to perform a functional analysis of the problems that covary with the depressed mood. This allows the clinician to specify target problems rather than to target the more general syndrome of depression. The behavioral approaches involve teaching clients/patients skills to increase positive events and to deal actively with negative events in their lives. Behavioral strategies include activity scheduling (Lewinsohn et al., 1984), self-control therapy (Rehm, 1984), stress-management techniques (Lewinsohn et al., 1984), problem-solving (Nezu, Nezu, & Perri, 1989), and social skills training (Bellack, Hersen, & Himmelhoch, 1981). Generally, these forms of behavior therapy have been demonstrated to be effective and to prevent relapse (Hoberman, 1990; Jarrett, 1990; Robinson, Berman, & Neimeyer, 1990).

Behavioral Marital Therapy

The rationale for marital therapy as a treatment for depression is based on the evidence that marital discord often is related to the onset, maintenance, and recurrence of depression (Barnett & Gotlib, 1988). Approximately 50% of couples seeking marital therapy have at least one spouse who is depressed (Beach, Jouriles, & O'Leary, 1985). Behavioral marital therapy (Beach et al., 1990; Jacobson & Holtzworth-Monroe, 1986) applies many of the components of the individual therapies to the couple. For instance, marital therapy focuses on increasing positive behaviors, decreasing negative behaviors, and improving communication and problem-solving skills. It also includes some more cognitive components such as correcting misperceptions, reframing, making reattributions, and examining the couple's goals and expectations. Behavioral marital therapy has performed as well as Beck et al.'s (1979) cognitive therapy for depression when treating clients/patients who are both depressed and maritally distressed (Jacobson, Dobson, Fruzzetti, Schmaling, & Salusky, 1991; O'Leary & Beach, 1990). Behavioral marital therapy seems to have a two-pronged effect for distressed couples in that it is as effective as cognitive therapy in decreasing the symptoms of depression, and it also increases marital satisfaction.

Interpersonal Therapy

According to this model, depression must be viewed in an interpersonal context, as relationships with others is seen as the primary area of dysfunction in depressives. Interpersonal therapy (e.g., Klerman, Weissman, Rounsaville, & Chevron, 1984) targets grief, role transition, role disputes, and interpersonal deficits in the depressed individual. This approach emphasizes the teaching of specific communication and social skills to counteract interpersonal deficits or disputes in one's personal or work life. There is also some emphasis on modifying the unrealistic expectations about relationships that often stem from problematic relationships in the past. A growing body of research supports interpersonal therapy's effectiveness in reducing the symptoms of depression and in preventing relapse (Frank,

Kupfer, Wagner, McEachran, & Cornes, 1991; see Jarrett, 1990, for a review).

Experiential Therapy

This model assumes that depression is a secondary response to the clients'/patients' difficulties in experiencing and expressing emotions, thoughts, and actions that pertain to key areas of distress in their lives. One such approach is Focused Expressive Psychotherapy (Daldrup, Beutler, Engle, & Greenberg, 1988). Here, therapists encourage clients/patients to take part in a number of exercises that are intended to evoke emotions that are typically suppressed (e.g., awareness exercises, two-chair dialogue, directed fantasy). The heightened awareness and increased capacity for self-expression that the clients/patients achieve are hypothesized to help them to come to terms with feelings, such as grief and resentment, while also opening up new areas of opportunity and fulfillment in a less restricted life. Although a recent development, one study has demonstrated that this approach was as effective as cognitive therapy in relieving the symptoms of depression (Beutler, Engle, Mohr, Daldrup, Bergan, Meredith, & Merry, 1991).

Psychodynamic Therapy

The psychodynamic approach (e.g., Luborsky, 1984; Strupp & Binder, 1984) views loss, chronic conflict, and lack of self-esteem as central themes in depression. According to this approach, changes in depressogenic thinking or environmental management alone may not succeed in altering chronic conflicts or profound fears of loss of love. In these cases, a deeper and more long-term approach is purportedly needed to tap unconscious memories or schemata. The aim is to resolve intrapsychic conflict related to significant others in the client's/patient's present and past so as to reorganize the client's/patient's personality, rather than just provide symptomatic relief. Karasu (1990) outlines the successive goals in treating the depressed patient: (1) to provide symptom relief through cathartic expression of suppressed aggressive feelings, (2) to lower superego demands and perfectionistic standards, thereby reducing feelings of guilt and inadequacy and raising self-esteem, (3) to make interpretations to

help clients/patients better understand their narcissistic wishes for love and excessive expectations in significant relationships, and (4) to uncover and recreate earlier conflicts from which the current disorder derives. With some resolution of conflictual feelings, the client/patient can search for more gratifying, realistic ways to achieve love and a sense of worth and gradually form a permanent foundation for preventing future depressive episodes.

In a recent meta-analysis of short-term psychodynamic therapies, Svartberg & Stiles (1991) found that for the diagnostic category of depression, these therapies were significantly less effective than other therapies, especially Beck's (1979) cognitive therapy. However, the number of studies included was small and most clinical trials use symptom reduction as the measure outcome, which is not the only goal of the psychodynamic approaches. We believe that the psychodynamic model is very useful in conceptualizing a case and that several of the techniques from that model can be especially helpful in the more chronic and recurrent cases that are likely to involve personality restructuring.

Biological Treatments

We also acknowledge the importance of understanding the biochemical components of depression, including the application of pharmacotherapeutic agents in treatment. While a review of the biological treatments for depression is beyond the scope of this chapter, the reader is referred to Shelton, Hollon, Purdon, and Loosen (1991) for an excellent review of this literature and a discussion of when and how to integrate biological and psychological treatments.

THEORETICAL AND CONCEPTUAL POSITION

The aforementioned models of depression acknowledge its complexity, yet each orientation emphasizes one particular aspect of functioning as dominant (e.g., cognition, behavior, interpersonal relatedness, suppressed emotions, intrapsychic conflict) and has developed a psychotherapy to target that area. Indeed, the aspects of functioning targeted by each of the psychotherapies have been found to be important factors in the course of depression. However, no single aspect has been demonstrated to be the predominant feature of the disorder, nor has one form of psychotherapy been found to be consistently superior to the other therapies that have been examined in clinical trials (Jarrett, 1990; Robinson *et al.*, 1990). We are not referring to psychodynamic therapy, as there are too few studies that have compared it with other therapies and because most studies use outcome measures that do not consider the goals of the psychodynamic approach.

The *homeostasis model* of depression has been proposed in various forms by a number of writers (Akiskal & McKinney, 1973; Beitman, 1987; Coyne, 1976; Craighead, 1980; Karasu, 1990) as a way to understand the complexity of depression. Depression is hypothesized to involve many different components of the client's/patient's functioning that form complex causal chains and cycles that maintain the dysphoric homeostasis (see Beckham, 1990, for a review). This conceptualization suggests that there are multiple points of dysregulation and therapeutic entry in the depressive syndrome and may explain why such a variety of treatments have an impact on its remediation.

Beckham (1990) views therapy as an attempt to alter one or more of the maintaining conditions, thereby disrupting the system and shifting it to a more healthy equilibrium. He contends that if psychotherapy alters one element of the depressive homeostasis, this effect quickly spreads to the other elements in the system. Similarly, Beitman (1987) describes a "deviation amplifying process" in which therapy creates a deviation in the system that then "snowballs" to other areas. Therapy is especially potent if it targets a "critical link." For example, when a client's/patient's depressive episodes seem to coincide with the ups and downs of her marital relationship, marital therapy can be employed to teach better communication and problem-solving skills. These skills may improve not only her relationship with the spouse, but also interactions with her friends and co-workers, thus increasing her sense of self-efficacy and social support. This, in turn, is likely to lead to feelings of greater satisfaction in life, which may impact positively on the client's/patient's behaviors toward her spouse.

The elements of the depressive homeostasis have not been specified, but we believe they are likely to be the variables that researchers have identified as influencing the course of depression. We present an integrative approach based on an assessment of these variables and the tailoring of treatment interventions to the profile of strengths and weaknesses identified for that individual.

A number of psychotherapists have applied the notion of reciprocal maintaining processes in their therapy approaches. For example, such an approach is similar to Wachtel's (1977) notion of cyclical psychodynamics and Safran and Segal's (1990) cognitive-interpersonal cycles. Other approaches (e.g., Beutler & Clarkin, 1990; Hoberman, 1990; Karasu, 1990; Lazarus, 1971) have applied the concept of developing a client/patient profile. Our approach is different from these approaches in that we emphasize the importance of basing treatment selection on (1) an assessment of a broad range of variables that have been identified in the research as affecting the course of depression, (2) a conceptualization of the principles of change that could facilitate the client's/patient's recovery, and (3) an awareness of the psychotherapies from a number of orientations that have been demonstrated to be effective in the treatment of depression. In order for this strategy to be effective, the therapist must gather a great deal of information about the individual, so that a comprehensive formulation of the client's/patient's depressive homeostasis—in the form of a profile of strengths and dysfunctions—can be derived.

THE TECHNIQUE AND PROCESS OF PSYCHOTHERAPY

One of the hallmarks of integrative therapy is its attention to the specific needs of the client/patient. There is no single "true" package for the heterogeneous disorder of major depression. Instead, integrative psychotherapy is a process of clinical thinking and decision-making (Beutler & Clarkin, 1990). We hope to elucidate the means by which therapists can draw from a variety of extant psychotherapy models in order to facilitate a more comprehensive understanding of the client/patient, as well as to generate more potentially fruitful points of intervention than would be possible within the strict confines of any given model of psychotherapy. We also endeavor to show a healthy respect for an empirical approach to therapy, while at the same time demonstrating that this is not incompatible with the all-important use of clinical intuition and artistry.

Assessment and Conceptualization

A thorough assessment is essential to an integrative approach so that the treatment can be tailored to the individual client/patient. The goal of the assessment is to develop a comprehensive description of the factors that influence the client's/patient's depression, rather than to solely target the symptoms of depression.

We suggest that this information be organized in two ways. First, a timeline can be developed that visually depicts the course of the individual's depression and other Axis I disorders, the history of suicidal gestures or attempts, and the life stressors associated with these. This first level of assessment puts the current episode of depression in historical context and represents a linear perspective. For example, the timeline may help a client/patient to see that he has a long history of panic attacks following high levels of stress, and that his depressive episodes tend to occur after the panic attacks become more frequent and interfere with his functioning. At this point, he views the panic as ruining his life, humiliating him, and demonstrating to the world that he is weak and a failure. When these thoughts predominate, he becomes suicidal. This description of the timing of the disorders, the stressors associated with them and with suicidality (if applicable), gives the client/patient and the therapist a way of understanding the relevant patterns and sequence of events that are so important in relapse prevention. We recommend that the clinician create the timeline to make sure that it is used to show connections, rather than for clients/patients to note how many times they have been depressed or how miserable their lives have been. This is especially likely to occur with depressives because of their pervasive patterns of negative thinking.

The second stage of the assessment yields the information with which to construct a profile of the strengths and dysfunctions that maintain the current depressive homeostasis for that individual. We suggest assessing the role of each of the psychosocial factors that we reviewed as factors influencing the course of depression. Other client/patient variables that we deem important are: Affective regulation and processing, impulse control, defenses, sense of identity, and sources of self-esteem. Assessment is an ongoing process and the model will undoubtedly be expanded as more is revealed in the course of therapy.

Other relevant background information to gather should include: (1) previous treatments, responses to treatments, and compliance; (2) reports from mental health professionals who have worked with the person, and (3) interviews with family members or people who know the client/patient well, especially regarding the client's/patient's premorbid functioning. The checklist included in Table 1 can be used as a guideline in the assessment phase of treatment.

Treatment Selection
and the Process of Therapy

Once the therapist has created the timeline and clinical profile for that individual, these can be shared with the client/patient so that he or she can better understand the depressive syndrome and can collaborate with the therapist in setting treatment goals. All of this information considers the whole person, but also can be overwhelming to the client/patient and to the therapist if priorities are not established. Initially, two or three areas of functioning can be selected to serve as the centerpiece of therapy. The first goal is symptom reduction and then the therapist can begin to improve the client's/patient's general mental health and work toward relapse prevention, provided the individual wants to continue therapy and has the resources to do so (Thase, 1990).

The client's/patient's level of premorbid functioning is an important consideration in treatment formulation. According to Beckham's (1990) conceptualization of the homeostatic model, the effects of therapy are most likely to spread in those individuals with relatively healthy premorbid functioning. In these cases, the therapist can target one element and disturb the homeostasis, so that well-established healthy behaviors reemerge. He contends that the optimal place to start treatment is in the area of functioning where

Table 1. Guidelines for Assessment

Timeline

1. History of depressive episodes (including previous contact with mental health professionals, treatment response, and compliance)
2. History of other Axis I disorders, as well as Axis II and Axis III disorders
3. History of suicidality (including precipitating factors, methods used, factors that prevented a successful attempt)
4. Major life stressors associated with the disorder(s) and with suicidality (assess past trauma)

Profile of strengths and dysfunctions
for the individual's depressive homeostasis

5. Cognitions: Attributional style, dysfunctional attitudes, hopelessness
6. Personality: Introversion-extroversion, interpersonal dependency
7. Identity: Sources of self-esteem, roles, conflict
8. Coping Skills: Problem-solving, affective processing and regulation, impulse control, defenses
9. Social skills
10. Relationships: Mate, family, general (e.g., work, friends)
11. Social integration
12. Interviews with relevant significant others, with eye toward assessing premorbid functioning

the client/patient has been the strongest in past and, therefore, where the homeostasis in most fragile. Similarly, Snow (1991) suggests that therapies can either capitalize on a client's/patient's strength or compensate for a particular deficiency. These views are consistent with the recent findings from the NIMH Collaborative Depression study (Elkin *et al.*, 1989) where better social adjustment at intake predicted a better and differential response to interpersonal therapy, and fewer dysfunctional attitudes were associated with a better and differential response to cognitive therapy (Sotsky *et al.*, 1991).

We also recommend targeting dysfunction in any of the psychosocial factors that we reviewed earlier as influencing the course of depression. A combined approach, whereby the therapist builds on the client's/patient's strengths and improves functioning in dysfunctional or deficient areas, may help to prevent relapse. For instance, a depressed woman who has good interpersonal skills and a strong social network may be having marital difficulties that over time have contrib-

uted to her sense of worthlessness and unlovability, social withdrawal, and to her depression. The therapist may help her to increase her social interactions, so as to give her experiences that contradict her feelings of being worthless and unlovable, but the problems in the marital relationship are likely to continue. In this case, it may be useful to encourage the couple to seek marital therapy, since behavioral marital therapy can alleviate both the symptoms of depression and improve marital satisfaction (e.g., Jacobson *et al.*, 1991).

Beckham (1990) also hypothesizes that the depressive homeostasis is more resistant to intervention in those with long histories of low self-esteem, ineffectual social functioning, or chronically dysfunctional families. In these cases, so many aspects of the client's/patient's life represent problem areas that there is no easily identifiable weak link in the depressive feedback loop. In such a system, changes in one domain may not be powerful enough to effect a therapeutic change in another. We also apply this principle to those with comorbid personality disorders, which are longstanding maladaptive and interpersonal patterns that can set the stage for depression.

A treatment-resistant depressive homeostasis is typified by the adult female client/patient who has had a history of being sexually abused throughout childhood. Since many of her problems may center around dysfunctional relationships, it is reasonable to hypothesize that the establishment of a warm, supportive, trusting therapeutic relationship may serve as a model for other relationships outside of therapy, thus breaking into a depressive cycle that is otherwise perpetuated by isolation or abuse. However, such a client/patient may have become extremely distrustful of others, and as a result will not easily collaborate with the therapist, regardless of the genuine good will that the therapist may demonstrate. Or, she may believe the sincere intentions of the therapist, but also firmly believe that she is a "bad" person, undeserving of the therapist's positive regard. This self-concept will impede interventions geared to break the cycle of depression. Therapy for those clients/patients with a relatively stable dysphoric homeostasis requires more intensive and broadly based interventions that aim to replace gradually the old behaviors and patterns with new ones.

We recommend involving the client/patient in establishing the target components and setting of therapeutic goals so that the individual does not become overwhelmed or lose motivation. Involvement in the process allows the person to feel in some control and to better understand the complexity of depression and the process of change. This can be used to challenge the common expectations of immediate improvement or no improvement.

The selection of techniques from this integrative perspective is based on a conceptualization of the strengths and dysfunctions that maintain the depressive homeostasis for a given individual. From this, the therapist can generate the principles of change relevant to that client/patient and select techniques that will effect these changes. This requires an awareness of the literature on the principles of the therapeutic change process and on the treatments that are effective in mobilizing these change processes. For instance, when the client/patient is both depressed and in a discordant marriage, interpersonal change is likely to facilitate a change in the symptoms of depression. In line with this, behavioral marital therapy has been demonstrated to have a two-pronged effect, improving the symptoms of depression and marital satisfaction. A person with negative interpersonal and self schemata and interpersonal difficulties is likely to benefit from Safran and Segal's (1990) cognitive-interpersonal approach because the therapist can work with an *in vivo* sample of the client's/patient's problems and access more affectively-laden ("hot") cognitions. This is consistent with a principle of change that emerges across orientations: Whenever possible, it is important to work with client/patients using *in vivo*, affectively-charged material to facilitate cognitive, affective, and behavioral shifts (for a review, see Goldfried & Hayes, 1989). This principle suggests the use of transference and countertransference in the therapy sessions, as well as affect-enhancing techniques, such as the gestalt two-chair technique (Greenberg, 1984; Perls, 1973) and variations of behavioral exposure therapy, when appropriate. We also recommend considering the client's/patient's personality style when selecting treatments and the most parsimonious way of combining treatments to target the most areas of functioning.

CASE EXAMPLE

Hale is a single, white male, aged 25, living near a major university. He had recently gained admission to a prestigious law school, but decided to defer his acceptance of their offer, following the onset of a significant depressive episode.

Assessment and Conceptualization

At the start of treatment, Hale underwent a comprehensive initial psychological assessment. (Note: We say "initial" because the assessment phase of therapy continues throughout the course of treatment, as new clinical material comes to light.) This evaluation was comprised of the following:

1. Self-report questionnaires (mailed to the client's/patient's home in advance of the first appointment) that focus on: (a) current life situation (school, work, relationships, etc.), and (b) historical information about the client's/patient's upbringing, culture, schooling, employment, medical and psychological health and treatment, patterns in important familial and romantic relationships, and social integration.

2. Structured diagnostic interview, using the Structured Clinical Interview for the DSM-III-R (SCID) (American Psychiatric Association, 1987).

3. Self-report depression inventories, such as the Beck Depression Inventory (BDI) (Beck, Steer, & Garbin, 1988) and the Hamilton Rating Scale for Depression (Hamilton, 1960) were used periodically throughout the course of therapy to measure therapeutic change and maintenance.

4. Structured clinical interview about current and past suicidality.

5. Open-ended interview to assess each of the variables listed in Table 1. A number of self-report inventories are available to assess these variables, but the clinician needs to balance a careful assessment with overwhelming the client/patient.

6. Hale's girlfriend also was included in two of the later sessions.

Based on Hale's initial assessment, the following information was obtained. His depression met DSM-III criteria for Recurrent Major Depression. He also had significant features of Obsessive-Compulsive Personality Disorder and Passive-Aggressive Personality Disorder, but did not meet the DSM-III-R criteria for either.

Hale reported two previous episodes of clinical depression: one at the age of 15, and another at the age of 18. The therapist (CFN) sought to determine what was happening in his life at these times. The first depression coincided with the older brother's leaving home to go to college, while he was left to work on his parents' farm and was discouraged from going to college. Parental pressures escalated, and they were especially unsympathetic and "ashamed" by his emotional problems. This was in sharp contrast to their outwardly expressed pride at the older brother's beginning college studies at an Ivy League school.

At the time of the second depression, Hale was starting his freshman year at the same school in which his brother was now a senior. While most of the family's attention was turned toward the brother's acceptance into medical school, Hale was silently vowing that he would one day achieve an advanced degree himself, and that he would *not* allow his family to chart the course of his life for him. When Hale confronted his parents with these sentiments, they blamed it on the influence of his "new, rich friends." They threatened to cut off his funding if he did not promise to return to the farm following graduation. This precipitated a full-blown clinical depression, and Hale was forced to take a lengthy medical leave of absence. Once again, he reported that the family felt stigmatized by his need for psychological attention and psychotropic medication. It was at this time that he began having suicidal thoughts, but he did not carry them out because he was determined to not let his parents "win." These suicidal thoughts recurred at times when Hale felt most invalidated by his parents.

Hale explained to his therapist that the symptoms of his current episode of depression came to the fore as he began to ponder the rigors of law school after his acceptance. He determined that he was lacking the emotional and intellectual skills that would be necessary to make the grade. The more he thought about this, the more sad, anxious, and hopeless he felt. This, in turn, confirmed his notion that he was not emotionally fit to survive the stressors that inevitably lay before him. Due to fear of failure, Hale asked for a deferment and continued working as a paralegal in

order to support himself financially, and to stay in the field in case he chose to begin his law school career the following year. At intake, he was not suicidal.

Hale had sought a psychiatrist for his first two episodes and received pharmacotherapy with positive effects. He complied with his medication regimen and attended all of his sessions with the psychiatrist. Since it had been nearly 10 years since Hale had seen the psychiatrist, it was not necessary to contact him. He decided to begin psychotherapy because this was his third episode of depression and he wanted to learn to prevent it.

As seen in Figure 1, all of this information can be depicted visually in the timeline that we described earlier. Although Hale had some Axis II features, these disorders generally do not lend themselves to a timeline because of their chronic course. However, they will be addressed in the development of his homeostatic model.

The following information was gathered to develop a profile of the strengths and weaknesses maintaining his current depressive homeostasis. Hale had grown up on a farm in rural New Jersey. He was the second son in a family of six children, raised as strict Baptists. The father was described as "distant, authoritarian, critical, and a harsh disciplinarian," while the mother was dubbed "controlling, though she could be caring." They were very sparing of praise, and Hale believed that he had worked hard all his life to gain but a meager amount of parental approval. He tried to do everything well to get his parents' approval, but began to feel that nothing that he did mattered. Relationships with siblings were termed "good," except for his relationship with his older brother, with whom things were "tense." His older brother seemed to get all of the parents' attention that he felt he could never get, no matter what he did. As a result, he felt that his parents did not love him because he was not as successful as his brother. If his own parents did not love him, he reasoned, nobody could.

Hale harbored a significant amount of anger. When asked if he was angry with his parents and his brother, he stated that he was furious, but that he could not express his feelings. When angry with his family, he felt guilty and was afraid that they would disown him if they knew how he felt.

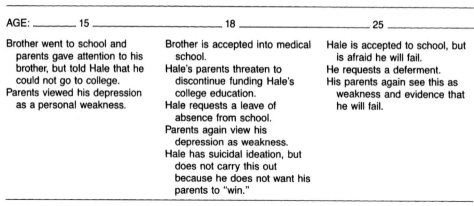

Figure 1. Hale's timeline.

Therefore, he communicated his anger indirectly and his parents viewed him as rebellious. He then tried even harder to control his anger and any positive feelings that he had for his family to avoid getting hurt. During his second depressive episode, Hale thought of trying to kill himself because then perhaps his parents would see how angry and hurt he was. These thoughts recurred when he felt invalidated and ridiculed by his parents, and contributed further to his feeling emotionally "weak" in their eyes.

In light of all of this conflict, it is not surprising that Hale had strongly mixed feelings about his identity and direction in life. Although he wanted to prove that he could be a success in the same manner as his brother, he felt that his persistence in pursuing a law degree might be a dreadful mistake. First, he had internalized his parents' critical view of him, and he believed deeply that he was a "weak" person. He therefore reasoned that he would not be able to meet the demands that law school and a career in law would present him. In fact, he even believed that he was admitted because of a clerical error and was dreading the day when he received the call that would confirm his belief. Second, even if he somehow "miraculously" graduated, he anticipated that he would become inextricably "caught between two worlds, belonging to neither." He expected that he would forever become the black sheep of his family, never again being able to return to his rural, religious life with his parents and their

community. At the same time, he determined that he would always be ill-equipped to compete with his colleagues, all of whom he saw as being decidedly more "cosmopolitan" and experienced in worldly affairs than he.

Hale noted that while in college, he had always done objectively well in school, although he dreaded exams, and often became run-down and ill during periods of academic pressure. He was afraid that if he failed, his parents would mock him and he would have to return to the farm and live the life that they demanded of him. He also thought that if he could do everything perfectly, his parents would give him attention, as they did his older brother. As a result, he became extremely anxious when studying, procrastinated, stay·d up all night, and ran himself down. This anxiety slowed him down and clouded his thinking, confirming his belief that he would not make it.

Although he had many acquaintances, he had few friendships, owing to his assumptions that if you get close to people they will hurt you, and that people did not think highly of him. He avoided people when he was depressed because he thought that the few people who did like him liked "Happy Hale" and would think less of him if they saw "Depressed Hale." Although he was involved in a romantic relationship at the time he entered therapy, he predicted that this soon would end because "Leslie fell in love with the Hale who was happy, not the person I am now."

She expressed her frustration because she constantly had to reassure him that she loved him and had no intention of leaving. She was Hale's primary source of support.

To prepare for people leaving him, Hale did not get close to people nor express positive emotions. To make matters worse, he put himself down before others did. His girlfriend and his two close friends gave him feedback on this maladaptive style, and he took this as proof that he was indeed socially defective. He ignored the positive feedback about his sardonic wit and how his friends missed him when he would withdraw from them.

The profile of strengths and weaknesses relevant to Hale's homeostatic model are described in Table 2. Based on this model, Hale and his therapist collaboratively worked on a list of goals for treatment. These included:

1. Improve his mood, sleep, and energy level.

2. Improve his relationships with his girlfriend and his friends.

3. Learn to view himself in a more confident and positive light by exploring some of his negative cognitions concerning his perceived weakness, incompetence, and feelings of being unloved.

4. Address his identity crisis.

5. Come to a firm decision on whether or not to go to law school.

6. Learn to explore his feelings (especially his anger) and cope with his perceived role in the family. At the very least, to be able to assert himself with his parents and ignore their harsh criticisms. At best, act as a catalyst to change the family system by expressing his feelings more directly.

Seeing that Hale's obsessive-compulsive personality features might continue to pose difficulties for him if left unaddressed, the therapist asked Hale if they could add two more goals.

7. Become more comfortable experiencing and demonstrating positive feelings for others.

8. Become more willing to make important decisions, even if he is not 100% certain that they are "perfect" decisions.

Table 2. Profile of Strengths and Dysfunctions for the Hale's Depressive Homeostasis

COGNITIONS	PERSONALITY
Maladaptive *Attributional Style*:	*Introverted*
(e.g., his acceptance into law school was a fluke, helplessness)	*Interpersonally Dependent*:
Dysfunctional Attitudes:	Needs constant reassurance
"I am weak because I am depressed"	Others must like/love him or he is worthless
"My parents don't love me because I am weak and stupid"	**IDENTITY**
"Because my own parents don't love me, nobody will"	*Sources of Self-Esteem*:
"I am going to fail"	Achievements and opinions of others
Hopelessness:	*Roles*: Black sheep of the family
Sought therapy to help himself	*Conflicts*:
Hopeless, but not suicidal	"Between two worlds"
	"Happy Hale," "Depressed Hale"
	"Passive Hale," "Angry Hale"
COPING SKILLS	**SOCIAL SKILLS**
Problem-Solving:	Good sense of humor, friends like him
Avoidance, procrastination, lowering expectations for himself	Awkward, self-effacing, guarded
Affective Processing and Regulation:	**RELATIONSHIPS**
Suppresses anger and positive feelings	*Mate*: Good, supportive, he needs reassurance
Impulse Control: No impulsive behavior, has not acted on suicidal thoughts	*Family*: Parents controlling, critical, rivalry with older brother
Defenses: Distance, isolation of affect, self-effacing	*General*: No problems at work, friends like him
	Social Integration: Low, one support

Treatment Selection
and the Process of Therapy

A close watch was kept on Hale's weekly responses on the Beck Depression Inventory (BDI). For the first four sessions, his scores hovered around 30, which is indicative of a severe level of depression in those who are so diagnosed. His sleep disturbance was particularly marked, with concomitant negative effects on his levels of energy and motivation. After discussing the pros and cons of taking medication, Hale and his therapist jointly decided that Hale would meet with a psychiatric consultant, who ultimately prescribed an antidepressant with somnolent qualities. All parties agreed that Hale might benefit best from a *combination* of psychotherapy and medication, as both physiological and somatic symptoms were quite prominent.

As therapy progressed, Hale and his therapist worked to conceptualize his problems from a number of different "angles," including behavioral, cognitive, experiential, interpersonal, psychodynamic, family systems, and psychobiological. Hale learned to appreciate the fact that his *internal* conflicts were every bit as important as his *interpersonal* conflicts with his parents, brothers, and peers. He began to understand how his role within his family system influenced his view of himself *outside* the home. He gained insight into the interrelations between his thinking patterns, his emotionality, and his overt actions. For example, he noticed that certain behaviors (going to see a movie with his housemates) could improve his mood, even if he had not "felt like" engaging in those behaviors in the first place. Related to this, he also learned that being physically active could increase his energy level. Additionally, Hale became adept at self-monitoring thoughts that exacerbated his mood and drained him of energy. He increased his self-awareness of positive feelings toward others, and realized that he avoided displays of such emotions out of a belief that a "weak" person such as he would be rendered even *more* vulnerable if others knew he was attached to them.

A significant breakthrough in understanding was achieved when the therapist helped Hale to assess his own "vicious cycles" (Beitman, 1987; Safran & Segal, 1990; Wachtel, 1977). For example,

his assumption that others would think negatively of him led him to call inappropriate attention to his own shortcomings. He had reasoned that being the first person to "call himself" on his problems would diminish the other person's negative view of him. In actuality, when he reexamined these interpersonal situations from memory and *in vivo*, he realized that his actions led to *awkwardness* in his interactions with others, leading them to see him as a "downer" and perhaps as too self-centered. Picking up on these negative feelings, Hale would take this as confirmation that he was socially defective, and would work that much harder to "correct" the situation by escalating his self-deprecation—and so, the vicious cycle would continue.

As these understandings were achieved, Hale's BDI scores diminished somewhat into the low 20s. Although his sleeping patterns were back to normal by the fifteenth therapy session (perhaps as a result of his medication), his BDI scores were still in the "moderately depressed" range, and many of the aforementioned goals were still as far away from Hale's grasp as when therapy began. In trying to understand the reason for this lack of progress, the therapist reflected on the case and realized that Hale had been avoiding many of his between-session assignments. Such assignments had included cognitive self-monitoring and rational responding regarding his sense of weakness, incompetence, and feelings of being unloved; generating and acting on ideas to break vicious cycles in interpersonal relationships, such as behavioral experiments in assertiveness, public displays of appropriate self-confidence, disinhibiting his positive statements toward family, friends, and girlfriend; and problem-solving with regard to his decision about law school.

Over time, the therapist noticed that he was working very hard with this client/patient, and enjoying the process less and less. He felt that Hale was demanding and critical, asking the therapist to justify all his suggestions and formulations to the "nth degree," to the point that the therapist became overly directive and vociferous in support of his own views and rationales. The therapist, upon observation of his own reactions, realized that he was thinking that "I'll have to work very, very hard with Hale, and he'll *still* be critical of me and of therapy. He won't appreciate my help and he won't change."

After pondering this, the therapist hit upon a potential hypothesis—namely, that Hale saw similarities between the therapist and his brother (after all, they were both professionals, of comparable age, and arguably in positions of "superiority" to the client/patient). The therapist's empathy for Hale grew almost immediately, while his dread for dealing with him in session diminished precipitously. The therapist chose to openly, but tactfully, address this hypothesis with Hale in the next session.

In order not to force an interpretation on Hale, which might exacerbate his resistance, the therapist carefully asked Hale if he would share his thoughts on how therapy was progressing to date. He made it clear that he valued Hale's opinions, and would take direction from them. In response, Hale was not as critical as he had been, but noted that he was fast arriving at the conclusion that only he could help himself—that the therapist was well-meaning, but not the person for the job.

At that moment, the therapist began to ask Socratic questions (cf. Beck, Shaw, Rush, & Emery, 1979) about other areas in Hale's life where this was true. After much discussion, Hale noted that as he grew up, his brother was always in charge of "keeping Hale in line," and "helping him out." The therapist asked Hale to close his eyes, relax, and imagine an actual memory when this had been particularly painful. Hale shed a few tears as he remembered a time when he passed a difficult geometry test after the brother had "tutored" him in an unsolicited and cursory fashion. When Hale returned home with his well-earned "A" proudly displayed, his father raved on and on about how wonderful the brother's teaching and coaching skills were.

When all was said and done in the therapy session, an important new understanding had been achieved. Hale believed that the therapist was "re-enacting the crime" mentioned above. Hale implicitly believed that his improvement in therapy would be a victory for the therapist (i.e., the older brother), thus giving Hale a powerful disincentive for changing in treatment, and an equally compelling motive for trying to "defeat" the therapist by remaining depressed.

Throughout this discussion, the therapist was vigilant in his expressions of support, humility, willingness to cooperate with Hale, and his *respect* for Hale. To Hale, these were the missing ingredients in his relationships with family members. Hale and his therapist agreed that the type of interpersonal overgeneralization between brother and therapist might occur in other relationships as well, and might reoccur in the therapeutic relationship under times of stress. From this point forward, the tug-of-war between client/patient and therapist lessened considerably, and Hale engaged in between-session assignments (of his own choosing) to a significantly greater extent.

Wachtel and Wachtel (1986) present convincing arguments regarding the value of obtaining therapeutic information from important people in the client's/patient's life. This was borne out in the therapy with Hale. Sessions 27 and 28 included Leslie, his girlfriend. Her role was to provide feedback that would highlight how she and others felt and thought about Hale. The therapist's job was to openly compare this to the content of Hale's previously stated assumptions on this matter. Hale's responsibility was to reconcile any inconsistencies between the two reports.

Not surprising, but most helpful, was the fact that Leslie provided viewpoints that were diametrically opposed to some of Hale's most self-defeating attitudes about himself and others. With heartfelt sincerity, and using an array of concrete examples to support her claims, Leslie provided information suggesting that her love for Hale was based on him as a whole person, not just the "happy Hale." The fact that she was still with him eight months after he had predicted she would leave him supported this assertion. Furthermore, Leslie challenged Hale's view that he had lost favor in his college friends' eyes because he had not yet entered law school. In fact, she reported, many of them were urging her for all of them to get together socially, as they missed Hale's company.

Hale's first inclination was to dispute Leslie's statements. However, earlier the therapist had Hale articulate the respect and faith he had in Leslie's judgment, so that he was forced to consider her complimentary comments more favorably. These two sessions were prime movers in helping Hale to take more interpersonal risks between sessions. His relationship with Leslie solidified (he even met her parents for the first time), and his social calendar gradually filled up.

At this point, Hale was ready to address his identity conflicts. The two-chair technique was used to help Hale separate what he wanted from what he thought his parents wanted. This technique was chosen because he was so intellectualized and had isolated his angry feelings and sense of self. Through this process, he was able to access his anger toward his parents for not accepting him and for telling him that he would "just get by" in life, while they openly adored his older brother. He also expressed his anger toward the side of himself that suppressed his needs and tried to please everybody. The angry side of himself then began to express firmly that he did not want to be a farmworker and that he wanted to be a lawyer. He told himself that he was intelligent, hard-working, and had the potential to be a good lawyer. At the end of the session, Hale was surprised to see this part of himself and reported feeling relieved and strong. He had known what he wanted all along but was afraid that he would fail and that he would disappoint his parents by not working on the farm.

At session 35, Hale announced that he had decided to enter law school, which would begin in two months. His mood had improved considerably, he had begun tapering off the medication under the psychiatrist's supervision, and many of his goals were at least partially achieved. Hale requested that therapy sessions be held less frequently, and that formal therapy be terminated when the first semester began. His rationale was that therapy had given him a "jump start," and now he wished to carry out the majority of the work himself. The therapist agreed, making sure to leave the door open for Hale to return for booster sessions during the course of the school year. Hale was given the profile of strengths and weaknesses related to his homeostatic model to allow him to see the progress that he had made and to remind him of old patterns that he would need to keep an eye on to prevent relapse. His procrastination, perfectionism, and fears of failure were reviewed, as were strategies to counteract them. Hale was also encouraged to continue to improve his relationship with his parents.

Hale's BDI scores for the final five sessions (36–40) were consistently below a score of 6 (negligible symptoms). At follow-up, 4 months later, he was still feeling good about himself and about his life. He proudly reported on his success in getting through a stressful semester, on his ever-diminishing social self-consciousness, his strong relationship with Leslie, and an improvement in his coping skills when he would go home to the farm for holiday get-togethers. Hale expressed his satisfaction with therapy, and with the therapist, yet another example of his improvement, as he so rarely had expressed positive feelings toward others in the past. At the time of the writing of this chapter, it has been eighteen months since Hale's most recent check-up session.

CONCLUSIONS

A homeostatic model of depression is the foundation of the integrative approach that we present. What this integrative approach demonstrates is that there is no single, simple treatment for the depressive syndrome. However, by evaluating an entire spectrum of psychosocial variables, in the present and in the past, therapists have an opportunity to come to a more complete understanding of each individual depressed client/patient, and to apply a wide range of interventions that have clear conceptual rationales and testable outcomes.

The next stage is to conduct aptitude-treatment interaction (ATI) research. The goal of the ATI strategy is to provide more empirically-based guidelines for matching client/patient types to different therapies, so as to increase treatment efficacy (for a review, see the special section of the *Journal of Consulting and Clinical Psychology*, April, 1991). Process research across therapies will contribute a growing body of knowledge on the principles of change that are so important in treatment formulation from an integrative perspective. Finally, we suggest that researchers include each of the specific targets of treatment (e.g. maladaptive schemata, intepersonal functioning) as measures of outcome, in addition to the standard measures of self-reported improvement in depression. We look forward to being a part of this exciting movement in psychotherapy and psychotherapy research.

REFERENCES

Abramson, L. Y., Metalsky, G. I., & Alloy, L. B. (1989). Hopelessness depression: A theory-based subtype of depression. *Psychological Review, 96,* 358–372.

Akiskal, H. S., & McKinney, W. T. (1973). Depressive disorders: Toward a unified hypothesis. *Science, 182,* 20–29.

American Psychiatric Association. (1987). *Diagnostic and statistical manual of mental disorders* (3rd ed. rev.). Washington, DC: Author.

Arkowitz, H., & Hannah, M. T. (1989). Cognitive, behavioral, and psychodynamic therapies. In A. Freeman, K. M. Simon, L. E. Beutler & H. Arkowitz (Eds.), *Comprehensive handbook of cognitive therapy* (pp. 143–167). New York: Plenum Press.

Barnett, P., & Gotlib, I. (1988). Psychosocial functioning and depression: Distinguishing among antecedents, concomitants, and consequences. *Psychological Bulletin, 104,* 97–126.

Barry, W. A. (1970). Marriage research and conflict: An integrative review. *Psychological Bulletin, 73,* 41–54.

Beach, S. R. H., Jouriles, E. N., & O'Leary, K. D. (1985). Extramarital sex: Impact on depression and commitment in couples seeking marital therapy. *Journal of Sex and Marital Therapy, 11,* 99–108.

Beach, S. R. H., Sandeen, E. E., & O'Leary, K. D. (1990). *Depression in marriage: A model for etiology and treatment.* New York: Guilford.

Beck, A. T. (1976). *Cognitive therapy and the emotional disorders.* New York: International University Press.

Beck, A. T. (1983). Cognitive therapy of depression: New perspectives. In P. M. Clayton & Y. E. Barrett (Eds.), *Treatment of depression: Old controversies and new approaches* (pp. 265–290). New York: Raven Press.

Beck, A. T., & Steer, R. A. (1990). Dr. Beck and Dr. Steer reply [Letter]. *American Journal of Psychiatry, 147,* 1577–1578.

Beck, A. T., Rush, A. J., Shaw, B. F., & Emery, G. (1979). *Cognitive therapy of depression.* New York: Guilford.

Beck, A. T., Steer, R. A., & Garbin, M. G. (1988). Psychometric properties of the Beck Depression Inventory: Twenty-five years later. *Clinical Psychology Review, 8,* 77–100.

Beck, A. T., Brown, G., & Steer, R. A. (1989). Prediction of eventual suicide in psychiatric inpatients by clinical ratings of hopelessness. *Journal of Consulting and Clinical Psychology, 57,* 309–310.

Beckham, E. E. (1990). Psychotherapy of depression research at a crossroads: Directions for the 1990s. *Clinical Psychology Review, 10,* 207–228.

Beitman, B. D. (1987). *The structure of individual psychotherapy.* New York: Guilford.

Bellack, A. S., Hersen, M., & Himmelhoch, J. (1981). Social skills training compared with pharmacotherapy and psychotherapy in the treatment of unipolar depression. *American Journal of Psychiatry, 138,* 1562–1567.

Beutler, L. E., & Clarkin, J. F. (1990). *Systematic treatment selection: Toward targeted therapeutic interventions.* New York: Brunner/Mazel.

Beutler, L. E., Engle, D., Mohr, D., Daldrup, R. J., Bergan, J., Meredith, K., & Merry, W. (1991). Predictors of differential response to cognitive, experiential, and self-directed psychotherapeutic procedures. *Journal of Consulting and Clinical Psychology, 59,* 333–340.

Blatt, S. J., D'Afflitti, J. P., & Quinlan, D. M. (1976). Experiences of depression in normal young adults. *Journal of Abnormal Psychology, 85,* 383–389.

Brown, G. W., & Harris, T. (1978). *Social origins of depression.* London: Free Press.

Brown, G. W., Adler, Z., & Bifulco, A. (1988). Life events, difficulties, and recovery from chronic depression. *British Journal of Psychiatry, 152,* 487–498.

Coyne, J. C. (1976). Toward an interactional description of depression. *Psychiatry, 39,* 28–40.

Coyne, J. C. (1990). Interpersonal processes in depression. In G. I. Keitner (Ed.). *Depression and families: Impact and treatment* (pp. 31–53). Washington DC: American Psychiatric Press.

Coyne, J. C., Kahn, J., & Gotlib, I. H. (1987). Depression. In T. Jacob (Ed.), *Family interaction and psychopathology* (pp. 509–534). New York: Plenum Press.

Craighead, W. E. (1980). Away from a unitary model of depression. *Behavior Therapy, 11,* 122–128.

Craighead, W. E., Kennedy, R. E., Raczynski, J. M., & Dow, M. G. (1984). Affective disorders-unipolar. In S. M. Turner and M. Hersen (Eds.), *Adult psychopathology: A behavioral perspective* (pp. 184–244). New York: Wiley.

Daldrup, R. J., Beutler, L. E., Engle, D., & Greenberg, L. S. (1988). *Focused expressive psychotherapy: Freeing the overcontrolled patient.* New York: Guilford.

DeRubeis, R. J., Evans, M. D., Hollon, S. D., Garvey, M. J., Grove, W. M., & Tuason, V. B. (1990). How does cognitive therapy work? Cognitive change and symptom change in cognitive therapy and pharmacotherapy for depression. *Journal of Consulting and Clinical Psychology, 58,* 862–869.

Elkin, I., Shea, T., Watkins, J. T., Imber, S. D., Sotsky, S. M., Collins, J. F., Glass, D. R., Pilkonis, P. A., Leber, W. R., Docherty, J. P., Fiester, S. J., & Parloff, M. B. (1989). National Institute of Mental Health Treatment of Depression Collaborative Research Program: General effectiveness of treatments. *Archives of General Psychiatry, 46,* 971–982.

Evans, M., Hollon, S. D., & DeRubeis, R. J. (1989). *Differential relapse following cognitive therapy, pharmacotherapy, and combined cognitive-pharmacotherapy for depression: A two-year follow-up of the CPT project.* Manuscript submitted for publication.

Frank, E., Kupfer, D. J., Wagner, M. S., McEachran, A. B., & Cornes, C. (1991). Efficacy of interpersonal psychotherapy as a maintenance treatment of recurrent depression. *Archives of General Psychiatry, 48,* 1053–1059.

Goldfried, M. R. (1980). Toward the delineation of therapeutic change principles. *American Psychologist, 35,* 991–999.

Goldfried, M. R., & Hayes, A. M. (1989). Can contributions from other orientations complement behavior therapy? *Behavior Therapist, 12,* 57–60.

Goldfried, M. R., & Newman, C. F. (1986, August). *A look at what therapists actually do.* Paper presented at the annual meeting of the American Psychological Association, Washington, DC.

Gotlib, I., & Hooley, J. M. (1988). Depression and marital distress: Current status and future directions. In S. Duck (Ed.), *Handbook of personal relationships* (pp. 563–570). New York: Wiley.

Greenberg, L. S. (1984). A task analysis of intrapersonal conflict resolution. In L. N. Rice & L. S. Greenberg (Eds.), *Patterns of change* (pp. 67–123). New York: Guilford.

Guze, S., & Robins, E. (1970). Suicide and primary affective disorders. *British Journal of Psychiatry, 117,* 437–438.

Haaga, D. A. F., Dyck, M. J., & Ernst, D. (1991). Empirical status of cognitive theory of depression. *Psychological Bulletin, 110,* 215–236.

Hamilton, M. (1960). A rating scale for depression. *Journal of Neurology, Neurosurgery, and Psychiatry, 23,* 56–62.

Hammen, C., Ellicott, A., Gitlin, M., & Jamison, K. R. (1989). Sociotropy/autonomy and vulnerability to specific life events in patients with unipolar depression and bipolar disorders. *Journal of Abnormal Psychology, 98,* 154–160.

Hayes, A. M. (1990, November). *A comparison of three psychotherapies for depression: The search for mechanisms of change* (Chair). Symposium conducted at the meeting of the Association for Advancement of Behavior Therapy, San Francisco.

Heppner, P. P., Baumgardner, A., & Jackson, J. (1985). Problem solving self appraisal, depression, and attributional style: Are they related? *Cognitive Therapy and Research, 9,* 105–113.

Hoberman, H. M. (1990). Behavioral treatments for unipolar depression. In B. B. Wolman & Stricker, G. (Eds.), *Depressive disorders: Facts, theories and treatment methods* (pp. 310–342). New York: Wiley.

Hollon, S. D., Shelton, R. C., & Loosen, P. T. (1991). Cognitive therapy and pharmacotherapy for depression. *Journal of Consulting and Clinical Psychology, 59,* 88–99.

Hooley, J. M. (1990). Expressed emotion and depression. In G. I. Keitner (Ed.), *Depression and families: Impact and treatment.* (pp. 57–83). Washington DC: American Psychiatric Press.

Hooley, J. M., & Teasdale, J. D. (1989). Predictors of relapse in unipolar depressives: Expressed emotion, marital distress, and perceived criticism. *Journal of Abnormal Psychology, 98,* 229–235.

Jacobson, N. S., & Holtzworth-Munroe, A. (1986). Marital therapy: A social learning/cognitive perspective. In N. S. Jacobson & S. Gurman (Eds.), *Clinical handbook of marital therapy.* New York: Guilford.

Jacobson, N. S., Dobson, K., Fruzzetti, A. E., Schmaling, K. B., & Salusky, S. (1991). Marital therapy as a treatment for depression. *Journal of Consulting and Clinical Psychology, 59,* 547–557.

Jarrett, R. B. (1990). Psychosocial aspects of depression and the role of psychotherapy. *Journal of Clinical Psychiatry, 51,* 26–35.

Karasu, T. B. (1990). Toward a clinical model of psychotherapy for depression: II: An integrative and selective treatment approach. *American Journal of Psychiatry, 147,* 269–278.

Keitner, G. I., & Miller, I. W. (1990). Family functioning and major depression: An overview. *American Journal of Psychiatry, 147,* 1128–1137.

Klerman, G. L., Weissman, M. M., Rounsaville, B. J., & Chevron, E. S. (1984). *Interpersonal psychotherapy of depression.* New York: Basic Books.

Lazarus, A. A., (1971). *Behavior therapy and beyond.* New York: McGraw-Hill.

Lewinsohn, P. M., Antonuccio, D. O., Steinmetz, T. L., & Teri, L. (1984). *The coping with depression course.* Eugene, OR: Castalia Publishing.

Luborsky, L. (1984). *Principles of psychoanalytic psychotherapy: A manual for supportive-expressive treatment.* New York: Basic Books.

Nezu, A. M., Kalmar, K., Ronan, G. F., & Clarijo, A. (1986). Attributional correlates of depression: An interactional model including problem solving. *Behavior Therapy, 17,* 50–56.

Nezu, A. M., Nezu, C. M., & Perri, M. G. (1989). *Problem-solving therapy for depression: Theory, research, and clinical guidelines.* New York: Wiley.

O'Leary, K. D., & Beach, S. R. H. (1990). Marital therapy: A viable treatment for depression and marital discord. *American Journal of Psychiatry, 147,* 183–186.

Paykel, E. S. (1919). Recent life events in the development of the depressive disorder. In R. A. Depue (Ed.), *The psychobiology of depressive disorders: Implications for the effects of stress.* New York: Academic Press.

Perls, F. (1973). *The gestalt approach and eye witness therapy.* Palo Alto, CA: Science and Behavior Books, Bantam Edition.

Rehm, L. P. (1984). Self-management therapy for depression. *Advances in Behavior Research and Therapy, 6,* 83–98.

Renne, K. S. (1970). Correlates of dissatisfaction in marriage. *Journal of Marriage and the Family, 32,* 54–67.

Robins, C. J., & Hayes, A. M. (in press). The prediction of depression. In G. Buchanan & M. E. P. Seligman (Eds.), *Explanatory style.* Hillsdale, NJ: Lawrence Erlbaum.

Robinson, L. A., Berman, J. S., & Neimeyer, R. A. (1990). Psychotherapy for the treatment of depression: A comprehensive review of controlled outcome research. *Psychological Bulletin, 108,* 30–49.

Rush, A. J., Beck, A. T., Kovacs, M., Weissenburger, J., & Hollon, S. D. (1982). Comparison of the effects of cognitive therapy and pharmacotherapy on hopelessness and self-concept. *American Journal of Psychiatry, 139,* 862–866.

Rush, A. J., Weissenburger, J., & Eaves, G. (1986). Do thinking patterns predict depressive symptoms? *Cognitive Therapy and Research, 10,* 255–236.

Safran, J., & Segal, Z. V. (1990). *Interpersonal process in cognitive therapy.* New York: Basic Books.

Shelton, R. C., Hollon, S. D., Purdon, S. E., & Loosen, P. T. (1991). Biological and psychological aspects of depression. *Behavior Therapy, 22,* 201–228.

Simons, A. D., Murphy, G. E., Levine, J. L., & Wetzel, R. D. (1986). Cognitive therapy and pharmacotherapy for depression: Sustained improvement over one year. *Archives of General Psychiatry, 43,* 43–48.

Snow, R. E. (1991). Aptitude-treatment interaction as a framework for research on individual differences in psychotherapy. *Journal of Consulting and Clinical Psychology, 59,* 205–216.

Sotsky, S. M., Glass, D. R., Shea, T., Pilkonis, P. A., Collins, J. F., Elkin, I., Watkins, J. T., Imber, S. D., Leber, W. R., Moyer, J., & Oliveri, M. E. (1991). Patient predictors of response to psychotherapy and pharmacotherapy: Findings in the NIMH Treatment of Depression Collaborative Research Program. *American Journal of Psychiatry, 148,* 997–1008.

Strupp, H. H., & Binder, J. (1984). *Psychotherapy in a new key.* New York: Plenum Press.

Svartberg, M., & Stiles, T. C. (1991). Comparative effects of short-term psychodynamic psychotherapy: A meta-analysis. *Journal of Consulting and Clinical Psychology, 59,* 704–714.

Swann, W. B., & Predmore, S. C. (1985). Intimates as agents of social support: Sources of consolation or despair? *Journal of Personality and Social Psychology, 49,* 1609–1617.

Thase, M. E. (1990). Relapse and recurrence in unipolar major depression: Short-term and long-term approaches. *Journal of Clinical Psychiatry, 51,* 51–57.

Wachtel, P. L. (1977). *Psychoanalysis and behavior therapy: Toward an integration.* New York: Basic Books.

Wachtel, E. F., & Wachtel, P. L. (1986). *Family dynamics in individual psychotherapy.* New York: Guilford.

Weissman, M. M., & Myers, J. (1978). Affective disorders in a U.S. urban community: The use of the Research Diag-nostic Criteria in an epidemiological survey. *Archives of General Psychiatry, 35,* 1304–1311.

Weissman, M. M., & Paykel, E. S. (1974). *The depressed woman.* Chicago, IL: University of Chicago Press.

Whisman, M. A., Miller, I. W., Norman, W. H., & Keitner, G. I. (1991). Cognitive therapy with depressed inpatients: Specific effects on dysfunctional cognitions. *Journal of Consulting and Clinical Psychology, 59,* 282–288.

CHAPTER 22

Psychotherapy Integration with Character Disorders

Jerold R. Gold and George Stricker

INTRODUCTION

The psychotherapy of character and personality disorders has received an exceptional amount of attention in the last two decades. The tenacity, pervasiveness, and severity of this type of psychopathology make it particularly difficult to approach in any narrow or traditional manner. We will present a model for understanding and treating character pathology that is derived from psychodynamic theories, but that integrates concepts and techniques from cognitive and behavior therapies.

Character or personality disorders are conditions in which the person's enduring patterns of behavior, thought, and relatedness are inappropriate or maladaptive. The ways that the patient structures and interprets experience are stereotyped, idiosyncratic, rigid, or excessively vague and variable. Affects, fantasies, and mo-

tives are experienced in overly free or in highly restrictive ways, and are poorly integrated into the person's conscious experience. The patient's overt behavior may be marked by exaggerations of certain types of interaction (dependency, aggression) or by a lack of other modes of relating (intimacy, empathy.) Such patterns of functioning are entrenched and repetitive, regardless of the objective situation or of the specific inner state with which the patient is faced.

The mental representations of the self and of others are distorted by affective and cognitive exaggerations, omissions, and misperceptions. This results in a private "inner world" of relationships with others and with the self which deviates to some degree from the observable qualities and characteristics of the persons with whom the patient interacts.

Adults disorders of character are understood to be the complex consequences of developmental deviations. By this we mean that early experiences of inconsistent, failed, or incompetent parenting cause the child to approach himself or herself and others in ways that produce skewed, maladaptive, and dysphoric interpersonal, cognitive, and motivational structures and processes. Such patterns remain unchanged into adult life and are then identifiable as pathological character traits.

Jerold R. Gold • Doctoral Program in Clinical Psychology, Long Island University, Brooklyn, New York 11201. George Stricker • Derner Institute of Advanced Psychological Studies, Adelphi University, Garden City, New York 11530.

Comprehensive Handbook of Psychotherapy Integration, edited by George Stricker and Jerold R. Gold. Plenum Press, New York, 1993.

The approach to psychotherapy integration with character disordered patients takes as its basis a developmental, psychodynamically oriented framework. We believe that this theoretical model is the most encompassing and most suitable for understanding the etiology of these disorders, as well as in working with the largely unconscious representations of self and of others that are at the core of character pathology. However, unlike standard psychodynamic approaches, we attempt to integrate behavioral and cognitive concepts and techniques at the theoretical level and in clinical practice. Such additions to the therapy are necessary because interpretive methods are limited in their impact upon many of the overt symptoms and character traits that are presented by these patients. Such phenomena often become extreme impediments to psychodynamic exploration, and serve also to promote and maintain the patient's distress and maladaptive way of life. Intervention in the behavioral and cognitive manifestations of character pathology can synergize powerfully with interpretation and developmental reconstruction, thus leading to a therapy that is more broadly applicable than any of its constituent parts.

THEORETICAL AND CONCEPTUAL POSITION

The psychodynamic theories of character development suggest that an individual's enduring ways of thinking, feeling, and of construing the self and others, are established in the first few years of life (Kohut, 1971; Reich, 1949; Winnicott, 1971). Early interactions with parents and other significant adults that give rise to anxious or otherwise dysphoric experiences can lead to permanent skewing of the way the child views particular persons and the affects, fantasies, and motives which were associated with those painful encounters. When such painful interactions dominate the child's early life, the representations (or schemata) of the self and of others become narrow and marked by the limitations and dysphoria of those encounters. For example, the child of angry, critical, and contemptuous parents may come to expect all relationships to be based on humiliation and failure to please the other, or may identify with the parent and view others as he viewed himself as a child. These representations usually are unconscious and multiple in nature, but they are the dominant psychological structures in the child's ongoing interpretation and structuring of experience. As a result, conscious cognitive structures, the patterns of behavior and of interacting with other people, are limited and distorted by earlier events and relationships. Social learning of a corrective and positive nature is difficult, if not impossible, because the patient does not seek out, and cannot assimilate, information about himself or herself or about others that does not correspond to his or her unconscious prototypes. The patient whose unrealistically poor self-esteem is unaltered or accentuated by successes is an example of these concepts: the achievements are debased or brushed away consciously because the "truth" about the person exists on an intrapsychic level, and is inconsistent with the facts of his or her external life.

Character pathology may be assessed and described through a "three-tier" model of personality functioning (Stricker & Gold, 1988). These tiers refer to different types or levels of psychological experience that are believed to be dynamically interrelated in a circular manner. Causation in this model is believed to be multidirectional in that any psychological phenomenon in any of the tiers can be either a resultant or a cause of a variable at another level of experience. This is in contrast to the traditional psychodynamic position that holds that behavior and conscious cognitive processes inevitably and exclusively are caused by unconscious motivational processes. Like Wachtel (1977; Gold & Wachtel, Chapter 5, this volume), we believe that the way a person thinks, behaves, and interacts with others has as much to do in maintaining and prolonging character pathology as do unconscious conflicts and inclinations. Of particular importance to the method of therapy that is to be described are the ways in which behavior and cognition can be modified to allow developmental deviations to be corrected or ameliorated.

The three tiers are constructs that are used for classifying, assessing, and locating different aspects of character pathology. Overt behavioral problems are located in Tier 1, deviant or maladaptive conscious cognitions and affects in Tier 2, and unconscious motives, conflicts, representations and schemata in Tier 3.

Character disordered patients display disturbed interpersonal and adaptive behavior on a manifest level. Such disturbances of conduct usually are repetitive and somewhat independent of the specific context or relationship. That is, the person behaves in a stereotyped and unobservant way, guided more by internal issues and needs than by an ongoing assessment of the situation. These entrenched interaction patterns differ in kind from patient to patient and from diagnosis to diagnosis. Maladaptive conduct may be overly aggressive or passive, isolating, avoidant, dependent, self-involved, self-effacing, erratic, or compulsive. There are other specific types of behaviors that may be part of these disorders as well, but the key point here is that it is the presence of such fixed patterns of action and conduct that are typical of character pathology.

The phenomena assigned to Tier 2 include the content and the structure of the person's conscious cognitive and affective life. Maladaptive and inaccurate beliefs about the self, other people, and the world are types of Tier 2 issues, as are the affects that are associated with such thoughts. Overly harsh self-critical ideas, hopelessness, phobic and other anxiety-generating thoughts, rigid moral attitudes, or unrealistically inflated perceptions of self-worth and personal power are a few examples of this type of cognitive material.

Tier 2 also includes structural cognitive issues similar to those described by Shapiro (1965) in his work on neurotic styles. Character disorders are marked by rigid and fixed ways of processing external information, and of reacting to and integrating internal affective and motivational states. These cognitive and perceptual structures cause the person to exaggerate, skew, avoid, or distort external information and inner experience in patterned modes that are recognizable and repetitive for each patient. Similar to these structural issues are fixed beliefs about particular interpersonal experiences (e.g., intimacy, sexuality, separation, or hostility) that make those experiences overly accessible or to be avoided.

Pathological conditions traditionally referred to as "ego deficits" also often are considered to be Tier 2 issues. Such deficits include difficulties with reality testing and consensually validated thinking, problems with impulse control and frustration tolerance, and related adaptational problems. These deficits often have overt behavioral manifestations that are included in Tier 1. Such deficits usually are based on failures of development that left gaps in the requisite cognitive skills that underlie adaptive behavior. For example, the "ego function" of impulse control requires the person to anticipate consequences, to remember to tell himself that he can wait, and to be able to believe that he can tolerate any discomfort associated with not acting.

Tier 3 is the location of those issues that have been the primary concern of psychoanalytic approaches to character pathology, though recent cognitive work (cf. Beck, Freeman, & Associates, 1990) has emphasized nonconscious factors as well. Here we refer to unconscious motivations and conflicts, as well as to enduring ways of representing the self and other persons, separately and in relationship to each other. Motives and conflicts generally are contained within and are expressed in the context of these internalized relationships. Such unconscious representations are called "objects" in psychodynamic theory, whereas in cognitive theory the term *schema* is preferred. Both constructs refer to variables that exist outside of patients' awareness, but which structure and govern their conscious perceptions of, and emotions and behavior toward, themselves and other people. In character pathology, the images of self and other are inconsistent with the persons in the patient's life, and with whom the patient actually may be. Instead, his representation of himself may be distorted, incomplete, fantastic, or debased, and such pathology can and does apply to his schemata of others. For example, a patient may unconsciously perceive himself to be omnipotent and deserving of adulation from others, all of whom he perceives as inferior, although in his actual encounters he is far from unique. Most patients will harbor a variety of such problematic representations that may contradict or be in conflict with each other, and that may be far removed from the person's manifest behavior and consciousness. Pathogenic schemata or representations are considered to be remnants of early developmental experiences that later relationships could not or did not ameliorate.

As may be inferred from our descriptions of the three tiers, any psychological event can, and usually is, located across all three levels of experience. Most clinically relevant events have overt behavioral, cognitive, and dynamic elements. We believe that the directionality of influence between the tiers is multiple and circular. Frequently, character pathology evolves from the "depths upward": an experience activates an unconscious image of the self and of an important relationship that is superimposed upon the current interaction, with disturbances of cognition and behavior as consequences of that unconscious substitution. However, a particular behavior or thought may also start a pattern of interaction that then elicits and confirms a dynamic issue, keeping archaic and maladaptive self and object representations intact. Interaction patterns and cognitive structures develop and are formed in the same developmental experiences as unconscious representations. These modes of action and thought will lead the person to find and perpetuate relationships that inhibit chances for the growth of new representations while "proving" the validity of older schema. For example, a patient who chronically thinks ill of himself or herself may behave in a passive and weak way with others, thus inviting hostility, criticism, and abuse, and ultimately reinforcing certain negative representations of the self and of others.

The tiers are dynamically related in other important ways. Character traits (thoughts, perceptions, behaviors) can become the meaningful equivalent of the self or of another person, as the patient develops an unconscious relationship with such characteristics. When this occurs, cognitive and behavioral interventions may be experienced as attacks on the identity of the patient or on an important unconscious object relationship. Similarly, defenses and resistances can be understood to be the Tier 1 and Tier 2 manifestations of an unconscious conflict or relationship. In both cases, the patient has strong needs or desires to keep thinking and behaving in pathological ways, despite their effects on his life and on the treatment. This is particularly apparent when the defense or character trait has been effective in avoiding anxiety or some other uncomfortable experience, or is a symbolic part of an attachment to an unconscious relationship or image of the self. Work on these phenomena can proceed from any of the three tiers, but will be most effective when the meaning of the behavior or thought is understood completely and the selected interventions are presented and used in ways that are experienced as benign and acceptable to the patient.

This is possible only when the unconscious dangers we have just outlined are understood by both parties.

The character disordered patient suffers greatly from self-imposed constrictions and restrictions of experience and learning. Problems at each tier keep the person from learning how to relate to himself or herself and to others in new and more positive ways. Often, a behavior, cognitive structure, or unconscious schema cannot be given up because the person has no other way to behave, think, or structure experience. Although the person may be aware of the negative effects of certain thoughts or behaviors, he or she may prefer to continue functioning in those ways because of greater discomfort with the ambiguity and awkwardness of not having any familiar tactics on which to rely. Also, changes in cognition and behavior often are experienced as threats to a fragile sense of identity and of individuality. The prospect of change then will be perceived as a threat: the patient will be left selfless or will cease to exist if his or her pathology is abandoned. New representations of the self and of others sometimes cannot be constructed until and unless the patient behaves differently and is conscious of the changes in his or her behavior. Unconscious representations are built up of memories and perceptions of the self in interaction with others. When an old representation is explored and abandoned, the patient does not necessarily have at his or her disposal the requisite and new interactional and cognitive strategies that would be the bases for corrective representations. When the therapist considers interventions at any of the tiers, the consequences at the other must be considered with regard to lags and gaps with which the patient is left.

As we will describe in more detail, character pathology may be targeted for intervention according to the tier in which it appears in either simple or complex ways. Simply, some problems may respond to interventions aimed at the dominant tier (a Tier 1 problem to a behavioral technique, Tier 2 to cognitive intervention, and Tier 3 to interpretation). However, because of the possibility that problems in one tier may be reinforced and maintained by problems in another, more complex strategies may be necessary. These require the assessment of the interrelationships between the tiers for any given phenomena, and a plan of intervention that takes these dynamic relationships into account. Frequently, it is necessary to change the patient's action patterns or cognitive structures in order to promote psychodynamic exploration, insight, and restructuralization of representations. At other points, behavioral or cognitive change occur without antecedent insight and representational changes.

CLINICAL AND THEORETICAL ANTECEDENTS

This approach to character pathology is based upon the psychoanalytic studies of such writers as Reich (1949), Winnicott (1971), Kohut (1971), and Kernberg (1975). Although differing in the specifics of their ideas, these authors share a concern with the critical role of early experience in shaping the structure of the person's behavior, cognition, and patterns of relatedness. In the writings of the last three authors, we have found crucial ideas about the etiology and treatment of impairment in self and object representations, which figure in the long-term, exploratory psychodynamic framework of our integrative treatment. Other dynamic writers who have influenced our thinking include Shapiro (1965), who did work on cognitive styles and psychopathology, and Alexander and French (1946), who recognized that new and corrective experiences were as necessary to psychoanalytic psychotherapy as was insight. The three-tier model of character pathology was originally presented by Stricker and Gold (1988).

Among students of psychotherapy integration, Wachtel (1977; Gold & Wachtel, Chapter 5, this volume) stands out as a major influence on the theory and method presented in this chapter. His cyclical psychodynamic theory of personality is echoed by our suggestion of the circular and multidirectional relationships between phenomena in the three tiers of experience. Clinically, Wachtel's (1977) explorations of an integrated dynamic and behavioral psychotherapy were elemental in our attempts to expand our work with character pathology.

Other integrative work that is related to this model include that of Ryle (1990; Chapter 7, this volume), Safran and Segal (1990), and Gold (1988, 1990, 1991).

THE TECHNIQUE AND PROCESS OF PSYCHOTHERAPY

Our work with character disordered patients is based on extensive inquiry into the three tiers of experience in a nondirective and free flowing way. Patients are encouraged to speak freely about whatever is of greatest concern to them at any given moment. It is the therapist's task to listen closely and carefully to patients' communications and their reports of their interactions with themselves and with others. In doing so, the therapist will identify repetitive and problematic behavior patterns, dysfunctional cognitive contents and structures, unconscious conflicts, and deviant representations and objects relationships. The identification of a particular issue in one tier will lead to exploration of the interrelationships between that variable and experiences in the other tiers of experience. The circular patterns of action and thought that reinforce and maintain dynamic conflict and pathological object and self representations are identified and explored. Similarly, the ways that unconscious images and inclinations are expressed and symbolized by thoughts, perceptions, and behaviors are noted and become the locus of intense inquiry.

When a problem area is understood in its unconscious, conscious, and behavioral manifestations, formal intervention begins. Because this therapy is based primarily on a developmental, psychodynamic model, we aim at assisting the patient in the task of expanding self-knowledge and self-awareness by developing *insight* into his or her dynamic conflicts, unconscious object relationships, and developmental deviations. We actively attempt to modify the patient's behavior and cognitive functioning when such intervention seems advantageous. In addition, we have found that certain developmental problems and difficulties in self and object relatedness best can be dealt with through a combination of psychodynamic understanding and active intervention based on modifications of behavioral and cognitive techniques. This last type of intervention requires the construction of operational definitions of unconscious, intrapsychic processes in behavioral and cognitive terms.

We now will proceed with more extensive discussions of the interventions that we have just mentioned.

Interpretation and Insight

The unstructured inquiry that serves as the framework of this therapy allows the patient to speak of any topic that crosses his or her mind. From the patient's dreams, random thoughts, memories, fantasies, and images come the therapist's inferences that serve as the basis of interpretation and insight. We aim at broadening the patient's awareness of his or her motivations, conflicts, and inner representations of the self and of other in three ways. The first two uses of insight and interpretation are traditional and would be found in any psychodynamic psychotherapy. The first use of insight includes assisting in a developmental, historical reconstruction of the significant relationships and experiences that warp and distort the patient's current dealings with himself or herself and with others. The second and related group of interpretations are meant to create for the patient an appreciation of his or her current motives, conflicts, and intrapsychic vulnerabilities as they are expressed in behavior, thoughts, affects, and symptoms. The last and more integrative type of interpretative work includes interpretations of the ways in which the patient's cognitive and behavioral functioning reinforces and promotes his or her maladaptive modes of self and object representation. Included in this type of interpretation is consideration of the ways that the patient finds and creates unwitting "accomplices in psychopathology" (Wachtel, 1977) who will encourage the status quo while inhibiting or punishing new ways of relating, thinking, or feeling.

Insight is a critical variable in this therapy. Expanded self-awareness and an ability to understand the effects of one's actions on other aspects of experience often will cause maladaptive behaviors, thoughts, and representations to become less automatic and inflexible. As this loosening of character takes place, persons gain more conscious control over their life and begin to perceive themselves differently. However, insight rarely is effective enough to be the single type of intervention that is necessary in the psychotherapy of character pathology. We have learned to utilize active interventions of a behavioral or cognitive nature in at least four circumstances. The switch from an exploratory approach to a more ameliorative or didactic technique is dictated largely by clinical necessity. Several recurring and extremely important clinical situations that are typical of the process of therapy with these patients can be handled best by such an integrative move. However, the shift from one technique to another is not devoid of meaning at conscious and unconscious levels, and these issues are of necessity an intrinsic part of the work. At times, inquiry into these meanings may be postponed until after the behavioral or cognitive technique has been attempted. With other patients, or at other points in any given therapy, the exploration of the patients' concerns about a new technique, and the meaning of the technique in terms of the therapeutic relationship, must precede any active work. The dynamic exploration of the idiosyncratic meanings of cognitive and behavioral interventions helps to ensure a more real and "seamless" integration of the analytic and cognitive-behavioral components of this therapy (Wachtel, 1991).

Cognitive and Behavioral Interventions

Resolving Resistive and Defensive Situations. Active intervention often becomes advantageous when the therapeutic inquiry has bogged down or become "stuck" in an area of resistance. Frequently, we find that a specific symptom, cognitive pattern or content, or action pattern has become a powerful and intractable distraction or focal concern that makes symbolic and depth-oriented exploration impossible. In these circumstances patient and therapist find that what little insight is available about the sources of the resistance is felt to be stale, overly intellectual, and of little help. In fact, the patient's behavior and thoughts may reinforce the unconscious issue and any conflicts associated with it, thus promoting any defensive efforts. Direct intervention via cognitive restructuring, imagery, relaxation, or other appropriate behavioral techniques may end this impasse. Frequently, more deeply felt and spontaneous insights may be the result of such overt changes. Once defenses and resistances have been relaxed or abandoned, the patient may gain greater access to the unconscious issues that prompted these actions.

Active interventions often are critically important when the patient's interpersonal relationships are reinforcing of any of his or her pathology. The influence of other people in the patient's life often is more powerful and pervasive than any amount of interpretation. If a state of resistance within the therapy can be linked to issues that are generated and maintained by external relationship problems, then interventions aimed at teaching the patient to interact differently with others may be invaluable in moving the therapy along.

When a defense, symptom, relational pattern, or character trait is unconsciously perceived as a part of the self or of an archaic tie to an object, direct intervention in those phenomena is likely to be ineffective or to promote heightened anxiety and resistance. When this occurs, all is not lost. Inquiry into the meaning of the active interventions often can be an aid in understanding the sources of the previous resistive situation. As this inquiry proceeds, the patient may come to perceive the loss of a problem in a more positive way, allowing either interpretative work or active interventions to be utilized. Such situations occur frequently in the treatment of character pathology, which is why we have found it to be better in most cases to start in an exploratory fashion rather than by addressing the symptoms immediately and directly.

Correcting Developmental Deficits. A second clinical situation in which the integration of active interventions is optimal is at those times in the therapy when the inquiry has uncovered and explored a developmental deficit that is not fully responsive to interpretation. Such deficits often require interventions that provide new experiences in the tiers of overt behavior and of cognitive processing of experience in order to provide raw materials out of which new internal structures and self- and object representations can be built. Traditional psychoanalytic theories argue that such intrapsychic changes are the results of identification with the analyst and of the mutative internalization by the patient of the analyst's interpretations, empathic and genuine responsiveness, and of new ways of thinking and acting that are tried out in the analytic setting (see, for example, Winnicott, 1971; or Kohut, 1971). We do not disagree with these ideas but hesitate to rely on them exclusively, as their mechanisms are poorly understood and such relational phenomena usually occur serendipitously rather than being planned for or consciously initiated. The efficiency of these mechanisms is questionable and

some significant areas of relatedness are likely to remain untouched. As a result, we attempt to find active and replicable methods for adapting behavioral and cognitive techniques to the task of filling in "gaps" or modifying deviant images of the self or of others.

Such goals can be accomplished in two ways. First, cognitive and behavioral measures can be used to shape new patterns of interaction and of thought that will yield new feedback from other people and from patients' observations of themselves in action. Such feedback often causes patients to question old images of self and others at an experiential and affective level that is not reached by insight alone. As the person constructs new images, it is much easier and less anxiety-provoking to consider letting go of old ones. Many patients with severe character pathology cling to their pathological introjects and self representations because of their fears that their inner worlds will be empty if such ties are cut. When the patient has a choice of adaptive replacement images, these fears sometimes are bypassed or are tempered by hope. Frequently, the new feedback about the self and others generated by active techniques is ignored, disbelieved, or repressed. At these times, interpretive work is utilized concurrently with the other interventions to uncover and resolve the dynamic and cognitive sources of such resistive activity.

Successful use of cognitive-behavioral procedures may have the effect of enhancing the patient's self-esteem and sense of mastery and competence. In changing his own behavior and in obtaining relief from his suffering the patient changes his relationship to, and representation of himself, and also may allow himself to become open to new images of, and responses from, other people.

Another way that cognitive-behavioral measures have been used to correct developmental deficits has been termed *combinatory integration* (Gold, 1988; 1991). This involves defining a problem in relatedness or in self-integrity in behavioral, cognitive, or perceptual terms. Once this is accomplished, patient and therapist create new experiences that address and correct the deficit. Much of this work has relied on guided imagery and related techniques for creating scenarios in which the patient perceives himself living in ways which require new and beneficial self and object representations. For example, many patients with "narcissistic" or "borderline" character disorders have poorly defined representations of the self that merge or overlap with representations of other people. As a result, independent action often is difficult, and such patients frequently cannot differentiate between thoughts, feelings, and inclinations that are their own and those that actually belong to someone else. One such patient, during the course of dynamic inquiry, identified a problem in differentiating himself from his mother. He perceived himself to be a part of a "one headed but two bodied person. It's really her head that controls us both." Interpretation was useful in making this merged representation conscious, and in helping the patient to understand its etiology and the effects of this sense of himself on his current relationships and experiences. However, repeated discussion of this issue did not lead to much change in it. Using his image of one head with two bodies attached, the therapist suggested that gradually changing the image might lead to other useful changes for the patient. The patient agreed to this, and together they worked on developing an image in which a second head budded out of the neck of the person, and came to have the features of the patient. As the head became fully developed and attached, the image came to include a gradual separation of the two bodies, until each existed as a fully functioning person.

This guided imagery took place over several weeks and alternated with exploration of its dynamic meaning for the patient, in relationship to his past and ongoing relationship with his mother. Much effort also was spent in exploring the meaning of these changes in terms of the therapeutic relationship, and with regard to the changes in the patient's thoughts and behavior in and out of sessions.

Cognitive-behavioral techniques also can be designed or modified to address problems in the self and in object relatedness. For example, many patients suffer from overly critical and severe attitudes toward themselves that reflect the internalization of hostile, attacking images of their parents, and an absence of a parental image that is soothing and comforting. Cognitive therapy is very effective in teaching people to modify their inner dialogue to include "calming self statements" (Beck, 1976). This type of technique can

be expanded by interpretation and imagery to be the core of building in new and benign parent images.

Enhancing the Therapeutic Alliance. Cooperation between patient and therapist in working toward the patient's progress and health is believed to be a necessity by therapist of most orientations, and there has been recent and important scrutiny of the ways this cooperation or alliance is ruptured and repaired (Gold, 1990; Safran & Segal, 1990). The establishment of a positively toned and collaborative relationship is both extremely critical and extremely difficult in working with character disordered patients. Character pathology is defined by deviant patterns of perceiving and responding to other people, and the therapist is not excluded from this. The patterns of relatedness which bring the patient to therapy contain the seeds of the therapy's destruction as well as offering the therapy a microcosm of the patient's interpersonal and intrapsychic life for direct study and intervention. If handled correctly, these destructive trends can be turned toward major changes in character and in relatedness.

The internal structures and representations of the self and others as capable of offering and receiving nurturance, affection, and care are damaged or missing for this group of patients. This deficit causes the patient to lack the expectable positive set that is the prototype or backbone of a beginning therapeutic alliance. Most patients with character disorders come to psychotherapy with a history of disappointment and failure in establishing and maintaining viable, intimate, and worthwhile relationships, and most are wary of hope, optimism, openness, and trust. In addition, many character-disordered patients are hypersensitive to rejection and other real and imagined slights, imperfections, and errors on the part of the therapist, leading to frequent and intensely emotional ruptures of the therapeutic alliance. To complicate things further, the same internal structures and cognitive sets that predispose these patients to alliance ruptures make these ruptures most difficult to repair. Patients whose pessimism, distrust, paranoia, hopelessness, or powerlessness have been evoked by some aspect of the therapeutic interaction are least likely, able, and willing to hear what the therapist has to say in the attempts to correct a rupture, particularly if the therapist continues to work in the same way that caused that rupture.

Accurate, sensitive, and timely interpretation, offered in a respectful, warm, and empathic context, are a key part of establishing and repairing a therapeutic alliance. However, we have found that integrating cognitive-behavioral procedures into the therapy sometimes is extremely helpful in establishing a collaborative interaction and in repairing breaks.

Suggesting an active intervention at or near the beginning of therapy has several advantages other than the potential for Tier 1 or Tier 2 change. Active interventions usually are more obviously pragmatic, comprehensible, and immediately gratifying, than is the slow paced, somewhat mystifying, and painful process of dynamic and developmental inquiry. Cognitive-behavioral measures introduced early in the process may become the basis for constructing the patient's perception of the therapist as helpful, concerned, and caring, and may lead to changes in the patient's self image and of others as well. Change begets more change, and with it the therapist builds the core of cognitive sets such as trust, hope, and optimism around which a viable therapeutic alliance may be built. Exclusive reliance on dynamic exploration and methods may be too depriving and frustrating for many character-disordered patients. It also may activate negative images of others who were withholding, mystifying, and exploitative, which cannot always be worked through via transference interpretations. However, a direct assault upon the entrenched symptoms, which are supported by a rich dynamic fabric, can lead to resistance. It is this extremely tricky situation which calls for an integrated approach.

The provision of relief from a troubling symptom or interaction pattern at any point during the therapy may reinforce the alliance by reinforcing or restoring hopefulness, trust, and faith in the therapist and in the therapy. As importantly, some of the dynamic and interpersonal issues that may cause a rupture of the collaboration may be corrected by a shift from dynamic exploration to active intervention. Many ruptures are caused by inadvertent wounds to the person's self-esteem caused by something the therapist said or did. Interpretation of these injuries often sets things back on the right track, but occasionally inquiry becomes impossible due to the intensity of the break, or because interpretative efforts take on a negative and attacking meaning to the patient. Addressing the problem on a cognitive or behavioral level (e.g., reinforcing the patients' expression of their hurt and anger through assertiveness training, or helping them to test the accuracy of their conscious beliefs) may defuse the situation and allow the patients to again perceive the therapist in a more positive and benign way.

Active Intervention in Treatment Destructive Situations. The psychotherapy of more severely disturbed character-disordered patients often is marked by crises, sudden and severe exacerbation of symptoms, and by the need for containment and management of the patient. Borderline, schizoid, and narcissistic patients typically have little tolerance for painful affects, memories, and for symptoms such as anxiety or depression. Yet, insight-oriented, developmentally based psychotherapy is built upon procedures that uncover and expose these patients to those experiences and emotions from which they have been attempting to escape all of their lives. Character-disordered patients often turn to drugs, alcohol, sex, religion, self-mutilation, aggression, or suicide when faced with such pain. Many discussions of therapy with such patients (see, e.g., Kernberg, 1975) suggest that adjunctive measures such as hospitalization or medication frequently are necessary as limit-setting measures or as reactions to decompensation.

We have found that many such crises and iatrogenic symptoms can be prevented or lessened by anticipating the patient's difficulties in tolerating the affects stirred up by exploration, and by working behaviorally and cognitively to build affect tolerance, the ability to tolerate frustration, and the ability to soothe and comfort oneself. Relaxation procedures, meditation exercises, calming and soothing self-statements, soothing imagery, or hypnosis are just some of the active techniques that can increase the patient's ability and capacity to bear pain. These techniques are suggested as the dynamic inquiry proceeds, and usually are prompted by the therapist's observations of, or the patient's reports of, more than moderate levels of discomfort. The appearance of resistance or a negative shift in the therapeutic relationship often are signals that too much is happening and that the patient requires assistance in tolerating what has been learned, or what is about to be uncovered.

The cognitive and behavioral measures used to build affect tolerance also are very helpful in situations where the person is self medicating through alcohol or drugs, or is engaging in ritualistic and destructive activities to avoid feelings, memories, or other insights. Such behaviors can be given up more easily if the patient is offered a viable alternative: the relaxation provided by alcohol or marijuana may be less attractive when the patient is taught to meditate or to use imagery or deep muscle relaxation, as one example. Another example is provided by the patient who reacted to sadness and loss by cutting himself ritualistically, finding the physical pain to be more tolerable than the emotional discomfort. He gradually was able to stop cutting as he learned to comfort and reassure himself through cognitive restructuring, and as he learned how to talk about his pain (through behavior rehearsal and other *in vivo* exercises) with people who would be sympathetic and interested.

Most character-disordered patients have long histories of turning to substances or to maladaptive behavior when in pain, and these choices frequently are the source of shame, guilt, and self-hatred, as well as a sense of inferiority, and weakness. When the patient is taught to cope with pain in prosocial and adaptive ways, beneficial feedback from others and from his observations of his own behavior result. This feedback can be hugely important in helping the patient to build self-esteem and an image of himself as competent, powerful, and healthy. As we have suggested, provision of new and helpful experience also goes a long way in helping the patient to establish and maintain a positive therapeutic alliance, and is useful in building and consolidating new and benign interpersonal schemata.

THE THERAPEUTIC RELATIONSHIP

We view the therapist—patient interaction as a crucial source of dynamic data and as an arena for learning new behavioral and cognitive skills. As we have emphasized repeatedly, much therapeutic effort is spent in attempting to build and maintain a viable therapeutic alliance between the two participants. We now will describe the other relational aspects of our integrative approach.

Therapeutic Stance

Like other students of psychotherapy integration who have psychodynamic leanings (e.g., Gold & Wachtel, Chapter 5, this volume; Ryle, 1990, Wachtel, 1977; Wachtel & Wachtel, 1986), we have abandoned the classical psychoanalytic stance of neutrality and have adopted a model of participant-observation (Sullivan, 1953). We believe that it is impossible to avoid influencing or being influenced by the patient, and that such mutual impact is best construed and approached as inevitable, acceptable, and as the source of useful data for exploration and intervention.

The therapeutic stance that we advocate is one of availability, interest, and activity. We aim to further understanding of unconscious processes by listening respectfully and quietly at times, but recognize the contextual nature of such phenomena (Wachtel, 1977). Therefore, we do not believe that active interventions, advice, or support interfere with dynamic exploration or yield tainted forms of intrapsychic data.

A didactic and supportive relationship with a real and available person often is among the most critical variables in the treatment of character disorders. Such patients come to therapy with a history of ineffective and maladaptive parenting and are in need of new figures for identification, as well as, at times, someone who will initiate and support new learning in a warm and structuring manner. Neutrality can serve only to reinforce and promote internal representations of others as unavailable and uncaring, and will keep the person in the position of feeling ineffective and incompetent.

Transference and Countertransference

All patients will engage the therapist in ways that reflect their learning histories, dynamic conflicts, internal representations, character structures, and patterns of relatedness. Character-disordered patients are no exception, but do differ in the intensity of such transferences, and in their readiness to construe transferences as real or factual. Also, the transference is a prototype of what brings the patient to treatment. As a result, we have found that careful exploration of, and intervention in, the transference reactions, and the complementary countertransference binds, are an elemental part of this work.

We understand transference in a way that is similar to the contextual, constructionistic theories held by Gill (1982), Levenson (1983), Safran and Segal (1990), and Wachtel (1977). In this view, the patient's transference reactions are understood to be an amalgam of his enduring intrapsychic structures and interpersonal patterns with some reality-based behaviors and characteristics of the therapist. Repetitive cycles of relatedness are evoked by the unique interaction of the two participants, and these interactions contain elements from the patient's past (motives, thoughts, object representations) as well as veridical perceptions of who the therapist is and how he or she has actually reacted.

Countertransference reactions are understood also as contextual, combining aspects of the unique personal history of the therapist with specific feelings, behaviors, and thoughts that are evoked by the individual patient. Countertransference reactions, and enactment of certain roles with the patient, are inevitable and should be subjected to silent scrutiny by the therapist in order to understand the patient's developmental history, and the ways that he or she creates accomplices in his or her vicious circles (Gold & Wachtel, Chapter 5, this volume; Wachtel, 1977). Where appropriate, countertransference and the therapist's awareness of his enactments are discussed with the patient, though this is done conservatively.

The repetitive circles of transference and countertransference are used as *in vivo* samples of the patient's way of living at all three tiers of experience. Difficulties at any tier can be addressed by interventions appropriate to the behavioral, cognitive, or dynamic component of the interaction that is the current focus of the therapy. Although much of our work in this area is dynamically oriented, we have found that approaching transference phenomena on a behavioral or cognitive level is very helpful. Cognitive interventions are particularly useful in helping the patient to sort out the reality-based part of his perceptions

from the redundant, structural pieces. Behavioral interventions are useful in helping the patient to learn new social and interactional skills that can supplant old patterns and to learn to manage the anxiety and other discomforts that may be the source of transference reactions.

Pitfalls, Indications, and Contraindications

The therapist who works with character-disordered patients with this integrative approach needs to be aware of certain tricky issues that are inherent. First, in moving between Tiers 1, 2 and 3, too rapid shifts can limit the breadth and depth of work done at each. Rapid and superficial scanning of data at Tier 3 may reflect countertransference issues that find easy shelter in an overreliance on work at Tiers 1 and 2. Similarly, ignoring Tier 1 and 2 problems in favor of exclusive work at Tier 3 may reflect other countertransferential issues.

This approach requires the therapist to be familiar with, and competent in, concepts and techniques drawn from three types of therapy. Also required is a greater belief in the powerful interrelationships between the three levels of experience than most therapists are trained to have. Personal therapeutic or theoretical biases may be communicated to the patient and thus may negatively influence the patient's ability to use interventions at any level.

We believe that this integrative therapy is the treatment of choice for the majority of character-disordered patients. It may not be indicated with those patients whose pathology would interact badly with work at any particular tier. For example, patients who suffer almost exclusively from identity diffusion might find cognitive and behavioral interventions to be a way of enacting their issues of pseudocompliance and overidentification. Patients with severely oppositional and antiauthoritarian character structures could find the didactic elements of work at Tiers 1 and 2 to be too tempting as targets for their rebellion and hostility. Very fragile patients, and those with very limited capacity for introspection and delay of gratification, might be better served with a therapy which emphasizes, or is exclusively concerned with, work at the behavioral and cognitive levels. With these types of patients, there is room for the omitted tier, but only after some delay and extensive work in the preferred tiers.

CASE EXAMPLE

The psychotherapy that will be presented here was conducted on a twice a week basis for several years. As it is impossible to present this work in its entirety, we will focus on the points in the treatment that are most illustrative of the approach to psychotherapy integration that we have discussed thus far.

Michael was a 28-year-old married man who came to therapy at the urging of his wife. He complained of vague and moderately severe anxiety symptoms, mild but chronic depression, and of a sense of uncertainty about who he was and where his life was going. He focused heavily on his occupational difficulties. He had been "almost successful" in a number of careers: rock musician, photographer, junior executive, and printing apprentice. He currently was self-employed in a computer consulting business that he was trying to get off the ground. He reported being happily married but said that his sexual relationship with his wife had virtually ended and that he had very little sexual desire, though he loved and respected her.

The first phase of the therapy involved a broad inquiry into all relevant experiences necessary to complete an assessment at Tiers 1, 2, and 3.

Tier 1 (overt behavior) was marked by repetitive patterns of starting projects and then abandoning them (a primary source of his vocational problems), by impulsive and hasty actions and choices, by the use of alcohol and marijuana to cope with unpleasant affect, and by patterns of interaction wherein Michael took care of other people to an excessive and extraordinary degree.

Tier 2 (conscious cognition and affect) contained rigid and moralistic demands for control over himself, other people, and the environment, and thoughts and images of punishment and catastrophe if he did not live up to these expectations. He also thought in terms of "shoulds" and "musts" when it came to other people and therefore almost always was disappointed and angry with himself and with others. His compulsive giving to other people yielded a conscious sense of pride and ideas about being better than other people, but he also suffered from doubts and worries about his self-worth. He was vaguely aware of the resentment and feeling of being exploited that taking care of others generated in him, but these affects were intolerable and caused him much anxiety and guilt.

Tier 3 (intrapsychic representations) had been shaped by Michael's relationships with a depressed and possibly psychotic father, and a rageful and narcissistic mother. The father had abandoned a promising career in publishing to move their family to a small town in the South where they lived in isolation and poverty, and suffered from extreme ethnic and religious discrimination that often turned violent. Mother clung to the patient (her eldest child) as her "Joy" who was to save the family and fulfill her ambitions. Michael's inner world was composed of fragmentary and conflicting identifications with these parents and with the images that had been projected onto him. He unconsciously was caught between a sense of grandiosity and omnipotence, and a sense of himself as insane, helpless, and doomed to failure. The narcissistic role of "Joy" brought with it a sense and image of a Christlike figure who suffered as he saved.

The assessment also revealed the multidirectional relationships between issues at the three tiers. Michael's psychodynamic issues were symbolized and expressed in his behavior and thoughts, but the way he acted and understood his experiences also confirmed and reinforced his self and object relationships. For example, each time someone unwittingly accepted his help, their happiness confirmed for him that it was his role in life to gratify others and to suffer in turn. When his behavior and cognitive difficulties caused him to fail at work, it was confirmation that he could not separate from, or be different than, his father.

The early phases of the inquiry were marked by Michael's enacting his role as the "joy" with the therapist. He was jocular, entertaining, and full of praise and good spirits. He offered his help with the therapist's computer system, suggested movies to see and music to listen to, and in general avoided looking deeply into his own behavior and psyche. Interpretation of these actions was not useful as they caused Michael to feel criticized and rejected. His behavior was supported by his ideas about his role in life and the "shoulds" and "musts" that governed his giving and care-taking. This pattern of interaction became a resistance that required resolution if an effective alliance was to be established.

A combination of cognitive and behavioral techniques were used to work with this problem, informed and at times supplemented by interpretation of the developmental and object relational meanings of Michael's caretaking. He was asked to role play with the therapist in order to try out new ways of behaving, and to help him to understand the impact of his behavior on the therapist and on himself. Imagery and written work was used to help him to assess the consequences of helping someone else who was supposedly there to help him. A technique that was particularly powerful was a combination of role playing and imagery. The therapist helped Michael to develop a scenario of the therapist's being totally dependent upon, and grateful to, Michael for his constant and total care and devotion. As these exercises proceeded, Michael became more aware of the anger, sadness, and hurt that his current way of life caused him. He also became more interested in learning new ways to go about things, and began to accept the pain of giving up a defensive and idealized image of his parents that had developed as a response to their pathology.

The result of this extended period of integrative work was that Michael began seriously to consider that the therapist did not need or want his help, and that the therapist could and would be interested in giving to, and helping, him. This set off a string of changes at all three tiers as Michael began to approach his character pathology and all of its manifestations from a new perspective.

This work was followed by a long period of dynamic and developmental investigation. A second integrative phase was initiated by Michael's return from a visit to his family. His flight home was marked by sudden and severe panic and claustrophobia, which continued unabated when he reached his home. He resorted to drug and alcohol use to manage these affects. In sessions, he was so panicked and distraught that little or no inquiry could be accomplished. Relaxation, calming imagery, meditation, and coping cognitive strategies were suggested, practiced, and assigned with the result that Michael's anxiety was

resolved after about 10 days. The resolution of these symptoms did not obviate the need for self-medication, and, in fact, this behavior seemed to intensify when he became less anxious. It became apparent that powerful dynamic issues had been evoked by Michael's visit. As these issues were interpreted, they were met by some relief, intermingled with anger and resentment toward the therapist. Exploration of these emotions led to the discovery that Michael felt he would be unable to tolerate the memories, emotions, and images that his visit had stimulated. In addition, he believed that if he gave up the ties to his parents and to the self that had developed in those relationships, he would have nothing left inside. These issues were dealt with by a combination of affect tolerance exercises, and with imagery and cognitive work, in which the patient was aided in using the facts of his life to build up an image of himself that he believed was positive, realistic, and free of compulsive giving. He then worked on a series of graded exercises in session and without where he tried out new roles with other people. These roles were based on the evolving new self-image which he was constructing in therapy, and involving changing old relationships, or starting new ones, in a way that his needs and interests were not self-excluded. As these tasks were accomplished, his substance abuse ended, and he was able to gradually move into another extended phase of dynamic work.

The final integrative phase of note occurred when the patient became ill with gallstones. This illness had a sudden and severe onset and required immediate surgery. His recuperation was marked by severe anxiety, and by postsurgical paranoia about his wife, friends, and the therapist. These reactions were found to be projections of his anger at himself for failing and for not being in total control of his body and his life. This was particularly painful for him as he had recently experienced much success in his business. Unconsciously, he seemed to equate this illness with being identical to his father, who became depressed and unavailable after professional success, to the point of destroying his career. Interpretive work helped Michael to understand the unconscious identification that had been activated. This was accompanied by cognitive and imagery exercises aimed at helping him to discriminate between his father and himself.

These examples (and there were many other integrative parts of this extended therapy) were typical of the interplay between dynamic understanding and active intervention that is inherent in this method of therapy.

CONCLUDING COMMENTS

The diagnostic and assessment framework of dynamically interrelated tiers of experience is useful not only with character pathology but with any patient who presents for individual psychotherapy. It is a structural model that does not prescribe the content of any individual's experiences. Instead, it offers the therapist a flexible and reliable way of conceptualizing what ails the person, and is an invaluable aid in selecting interventions.

Our training and experience lead us to integrate cognitive, behavioral, and imagery-based techniques into the developmental psychodynamic bedrock of this approach. Techniques drawn from other schools of psychotherapy probably will be compatible with that dynamic underpinning, and will enrich and expand this approach.

REFERENCES

Alexander, F., & French, T. (1946). *Psychoanalytic therapy*. New York: Ronald Press.

Beck, A. T. (1976). *Cognitive therapy and the emotional dis-* orders. New York: New American Library.

Beck, A. T., Freeman, A., & Associates. (1990). *Cognitive therapy of personality disorders*. New York: Guilford.

Gill, M. M. (1982). *The analysis of transference, Vol. 1*. New York: International Universities Press.

Gold, J. R. (1988). An integrative approach to psychological crises of children and families. *Journal of Integrative and Eclectic Psychotherapy, 7*, 123–137.

Gold, J. R. (1990). The integration of psychoanalytic, interpersonal, and cognitive approaches in the psychotherapy of borderline and narcissistic disorders. *Journal of Integrative and Eclectic Psychotherapy, 9*, 49–68.

Gold, J. R. (1991). Repairing narcissistic deficits through the use of imagery. In R. Kunzendorf (Ed.), *Mental imagery* (pp. 227–232). New York: Plenum Press.

Kernberg, O. (1975). *Borderline conditions and pathological narcissism*. New York: Jason Aronson.

Kohut, H. (1971). *The analysis of the self*. New York: International Universities Press.

Levenson, E. A. (1983). *The ambiguity of change*. New York: Basic Books.

Reich, W. (1949). *Character analysis*. New York: Noonday Press.

Ryle, A. (1990). *Cognitive-analytic therapy: Active participation in change*. Chichester, England: Wiley.

Safran, J., & Segal, Z. (1990). *Interpersonal processes in cognitive therapy*. New York: Basic Books.

Shapiro, D. (1965). *Neurotic styles*. New York: Basic Books.

Stricker, G., & Gold, J. (1988). A psychodynamic approach to the personality disorders. *Journal of Personality Disorders, 2*, 350–359.

Sullivan, H. S. (1953). *The interpersonal theory of psychiatry*. New York: W. W. Norton.

Wachtel, P. L. (1977). *Psychoanalysis and behavior therapy: Towards an integration*. New York: Basic Books.

Wachtel, P. L. (1991). Towards a more seamless integration. *Journal of Psychotherapy Integration, 1*, 32–41.

Wachtel, E. F., & Wachtel, P. L. (1986). *Family dynamics in individual psychotherapy*. New York: Guilford.

Winnicott, D. W. (1971). *Maturational processes and the facilitating environment*. New York: International Universities Press.

CHAPTER 23

Psychotherapy with Substance Abusers

Nicholas A. Cummings

Psychotherapy with non-abstinent substance abusers is difficult, if not impossible, as all understanding is soluble in alcohol or drugs. (Cummings, 1979)

INTRODUCTION

Psychotherapy with substance abusers as we know it today is a phenomenon of essentially the decade of the 1980s. It has grown largely outside the direct contributions of psychiatry and psychology as disciplines. In fact, not too long ago those psychotherapists who specialized in the treatment of substance abuse were not accorded the same degree of respectability as those psychotherapists who treated the mainstream of psychological conditions. It was to elevate substance abuse specialization into mainstream psychotherapy that I chose to make psychotherapy with addicts the topic of my presidential address (Cummings, 1979) to the American Psychological Association (APA). My goal was partially realized as

Nicholas A. Cummings • American Biodyne and the Foundation for Behavioral Health, South San Francisco, California 94080.

Comprehensive Handbook of Psychotherapy Integration, edited by George Stricker and Jerold R. Gold. Plenum Press, New York, 1993.

widespread demand resulted in the address going into the seventh printing by the APA. The twelve-step philosophy received for the first time a psychological foundation. However, outpatient application with substance abusers was deemphasized in favor of the 28-day hospital program which exploded in the following decade into a $40 billion annual industry (A. Foster Higgins, Inc., 1990), which generated an acrimonious debate that is just now being resolved in favor of outpatient treatment.

This controversy on the efficacy of inpatient versus outpatient treatment has been so heated that it has obscured three facts. First, inclusion of substance abuse treatment as a covered benefit in health insurance is a relatively recent phenomenon, primarily of the last 20 years. Second, the large-scale hospitalization of addicted persons is a very recent phenomenon, essentially of the past decade and in current numbers only in the past 5 years. Third, inpatient and outpatient treatment is not a difference of treatment modalities, but a difference in settings. In view of these considerations, it may be worthwhile to review the developments in substance abuse treatment over the past quarter of a century (Cummings, 1991).

HISTORICAL PERSPECTIVE

Thirty years ago no major health plan in the United States reimbursed for the treatment of substance abuse. The medical consequences of alcoholism, such as cirrhosis of the liver, were covered, but the treatment of alcoholism itself was not. Even medical detoxification coverage was essentially absent. The wealthy went to plush private sanitoriums where they paid out-of-pocket and their alcoholism was disguised by a medical diagnosis, such as pneumonia, while they were "dried-out." Poor alcoholics detoxified each other by use of what was termed a "hummer": The alcoholic detoxing the other alcoholic would ration small amounts of alcohol sufficient to prevent delirium tremens or other sequelae of withdrawal. In between was the middle class who could afford out-of-pocket expenses sufficient to dry-out in small motel or guest house settings operated by recovering alcoholics with little or no medical supervision. The technique was primarily that of the hummer, with a strong helping of Alcoholics Anonymous philosophy thrown in during the few days the alcoholic was drying out.

The most conspicuous addicts were the chronic public inebriates who for the most part were remanded to the criminal justice system. A few of the more progressive states had provisions in their Welfare and Institutions Codes for the involuntary commitment of chronic inebriates to the state hospitals in programs that were set apart from those provided for the mentally ill. Most of these programs were on locked wards intended to enforce several weeks of abstinence. Treatment was mostly aversive conditioning: The patient was served cocktails in rapid succession in a simulated barroom setting, and after having been given Antabuse. Following what would be 48 hours of excessive vomiting and other unpleasant physical symptoms, the patient was given Antabuse and again ushered into the simulated barroom for drinks. This was repeated a prescribed number of times under the hypothesis that an aversive reaction to the consumption of alcohol would be created. Not surprisingly, the technique did not work and did not survive the state hospital era.

A unique program for heroin addicts was operated by the federal government at Lexington Barracks. With the guarantee of anonymity, the addict could enter the program for several weeks and under an assumed name while withdrawing from heroin. These heroin addicts seldom entered Lexington Barracks with the intent of going straight. Rather, they wanted to reduce the required daily quantity of heroin to which they had built-up so as to make their addiction more affordable. This, of course, was impossible. Shortly after leaving the facility, the addict rapidly returned to the level of drug tolerance previously achieved. This pioneering program was regarded as a success by no one, and after several decades it was closed when the federal government began licensing experimental methadone programs.

In the 1960s health plans began to include mental health and chemical dependency treatment (MH/CD) benefits, and by the 1970s most plans were characterized by including such benefits. However, most hospitalization was for medical detoxification, not for rehabilitation, something that was to change drastically in the decade of the 1980s. For most of the health plans, it was simple to adopt the 30-day hospital benefit that had become standard in medicine and surgery, and reject recommendations for 60- and 90-day benefits. Some fewer health plans, however, did adopt 60- and 90-day benefits, with others compromising at 45 days.

As a result of these insurance benefits the decade of the 1960s saw the emergence of a new industry: Chains of private chemical dependency hospitals with formulated 28-day inpatient programs that dove-tailed with the general indemnity benefit. There were also 45-, 60-, and 90-day programs for those holding health policies with more liberal benefits, but the 28-day program which included both detoxification and rehabilitation in a hospital setting became standard. In this manner, the field of substance abuse treatment unfortunately adopted the acute care model rather than the rehabilitation more appropriate to chronic conditions such as addiction.

In the beginning, there was little concern on the part of the insurance industry as relatively few persons filed for this inpatient benefit. The emergence of employee assistance programs (EAP's) did much to accelerate the use of the CD hospital benefit as EAP counselors made certain the employee took full advantage of available benefits. In some industries, such as the auto workers, inpatient rehabilitation became the preferred mode, with health economists taking note of the "revolving door" nature of these programs as early as the 1970s (Gallant *et al.*, 1973).

The giant leap in the use of inpatient CD rehabilitation programs occurred following the enactment by the Congress in 1985 of Diagnosis Related Groups (DRG's) in Medicare and Medicaid. Reimbursement to hospitals was no longer on a cost plus 15% basis, but on a schedule of a set number of days for each of over 300 DRG's. Seemingly overnight the occupancy rate of medical and surgical beds dropped drastically. Hospitals were in financial trouble until it was noticed that DRG's did not apply to MH/CD. By 1986, most hospitals converted empty beds to CD units and entered into aggressive multimedia advertising to market these newly proliferated programs. They were inordinately financially successful as the treatment of CD conditions in the United States increased in cost an average of over 40% for each of the succeeding 4 years.

The decade of the 1990s has seen the reversal of this reliance on inpatient rehabilitation with the first 2 years seeing a reduction of 15% and 25% successively in inpatient CD utilization. It is predicted that this new downward trend, based on a large body of outcome research, will continue. This impact of research on public policy in such a short time is unprecedented, and was reviewed by myself (Cummings, 1991).

INPATIENT VERSUS OUTPATIENT TREATMENT

In 1983, the Congressional Office of Technology Assessment (OTA) (Saxe, Dougherty, Esty, & Fine, 1983) released a report on the effectiveness of outpatient versus inpatient treatment of alcoholism and unleashed a storm of controversy. This review of the extant research revealed that although high-cost treatments, such as hospitalization, were probably justified by cost-benefit analysis, there was a substantial body of evidence that indicated less costly outpatient care was equally effective. Several years earlier, Cummings (1979) published the results of a 7 year Kaiser-Permanente study which showed that 95% of addicts

could be effectively treated outside an inpatient setting. These findings generated not a ripple of protest inasmuch as the for-profit sector of substance abuse treatment was still in its infancy and had not yet become a part of the giant Mental Health Complex (Duhl & Cummings, 1987), which was to be the case just a few years later.

The OTA report admitted that most of the studies upon which the conclusions were based were uncontrolled, and that the conclusions could be regarded as only tentative. It argued, however, that there was sufficient evidence, even if not adequately controlled, to at least call into question the ultimate cost-effectiveness of inpatient care. Three years later, Miller and Hester (1986) reviewed both the original uncontrolled studies and the more recent controlled studies and announced some startling conclusions. Whereas a host of confounding factors in the uncontrolled studies render their data inconclusive, the 26 controlled studies consistently reported no statistically significant differences between treatment settings or differences in intensity of treatment. They pointed out that these findings are consistent with the overall literature on inpatient psychiatric care (Kiesler, 1982).

Five years after its initial report, the OTA updated its findings (Saxe & Goodman, 1988), this time focusing on the controlled studies that had emerged. They reaffirmed their initial finding that both inpatient and outpatient treatment have demonstrable effectiveness, but there is no evidence to suggest that inpatient treatment is better than outpatient treatment. They addressed public policy issues and flatly stated,

the data strongly suggest that to the extent we have developed a system of providing care for alcoholism that rests on inpatient treatment, we are greatly overspending. Such overexpenditures have the result of inflating the necessary costs of alcoholism treatment and, perhaps, denying treatment to those who are unwilling or cannot afford inpatient programs. (p. 3)

It may be worthwhile to consider in some detail the complexity of the question, and to review a number of these controlled studies.

CONTROLLED STUDIES

Some of the problems inherent in studying the efficacy of inpatient versus outpatient treat ment include the following: Length of hospital stay can be influenced by motivational variables, severity of the problem, coercion, and appropriateness of client-treatment match (Miller, 1985; Miller & Hester, 1987a,b); clients judged as unmotivated may be terminated early by the staff (Holser, 1979) or even not referred for lengthy care (Sheehan, Wieman, & Bechtel, 1981). Studies controlling for confounding variables necessarily employ random assignment to control and experimental groups, such as those that follow.

In one of the most cited studies in substance abuse (Edwards *et al.*, 1977), 50 alcoholics seen in inpatient and outpatient care, and 50 alcoholics randomly assigned to receive only an evaluation and a single-counseling session were followed-up 1 year and 2 years after treatment. No significant differences were found between groups on any measure of improvement. In another study (McCrady, Longabaugh, *et al.*, 1986), no significant difference in improvement was found between patients randomly assigned to either inpatient or day care. Chapman and Huygens (1988) compared inpatient, outpatient, and single confrontational interview situations and found no differences in outcome. The confrontation was in the presence of the patient's spouse, family member, or close friend. As reported by the OTA (Saxe & Goodman, 1988), Newton and Bowman randomly assigned alcoholics following detoxification to after care alone, or 25 days inpatient treatment plus after care. No significant differences were found at 2-, 4-, 7-, 10-, or 13-month follow-ups. In a similar study (Mosher, Davis, Mulligan, & Iber, 1975), 200 alcoholics were randomly assigned to receive or not receive 30 days of detoxification and inpatient treatment. No significant differences were found in abstinence, work status, drug use, or anxiety on 3- and 6-month follow-ups.

The dangers of detoxification are often cited to justify hospitalization. Indeed, delirium tremens can be a severe form of alcohol withdrawal, and withdrawal from several drugs can result in convulsions (e.g., alcohol, barbiturates, benzodiazepines). A number of controlled studies indicate that only a small number of addicts need to detoxify in the hospital (Feldman, Pattison, Sobell, Graham, & Sobell 1975; Hayashida *et al.*, 1989; O'Briant, Petersen, & Heacock, 1977). Annis

(1987), in reviewing the literature, concluded that 90% of addicts cannot only be detoxified outside of the hospital, they need no medication to do so. Annis further concluded that hospitalization should be reserved for those relatively few patients who need management of *medical* sequelae.

Neither length of hospital stay nor duration of outpatient treatment correlates with successful outcome. A number of studies (Mosher *et al.*, 1975; Pittman & Tate, 1972; Page & Schaub, 1979; Walker, Donovan, Kivlahan, & O'Leary, 1983; Willems, Letemendia & Arroyave, 1973) comparing hospital stays from 1 to 7 weeks found no advantages in longer over shorter stays. Similarly, length of outpatient care does not increase improvement (Powell, Penick, Read, & Ludwig, 1985; Robson, Paulus, & Clarke, 1965; Smart & Gray, 1978). Even more startling are studies that indicate 6 to 18 weeks of outpatient therapy was no more effective than self-help with minimal therapist contact (Buck & Miller, 1986; Miller, Gribskov, & Mortell, 1981; Miller & Baca, 1983).

Matching addicts to treatment on the basis of clinical dimensions has been the focus of several studies, and these have yielded the only demonstrable positive results for the variable of intensity. In general, more severe and less socially stable alcoholics do better in either inpatient or more intensive outpatient treatment, whereas less severe and more socially stable alcoholics do better in outpatient care, and even less intensive outpatient treatment (Annis, 1987; Kissin, Platz, & Su, 1970; McLachlan & Stein, 1982; McLellan *et al.*, 1983; Orford, Oppenheimer, & Edwards, 1976; Smart, 1978; Stinson, Smith, Amidjaya, & Kaplan, 1979; Willems *et al.*, 1973). But as Miller and Hester (1987b) point out, when heterogeneous populations of alcoholics are averaged together, no significant advantage of inpatient over outpatient treatment emerges. They conclude that brief hospitalization may be warranted for severe pharmacologic dependence, suicidality, or homelessness, but for most patients outpatient treatment is as effective as inpatient.

Miller and Hester (1987a) reviewed five controlled studies evaluating partial hospitalization (day care or halfway house) and found no advantage for inpatient versus partial residential treatment. They also found only one study (Stinson *et al.*, 1979) that compared inpatient settings with a high density of staff to low density of staff, with the surprising finding that the latter had a statistically significant advantage in measures of abstinence over the former. It was as if the greater self-direction induced by the lower staff density carried into the patient's life after release from the hospital.

There is now a plethora of evidence indicating that inpatient care is no more effective for most addiction patients than outpatient treatment, and when one compares the difference in cost, the advantage is decidedly on the side of outpatient care. Yet the community continues to clamor for inpatient care for a number of reasons. First, the addict is looking for a magical "fix" of the problem in a setting where responsibility, self-initiation, and pain will be minimized. The family also wants a vacation from the addict who by the time of presentation for treatment has been the source of familial disruption or chaos for weeks, months, or years. Similarly, the employer who has felt the economic pinch of the high cost of healthcare as well as the loss of productivity from addicted employees and those fellow employees they disrupt, wants the addict out of the workplace until recovered. For all these, inpatient setting is the obvious solution, for while the patient is away for 28 days all concerned can cherish the illusion that something is being done to forever fix the problem.

OTHER CONTROVERSIES

The preceding decade has seen an emerging consensus on a number of other controversies that have hampered the development of integration in the psychotherapy of substance abusers. These have been summarized in the report to the Congress by the Secretary of Health and Human Services (Sullivan, 1990).

1. There are both physiological and psychological aspects to addiction, and although in the initial detoxification the former may be the primary focus, in the long range the latter may be the more compelling aspect.

2. There is no such thing as a single personality that leads to addiction, and a number of conditions may place the individual at risk. Among these are phobias, protracted anxiety states, and chronic depression because of the temporary relief that the drug or alcohol induces, as well as the expected array of personality disorders. The characteristics ascribed to the addicts, such as denial, obstinacy, lying, irritability, hostility, poor object relations, and mild paranoia are the result of the addiction, not its cause.

3. One of the body's methods of dealing with noxious agents, of which alcohol and drugs are a type, is to involve tissue changes with increasingly more cells involved. This is called alcohol or drug tolerance, so that with sustained use it takes more and more of a drug to produce the desired effect. Axiomatically it can be stated that the highest level of tolerance becomes the minimum daily requirement for life. It may take an alcoholic 10 years to build to a quart of whiskey a day, but once that is reached, even though he or she may be dry for 5 years, when drinking behavior resumes it is only a matter of days or a few weeks before the alcoholic is ingesting a quart of whiskey a day. This phenomenon is clearly seen in heroin addiction where even after years of abstinence, the weight of "the monkey" achieved before quitting becomes the amount of heroin required within hours, and one that would have been a lethal dose in the early stages of addiction. The tissue changes are readily seen in calorie addiction. Once an adipose (fat) cell is created it is never eliminated. One loses weight by emptying these cells, but they remain like so many empty "baggies" crying to be refilled (Cummings, 1979).

4. In spite of the intense interest in finding a genetic marker, especially for alcoholism, it is unlikely that such a single gene will emerge. On the other hand, a number of heritable predispositions that do not cause alcoholism, but may increase or decrease the likelihood have already been discovered with more future discoveries being probable. It is difficult for most psychotherapists to comprehend the difference between an inherited trait and a heritable predisposition, and two examples might be helpful, one that increases the risk and one that decreases such risk.

The first step in a complicated series of enzyme changes following the absorption of ethyl alcohol is the breakdown of the alcohol by the enzyme alcohol dehydrogenase into acetylaldehyde. In most persons the breakdown into acetylaldehyde occurs at a steady pace, and since acetylaldehyde is more intoxicating than the alcohol itself, the individual receives the first signs that he or she has had enough to drink: dizziness, stomach queasiness, slurred speech, unsteady gait. These uncomfortable feelings are such that most people will refrain from drinking further. However, some persons have an inherited slow acting, or low volume alcohol dehydrogenase and do not receive these early signs of intoxication. Such persons seem to drink a great deal without discomfort or indications of being drunk, only to suddenly become very drunk and even pass out once the large intake of alcohol is converted to acetylaldehyde. Individuals with slow acting, or low volume alcohol dehydrogenase have several times the probability of becoming addicted, as most persons drink to feel relaxed and euphoric, and these individuals need to imbibe a great deal to reach the state, which unfortunately, when it appears, comes in exaggerated form.

A heritable trait which markedly reduces the probability of becoming addicted to alcohol is the "Asian flush," so named because it is frequent in but not limited to Asian populations. This is an allergic response to alcohol that produces such uncomfortable cardiovascular and gastrointestinal responses that the person is very reluctant to drink even the small amounts of alcohol that inevitably result in this discomfort. As these conditions illustrate, they are not genetic markers that result in alcoholism or lack of it, but are predisposing causes that increase or decrease the probability. As one example, a person with slow acting alcohol dehydrogenase may be a devout Mormon who has never taken a drink of alcohol, and for whom the heritable slow acting enzyme is irrelevant. On the other hand, the best known predictor of addictive behavior is the son or daughter of an alcoholic. This predictor embodies all factors: physiology and learning, as well as possible heritable conditions (Sullivan, 1990).

TREATMENT MODALITIES

As indicated above, the inpatient versus outpatient controversy is one of difference in setting, not treatment modalities. Treatment modalities cluster around four philosophies: Medical, psychoanalytic, behavior modification, and twelve-step. Any of these may be found in hospitals and in outpatient programs.

Medical Model

The medical model of treating addiction potentially addicts a person to a stronger drug to get off the drug to which the person was previously addicted (Cummings, 1979). Just as in the 1910s heroin was introduced as a "cure" for morphine addiction, methadone is used to get addicts off heroin, benzodiazepines and anxiolytics are used to get alcoholics off alcohol, and amphetamines are used to control calorie "addiction." This model sees addiction as a physical craving that must be interrupted by chemical means. Most psychiatrists, as well as physician addictionologists, and especially those who have hospital-based practices, subscribe to this model. Addiction is seen as physiological, and possibly even genetic. It is one example of the disease model of addiction, and is compatible with the physician's training and armamentarium.

The medical model is vehemently opposed by the twelve-step philosophy which, curiously, is the other major disease model of addiction. The criticism contends that the medical model plays into the patient's desire for a quick fix without self-responsibility for continued addictive behavior, and further reinforces the addict's belief that all solutions to problems are chemical in nature.

An integrated twelve-step model would include pharmacology, but in practice the medical model and the twelve-step philosophy tend to become polarized.

Psychoanalytic Model

The psychoanalytic model, which essentially strives to elicit insight into the underlying conflicts that lead to addiction, is out of favor in CD treatment circles. Until the recent era, however, individual psychoanalytically oriented psychotherapy was the usual approach to treatment by independently practicing psychotherapists. It is the opposite of the disease model. It sees addiction as a set of unconscious emotional conflicts rooted in development that predispose the individual toward addictive behavior.

This model is criticized as lacking the confrontation needed to break through the addict's denial, and even abetting the avoidance of the problem by not addressing it directly. In fact, there is consensus that insight is perhaps the least effective approach, unfortunately leading most CD psychotherapists to abandon interest in insight therapy altogether, thus throwing out the baby with the bathwater (Cummings, 1979, 1991).

As a unique application of insight therapy, Peele (1978) sees all addictions as "love addiction," with the understanding of one's fear of commitment as the cornerstone to conquering one's addiction.

Behavioral Model

This is the traditional psychological model. Based on behaviorism, and more recently on cognitive behaviorism, it holds that addictive behavior can be controlled and that an addict can be restored to being a social user. The latter aspect, disputed by the overwhelming majority of CD treatment experts, became discredited with the research of Mark and Linda Sobell which purported to have turned addicts into social (controlled) drinkers, and which a follow-up of the original population by researchers at the University of California at Los Angeles (UCLA) alleged was fraudulently reported. The subsequent researchers found that the subjects had not controlled their drinking and most had died of alcohol-related complications. The few who were still alive had become abstinent by their own initiative (Cummings, 1991).

Most psychologists are still trained in the behavioral model of the treatment of addiction. It holds that addiction is a constellation of learned behaviors that can be modified and is the direct opposite of the disease model. Notwithstanding the basic goal of controlled drinking, which most CD experts see as flawed, cognitive behavioral techniques are extremely useful in an integrated model of CD psychotherapy.

Twelve-Step Model

In the 1930s Bill Wilson founded Alcoholics Anonymous (AA) with its disease model which states that there is no "cure" for alcoholism and

that abstinence is the only response to addiction. Therefore, sober alcoholics are "recovering alcoholics," for whom there are twelve steps to this recovery. Originally AA was a self-help movement, but as more and more recovering alcoholics became alcoholism counselors, the twelve-step philosophy has become the dominant modality in CD programs. Most experts regard its basic philosophy of abstinence and recovery as the most effective approach.

Within the last two decades the AA philosophy has been expanded to include Narcotics Anonymous (NA), Cocaine-Abusers Anonymous (CA), Gamblers Anonymous (GA) and Overeaters Anonymous (OA). Even more recently the twelve-step modality has been stretched to include conditions upon which there is disagreement as to whether they are really addictions (e.g., sex and love addictions, compulsive spending, and compulsive shoplifting). And within the past two or three years there has been proliferation of absurd proportions, with a count of over 275 different conditions to which the twelve-step philosophy is purportedly applied (Andrews, 1991).

At the present time the twelve-step movement is characterized by a religious zeal which attempts to guard the purity of the model, while at the same time allowing it to commercialize. In a sense, the movement has been a victim of its own success. Most CD programs have essentially been captured by recovering addicts, lending to a two-caste system with some disdain or distrust of psychotherapists who themselves are not recovering addicts.

In delineating the twelfth step as maintaining abstinence by helping others achieve sobriety, the founder of AA saw this as a volunteer endeavor, and he worried that the trend for recovering alcoholics (and other addicts) to become *paid* counselors had the potential of corrupting the twelve-step philosophy. He expressed the concern that this could lead to commercialism, and he foresaw what seemed so unlikely when he expressed his fear: crass television commercials huckstering expensive recovery programs (B. Wilson, personal communication, May 1978). The founder of AA did not live long enough to see his innermost fear materialize, but the rest of us have.

TOWARD PSYCHOTHERAPY INTEGRATION

The challenge to any integrated model of psychotherapy with substance abusers is to maintain the effectiveness of the twelve-step philosophy, especially its emphasis on sobriety and recovery, and at the same time purge it from its almost fanatic zeal and move it toward sound psychological professionalism. Clinical skills need to be honed and psychological constructs sharpened. Psychodynamics, behavioral techniques, and systems theory can all serve to augment the twelve-step model and render it more effective. It is no longer sufficient to rely on confrontation, zeal, and exaggerated claims (Shain, 1991). To the extent addiction is a disease, it is a disease somewhat analogous to diabetes: it is the patient's responsibility to stay away from sugar or, in the case of the addict, from mind-altering drugs.

Onion and Garlic

Although psychodynamically oriented psychotherapy has had disappointingly a lack of success as a technique with addicts, an appreciation of psychodynamics accords the therapist virtually a road map to understanding addictive behavior. In dealing with addicts and other very difficult patients, the metaphor of the Onion-Garlic Chart (see Table 1), based on psychodynamics, has proven useful. Consider what happens when we eat onions for lunch and return to the office. Our co-workers are not aware of the onion, but all afternoon, every time we swallow we taste the onion. On the other hand, had we eaten garlic for lunch, we would no longer be aware of the garlic, but all our co-workers would move away from us. In short, onion persons suffer, while garlic persons make everyone else suffer. All of our patients predominantly fall into one or the other category.

In addition, patients can be divided as to whether they are capable of achieving insight or whether uncovering therapy will be helpful, versus those for whom uncovering would be deleterious. Thus, the Onion-Garlic Chart is a fourfold table.

As shown in Table 1, addicts are always garlic and are capable of profiting from understanding themselves. The problem has been that therapists

Table 1.   Onion-Garlic Chart

Analyzable	
Onion (repression)	Garlic (denial)
Hysteria	Addictions
Anxiety	Neurotic character
Phobias	disorders
Organ neuroses	Personality disorders
Obsessive-compulsive	Impulse neuroses
Depression	Hypomania
	Narcissistic personality
	Borderline personality
Nonanalyzable	
Onion (withdrawal)	Garlic (withdrawal)
Organ psychoses	Impulse schizophrenia
Obsessional schizophrenia	Mania
Psychotic depression	Paranoia

Note: The narcissistic personality and the borderline personality have much in common (garlic attitude, addictions, perversions, poor reality testing, weak ego strength). The narcissistic personality will be differentiated by its extreme and pervasive vulnerability. The narcissistic personality will eventually respond to insight. The borderline personality will deteriorate with uncovering therapy.

have attempted insight before the garlic has been effectively addressed. Psychotherapists are inherently caregivers. This is one reason why we have become psychotherapists. We want to alleviate suffering, and we are adept at reducing the guilt of the neurotic as seen in the upper left quadrant of the Onion-Garlic Chart. But applying the same techniques to garlic patients (addicts, personality disorders) is like pouring gasoline onto a fire. And because we want to alleviate suffering, a psychotherapist can always find that sliver of onion in every bunch of garlic, ignore the latter and rush to treat the former. The result is therapeutic failure.

Dual diagnoses are popular now in many circles because they permit a treatment program to treat two conditions simultaneously and bill for both. In point of fact, there is no such thing as an addict who behind the addiction does not have a profound psychological condition that needs to be addressed. For example, an agoraphobic (onion) becomes addicted to alcohol or iatrogenically to Valium because one or the other enables the afflicted to leave the house. But once addicted, the patient is now garlic. Therapeutic failures with addicts can be minimized if the therapist bears in mind the axiom "always treat garlic before onion." Once the addiction is in recovery, the agoraphobia may now be treated. On the other hand, there are many addicts who, once in recovery, manifest more garlic (e.g., borderline personalities, neurotic character disorders, personality disorders). The therapist continues to apply the therapeutic techniques now applicable to the underlying garlic.

It is important to note that in the type of patient whose addiction is now in recovery and whose onion is being treated, this patient will frequently manifest vestigial garlic behavior. In AA this is called the "dry drunk"; even though the patient is dry, he or she begins to manifest the denial associated with being wet. When garlic behavior in the now onion patient appears, it is important that the therapist adhere to the axiom of "garlic before onion" and temporarily suspend onion treatment in favor of garlic treatment. Failure to do so will often result in the patient's relapse into abuse of his or her substance.

Phase I: The Presentation

No addict presents to a psychotherapist in order to receive psychotherapy which will lead to abstinence. The addict is there for the therapist to fix something with the spouse, lover, boss, police, probation officer, or judge, or to be taken back to the halcyon days when the chemical merely resulted in euphoria and not trouble. If the therapist does not understand this, therapy will not even get started. Occasionally, even after 35 years of treating addicts, I will see a patient for the first time who will sound so sincere as to appear to be the exception. At such times, the therapist should count to 10, and if the patient is still regarded as sincerely seeking to go clean, the therapist should now count to 100. Denial in addiction is so pervasive, that it never stops. As one recovering patient who was reflecting back on his denial during the first sessions with the therapist put it, "Even when I was telling the truth I was using the truth to set up the next lie."

These initial sessions are critical. The naive therapist will lose the patient, but so will the therapist who, in an effort not to be conned, pounces on the patient and prematurely confronts the denial. Most patients are lost to treatment

during this initial critical period. The goal of the initial sessions is to bond with the patient, since interventions which precede the bonding will be ineffective. Often, this involves a fine line between doing all the things that will facilitate bonding (listening with concern and empathy, not challenging the patient's veracity) and not appearing so naive or gullible in the face of the patient's denial that the therapist loses credibility.

The initial session(s) is also the place where a triage is made, with those who may need medical detoxification in the hospital because of the physical complications of the substance abuse (impending delirium tremens, risk of convulsions, and other sequelae) versus those who can be withdrawn or titrated on an outpatient basis. In this integrated model, rehabilitation ideally takes place on an outpatient basis, and inpatient (hospital) rehabilitation is appropriate for those patients who have previously failed at all outpatient attempts. A note of caution is indicated: the converse is not necessarily true that someone who has failed several inpatient rehabilitation settings should receive another admission to the hospital. In my experience, such a patient might well succeed in the first outpatient program because even after several hospitalizations it was in the outpatient setting that he or she took self-responsibility for the first time.

The successful treatment of substance abuse requires a continuum of care with skillful triage to each sector. A continuum will include the following:

A. Detoxification

1. Inpatient medical detoxification, 3 to 4 days (10%–15%).
2. Outpatient medical titration (30%–35%).
3. Outpatient "cold-turkey" under intense psychotherapeutic and community support (40%–50%).

B. Rehabilitation

1. In a hospital setting (5%–10%).
2. In an intensive outpatient (IOP) seting of several hours a day for 6 months (25%–35%).
3. In outpatient group and individual psychotherapy for 5 months (50%–60%).

Triaging to the appropriate program for each patient during the initial session(s) is, along with the quality and effectiveness of these programs, an important determinant in the successful or unsuccessful outcome of treatment. In addition to the programs above, psychotic drug addicts need their own special programs. It is further recommended that patients with Borderline Personality Disorder be put in groups with only other borderline patients, as they will turn a mixed group into chaos as they split the members.

Phase II: The Motivation and the Therapeutic Contract

The greatest ally a therapist has is a boss, spouse, or judge who has had it with the patient. During bonding and in succeeding sessions, it is important that the patient's discomfort with his or her problem or the anxiety level are kept fairly high, for once the addict feels comfortable again he or she will drop out of treatment. Therefore, it is especially important to refrain from rushing in to rescue the patient or fix the problem. An optimal level of anxiety and discomfort will facilitate bonding and enhance motivation. One of the reasons that inpatient rehabilitation is often a revolving door is that the hospitalization results in diminished anxiety and discomfort, and the patient's problem may go away (e.g., the boss, spouse or judge feels sorry for the poor patient who is so sick that hospitalization is required).

The primary goal in the second phase is to motivate the patient to initial abstinence so that psychotherapy can really begin. This will involve confronting the denial, but this confrontation must be skillfully performed. It should not be a blunt instrument. The one exception might be ex-convicts whose addiction resulted in prison, or possibly sociopaths who have manipulated several previous programs. For such individuals, blunt confrontation and the leverage of their legal problems may be the most efficacious avenue. With most others, however, the confrontation should reflect the utmost clinical skill.

Shain (1991) has expanded the array of confrontation skills from the most subtle to the obvious. Cummings (1979) in a unique application of confrontation utilizes the addict's own characteristic obstinacy to challenge and motivate the patient. In this technique the therapist skillfully verbalizes the patient's own denial, while at the same time withholding treatment as something not worthwhile for that particular addict. Examples are: "You can beat this yourself"; "You have been conning your wife for over 10 years and with a little effort you could con her into taking you back"; "Your boss is a softy and we can figure out a way to get him to rescind his firing you again." Here the therapist verbalizes the patient's covert beliefs, resulting in the patient's beginning to talk like the therapist (e.g., "I can't continue to fool myself, my wife or boss deserve better"). But whatever technique is used to confront the patient and break through the denial, here is another instance where clinical skill, not just good intentions, is required.

In the successful confrontation, the patient's implicit contract for coming into treatment (e.g., fix me; get my wife back) is identified and discussed, and an explicit therapeutic contract is agreed upon. This includes the agreement to enter a 5-month group therapy program wherein only 3 relapses (falls) are permitted, and after the fourth relapse the patient is excluded from treatment and cannot re-enter treatment until after the group of which he or she was a part concludes the treatment program. Attendance is mandatory as is abstinence; imbibing in a mind altering drug or an absence each constitute one fall. The patient is allowed up to 5 individual sessions to be used only in critical need so that individual sessions do not drain from the group energy and commitment. Fraternization among group members outside the group is forbidden so that there will be no subgroups. Friends, co-workers or relatives are not placed together in the same group. These rules become part of the therapeutic contract which is rendered in writing so that there is absolute clarity as to what has been agreed.

Many patients do not respond to the confrontation or the challenge, no matter how skillfully presented. These patients may be highly resistant because they are simply not ready to confront their denial. In AA terms, they have not bottomed-out. For these patients a psychoeducational, open-ended preaddictions group can make a significant difference. In one study (Cummings, 1991) the number of persons entering the outpatient addictions program was doubled by having made available such a nonthreatening psychoeducational program.

Phase III: Group Therapy— Withdrawal

As the group therapy begins, although clean, the patients are still experiencing withdrawal. They complain of restlessness and insomnia. Depressions or phobias emerge. Usually articulate, if not glib patients have difficulty expressing themselves. Social ineptitudes previously masked by chemicals become painfully apparent. And, for some curious reason, all of the mistakes, procrastinations and neglects resulting from years of substance abuse choose this time to come home to roost.

These patients need a great deal of support. In addition to the therapist being there for them, they are urged to participate in AA, NA, CA, GA, and OA, and one or even two meetings a day for the first several weeks is not an unusual regimen in this stage. Although the physical withdrawal improves in 60 days, there is a markedly noticeable improvement in 6 months and again another after about 1 year. The later improvements would seem to represent improvement in psychological rather than physical withdrawal.

During Phase III, the patient's withdrawal will improve only to have this improvement followed by a marked regression. The patients will variously describe depression and other uncomfortable physical symptoms of withdrawal characteristic of having just come off a prolonged binge, yet the patient has been clean. AA has named this the "dry drunk," or the "dry hangover." The purpose is to make the addict so uncomfortable so he or she will exclaim to himself or herself, "If I'm going to feel this badly without the chemical, I may as well go back to my chemical and at least enjoy the first part of the binge–hangover cycle." A dry hangover usually lasts days or a couple of weeks. Some few patients have reported experiencing it for as long as 2 months. It disappears as rapidly as it emerged once the addict makes the decision not to resume the chemical no matter how intense the discomfort becomes.

Phase IV: Group Therapy— The Games

Overlapping the withdrawal phase, the phase called "The Games" begins. All addicts play games, and they cannot go from destructive games to no games. Phase IV has as its goal the teaching of constructive games.

One of the major games is called "rescue" and differs from actually helping someone in need. All addicts become the focal point of everybody who has a problem. They are called on the phone day and night by friends who tell them their troubles. They play the rescue game no matter how undeserving the person. They attempt to rescue them because when they themselves mess up and are undeserving, they can then feel entitled to be rescued.

The "rubber ruler" is one of the most frequent games and can take many forms. It can consist of telling the bartender to leave the olive out of the martini, with all kinds of jokes about how many cubic centimeters of gin the olive displaces. The real reason is that after seven martinis, the alcoholic does not want to look at an ashtray and see seven toothpicks, because he or she wants to walk out of the bar and say that only three martinis were consumed.

The foodaholic will believe that the giant-sized bag of potato chips he or she just demolished was only ¼ full, when it was really ⅞ full. The rubber ruler can be either stretched or compressed. An addict will often be convinced he or she has been clean for 1½ months when it has only been about 10 days.

The "vending machine" is an interesting game that alcoholics play. It says, "I have been a good boy, I have been a good girl. Why isn't life making it easy for me?" It begins in childhood when our parents forgive our F in spelling because we did so well in Sunday school two days earlier, even though the two are totally unrelated. Alcoholics continue such childish expectations and demand miracles after having been dry for 2 or 3 weeks. Because they have been good, addicts expect life to open up and give them all they want: a better job, a better lover, freedom from their probation officers, instant health.

Another common game is "self-pity," and no addicts will resume their addiction until they first get themselves into the vortex of self-pity that makes the thing possible. Addicts like to refer to it as the "pity-pot." Self-pity can be justified by a cross word from a boss, a nagging spouse, or a so-called sick society. All of these become excuses to resume drug activity. In fact, addicts quite frequently precipitate crises in order to justify their addiction, a common ploy being to incite a previously nagging spouse to begin nagging again as an excuse to end a period of sobriety.

In all of these games one sees the addict's careful point-counterpoint in which guilt, justification, absolution, and punishment abound in complex acting-out patterns that assure the continuation of the addictive life-style. From morning-after remorse to contrition when arrested for drunk driving, the addict not only is full of good intentions but manages to suffer in such a way that he or she can continue to view himself or herself as blameless and misunderstood. So the addict settles for what Peele (1978) called "comfortable discomfort." He or she becomes a kind of successful loser who alternates between elation at having fooled the world and depression at the discovery of his or her low self-esteem and lack of self-confidence.

The addict is adroit at playing the "feeling game," so the unwary therapist may be fooled into accepting the counterfeit feelings as genuine insight, just as the addict's friends have been fooled for years. In fact, everyone has had the experience of being shocked to learn that a friend or neighbor who was known for sincerity, concern, and honest feeling turned out to be an addict who had neglected his or her family for years. The therapist would do well to employ only positive changes in behavior over suitable periods of time as the real yardstick to insight or understanding.

The "file card" is an important game because it is an unconscious determination to resume drinking at a certain point in time, or once certain conditions have been fulfilled. In *While Rome Burns*, Alexander Woollcott has one of his characters telephone his hostess of the night before to apologize for missing her dinner party, saying, "On the way to your home I was taken unexpectedly drunk." No one is taken unexpectedly drunk. Rather, one plants a decision in the back of one's mind to the effect that if my wife nags me the 20th time or if my boss makes me work weekends, I deserve a drink. Once the event happens, the addict begins to drink, or pop pills, without having to arrive at any further conscious decision, in such a way that the file card, once filed, is automatic although forgotten.

Alcoholics are perfectionists. If one were an unscrupulous employer one would hire nobody but primary alcoholics. Without their knowing it, they would not be expected to work on Mondays because they would be recovering from their hangovers, and they would be expected to miss work on Fridays because they could not hold off for the weekend and would begin drinking on Thursday night. But on Tuesdays, Wednesdays, and Thursdays, the employer would get two weeks worth of work out of them. They are perfectionists, but their perfectionism is part of the game that feeds their life-style and justifies addiction.

In playing "musical chairs" the addict, while remaining technically clean, substitutes another substance and essentially keeps the addiction alive. If the new substance is not made part of the abstinence contract, right after the program is concluded the abuser will return to the primary substance and to an addictive way of life. Food, gambling, and prescription drugs are among the favorite substitutes.

Every addict believes inwardly that he or she is a "special person." It seems paradoxical this belief would be held in parallel with the overwhelming inferiority that addicts feel, yet they exist side by side and feed on each other. The special person is so exalted that the addict never achieves the dizzy height. Consequently every achievement pales in the face of the special person so that the addict never has the solid sense of achievement. The inferiority complex looms even larger because it is never counter-balanced by the inner reward of having done something well. So the addict approaches his or her special person only when high on chemicals. This only intensifies the crash when sober and increases the reliance on drugs to feel adequate.

A particularly insidious form of "special person" is the belief "I am the exception to the rule. I will go from addiction to social user." Every addict subjects himself or herself to the *test*. In this game the alcoholic has one drink to prove he or she can stop. This test may be repeated several times, and passed each time. Eventually the compulsive behavior will return en masse. This is because the test convinces the patient that he or she is not an addict and can relax vigilance. One alcoholic went to a bar after work each night for just one drink to prove he could do it and stop. He succeeded for 8 nights. On the ninth night, he closed the bar and continued into a 3-day binge. The number of ways to play "the test" are infinite, and the addict will always "prove" initially that he or she is not addicted.

Phase V: Group Therapy— The Working Through

With the mastery of the destructive games and before the substitution of positive or healthy games, the group members suddenly become zealots. This is the "holier-than-thou stage" out of which many reformed drunks never emerge. It is important that this highly authoritarian outlook be understood and ameliorated, for during this phase the addict becomes merciless toward a fellow group member who may have a fall. Such an outlook toward the world can lead only to new kinds of problems in living.

Once this is worked through, and about halfway through the 20 group sessions, the group members become depressed. They realize there is no shortcut, only hard work ahead. The fanaticism disappears, but so does the enthusiasm that carried the client thus far. It is as if the energy goes out of the group, and each group member settles into a profound depression that places him or her at risk. It is interesting that few clients have falls during this period; most of the falls have occurred in Phase II, when most of the testing of the limits is being acted out. Furthermore, the therapist's vigilance is alerted at this period, and the group members who have now been working together for several months accept the assurance that once this depression is weathered, better days are coming.

Phase VI: Group Therapy— Self-Responsibility

In the final phase, the client seems to finally accept responsibility. This is in the form of a conviction, heretofore aggressively resisted, which concludes that abstinence is for life, not the 6 months of the group program. With the acceptance of this fact comes a kind of peaceful resolution with oneself and a sense of mastery.

This phase appears just at the point when the addict despairs that he or she will never emerge from the profound depression. It happens suddenly, and clients describe it as an experience

similar to learning to type or mastering a foreign language: proficiency is preceded by a seemingly interminable period of more or less mechanical struggling. Then one day one is typing or speaking the language. In our case, the addict has made the decision to go one day at a time, and that recovery is for life. The client is no longer subject to panicky mood swings that send him or her scurrying for the bottle, the needle, or the pill.

The key ingredient has been the therapist, whose unrelenting firmness, fairness, and honesty have provided a role model and whose deep commitment and concern have ameliorated the client's chronically low self-esteem and interpersonal distrust, so aptly described by Chein as quoted by Cummings (1979, p. 1128).

THE CASE OF MARLA

Marla, a 38-year-old, single woman who had been living with her fiancé for almost 3 years, had been in treatment for agoraphobia for 14 months when she was admitted to a detoxification hospital unit following a 6-day binge on alcohol and Valium. In the over a year she had been in treatment, her psychotherapist was unaware that Marla had a severe substance abuse problem. Twice Ron, the fiancé, hinted at it to the psychotherapist. Marla responded with convincing denial, and the therapist, in a manner characteristic of many of her colleagues, chose to ignore the warning signs and avoid the acrimony that would surely have followed had she not done so.

Marla was engaged to be married to her live-in boyfriend when she suffered severe injuries in an automobile accident which necessitated several reconstructive bone surgeries over the following year. The wedding was postponed 3 times over the next 2 years, and Ron was becoming discouraged after a period of impatience.

Following the accident the patient became phobic while driving and soon she could not drive at all. This interfered with a very successful business she had founded and developed. Marla was a public accountant who serviced an impressive number of very small businesses. Routinely, once a month, she would pick-up the general ledgers of her clients, take them to her office in her home, and reconcile the books and prepare necessary tax and other forms. Her new inability to drive created a hardship. Ron would have to take time from the automobile service station he owned and managed to drive Marla to her clients' businesses. As matters between them became more strained and Ron insisted they marry and live on his quite adequate income, Marla progressed from the phobia of driving to an inability to leave the house at all unless Ron was with her. She had become agoraphobic.

Her psychotherapist, a specialist in agoraphobia, treated Marla in group and individual therapy without any progress whatsoever. The psychotherapist seemed to ignore the fact that Marla did not demonstrate the behavior characteristic of agoraphobics: compliant, perfectionistic people-pleasing; in other words, the epitome of "onion" behavior. To the contrary, she was defiant, argumentative and seldom did her desensitization assignments; in other words, her behavior was "garlic," and consistent with her unrecognized substance abuse problem.

Once hospitalized for detoxification following her potentially lethal Valium and alcohol binge, her addiction was addressed. After several attempts at denial, she discussed for the first time a history of alcoholism beginning at age 11. In college she learned to hold her drinking behavior in check until the weekends by substituting large daily doses of Valium which she obtained from several physicians, each of whom thought he was the only one prescribing the medication. Once abstinent for several months, she was now ready to grapple with her phobias.

Marla's phobias began in the first grade with a full-blown school phobia. Her intense competition with her little brother, who she was sure would capture mother's affection while Marla was at school, was never really addressed by the school psychologist. Her phobia grew and interfered with learning, but she attended school as she was forced to do. At age 11, she discovered that alcohol dissolved her phobia, and she spent the remainder of her childhood and adolescence getting hold of enough alcohol to make life tolerable. By the time she got to college, her drinking was out of control. The discovery of Valium allowed her to become a weekend binge drinker, and enabled her to complete college. The phobias were now all but forgotten, buried deep in an addictive life-style.

The automobile accident occurred just as Marla was struggling with her terror of making a marriage commitment to Ron. She had chosen a man just like her little brother, then proceeded to punish him for being like her brother. In all ways she competed with him, defeating and belittling him at every opportunity. The resurgence of severe phobic behavior enabled her to both postpone the commitment of marriage, and at the same time to tie her to the ambivalent relationship part of her needed, and the other part wanted to leave.

Marla has been abstinent 3 years and she no longer is phobic. She continues her recovery from alcohol and Valium addiction. The important point is that the understanding of her phobic (onion) behavior was not possible as long as it was covered by addiction (garlic).

REFERENCES

Andrews, L. M. (1991, June). *Spiritual issues in treatment.* Keynote address presented at the Annual Meeting of the Employee Assistance Society of North America (EASNA), Atlantic City.

Annis, H. (1987, October). *Effective treatment for drug and alcohol problems: Do we know?* Paper presented at the Annual Meeting of the Institute of Medicine, National Academy of Sciences, Washington, DC.

Buck, K., & Miller, W. R. (1986). *Minimal intervention in the treatment of problem drinkers: A controlled study.* Unpublished manuscript as quoted in Miller, W. R. and Hester, R. K. Inpatient alcoholism treatment. *American Psychologist, 41,* 794–805.

Chapman, P., & Huygens, I. (1988). An evaluation of three treatment programs for alcoholism: An experimental study with 6 and 18 month follow-ups. *British Journal of Addiction, 83,* 67–81.

Cummings, N. A. (1979). Turning bread into stones: Our modern antimiracle. *American Psychologist, 34,* 1119–1129.

Cummings, N. A. (1986). The dismantling of our health system: Strategies for the survival of psychological practice. *American Psychologist, 41,* 426–431.

Cummings, N. A. (1988). Emergence of the mental health complex: Adaptive and maladaptive responses. *Professional Psychology: Research and Practice, 19,* 308–315.

Cummings, N. A. (1991). Outpatient versus inpatient treatment of substance abuse: Recent developments in the controversy. *Contemporary Family Therapy, 13,* 5.

Duhl, L. J., & Cummings, N. A. (1987). The emergence of the mental health complex. In L. J. Duhl & N. A. Cummings (Eds.), *The future of mental health services: Coping with crisis* (pp. 1–13). New York: Springer.

Edwards, G., Orford, J., Egert, S., Guthrie, S., Hawker, A., Hensman, C., Mitcheson, M., Oppenheimer, E., & Taylor, C. (1977). Alcoholism: A controlled trial of "treatment" and "advice." *Journal of Studies on Alcohol, 38,* 1004–1031.

Feldman, D. J., Pattison, E. M., Sobell, L. C., Graham, T., & Sobell, M. B. (1975). Outpatient alcohol detoxification: Initial findings on 564 patients. *American Journal of Psychiatry, 132,* 407–412.

Gallant, D. M., Bishop, M. P., Mouledoux, A., Faulkner, M. A., Brisolara, A., & Swanson, W. A. (1973). The revolving-door alcoholic: An impasse in the treatment of the chronic alcoholic. *Archives of General Psychiatry, 28,* 633–635.

Hayashida, M., Alterman, A. I., McLellan, A. T., Obrien, C. P., Purtill, J. J., Volpicelli, J. R., Raphaelson, A. H., & Hall, C. P. (1989). Comparative effectiveness and costs of inpatient detoxification of patients with mild-to-moderate alcohol withdrawal syndrome. *New England Journal of Medicine,* February 9, 358–365.

A. Foster Higgins, Inc. (1990). Health care costs in the 1980s *Medical Benefits, 8*(9), 1–2.

Holser, M. A. (1979). A socialization program for chronic alcoholics. *International Journal of the Addictions, 14,* 657–674.

Ito, J. R., & Donovan, D. M. (1987). Aftercare in alcoholism treatment: A review. In W. R. Miller & N. Heather (Eds.), *Treating addictive behaviors: Processes of change.* New York: Plenum Press.

Kandel, E. R. (1976). *Cellular basis of behavior.* San Francisco: Freeman.

Kiesler, C. A. (1982). Mental hospitals and alternative care: Noninstitutionalization as potential public policy for mental patients. *American Psychologist, 37,* 349–360.

Kissin, B., Platz, A., & Su, W. H. (1970). Social and psychological factors in the treatment of chronic alcoholism. *Journal of Psychiatric Research, 8,* 13–27.

McCrady, B., Longabaugh, R., Fink, E., Stout, R., Beattie, M., & Ruggieri-Authelet, A. (1986). Cost effectiveness of alcoholism treatment in partial hospital versus inpatient settings after brief inpatient treatment: 12 month outcomes. *Journal of Consulting and Clinical Psychology, 54,* 708–713.

McCrady, B., Noel, N., Abrams, D., Stout, R., Nelson, H., & Hay, W. (1986). Comparative effectiveness of three types of spouse involvement in outpatient behavioral alcoholism treatment. *Journal of Studies on Alcohol, 47,* 459–467.

McLachlan, J. F. C., & Stein, R. L. (1982). Evaluation of a day clinic for alcoholics: *Journal of Studies on Alcohol, 43,* 261–272.

McLellan, A. T., Luborsky, L., Woody, G. E., O'Brien, C. P., & Druley, K. A. (1983). Predicting response to alcohol and drug abuse treatments; Rule of psychiatric severity. *Archives of General Psychiatry, 40,* 620–625.

Miller, W. R. (1985). Motivation for treatment: A review with special emphasis on alcoholism. *Psychological Bulletin, 98,* 84–107.

Miller, W. R., & Baca, L. M. (1983). Two-year follow-up of bibliotherapy and therapist-directed controlled drinking training for problem drinkers. *Behavior Therapy, 14,* 441–448.

Miller, W. R., Gribskov, C. J., & Mortell, R. L. (1981). Effectiveness of a self-control manual for problem drinkers with and without therapist contact. *International Journal of the Addictions, 16,* 827–837.

Miller, W. R., & Hester, R. K. (1986). Inpatient alcoholism treatment. *American Psychologist, 41,* 794–805.

Miller, W. R., & Hester, R. K. (1987a). Matching problem drinkers with optimal treatments. In W. R. Miller & N.

Heather (Eds.), *Treating addictive behaviors: Processes of change.* New York: Plenum Press, 272–288.

Miller, W. R., & Hester, R. K. (1987b). The effectiveness of alcoholism treatment methods: What research reveals. In W. R. Miller & N. Heather (Eds.), *Treating addictive behaviors: Processes of change.* New York: Plenum Press, 102–114.

Mosher, V., Davis, J., Mulligan, D., & Iber, F. L. (1975). Comparison of outcome in a 9-day and 30-day alcoholism treatment program. *Journal of Studies on Alcohol, 36,* 1277–1281.

O'Briant, R., Petersen, N. W., & Heacock, D. (1977). How safe is social setting detoxification? *Alcohol Health and Research World, 1*(2), 22–27.

Orford, J., Oppenheimer, E., & Edwards, G. (1976). Abstinence or control: The outcome for excessive drinkers two years after consultation. *Behavior Research and Therapy, 14,* 409–418.

Page, R. D., & Schaub, L. H. (1979). Efficacy of three-versus five-week alcohol treatment program. *International Journal of the Addictions, 14,* 697–714.

Peele, S. (1978). Addition: The analgesic experience. *Human Nature,* September.

Pittman, D. J., & Tate, R. L. (1972). A comparison of two treatment programs for alcoholics. *International Journal of the Addictions, 18,* 183–193.

Powell, B. J., Penick, E. C., Read, M. R., & Ludwig, A. M. (1985). Comparison of three outpatient treatment interventions: A twelve-month follow-up of men alcoholics. *Journal of Studies on Alcohol, 46,* 309–312.

Robson, R. A. H., Paulus, I., & Clarke, G. G. (1965). An evaluation of the effect of a clinic treatment program on the rehabilitation of alcoholic patients. *Quarterly Journal of Studies on Alcohol, 26,* 264–278.

Saxe, L., & Goodman, L. (1988). *The effectiveness of outpatient vs. inpatient treatment: Updating the OTA report* (Health Technology Case Study 22 Update). Washington, DC: Office of Technology Assessment.

Saxe, L., Dougherty, D., Esty, K., & Fine, M. (1983). *The effectiveness and costs of alcoholism treatment.* (Health Technology Case Study 22). Washington, DC: Office of Technology Assessment.

Shain, M. (1991, June). *A better look at constructive confrontation.* Paper presented at the Annual Meeting of the Employee Assistance Society of North America (EASNA), Atlantic City.

Sheehan, J. J., Wieman, R. J., & Bechtel, J. E. (1981). Follow-up of a twelve-month treatment program for chronic alcoholics. *International Journal of the Addictions, 16,* 233–241.

Smart, R. G. (1978). So some alcoholics do better in some types of treatment than others? *Drug and Alcohol Abuse, 3,* 65–76.

Smart, R. G., & Gray, G. (1978). Minimal, moderate and long-term treatment for alcoholism. *British Journal of Addiction, 73,* 35–38.

Smart, R. G., Finley, J., & Funston, R. (1977). The effectiveness of post-detoxification referrals: Effects on later detoxification admission of drunkenness and criminality. *Drug and Alcohol Abuse, 2,* 149–155.

Stinson, D. J., Smith, W. G., Amidjaya, I., & Kaplan, J. M. (1979). Systems of care and treatment outcomes for alcoholic patients. *Archives of General Psychiatry, 36,* 535–539.

Sullivan, L. (1990). *Alcohol and Health: Seventh special report to the U.S. Congress from the Secretary of Health and Human*

Services. Washington, DC: Department of Health and Human Services.

Walker, R. D., Donovan, D. M., Kivlahan, D. R., & O'Leary, M. R. (1983). Length of stay, neuropsychological performance, and aftercare influences on alcohol treatment outcome. *Journal of Consulting and Clinical Psychology, 51,* 900–911.

Whitfield, C. L., Thompson, G., Lamb, A., Spencer, V.,

Pfeifer, M., & Browning-Ferrando, J. (1978). Detoxification of 1,024 alcoholic patients without psychoactive drugs. *Journal of the American Medical Association, 239,* 1409–1410.

Willems, P. J. A., Letemendia, F. J. J., & Arroyave, F. (1973). A two-year follow-up study comparing short with long stay in-patient treatment of alcoholics. *British Journal of Psychiatry, 122,* 637–648.

CHAPTER 24

Organic Disorders

Mitchel Becker

The treatment of the brain-injured patient has primarily been shaped by the rapidly developing field of neuropsychology. In its earlier stages, neuropsychology focused on assessment of brain injury with particular interest in differential diagnosis. A more recent trend in neuropsychology emphasizes rehabilitation of the brain-injured patient (Boll, 1985). A holistic approach advocates treatment of the patient in the setting of his family, workplace, group, and community (Hoofien & Ben-Yishay, 1982). The therapies, intensive milieu, group therapy (Guggenheim & Lesser, 1990) and cognitive remediation are designed to teach the patient how to act, feel, and experience. The holistic intensive therapy was born out of a need to treat the vast array of impairments and life problems caused by severe brain injury. In my opinion, the pressing need for direct therapeutic interventions has overshadowed the patient's psychological hurt and conflict. Perhaps more importantly, all patients must have an emotional response to the dependent position of being taught and told in therapy how to be. The art of listening to the patient's experience of life and therapy, is

most masterfully explored by the psychoanalytic school of thought, is glaringly absent from the neuropsychological literature.

This chapter will propose a method of integrating accepted directive approaches with psychoanalytic method. The directive approaches offer direct change in many spheres of function. Psychoanalytic therapy provides the patient the emotional setting to work through the infinite emotions and experiences of being brain-injured and rehabilitated. The manner of integrating these two aspects of the therapy will be elaborated upon.

THEORETICAL AND CONCEPTUAL POSITION

The dominant theoretical approach to the treatment of brain injury is a "directive approach" in which specific deficits and impairments are directly ameliorated through an active intervention. Cognitive remediation treats cognitive impairments, behavior modification changes maladaptive behavior (Eames & Wood, 1985), and educational methods develop the patient's and family's understanding of the neuropsychological deficits (Mckinlay & Brooks, 1984).

This approach states that the specific and concrete problems of the brain-injured patient

Mitchel Becker • The National Institute for the Rehabilitation of the Brain Injured, Tel Aviv, Israel.

Comprehensive Handbook of Psychotherapy Integration, edited by George Stricker and Jerold R. Gold. Plenum Press, New York, 1993.

(herein called the *patient*) are a source of acute distress and their amelioration markedly improves the individual's quality of life. Furthermore, a strong case has been made in favor of sufficing with the above stated therapies and against the use of the psychoanalytic approach.

The patient's egocentricity or lack of self-awareness limits insight (Levin, Benton, & Grossman, 1982). High affective lability and impulsivity limit frustration tolerance. Passivity and apathy hinder initiative. Cognitive deficits in the areas of attention, concentration, memory, language reception, comprehension, and higher levels of thought, including processing, abstraction, organization, and problem-solving (Crosson, 1987; Lezak, 1978), minimize the ability to learn. These deficiencies have lead therapists to rule out insight-oriented therapies with the organically disordered patient. The psychoanalytic process seemed too nondirective, unstructured, and intellectually demanding.

Despite these reservations, it is my contention that psychoanalytic psychotherapy is integral to the rehabilitation of the brain-injured patient. After brain injury, the self experiences change in the manner of emotionally, cognitively, socially, and occupationally functioning and being. This phenomenologically different experience of self is not easily assimilated into the previous self-representation. Borrowing conceptions from self-psychology (Kohut, 1971), the changes caused by brain injury threaten the cohesiveness, continuity, and vitality of the individual's representational world.

The representational world is defined as the schema of "affectively colored configurations of self and object representations" which organize a patient's subjective experience (Stolorow, Atwood, & Ross, 1978, p. 247). Unworked through issues of acceptance of brain injury result in experiences of self as fragmented, guilt ridden, and in utter despair. Clearly, these experiences may manifest as rigid resistance to change in therapy. This resistance is best worked-through via psychoanalytic psychotherapy (Rhoads & Feather, 1972). Thus, I propose an integrated therapy called the *cyclic model* in which there is a cyclic shifting between direct intervention to change maladaptive patterns of thought and behavior and a psychoanalytic approach to work-through

resistance to change and help accept the brain injury.

CLINICAL AND THEORETICAL ANTECEDENTS

The "vicious circle" model of psychopathology is a product of Paul Wachtel's (1977) theoretical integration of psychoanalysis and behavior therapy. In Wachtel's writings, man is seen as being destined to repeat the same patterns of interaction with others throughout life. Although this theory strongly parallels Horney (1950) and Sullivan (1953), Wachtel's (1977) theory diverges from them in his conclusion, "that an understanding of the role of interpersonal events in perpetuating neurosis, implies a need for more *active intervention* by the therapist in order for neurotic patterns to change" (p. 41). The patient's current behavior and perception are instrumental in maintaining the presenting problems. For example, the individual who is unassertive because of fear of his own rage, presents an interpersonal style which generates rage.

Wachtel (1982) sees the use of transference and analysis of resistance as ways of clarifying and confronting the patient's style of being in the here and now. However, when the patient is relatively resistance free, the change must be stimulated and guided by behavioral technique. Similarly, Rhoads and Feather (1972) and Birk and Brinkley-Birk (1974) demonstrated how the psychoanalytic understanding of transference and resistance were crucial in the success of behavior therapy.

In contrast, others have seen behavior therapy as creating an availability for the psychoanalytic process (Glantz, 1981; Seagraves & Smith, 1976). Becker (1985) describes a cyclic-alternating integration of psychoanalysis and behavior therapy in which the two therapies reciprocally alternate in a figure–ground manner. Becker offers an integrative therapy in the treatment of severe personality disorders. The psychoanalytic work is designed to create and maintain a holding environment (Winnicott, 1965) or self-object bond (Kohut, 1971).

In summary, the brain-injured patient is treated via a direct focus on breaking vicious cycles of maladaptive behavior while working through resistance and transference to maintain the therapeutic bond.

THE TECHNIQUE AND PROCESS OF PSYCHOTHERAPY

Psychotherapy of the brain-injured patient constantly balances a focus on the work of awareness and acceptance of the brain injury and the need to cope with everyday living. These two issues are evident throughout the therapy in a figure–ground manner with each aspect of the therapy reciprocally benefitting the other. Acceptance prepares the groundwork for direct change, while successful change serves to strengthen and encourage the individual to engage in the process of self-awareness and acceptance. The work of psychotherapy can be seen as comprising these six elements: (1) establishment of the therapeutic alliance, (2) assessment, (3) defining the problem, (4) direct intervention, (5) the psychoanalytic work, and (6) the cyclic integration.

Establishment of Therapeutic Alliance

The therapist–patient relationship has its initial origins in an empathic understanding of the patient's current state of distress. This often strikes the most pressing issues of loss and metamorphosis of the self. The degree of acceptance is expressed in the manner that the patient presents the changes in his cognitive ability, relationships, and employment. The therapist's ability to simultaneously empathize with the loss and self-injury while not threatening the individual's psychological sense of integrity will determine the strength and stability of the therapeutic alliance. In this vain, the therapist may decide that this first stage of therapy, in which the patient–therapist bond is created, must be prolonged in its duration and that a thorough neuropsychological assessment is still too threatening.

In contrast, the establishment of a patient–therapist alliance involving emotional expression may be too threatening, in which case the therapist may quickly move to the neuropsychological testing. In general, on a conscious level, the patient is rather eager to receive feedback on his or her cognitive functioning and more defensive about personality changes. However, I have seen a number of patients who were psychologically invested in presenting themselves as emotionally disturbed to mask their cognitive impairments. It gradually became clear that for them the cognitive impairments were the most painful aspect of their injury. Thus, the fine balance between confrontation and respect for defenses must take into account that patient's emotional investment in the different aspects of self; cognitive, emotional, interpersonal, and occupational.

The issue of independence-dependence though a universally essential issue is of crucial importance with the brain-injured patient. A brain injury directly jeopardizes the individual's basic autonomy. The issue of dependence is almost always highly emotionally charged. The patient's organic impairments make him or her inherently prone to develop a strong dependency on the therapist. In contrast, the patient experiences a deep narcissistic injury over having his or her independence destroyed. The therapist's delicate dance in dealing with both the needs for dependence and affirmation of the patient's independence (despite very real limitations) will markedly determine the degree of success in establishing a therapeutic alliance and the durability of the relationship.

The two core issues presented in this section, loss and dependence, have mutually overlapping themes of acceptance of self. They directly relate to the basic vulnerabilities and frustrations of the injured self and thus will dictate the tone of the therapeutic relationship and will continue to accompany patient and therapist throughout the therapy.

Assessment

There is an extensive literature on neuropsychological assessment of brain injury and a separate rich literature on personality assessment. The object of this subsection is to delineate an integrative approach to these two crucial aspects of assessment.

When assessing the patient with documented brain injury, differential diagnosis between organic and personality disorder in my opinion becomes far less important. Instead, the psychological assessment is designed to *describe* how the brain injury affects the individual's capacity to cope with the daily demands of living. This integrative approach claims that changes in cognition affect personality, changes in personality affect cognition, and that traumatic brain injury is experienced by the self as a narcissistic injury. In this vain, it is essential to see cognition as an integral part of the individual's personality and vice versa. Therefore changes in either cognition or personality will frequently have a reciprocal change in the other. For example, memory loss for daily events (anterograde amnesia) may frequently be paralleled by a repressive style in which the patient selectively represses emotionally painful issues. Similarly, a right brain injury resulting in poorly processed and organized thought may result in an experience of self as fragmented. Patients suffering from an obsessive preoccupation with the events leading to an injury will frequently manifest as poor attention skills and memory dysfunction.

It is equally important in the assessment phase to understand how a specific injury affects the individual at his particular stage of life. Synthetic or organizational skill impairments can acutely affect an adolescent's task of crystallizing a sense of identity. On a personality level, defenses of denial (Prigatano, 1987) and isolation against intense vulnerability results in experiences of unintegrated islands of awareness, thus derailing the process of identity formation and cohesion.

Middle adulthood, in which the self-identity is already consolidated, revolves around the individual's need for mastery, accomplishment, and productivity. Being inactive and nonproductive, such as in the frontal lobe adynamia syndrome and in the impairment of the reticular activating system, causes intense guilt feelings from the highly critical ego-ideal and superego.

Late adulthood, frequently viewed as a period of dignity in which the individual reflects upon his past with pride, is disrupted by cognitive impairments which impair one's ability to remember and properly sequence past events. The lack of a sequential memory is experienced as a discontinuity between past and present resulting in existential meaninglessness, shame, and despair.

Premorbid personality is another factor of assessment (Bond, 1984). What is the fit between former personality and the organically induced changes? The larger the disparity between premorbid personality and postinjury personality, the more acute the intrapsychic turmoil. For example, a reserved individual who suffers a disinhibitive syndrome, an artist who suffers a right brain injury, a highly emotionally expressive individual who suffers a flattened affect, are individuals who will experience a deep narcissistic injury. The self is in disequilibrium, and is experienced as chaotic or fragmented, non-vital, lacking drive or noncontinuous in time.

Thus assessment incorporates premorbid personality, life stage, cognitive impairment, and degree of narcissistic injury to conceptualize a comprehensive picture of psychological function in which these different aspects of assessment interact with each other.

Defining the Problem

This phase flows directly from the assessment. It is composed of a series of sessions, following the neuropsychological assessment, in which the therapist provides feedback from the testing. The therapist aims to state the feedback in a manner that best reorganizes the patient toward the goal of confronting the loss suffered from the injury while simultaneously beginning steps toward rehabilitation. An empathic statement of the problem addresses the patient's distress while maintaining the homeostasis of self. As previously stated, successfully empathizing with the patient's self-injury reinforces the therapeutic alliance.

While I emphasize awareness of the patient's vulnerability, it is important not to underestimate the durability of the patient's psychological defenses. The patient is able to experience an explicit confrontation during a feedback session concerning painful changes in cognition and personality and to have no emotional response, having successfully defended himself or herself via denial (Prigatano, 1987) and cognitive confusion. Feedback should be provided in a manner to best compensate the patient's cognitive impairments. The patient is asked to self-evaluate each function before the therapist reports test results. In addition, when necessary, the patient is requested to summarize each section of the feedback.

The conclusion of the feedback phase is treatment recommendations. The selected goals should be a source of deep distress and yet have a good prognosis for change. The therapist takes a share of the responsibility to create an atmosphere of success which further strengthens the therapeutic alliance.

Direct Interventions

The types of direct interventions available to the therapist are selected from the vast armamentarium of the eclectic psychotherapist in response to the needs of the patient. The following are examples of using different direct interventions for specific problems.

Relaxation Training. The patient frequently presents with high anxiety. This may be in response to the actual traumatic experience of the brain injury, or performance anxieties related to feeling incompetent and helpless. Muscle relaxation training and guided imagery serve to distance the patient from his anxiety and thus achieve a sense of control. Guided imagery is creatively constructed in response to the patient's personality.

For example, a patient feeling trapped in obsessive thought over a car accident may be instructed to imagine "all the pictures of the accident (a detailed description of the accident) are slowly gathering in the sky, all your thoughts, feelings, worries and sensations (all elaborated) ever so slowly gathering, gathering and slowly falling into an immense fishnet. The net slowly catches everything and magically becomes lighter and lighter—the heavy load lightens. You, too, feel light, light as a bird, a bird that can slowly gather the net's strings and gradually lift the net in its mouth. You are flying over lands and seas. As you fly farther and farther, you can gradually allow the net to fall. The net falls and falls and you are freer and freer." The intense sense of burden and trauma are themes, frequently presented by most of the patients, which may be directly ameliorated by the relaxation training. Resistance to these exercises stems from issues of dependence and losing control which are related to the vulnerability of self experienced by the patient.

Social Skills Training. The broad area of social skills training is essential to the psychotherapy of the brain-injured patient. Patients may struggle with self-presentation, conversation skills, nonverbal communication, and intimacy. Maladaptive social behaviors, such as poor social judgment and impulsivity, are very frequently the family's presenting problems. Modes of treatment can vary between individual and group therapy (Guggenheim & Lesser, 1990). Heavy emphasis is placed on direct feedback to the patient on his or her behavior and its consequences. Role playing and *in vivo* exercises are used to provide an active experience of learning. Homework assignments are given to reinforce new behaviors learned in sessions.

One specific area of social skills training is assertiveness training. Patients who suffer from reduced social skills and self-esteem are frequently in need of assertive behavior. Assertiveness is differentiated from aggression and passivity (Lange & Jakubowski, 1976) frequently found in the brain-injured population. The patient is taught to communicate his or her need in a self-assertive manner that is neither hostile nor self-pitying. Often patients are assisted in reasserting their independence from significant others. In a quite natural way, a family's acute response to the patient's debilitated states of coma, disorientation, and physical limitation after brain injury is extreme protectiveness. The natural process of recovery from brain injury may not automatically be accompanied by changes in the interpersonal relationships with "caretakers." The patient must convince the caretaker that he or she is ready to assume more independence.

Family Therapy. Family therapy is indicated when the family system is unable or unwilling to allow the rehabilitative process to unfold (Mckinlay & Brooks, 1984). The family behavior is seen as preventing the patient from functioning at a maximum level due to either the family's overprotectiveness or denial of the patient's impairments. The overprotective family is helped to gain a neuropsychological understanding of brain injury and recovery with an empathic interpretation of the family's natural resistance to exposing the patient to potentially painful failure. The family denial is related to issues of loss and mourning. Often family denial parallels the patient's denial. Progress in working-through the issues of loss and change whether it is family or patient frequently results in reciprocal progress by patient or family.

Cognitive Remediation. The field of cognitive remediation is a vast area of neuropsychology which will not be elaborated upon in this chapter. Suffice it to say the cognitive remediation is integral to the patient's rehabilitation. In accordance with the patient's cognitive deficits, cognitive remediation may focus on attention, concentration, language, memory, learning, logical thinking, and organization.

In contrast to "preprogrammed" therapy in which the patient was required to fit himself or herself to the lesson, recent trends in cognitive remediation focus on the patient. The patient is asked to bring examples of daily cognitive dysfunction which cause personal distress. This approach is to achieve maximum motivation to confront the arduous anxiety-provoking work of cognitive remediation. In this sense, the cognitive remediation is only a part of an integrative approach. Thus, for example, a patient must achieve awareness and be in distress over his inability to remember specific tasks requested by his boss. The patient participates in discovering why he is not succeeding to perform the task. Analysis may reveal a severe deficit in automatic auditory memory. Then only with a maintained high motivation can the patient learn to "effortfully" commit the boss's instructions to memory by verbally repeating the instructions out loud in a socially acceptable manner.

Cognitive Therapy. Cognitive therapy (Beck, 1976; Ellis, 1962) is frequently the treatment of choice for the rigid thinking found in this population. Patients learn how their thinking perpetuates their maladaptive functioning and they are guided to perceive alternative approaches to chronic problems. Approaches to depression (Beck, 1967) are appropriate for helping patients who are ensconced in helplessness and in passivity.

Poor impulse control and impaired frustration tolerance can be treated with Meichenbaum's (1977) self-instruction technique. The treatment goal is to build up cognitive mediation between emotion or drive and behavior thus increasing the individual's capacity to distance, plan, and organize his or her behavior.

Work Placement. Work placement as well as other "heavy handed" interventions are easily interpreted by patients as a blow to their independence. Thus, careful consideration of the patient's state of independence must precede placement of a patient in the work place. Having said that, it is equally important to stress that helping a patient become employed can have enormous impact on the patient's sense of self. Oftentimes the work placement is the final stage of therapy marking the patient's improved social skills and acceptance of his or her lower level of vocational functioning. As in most interventions, there is a large continuum of degree of intervention. The therapist may only counsel, personally help the patient negotiate a work agreement with the employer, or refer the patient to a vocational placement worker.

The Psychoanalytic Work

All of the psychoanalytic work must be uniquely structured to compensate for specific cognitive limitations. The therapist must actively check with the patient to assure that the material is properly attended, processed, analyzed, remembered, organized, and integrated. Attention problems are compensated for by checking that the patient is "with" the therapist and the therapy material and by frequently asking the patient what he or she is thinking. Processing problems are approached by asking questions which force the patient to retrieve what was said in his or her own words. The patient is encouraged to "effortfully" or actively listen and process the material brought to the session by repeating and summarizing what is said. The patient is gradually expected to initiate these repetitions and summaries on his or her own accord. This is done in a socially natural communication, for example, "So let me see if this is clear to both of us" and "In other words we are saying." A more difficult achievement for the patient is the need to analyze and integrate the material. Here the therapist must be highly active in encouraging the patient to take interest in how the specific issue at hand might be related to other issues. Thus, although as in any psychoanalytic process, concepts, emotions and schemata are gradually built up by the patient, the working-through process is more repetitive and arduous with a "heavier hand" of the therapist guiding the speed and breadth of the process. Similarly, the therapist has other, non-conventional active roles in the psychodynamic process. This is primarily in response to the patient's passivity, an inclination to avoid difficult issues and rigidity. The therapist is often forced to decide upon the sessions' content or initiate a certain line of thought.

As previously stated, the patient's subjective experience of his or her brain injury is the central theme of the psychoanalytic work. The psychoanalytic setting enables the patient to discover his or her self-experience and come to terms with that experience. In essence, the latter goal of acceptance of the brain-injury must be preceded by an increased awareness of self. Using psychological defenses of avoidance, denial, repression, projection, and splitting, the patient fends off any awareness of the injured self. In the therapy, the patient brings himself or herself via description of daily experience, interpersonal relationships, dreams, and the therapist–patient relationship. Using psychoanalytic techniques of mirroring (Kohut, 1971) and clarification (Greenson, 1967), the patient's experience of self as manifested in behavior, emotion and thought is highlighted and magnified. The therapist may at times label an experience of the patient formerly not categorized or verbalized. The constant empathic mirroring and clarifying serves to affirm existence of parts of self previously unconscious and/or not processed.

The content of this awareness phase of the psychoanalytic work is in essence a working-through of the material already described from the assessment and defining the problem phases. The psychoanalytic process enables the patient to assimilate the new feedback at a pace that he or she can emotionally tolerate.

The achievement of increased self-awareness lays the groundwork for the next phase, coming to terms with this new awareness. The patient will then begin to bring different distresses of the self. The different states of self-disequilibrium, fragmentation, lost continuity, instability, and enfeeblement are accompanied by emotions of shame, guilt, and despair. The therapist uses interpretation to help the patient learn to accept the conflict ridden areas of self. It is my experience that the core conflict is between the old and new representations of self and other.

This conflict is, at times, at war proportions—each self fighting desperately to survive the other. The patient is encouraged to describe this war by bringing the dialogue between the selves into the therapy room. The therapist's interpretations attempt to explain the experience of self in disequilibrium in terms of the patient's stage of life when injured, premorbid level of psychological development, and type and severity of brain injury.

The patient whose self experience is one of fragmentation, meaninglessness, and dramatic change often presents with feelings of emptiness, shame, rage, and self-disgust. Once the patient has achieved an awareness of his or her current state he or she is helped to build insight into the causes. Interpretations may center around lost dreams for the future. The patient works-through rage and depression over the dreams that were cruelly snatched away. The emphasis on the future ultimately frees the patient to deal with the present. These intense feelings of a future doomed are most frequently found with adolescents and young adults in which the self-identity has not been crystallized. However, other populations such as narcissistic personality disorders unable to cope with the brain-injury present similar experiences of a chaotic fragmented self. The severe, right-hemisphere-injured patient is more prone to experience a fragmented representation of self, other, and world.

Cognitive deficits directly inhibit the capacity to consolidate different aspects of self. The synthesis of post with preinjured self is at times cognitively beyond the patient's capacity without the aid of the therapist. Interpretations are designed to integrate the different self experiences in a manner in which the defense of splitting is interpreted with the borderline patient (Kernberg, Selzer, Koenigsberg, Carr, & Appelbaum, 1989). The therapist emphasizes the origin (the cognitive deficit), the content (the old and the new self), and the motivation (the fear to confront loss).

Patients whose experience of self is dominated by instability in time and person and who are overwhelmed by feelings of guilt are responding to demands of the former self at the reduced capacity of the new self. Beyond the awareness of frustration and guilt over not functioning as desired, interpretations focus on the fear to reorganize and begin the rehabilitation process. The married parent in the middle of his most productive years suffers guilt feelings over not fulfilling his role of husband and father. He struggles with self-statements of "I am useless," "I am irresponsible," "I am cruel to others," and "I am selfish to languish in my own self-pride." Mature young adults with well developed ego and super-ego may present in a similar manner. Interpretations emphasize the state of entrapment; to act versus to be helpless, and the fear to act in a less than perfect manner. This may lead to internalized parent expectations. Personalities with rigid and high expectations are prone to this experience of self as guilt ridden and unstable. Brain injury resulting in the primary personality changes of rigidity and passivity serves to exacerbate the patient's capacity to creatively progress beyond his or her self-injury. In this case, interpretations center on the patient's difficulty to perceive alternatives.

Impaired function is considered by the patient as non-function. The patient is compelled to come to terms with marked reduced function. Working-through the acceptance of injury enables the patient to confront reality and build more appropriate expectations.

Feelings of despair and hopelessness are a product of the experience of self as enfeebled, stripped of power and vitality. The patient experiences life as terminated. His or her perspective of the past is blackened by an over-generalizaton of present hurt. In the language of selves, the new, weak, brain-injured self monopolizes not only present and future but even the past. This sense of a lost past is most characteristic of late adulthood. In this case, the therapist interprets the patient's life stage as highly instrumental in creating the despair. Coming to terms with the present hurt enables the patient to recover his or her past. Interpretations focus on the patient's need to retain the dignity of the past. The therapist aids the patient to rebond with the former self's past to create a place of security, comfort, and pride. With this step the patient begins or continues his or her rehabilitation.

Hysterical personality disordered individuals who throughout their lives struggled with issues of low self-esteem are prone to depreciate their past by globalizing their present distress. This type of patient needs to differentiate lifelong struggles and present coping with brain injury. It is important to stress that memory impair-

ment distorts and magnifies the experience of losing self in a continuum of time by blurring the boundaries between past and present.

Other cognitive impairments affecting the patient's capacity to differentiate between essential and nonessential information, and the processing of material further influence the tendency to blend past success with current dysfunction. When appropriate, the patient is urged to rebuild past representations of self at times even via photo albums and videos of the former self.

The ultimate work of acceptance of change is for the patient to assimilate the cognitive impairments and personality changes into a comprehensive self-representation. Change is seen as a part of the whole self in a dimension of time and identity and is not perceived as a foreign intruder ego dystonic to the self.

The Cyclic Integration

Working through resistance is the cornerstone of this integrative model. Resistance to the therapy and to change is the primary reason that the psychotherapy of the brain-injured patient cannot suffice with the directive therapies alone. Resistance is conceptualized on two levels. Primary resistance is the result of a disrupted therapist–patient bond. This resistance must be immediately attended to since it directly jeopardizes the psychotherapy. In this, the psychoanalytic work not only serves to create but more importantly to maintain a type of holding environment (Winnicott), 1965) or self-object bond (Kohut, 1971), which is essential to the efficacy of any behavioral intervention. It is therefore imperative to restore the therapist–patient bond. Patient and therapist review and analyze the previous interactions to track where the rupture in the bond occurred. The discord may be in response to transference issues in which the patient projects on the therapist unresolved conflicts with significant others in the past or present. Working through this transference phenomenon restores the holding environment.

In other instances, the patient is reaching to a difficult aspect of the "real relationship" (Greenson, 1967). The therapist may be overly directive in his determination to more highly structure the session to compensate for cognitive deficits. In contrast, attempting to respect the patient's need for control and independence, the therapist may be creating an intense confrontation with the patient's sense of vulnerability and helplessness. Thus, the patient–therapist dyad struggles with the desirability of freedom versus structure in which the psychoanalytic process is to be evolved. Even more powerful sources of disruption to the therapeutic bond are the directive interventions. Most of the directive interventions can cause the patient to experience the therapist as critical and unaccepting. The very fact that the therapist wants to change a thought, emotion, or behavior of the patient is interpreted as a rejection of that part of the patient. Thus, cognitive therapy, cognitive remediation, relaxation training, and assertiveness training are easily seen as non-acceptance. The therapist must then return to the issues of self. In essence the patient is projecting his or her own self-rejection onto the therapist. This often leads to insight into the patient's vulnerability and fear to change. Other issues provoked by the directive interventions are of control, power and dependency. The active intervention in which the therapist displays power or control over the patient is quite clearly a potentially threatening experience.

In essence the therapist is "doing something to" the patients as opposed to the anonymous, nonjudgmental, unconditional acceptance stance sought after (but never fully achieved) by psychoanalysis. When the patient has a negative response to the therapist's active intervention, there must be a halt in the directive intervention and an analysis of the disrupted bond.

Specific cognitive deficits and organic personality changes can also exacerbate the patient's reaction to a perceived empathic lapse on the part of the therapist. The patient's poor ability to see specific events as a single part of a whole relationship, the impulsivity, and the rigidity all contribute to an obsessive locked focus on the sense of being rejected, misunderstood, and insulted, and a disintegration of the patient–therapist bond. The therapist must actively help the patient reconstruct the past representations of the therapist, thus creating a more complete perspective to the relationship.

The secondary form of resistance is a resistance to the work of therapy—both the psychoanalytic work and the directive interventions. In either case, the therapist invites the patient to explore why the work at hand is threatening. This exploration can take place since the therapeutic alliance remains intact.

Gradually the patient discovers how the therapy threatened the self-homeostasis. The work of self-awareness and acceptance is clearly anxiety-provoking work and the resistance to such work is empathized with and further analyzed. Resistance to the direct interventions is primarily due to experiencing the directive intervention as an enacted confrontation of the patient's limitation. The hope to rehabilitate such deficits does not comfort the patient invested in denying the deficits. Defenses are analyzed leading to the work of accepting the brain-injured self. Successful resolution of the resistance may be manifested in the patient's initiating a return to the previously refused or unsuccessful assignment.

In summary, the integrated therapy consists of a cyclic shifting from one therapeutic stance to another in a figure–ground manner in response to the ebb and flow of motivation to change and resistance. After the establishing of the empathic therapeutic relationship via psychoanalytic technique, the therapy shifts to the directive interventions. These learning tasks are continued until resistance is encountered. The therapy then shifts to a psychodynamic analysis of resistance. Primary resistance, the disruption of the empathic bond, is addressed first and the bond is restored. Secondary resistance to the therapy itself is then worked-through. Resolution of resistance then ushers in the directive therapy.

CASE EXAMPLE

The following case study illustrates the integrated therapy approach. Mr. Z. is a married, 38-year-old father of three children. Prior to his injury, Z. was an individual successful in all endeavors. His father's favorite of ten sons, he was a well-respected cattle rancher who was frequently consulted professionally.

At the age of 34, Z. was head injured in a car accident with a loss of consciousness for 2 hours. After several hours of observation, he was discharged from the hospital. On three more occasions Z. reported back to the emergency room (ER), complaining of headache and dizziness and on each occasion was dismissed without treatment. On his fourth visit to the ER approximately 2 weeks from the accident, a hematoma was discovered and operated upon.

Attempting a return to work after a year of recuperation, Z. experienced himself as incompetent. In response to great difficulty at work, Z. entered a deep depression, attempted suicide, and was subsequently hospitalized for 2 weeks.

After two years of outpatient treatment in a psychiatric clinic, Z. was referred to the Recanati Rehabilitation Center for a neuropsychological assessment to assess the need for cognitive remediation. The former therapist described the process of the previous treatment as follows: After an initial improvement of obsessive suicidal ideation, Z. stagnated in a state of helplessness to improve his daily functioning.

The neuropsychological assessment indicated a below average level of current intellectual functioning with cognitive deficits in the areas of multichanelled attention, short-term memory, and higher levels of abstraction. The evaluation recommendation was psychotherapy with the addition of cognitive remediation when needed.

The initial phase of treatment was the establishment of an empathic patient–therapist relationship. This phase included an in-depth history taking including an analysis of Z.'s previous rehabilitation efforts. This process enabled the experience of empathy between patient and therapist with a primary focus on Z.'s sense of narcissistic injury—that he had lost a self-prepresentation of being a successful, confident, and caring person. Cognitive remediation was then introduced in the therapy. Simple attention was the first cognitive skill to be addressed. At the same time, relaxation training was begun. In both the cognitive remediation and the relaxation training, Z. was consistently distracted by his own internal dialogue of negative self-statements. In response to the resistance to the behavioral and cognitive work, the therapy shifted to a psychodynamic analysis of Z.'s subjective experience of these "distractions." Z. had allowed his many worries and problems to take over every moment of his life. This obsession with problems was analogized to a monster. He was assigned an imagery technique; to control a monster who was recklessly throwing bundles of problems at Z. He was instructed to say, "Sit still, I'll tell you what package to give." This behavioral

intervention enabled Z. to concentrate on the cognitive remediation and relaxation training sessions, and, most importantly, improved his attention and concentration at work and home.

In the following session, Z. reported an acute sense of helplessness to overcome his many problems and an overall sense of failure in the therapy. This resistance to further progress in the behavioral and cognitive work was responded to with a shift to the psychodynamic work. The primary resistance, that is, the endangered bond between patient and therapist was immediately addressed.

Clarification techniques revealed that Z. experienced the therapist as doubting the validity of his cognitive deficits. Further analysis of Z.'s interaction with the therapist revealed that similar interactions were repeated with others. Z. felt that others thought he was "acting" sick. This interaction had its origin in the emergency room where he was continuously told he was hypochondriacal and, finally, on his fourth visit having his subjective sense confirmed by "objective" scanners. This confrontation of Z.'s displacement of mistrust resulted in marked change of Z.'s motivation and functioning. Z.'s cognitive work became increasingly more consistent and efficient—being less hindered by internal dialogue. Z. was instructed to devote one hour per day to pleasant recreation with his wife. Z. reported positive results for several weeks. However, on the third week, Z. reported difficulty experiencing himself as a worthwhile, productive, and vigorous self. This resistance to internalizing a sense of a more healthy self was highlighted in a cognitive remedial task of pacing oneself with recorded instructions. Upon seeing objective improvement in his performance, Z. said "the tape must be slower this time" and quickly added "I know that must sound illogical." This led to further exploration of his reexperiencing the emergency room. Z.'s sense that other perceived him as an "actor" was in fact a projection of his own denial of cognitive deficits. Z. experienced his problems as emotional rather than cognitive since he conceived emotional problems as temporary and cognitive problems as permanent.

Z. was thus protecting his self from further injury. The clarification of these defenses and their motivation lead to increased positive goal-directed behavior designed to change dysfunctional patterns. Z. was assigned a social task: to inform friends of his cognitive impairments which had previously been kept secret. Z. complied with the task with positive results including a marked decrease in anxiety. The therapy then consistently shifted back and forth between a behavioral focus on informing others of his cognitive limitations (including co-workers) and a psychodynamic focus on the severe confrontation the self experienced upon admitting to himself that he was cognitively limited. This confrontation was experienced in a manner which prevented a sense of chaos and enfeeblement and fostered a sense of stability and vitality.

The process of Z.'s therapy can be described as follows: Z. experienced his cognitive impairments as a narcissistic injury. This sense of injury was on a continuum of severity from fragmentation and instability (during his acute depression), to instability and enfeeblement (during the initial stages of therapy), to enfeeblement (during the intermediate stages of therapy), to a painful and yet constructive acceptance of his cognitive limitations (at present).

The cultivation of a stable and vital self-representation with a concomitant diminishing sense of self-injury and a more trustworthy object representation was made possible by the complementary effect of a strong and stable therapeutic bond and the positive learning experiences provided by the cognitive and behavioral interventions.

CONCLUDING COMMENTS

There are two unique characteristics to this integrative psychotherapy. The first characteristic is treating patients experiencing a basic vulnerability of self. In this case, the brain-injured patient's vulnerability stems from the traumatic brain injury and dramatic changes in self. Similarly, the integrative model suggested in this chapter can be easily adapted to other patients who experience intense anxiety and vulnerability; personality disorders with and without cognitive deficits. The hallmark of the therapy is creation and maintenance of the holding environment or self object bond to facilitate the directive interventions. Restoration of that bond when disrupted

must always take top priority before resumption of any other intervention.

The second unique element of this integrative model is the attempt to combine neuropsychological understanding of the patient with the psychoanalytic work. Psychoanalysis ultimately strives to provide the patient with an etiological understanding of his problem. Although, psychoanalysis has increasingly emphasized the here and now, the patient's present style of being is seen as having developed in response to specific types of interpersonal relations with significant others of his or her childhood. Thus, the here and now presentation of self is ultimately anchored to an interpretation of early object relations. In contrast, the anchor for some of the brain-injured patient's style of being may be a cognitive deficit. The therapist interprets the patient's here and now presentation of self in terms of specific cognitive deficits. This manner of psychotherapy work is fitting for patients suffering organic deficits from birth.

The work focuses on how the cognitive deficits interfered in the development of self and object. Anchoring schema of self-behavior and emotion to specific organic limitation serves to organize the self around the new insight, experienced as empathic understanding of the patient by the therapist. In my opinion, many interpretations provided in psychotherapy mistakenly attribute maladaptive interpersonal relations to unempathic parents, when in fact the therapist is unempathically missing the neuropsychological impairment.

Much more research is needed to explore the impact of cognitive deficits both in born and acquired on personality development and experience of self in the here and now. Further understanding will enable us to integrate directive intervention with empathic understanding and thus minimize primary and secondary resistances.

With regard to the cyclic alternation between psychoanalytic work and directive intervention, it is quite clear that the therapist's shifting from one therapeutic stance to another has a major impact on the therapeutic relationship. Further clinical case study analysis may help reveal the patient's experience of these shifts and help us conceptualize the most effective manner of shifting from one stance to another.

REFERENCES

Beck, A. (1967). *Depression, causes and treatment*. Philadelphia: University of Pennsylvania Press.

Beck, A. (1976). *Cognitive therapy and the emotional disorders*. New York: International Universities Press.

Becker, M. (1985). *An integration of psychoanalysis and behavior therapy: A case study*. Unpublished doctoral dissertation. Yeshiva University.

Birk, L., & Brinkley-Birk, A. (1974). Psychoanalysis and behavior therapy. *American Journal of Psychiatry, 131*, 499–510.

Boll, T. J. (1985). Developing issues in clinical neuropsychology. *Journal of Clinical and Experimental Neuropsychology, 7*, 473–485.

Bond, M. R. (1984). The psychiatry of closed head injury. In N. Brooks (Ed.), *Closed head injury: Psychological, social and family consequences* (pp. 748–778). New York: Oxford University Press.

Crosson, B. (1987). Treatment of interpersonal deficits for head trauma patients in inpatient rehabilitation settings. *Clinical Neuropsychologist, 1*, 335–352.

Eames, P., & Wood, R. (1985). Rehabilitation after severe brain injury: A follow up study of a behaviour modification approach. *Journal of Neurology, Neurosurgery, and Psychiatry, 48*, 613–619.

Ellis, A. (1962). *Reason and emotion in psychotherapy*. New York: Lyle Stuart.

Glantz, K. (1981). The use of relaxation exercise in the treatment of borderline personality organization. *Psychotherapy: Theory, Research and Practice, 18*, 379–385.

Greenson, R. (1967). *The technique and practice of psychoanalysis (Vol. 1)*. New York: International Universities Press.

Guggenheim, N., & Lesser, R. (1990). Group therapy with brain injured adults. In E. Vakul, D. Hoofien, Z. Groswasser (Eds.), *Rehabilitation of the brain injured: A neuropsychological perspective* (pp. 61–67). London: Freund Publishing House.

Hoofien, D., & Ben-Yishay, Y. (1982). Neuropsychological therapeutic community rehabilitation of severely brain injured adults. In E. Lahav (Ed.), *Psychological research in rehabilitation* (pp. 87–99). Jerusalem: Israel Ministry of Defence Publishing House.

Horney, K. (1950). *Neurosis and human growth: The struggle toward self realization*. New York: Norton.

Kernberg, O., Selzer, M., Koenigsberg, H., Carr, A., & Appelbaum, A. (1989). *Psychodynamic psychotherapy of borderline patients*. New York: Basic Books.

Kohut, H. (1971). *The analysis of the self*. New York: International Universities Press.

Lange, A., & Jakubowski, P. (1976). *Responsive assertive behavior: Cognitive behavioral procedures for trainers*. Champaign, IL: Research Press.

Levin, H. S., Benton, A. L., & Grossman, R. G. (1982). *Neurobehavioral consequences of closed head injury*. New York: Oxford University Press.

Lezak, M. D. (1978). Living with the characterologically altered brain injured patient. *Journal of Clinical Psychiatry, 114*, 373–410.

Mahoney, M. J. (1974). *Cognition and behavior modification*. Cambridge, MA: Ballinger.

McKinlay, W. W., & Brooks, D. N. (1984). Methodological problems in assessing psychosocial recovery following severe head injury. *Journal of Clinical Neuropsychology, 6*, 87–99.

Meichenbaum, D. (1977). *Cognitive-behavior modification: An integrative approach*. New York: Plenum Press.

Prigatano, G. P. (1987). Personality and psychosocial consequences after brain injury. In M. J. Meier, A. L. Benton, & L. Diller (Eds.), *Neuropsychological Rehabilitation* (pp. 355–378). New York: Churchill Livingstone.

Rhoads, J. M., & Feather, B. W. (1972). Transference and resistance observed in behavior therapy. *British Journal of Medical Psychology, 45*, 99–103.

Seagraves, R. T., & Smith, R. C. (1976). Concurrent psychotherapy and behavior therapy: Treatment of psychoneurotic outpatients. *Archives of General Psychiatry, 33*, 756–763.

Stolorow, R. D., Atwood, G. E., & Ross, J. M. (1978). The representational world in psychoanalytic therapy. *International Review of Psychoanalysis, 5*, 247–256.

Sullivan, H. S. (1953). *The interpersonal theory of psychiatry*. New York: Norton.

Wachtel, P. L. (1977). *Psychoanalysis and behavior therapy: Toward an integration*. New York: Basic Books.

Wachtel, P. L. (1982). What can dynamic therapies contribute to behavior therapy. *Behavior Therapy, 13*, 594–609.

Winnicott, D. (1965). *The maturational processes and the facilitating environment*. New York: International Universities Press.

CHAPTER 25

Chronic Pain

ON THE INTEGRATION OF PSYCHE AND SOMA

Robert H. Dworkin and Roy C. Grzesiak

INTRODUCTION

Chronic pain is both a medical and a behavioral problem and it is accompanied by great personal suffering as well as substantial economic costs to society. In assessing the impact of chronic pain, Bonica (1990) estimated that in 1986 (the most recent year for which data were available), 97 million Americans suffered from chronic pain (e.g., back pain, headache, musculoskeletal, and neurological syndromes), 400 million days of work were lost, and the total cost was 79 billion dollars. The suffering caused by chronic pain is more difficult to quantify. Nevertheless, based on both research and clinical experience there is a consensus that "in addition to depression, patients develop associated chronic invalid behaviors . . . curtailment of social activity . . . become increasingly homebound, and their chief interaction with

Robert H. Dworkin • Departments of Anesthesiology and Psychiatry, College of Physicians and Surgeons, Columbia University, New York, New York 10032.   Roy C. Grzesiak • Departments of Anesthesiology and Psychiatry, New Jersey Medical School, Newark, New Jersey 07103.

Comprehensive Handbook of Psychotherapy Integration, edited by George Stricker and Jerold R. Gold. Plenum Press, New York, 1993.

others, in the home as well as out of it, is via the sick role" (Sternbach, 1984, p. 175).

In this chapter, we will present the rudiments of an integrative approach to psychotherapy for chronic pain patients. Our purpose at this point is to put forth some suggestions, using both theoretical and clinical examples, to illustrate why we think it is important to adopt a comprehensive and integrative approach to patients with chronic pain. This presentation is primarily clinical in nature; it does not address the more complex issues of metatheory, problems of combining insight and action theories, or some of the more pervasive relational issues involving transference and countertransference that are germane to integrated practice, whether it be with problems of living or problems of illness and pain. The integrated approach we will describe combines psychotherapeutic intervention with self-regulatory approaches and behavioral prescription within a psychobiological perspective. The psychotherapeutic interventions vary on a continuum from supportive to insightful-interpretive depending on patient needs. We use the term *psychobiological* to indicate that most chronic pain problems reflect two interacting processes: a failure to cope with early pain or discomfort, followed by increasing involvement and automaticity of both the underlying psychological and biological processes (Bakal, 1982). We believe that the psychological contributions to a chronic pain syndrome vary within a multifactorial matrix in which intractability often reflects developmental and psychosocial events, learned psychological responses, and ongoing psychobiological processes.

THEORETICAL AND CONCEPTUAL POSITION

Chronic pain has been defined in many ways (e.g., Crue, 1986; Loeser, 1982; Loeser & Black, 1975; Merskey 1986; Sternbach, 1974), and these definitions range from those that include psychological maladjustment among the criteria to those that require an absence of psychopathology. In this chapter, we will use the most inclusive approach to the definition of chronic pain, one based on the amount of time that the individual has suffered from pain. The Subcommittee on Taxonomy of the International Association for the Study of Pain has proposed that chronic pain is pain that persists beyond the normal time of healing and that three months is the "most convenient point of division between acute and chronic pain" (Merskey, 1986, p. S5).

This approach to the definition of chronic pain is atheoretical and reveals just how little is known about the etiology of chronic pain. Although the social and psychological consequences of chronic pain have been well described, the processes by which this disorder develops have not been identified. Because we believe that the way in which psychotherapists construe the development of a disorder plays a large role in determining psychotherapeutic process, we want to begin this chapter by demonstrating that at the present time there is no satisfactory evidence that psychological factors can *cause* chronic pain. This assertion may surprise some readers (and even some pain specialists) who may have assumed that if a physical basis for a disorder has not been found then the pathology must be psychological. The most unfortunate example of assuming that psychological factors play a causal role in chronic pain is the distinction between "organic" and "psychogenic" pain, which continues to be made in clinical practice. Several different factors probably contribute to the persistence of this distinc-

tion, among which are the need for some kind of explanation when physicians cannot adequately account for an individual's pain and the mistaken belief held by some psychotherapists that only pain that is psychologically determined can be ameliorated psychotherapeutically. However, chronic pain is a complex phenomenon, and this distinction is not only unnecessarily simplistic but is in many respects injurious to patients who are suffering from pain that is insufficiently understood.

Psychosocial Antecedents of Chronic Pain

The evidence that psychosocial factors play a causal role in the etiology of chronic pain is meager. Studies of patients who are already suffering from chronic pain and its deleterious effects cannot differentiate the antecedents of chronic pain from its concomitants and consequences (Dworkin, 1992). The confounding of potential antecedents of the development of chronic pain with its negative consequences is most obvious in considerations of the psychological aspects of this disorder. For example, it has frequently been reported that a substantial proportion of chronic pain patients suffer from depression (Dworkin & Gitlin, 1991; Romano & Turner, 1985), but studies of chronic pain and depression have not resolved whether the stress of living with chronic pain causes patients to develop a depressive disorder or whether depression causes an experience of chronic pain.

A large number of retrospective studies have been conducted that conclude that various psychological factors play a causal role in the development of chronic pain. However, the shortcomings of retrospective methods are well known and include several problematic assumptions. For example, in several recent studies that attempt to identify psychological precursors of chronic pain (Adler, Zlot, Hurny, & Minder, 1989; Gamsa, 1990; Gamsa & Vikis-Freibergs, 1991), it is assumed that individuals can accurately recall their childhood experiences, relationships with parents, and premorbid personality. Such reports by patients (or by anyone else, for that matter) are subject to numerous biases, not the least of which is that the chronic pain from which patients suffer may influence their recollections and/or their willingness to report such presumed antecedents of chronic pain. It is impossible to satisfactorily distinguish antecedents from consequences of chronic pain using such retrospective methods, and it is not surprising that different studies using these methods come to different conclusions about the importance of psychological factors in the etiology of chronic pain. Similarly, it is also not possible to conclude that psychological factors contribute to the development of chronic pain when measures of psychological functioning, such as the Minnesota Multiphasic Personality Inventory (MMPI), are used to examine patients who already have chronic pain and who therefore may have developed psychological distress as a consequence of their pain (Love & Peck, 1987; Watson, 1982).

Although the research that is currently available has not demonstrated that psychological factors can cause chronic pain, as psychotherapists we must consider the possibility that such factors have contributed to the development of chronic pain in our patients. In his book on somatoform disorders, Ford (1983) noted that 25% of the population utilize 50% of medical or health services. We would like to modify and extend that observation and apply it to chronic pain by stating that only a small percentage of individuals with persistent pain go on to become chronic pain patients. In attempting to account for this, George Engel (1951, 1959) developed the concept of the pain-prone patient. In contemporary pain literature one often sees a misinterpretation of this concept. Most notable is the interpretation of Engel's work as suggesting a single pain-prone personality type. That is not what Engel said and it is not what he implied. Rather, he was addressing the fact that individuals with chronic pain, strictly on the basis of clinical findings, seemed to share some common denominators in terms of early life experience. These early experiences, he believed, served as the foundation for an "individual psychic signature" that gave idiosyncratic meaning to the pain and served as the basis for a propensity to suffer. However, he did not confine this pain-proneness to a single personality type and felt that it could be found in a variety of personality styles, including schizophrenia. It is interesting to note how closely factorially derived chronic pain patient MMPI profiles (Bradley, Prokop, Margolis, & Gentry, 1978) and Sternbach's (1974) composite MMPI profiles seem to fit with the personality types referred to by Engel (1959).

Two recent reports provide retrospective data that are consistent with Engel's (1959) suggestion that early experiences play a role in perpetuating pain complaints. One involved facial pain (Harness & Donlon, 1988) and the other involved a controlled, retrospective attempt to confirm Engel's patterns of early developmental experience (Adler et al., 1989). In the latter study, the so-called psychogenic pain group had significantly more of the following experiences: (1) Parents who were verbally or physically abusive of each other; (2) parents who were physically abusive of the child; (3) child, deflecting aggression from one parent to the other onto him or herself; (4) parents who suffered from illnesses or pain; (5) ill parent of the same gender as the patient suffering from pain; (6) pain of patient and parent in the same location; (7) number of surgeries in adulthood; (8) disturbance in interpersonal relationships; and (9) disturbance of work life. Regarding disturbances in work life, Blumer and Heilbronn (1989) have suggested that a trait they call "ergomania" describes a conflicted work ethic that seems to characterize many chronic pain patients before the onset of their pain. These individuals have a history of excessive work performance, relentless activity, self-sacrifice, and the precocious assuming of adult responsibilities and roles. As clinicians, it has been our experience that a number of chronic pain patients seem to present with these elements of pain-proneness in their early histories. Recently, Ciccone and Grzesiak (1990b) presented a preliminary study comparing neck and back pain patients with controls and found significant differences with respect to work variables identified by Blumer and Heilbronn (1989).

Data of this sort are certainly consistent with the hypothesis that some individuals bring to the chronic pain experience a propensity to suffer that confounds and complicates their capacities to improve without psychological assistance, regardless of the presence or absence of continuing biological input. However, it is certainly also possible that individuals who are suffering from chronic pain and the disability and feelings of vulnerability it causes defensively experience or present themselves as premorbidly "ergomanic." It is only by means of prospective research on chronic pain that this confounding of cause and consequence will be resolved. Although the importance of prospective research on the development of chronic pain has been evident for some time, studying patients before and after the onset of chronic pain has been considered "an obviously impractical task" (Sternbach & Timmermans, 1975). This may not be so. Three recent studies have investigated the relationship between pain and depression prospectively (Dworkin, Hartstein, Rosner, Walther, Sweeney, & Brand, 1992; Turner & Noh, 1988; Von Korff, Le Resche, & S. F. Dworkin, 1990), and in each of these studies pain at a follow-up assessment was significantly predicted by depression at an earlier baseline assessment. These results constitute preliminary evidence that a psychological factor—that is, depression—may sometimes be a causal antecedent of chronic pain.

Psychosocial Concomitants of Chronic Pain

We have devoted so much attention to arguing that the extent to which psychological factors contribute to the etiology of chronic pain is presently unknown because the assumption that such factors cause pain often distracts therapists from other psychological aspects of the chronic pain experience. It is certainly possible that psychological factors sometimes cause or contribute to the development of chronic pain. But there can be little doubt that psychological factors are an integral component of a patient's ongoing experience of chronic pain, whatever its etiology. Psychological factors can intensify or inhibit pain and contribute to the many different characteristics of an individual's chronic pain syndrome in diverse ways. For example, recent research suggests that psychosocial factors may play a larger role in characterizing the chronic pain experience than biological processes (Rudy, Turk, Zaki, & Curtin, 1989; Turk & Rudy, 1987, 1988). Another, more specific, example is that depression has been found to be associated with treatment response, treatment compliance, pain intensity, disability, activity level, and coping in chronic pain patients (Dworkin & Gitlin, 1991).

From a clinical standpoint, it is of course necessary to consider many different aspects of a patient's experience of living with chronic pain.

Crue (1986) divides chronic pain patients on the basis of whether or not they are coping well with their pain. Although we find this a useful concept, it is often even more important to explore the patient's own report of how well he or she is coping and then to consider any discrepancies between this self-evaluation and the coping we have observed. In a discussion of psychotherapy for the chronic pain patient, it is also particularly important to address the issue of suffering. Unlike pain behavior—the overt behaviors that patients exhibit that have been hypothesized to respond to the shaping effects of reinforcement—suffering refers to the unique idiosyncratic meaning that the patient superimposes on the pain sensation. These idiosyncratic meanings may well have their origins in early experiences, given the evidence that parents and offspring of chronic pain patients seem to have an elevated risk of chronic pain and other illnesses and injuries (e.g., Chaturvedi, 1987; Katon, Egan, & Miller, 1985; Raphael, Dohrenwend, & Marbach, 1990; Violon & Giurgea, 1984). But these meanings also reflect more recent experiences and current interpretations of the experience of pain (Ciccone & Grzesiak, 1988; Turk, Meichenbaum, & Genest, 1983). The meaning of pain to most patients is undoubtedly a complex consequence of both developmental and current experiences, for example, the patient with chronic abdominal pain who experiences her pain as punishment for an abortion.

Is There a Theory of Chronic Pain?

There are a number of reasons why a model of chronic pain is valuable to the psychotherapist who treats chronic pain patients. A model allows the therapist to educate patients about the disorder from which they suffer. It also provides a consistent orientation for addressing many of the questions that some patients have about the role of psychological factors in their chronic pain syndrome. A model is also useful when psychotherapists need to discuss the role of psychological factors in chronic pain with other health professionals. And, most importantly, a model of chronic pain can provide the therapist with a perspective within which to evaluate the diverse psychological aspects of the chronic pain experience and the multiple therapeutic options that are available in an integrated psychotherapy.

Although many models of chronic pain can serve these purposes, we prefer a model that considers the development of a chronic pain syndrome to be the result of an interaction of both biological and psychosocial processes (Dworkin et al., 1992; Grzesiak, 1991). We find it easiest to talk to our patients, our colleagues, and ourselves in ways that are consistent with current knowledge, and so this model is not only based on chronic pain research but also has great heuristic potential.

The models of chronic pain that posit an interaction of biological and psychological factors have been termed *biopsychosocial* (Grzesiak, 1991), *diathesis-stress* (Dworkin et al., 1992; Turk & Flor, 1984), *psychobiological* (Bakal, 1982), and *biobehavioral* (Feuerstein, Papciak, & Hoon, 1987). In all such models, a biological vulnerability (the diathesis) is a necessary but not sufficient condition for the development of a disorder (cf. Meehl, 1962), which only occurs when various psychosocial processes are also present (the psychosocial, stress, or behavioral component of the model). With respect to chronic pain, the biological diathesis is likely to be complex, consisting of genetic factors as well as physiological vulnerabilities resulting from disease, injury, and possibly stress.

The psychosocial factors that must accompany this biological diathesis for chronic pain to develop are also likely to be complex. A valuable guide to choosing the types of variables to be considered within the psychosocial domain has been provided by the Dohrenwends and their colleagues (Dohrenwend & Dohrenwend, 1981; Dohrenwend, Shrout, Link, Martin, & Skodol, 1986). These authors propose that the "life-stress process" consists of three components—recent stressful life events, ongoing social supports, and personal dispositions (personality and psychopathology)—and suggest that these psychosocial factors can be antecedents of a variety of physical as well as psychological disorders. All competent therapists, whether they are integrative or not, consider these aspects of their patients' lives. With respect to chronic pain, it is also important to attend to the individual's responses to physical illness and symptoms. These responses have different components, including—but not limited to—somatization (Lipowski, 1988), abnormal illness behavior (Pilowsky, 1989), hypochondriasis (Kellner, 1986), and somatosensory amplification (Barsky & Wyshak, 1990).

It should be evident that this model of chronic pain is not a well-specified theory, but the approach does provide an orientation for the integrative therapist who is considering the origins of a patient's pain syndrome. However, this psychobiological approach to the etiology of chronic pain must be supplemented by a consideration of the diverse concomitants and consequences of a patient's chronic pain syndrome. The multiaxial approach to the assessment of chronic pain that has been proposed by Turk and Rudy and their colleagues (Rudy et al., 1989; Turk & Rudy, 1987, 1988) provides a valuable guide for this purpose. In this approach, the multiple psychosocial and behavioral aspects of a chronic pain syndrome are emphasized—for example, psychiatric disorder, coping style, pain behavior, responses of family members, and various kinds of social, physical, and occupational disability. That we have also considered some of these "consequences" of living with chronic pain to be potential "antecedents" of a chronic pain syndrome may serve as a useful reminder that a therapist must know a patient very well before it is possible to unravel the complex developmental fabric of premorbid antecedents, character style and symptoms, and maladaptive consequences.

Is an Integrative Psychotherapy for Chronic Pain Patients Necessary?

Given the large number of psychological interventions that have been proposed for the chronic pain patient (Holzman & Turk, 1986), it is important to consider whether another approach is warranted. Our belief that an integrative approach to the psychological treatment of chronic pain patients is necessary directly follows from the approach to the etiology and psychosocial consequences of chronic pain that we have described above. Chronic pain syndromes are disorders in which biology and psychology are intertwined (although patients do not think of their disorders in this fashion when they first come to us). Diverse and complex patterns of biological, psychological, and social factors constitute chronic pain, and these patterns vary over the longitudinal course of a chronic pain syndrome. The multifactorial and longitudinal complexity of chronic pain requires that a number of different treatment approaches—medical, psychological, rehabilitative—be available for the optimal treatment of pain patients, which is the rationale for a multidisciplinary team approach to the treatment of chronic pain. Based on the same reasoning, the psychologist or psychiatrist who is involved in the treatment of chronic pain patients should also have as large a number of treatment options available as possible. Integration can have two meanings in the psychotherapy of the chronic pain patient (as well as in the treatment of many other disorders). One involves the integration of different psychological approaches within the treatment of a single patient (what is typically considered an integrative psychotherapeutic approach), and the other involves the therapist's use of different techniques for different patients (in this latter use of the term *integration*, the integration may be thought of as existing within the therapist's repertoire, not in the treatment). We believe that both of these types of integration are necessary in the treatment of chronic pain patients. As we hope to demonstrate below, different chronic pain patients sometimes require very different therapeutic strategies, some of which are unimodal, but an integrative psychodynamic psychotherapy is the treatment approach we use most often and which we believe addresses both pain and suffering.

CLINICAL AND THEORETICAL ANTECEDENTS

Psychological services, including both assessment and treatment, are commonplace components of multidisciplinary pain management centers. However, the theory and practice of psychotherapy for chronic pain patients is not well developed. Both behavioral (e.g., Fordyce, 1976; Grzesiak, 1980) and cognitive (e.g., Ciccone & Grzesiak, 1984, 1988, 1990a; Eimer, 1989) approaches can be effective. Turk *et al.* (1983) have described a cognitive-behavioral treatment for chronic pain patients that has become the most widely accepted psychological intervention for this population. Although we believe that cognitive-behavioral modification constitutes an important, if not essential, component of the psychological treatment of chronic pain patients, we

believe that this therapeutic approach does not suffice for many chronic pain patients. Revealingly, the index of Turk *et al.*'s (1983) volume does not include the word transference, nor does it refer to antidepressant medication, two aspects of a more comprehensive and integrated approach to psychological intervention for chronic pain patients.

The way in which we attempt to integrate the cognitive-behavioral perspective within a psychodynamically informed psychotherapeutic approach to chronic pain may be described most easily by providing the central references of a recommended syllabus for supervisees. These include not only the Turk *et al.* (1983) volume, but also Wachtel's (1977) classic analysis of the integration of psychodynamic and behavioral approaches and Basch's (1980, 1988) developmental spiral and self psychological context for psychotherapy. Both of these approaches provide coherent perspectives within which therapeutic strategies such as behavioral prescription and relaxation training do not interfere with, and may even further, a spirit of psychodynamic inquiry and the unfolding of the psychotherapeutic relationship (see also Bellissimo & Tunks, 1984; Frank, 1990; Kutz, Borysenko, & Benson, 1985; Moss & Garb, 1986). Also relevant to the approach we discuss in this chapter are discussions of psychodynamic psychotherapy for chronic pain patients (e.g., Aronoff & Rutrick, 1985; Pilowsky, 1978, 1988; Pinsky, 1975; Pinsky & Malyon, 1978) and the work of authors who have combined cognitive and psychodynamic or interpersonal perspectives (e.g., Guidano & Liotti, 1983; Horowitz, 1988; Horowitz, Marmar, Krupnick, Wilner, Kaltreider, & Wallerstein, 1984; Shapiro, 1965). Combining these approaches in a model that enables behavioral principles and cognitive style to stand alongside psychodynamic processes affords the clinician both flexibility and clinical power. If psychological involvement in chronic pain is conceptualized as varying from minimal to maximal, as potentially involving cognitive, behavioral, affective, psychophysiologic, and intrapsychic (unconscious) components, and as playing a role as cause, consequence, and/or concomitant, then the value of being able to bring an integrative psychotherapy to bear on the chronic pain patient's pain and suffering becomes clear.

In our experience, some form of relaxation

training is an important component of the treatment of many chronic pain patients. Published protocols are widely available (e.g., Grzesiak, 1977; Turk et al., 1983), as are a variety of inexpensive cassette tapes. Relaxation training may be supplemented by hypnosis, which is an effective approach to deepening relaxation and extending its benefits. In addition, hypnosis appears to have beneficial effects beyond relaxation, and it provides a range of specific approaches that allow patients to reduce the sensory aspect of their pain as well as the suffering with which it is associated (Barber, 1982, 1990; Hilgard & Hilgard, 1983). Although we believe that biofeedback approaches can be an effective intervention in the treatment of chronic pain, current research suggests that they are no more effective than relaxation training (Roberts, 1987) and we typically do not find it necessary to use these methods.

In addition to these fundamental aspects of an integrated psychotherapy for chronic pain patients, it is also necessary for the therapist to become familiar with the psychiatric disorders that are commonly associated with chronic pain (e.g., Dworkin & Caligor, 1988; Dworkin & Gitlin, 1991), as well as with psychopharmacology (Gitlin, 1990), an often invaluable adjunct in the treatment of chronic pain patients (e.g., Atkinson, 1989; Monks, 1990).

THE TECHNIQUE AND PROCESS OF PSYCHOTHERAPY

Multidisciplinary treatment planning for the chronic pain patient must include a psychological intervention that is tailored to each patient's unique psychological state, including, for example, cognitive/perceptual style, affective state, behavioral dysfunction, psychophysiologic status, and, last but not least, more traditional concerns related to personality, character, and psychopathology. Recently, Turk (1990) has discussed the need to customize treatment for each patient; we are making a similar point but restrict ourselves to tailoring the various psychological components of intervention on the basis of clinical findings unique to each patient. We have carefully avoided using the phrase "psychotherapy for chronic pain." Psychotherapy is not for pain, it is for people.

First Contact: Educating the Pain Patient

Individuals suffering from chronic pain do not come to pain management clinics for psychotherapy, they come for pain relief. The mere idea of seeing a psychologist or a psychiatrist often causes negative reactions like "You think it is all in my head!" Therefore, the patient must be educated as to how psychological factors are important components of the pain experience. There are no clear guidelines available for educating patients about the importance of the multidisciplinary approach to chronic pain, which often includes an evaluation by a psychologist, a psychiatrist, or both. DeGood (1983) and Grzesiak (1989) have made suggestions concerning how to gently introduce psychological concepts within the context of multidisciplinary pain management. Psychological factors such as coping with the stress of chronic pain must be depathologized, the normal continuum of coping skills must be emphasized and, above all, the pain must always be appreciated as real. Oxman (1986) has suggested that not reassuring the patient about the possibility of pain relief often has the paradoxical effect of increasing rapport and fostering therapeutic alliance. Goldsmith (1983–1984) has suggested that resistance be utilized by downplaying the potential role of psychological factors during initial interactions, which will often enable pain patients to feel more comfortable revealing possible psychological contributions to their chronic pain syndrome.

There is a simple approach to describing the role of psychological factors in chronic pain that we find useful with the great majority of patients and which can also be used effectively by physicians making referrals for psychological treatment. In this approach, we begin by emphasizing that the reason the patient has been asked to see a psychologist is not because the pain is lacking a physical basis and "is all in the patient's head" (we add that we are not sure that we have ever seen such a thing, which is true). We continue by saying that psychologists are involved in the treatment of chronic pain for two reasons: because there are effective treatments, such as relaxation training and hypnosis, which psychologists have been trained to administer, and because many patients who are suffering from chronic pain find themselves in a vicious cycle which it is sometimes helpful to discuss with someone who is familiar with chronic pain. We then describe this vicious cycle, in which pain causes stress and tension (and, depending on what the patient has already revealed, depression, anxiety, or anger), which causes more pain, which causes more stress and tension, and so on. In our experience, most chronic pain patients not only agree with this characterization of their current life, but also then furnish examples of pain causing stress or stress causing more pain. Depending on the patient and the context of the referral, we may refer to this aspect of the psychological intervention as *counseling*, in order to minimize the resistance that is very common among chronic pain patients at this early stage of treatment.

The Early Sessions

With most chronic pain patients, we find it useful to begin therapy by asking the patient to tell us about themselves, beginning with their childhood. When giving the patient an overview of the treatment, we say that this typically takes about two sessions, and that the medical history should be described in detail beginning at the point in the patient's life at which health became problematic. We tell patients that even if we were present when their medical history was taken by a physician, hearing medical problems within the context provided by a life story is very helpful and gives us a much richer appreciation of what they have been going through. Typically, there is little resistance to this endeavor, although some patients race through their premorbid life, asserting that it has little to do with their chronic pain. There are no chronic pain patients, however, who are averse to describing in detail what their lives have been like since the onset of their pain or illness, and the patient's response to the open-endedness of these initial sessions provides a wealth of information.

During these initial sessions, the therapist must be alert to the possibility that the patient is suffering from a psychiatric disorder, for example, major depression, posttraumatic stress disorder, or panic disorder (Dworkin & Caligor, 1988; Dworkin & Gitlin, 1991). Sometimes, patients become defensive about discussing the symptoms of these disorders, believing that an acknowledg-

ment of such symptoms would suggest that their pain is caused by psychological factors. In some instances, this perception is based on previous evaluations. Although few health professionals would say to a patient "The pain is all in your head," many do say things like "We can't find a physical cause for your pain, so it must all be caused by stress or anxiety." Since almost no chronic pain patients want to be told that their pain is a result of such factors, they learn to be defensive about psychological symptoms and stress, sometimes denying them entirely.

We typically do not conduct a formal psychiatric evaluation, but rather attempt to assess the symptoms of potential psychiatric disorders within these initial sessions. Of course, if there is evidence of a psychiatric disorder and depending on the type of disorder, these sessions may become more focused on the assessment of psychiatric symptoms. Whether the patient is suffering from a psychiatric disorder or not, we find it possible to assess the symptoms of these disorders in chronic pain patients with tact and sensitivity. Questions that *sympathize* with the patient's experience often work well (e.g., "All of this has been going on for so long—how has it affected your spirits?" "It sounds like that was a horrible accident—do you find yourself thinking about it or dreaming about it?"). Similarly, questions that *normalize* the patient's experience are often more acceptable (e.g., "Many of our chronic pain patients say that stress makes their pain worse—do you have any things going on in your life that do this?" "When people suffer from chronic pain, they often find that they become especially anxious or frightened, sometimes in certain situations and sometimes for no reason at all—do you ever feel this way?"). Another approach is to imply that the symptoms are a result of the chronic pain which, of course, they may be (e.g., "Pain as bad as yours sometimes causes changes in a person's sex drive—has yours?" "Has the pain made it difficult for you to enjoy activities with your friends and family the way you used to?" "Do you find yourself staying home much of the time or avoiding certain activities, like driving your car?" "Are there any things that you are still able to enjoy in spite of the pain?"). Although asking about suicidal thoughts and impulses can seem difficult, especially if the patient has denied feeling depressed, it is very important to do so (e.g., "With all this going on, do you sometimes wonder whether life is worth living?" "Do you find that sometimes you are in so much pain that you have thoughts of killing yourself?").

With a few chronic pain patients, these initial life history sessions evolve directly into a psychodynamic psychotherapy in which there may be little need for the integration of cognitive-behavioral interventions. Although these patients do not typically experience relief of their pain during the early course of treatment, they prefer discussing their lives within the context of an insight-oriented psychodynamic therapy. Given that these patients have almost always been told that the therapist uses such cognitive-behavioral interventions as relaxation training and hypnosis, it is important to explore with the patient whether they are resisting the use of these techniques. Nevertheless, when our patients have directed us away from an integrative approach to their treatment and toward a psychodynamic psychotherapy, we have almost always followed. This does not reflect an anti-integrative bias, but rather our experience that relief of the suffering that accompanies chronic pain can often be achieved in tandem with relief of the non-pain related suffering that a patient brings to a psychotherapeutic relationship. For example, a 28-year-old man who was referred for multidisciplinary treatment of groin pain revealed during the initial medical evaluation that his mother had been diagnosed with manic-depressive illness and that he had not been in a relationship with a woman since college. Although nerve block injections brought some relief, his pain continued to interfere with athletic and sexual activity. However, he did not want to pursue relaxation training and devoted his psychotherapy sessions to discussions of his relationships with his divorced parents and with women. He terminated psychotherapy after five years of treatment, recently married, and has just published a book on the relationships that famous football coaches have established with the members of their teams. At the time of termination, the therapist did not know whether the patient still suffered from groin pain—the patient had only intermittently referred to his pain during the previous three years, each time saying that the pain clinic (by this he meant the psychotherapy)

"doesn't lessen your pain, it just teaches you how to ignore it."

Varieties of Integrative Psychotherapy with Chronic Pain Patients

The main point we hope to make regarding psychotherapy for chronic pain is, simply put, that therapeutic response dictates therapeutic direction. In psychological treatment planning for the chronic pain patient, we must be cognizant of the fact that there are individuals with chronic pain, even individuals who appear at tertiary pain management centers, who do not have significant psychological factors complicating their pain problem. Psychological evaluation, however accomplished, attempts to identify areas of disruption or dysfunction across affective, cognitive, behavioral, and psychophysiological domains. Sternbach (1974) and Bradley and associates (1978) were among the first to empirically demonstrate a lack of homogeneity in the personalities of chronic pain patients; unfortunately, such findings have not been translated into reliable and valid guidelines for individualized psychological interventions. On the basis of his or her initial assessment and the evolving therapeutic relationship, the therapist develops an intervention that takes into account the presence or absence of personality problems, character style, and psychopathology. Each individual with chronic pain brings to that problem a personality that is, of course, unique, and that also shares important features with other pain and psychotherapy patients.

After obtaining a sense of the patient based on the initial two or three sessions, we typically begin training in what have been termed *self-regulatory strategies*, that is, relaxation, hypnosis, and biofeedback. In our experience, psychotherapy is most effectively introduced to the chronic pain patient by beginning with approaches such as these. Patients are expecting this training to occur because we emphasized the effectiveness of these techniques when we initially described the psychologist's role in pain treatment to them. A first session of relaxation training (the self-regulatory strategy with which we most often begin) can be an abrupt shift from the less structured history sessions which it follows. We try to make the transition as smooth as possible by asking the patient at the beginning of the session whether he or she had any thoughts about the previous week's session and discussing these briefly and by then noting (and sometimes exploring) just how abrupt the transition to relaxation training will be. At this point, education is again extremely important, and we spend the remainder of this session discussing relaxation training with the patient and demonstrating its use, with a cassette tape that the patient will be given to take home.

In subsequent sessions, the patients' experiences practicing relaxation exercises on their own are discussed and additional tapes may be dispensed. Often, hypnosis and training in self-hypnosis are more easily and effectively introduced after the patient has been practicing this type of cassette-guided relaxation for one or two months. In any event, while the patient becomes more skillful at relaxation (or other self-regulatory strategies), the psychotherapy ("counseling") part of the treatment continues. As is true of all psychotherapy, there is a vast array of issues that the therapist and patient can discuss, but in this first month or two of treatment chronic pain patients typically focus on the negative impact of their pain on their relationships with family and friends, on work, and on their mood. Of course, in discussing these topics the therapist should be alert to developmental themes. Chronic pain patients are more willing to discuss their childhood and adolescence in the context of their current difficulties, and there are many themes that can be discussed in this fashion (for example, self-esteem, dependency, punishment).

Relaxation Training in Relatively Uncomplicated Chronic Pain. For some patients, the sensory aspects of chronic pain have caused minimal adverse effects on their lives. In such a psychologically uncomplicated case of persistent pain, psychological interventions may not be used or may be limited to one of the self-regulatory approaches. These techniques can be taught as coping skills that allow the patient to be less aware of pain and discomfort (Grzesiak, 1977; Grzesiak & Ciccone, 1988). The following case illustration is abstracted from Grzesiak (1977) and used with permission.

A 28-year-old male with flaccid paraplegia following a gunshot wound to the T(thoracic)-12

area was seen for relaxation training some two years after his injury. He reported almost constant mild pain sensations of an itching nature in his lower back at the level where sensation was lost. Additionally, he reported periodic sharp, severe pain in the sacral area, an area that had once had decubiti. During attacks of the sharp pain, he found it almost impossible to participate in his physical rehabilitation program and insomnia was a frequent concomitant. Propoxyphene hydrochloride and acetaminophen were prescribed on an as-needed basis for the pain. In the previous acute hospital setting, a psychologist had made a brief and unsuccessful attempt to modify the pain through relaxation training.

During the first session, a muscle relaxation technique was applied down to the abdominal level in conjunction with a meditation-like technique (for details, see French & Tupin, 1974; or Grzesiak, 1977). The patient's subjective report after the session was that his body felt relaxed and that his mind was in a pleasant state, but that he was aware of pain sensations in the background. He was encouraged to practice the technique independently. He was seen again the next day and then for a total of five formal training sessions within a 2-week period. He practiced the relaxation-meditation nightly and he reported that he was growing more successful in altering the experience of pain. According to the patient, the relaxation procedure "mellowed" the pain and he said "I can live with it now." Staff observations indicated a better program attendance and a marked decrease in pain complaints. This particular patient was on a rehabilitation program consisting of physical therapy, occupational therapy, recreation, and vocational evaluation at the time of treatment, but he was not in psychotherapy and there were no changes in medication. The patient was followed for almost 4 years and he continued to report success in using relaxation to modify his experience of pain.

This patient demonstrates the uncomplicated application of relaxation training for the modification of the sensory aspects of pain in an individual who was not believed to have significant psychological factors associated with his chronic pain. The rationale for using relaxation or self-hypnotic procedures in cases of this sort has been spelled out by a number of practitioners (e.g., Barber, 1990; Grzesiak, 1977; Grzesiak & Ciccone,

1988; Lichstein, 1988); this approach can also be beneficial with patients suffering from acute pain and postoperative pain (Chapman & Turner, 1986; Hartstein & Dworkin, in press). In the case reported above, the clinician was alert to the possibility of unconscious or covert messages that would indicate that suffering was part of the clinical picture in addition to pain sensation, but no evidence of this appeared (or else it was missed by the psychotherapist).

Sometimes relaxation training will go awry because personality or character issues interfere with the patient's ability to become relaxed in the therapist's presence. For example, a 30-year-old single female professional was referred by her orthopedic surgeon for anxiety. She appeared extremely nervous and, despite her apparent best efforts to cooperate, was quite guarded in her presentation. After explaining the rationale of relaxation training, the psychotherapist began the training. When the therapist stated: "O.K., the first thing I want you to do is to make yourself comfortable in the chair and then close your eyes," the patient responded by becoming overtly anxious and she was unable to close her eyes. An alternate method of having her focus on a small dot on the wall across from where she was sitting failed as well. She relayed some of this anxiety to her concerns that the therapist was male and hinted that she had had marked difficulties with men throughout her life.

The value of having an integrative approach toward psychotherapy with chronic pain patients is illustrated by this brief anecdote. Although this young woman certainly needs anxiety management, the sources of her anxiety are not to be found in her reaction to pain. Her pain is complicated by conflict and suffering, a suffering that is uniquely hers and inextricably linked to her psychological development. The avenues for dealing with conflict of this sort do not lie in anxiety or pain management techniques but rather in a psychotherapeutic inquiry, one which considers psychodynamic and relational issues.

Psychiatric Disorder and Chronic Pain. As we have suggested above, a substantial percentage of chronic pain patients have a psychiatric disorder, and this possibility must be evaluated with all patients. Many chronic pain patients, in resisting psychological evaluation and intervention, argue

that their psychological distress would disappear if only their pain syndrome was treated effectively. Treatment of chronic pain may alleviate a psychiatric disorder in some instances (Maruta, Vatterott, & McHardy, 1989), but when a pain syndrome and a psychiatric disorder occur together it is usually necessary to treat these disorders concurrently for any lasting relief from chronic pain to occur. The following case makes this clear.

A 38-year-old divorced mother of two was referred for multidisciplinary pain treatment by an orthopedic surgeon whose diagnostic impression was "mechanical low back syndrome with significant supratentorial component as well as probable secondary gain" ("supratentorial" is a medical euphemism for psychogenic). The patient's pain had begun one year before when she opened the bottom drawer of a file cabinet at work and it fell on her; all of the drawers opened out into her and the cabinet pinned her against the wall. She remembers hitting her head against the wall, but does not remember losing consciousness. The patient suffered multiple bruises of her right arm and leg, was seen briefly in the company infirmary, and was sent home with a diagnosis of concussion. Over the course of the year following the accident, headaches and back, leg, hip, and knee pain continued and the patient required a cane for walking. She continued to work throughout this time but her performance deteriorated and she was demoted. The patient was evaluated by numerous physicians, but physical therapy, nonsteroidal anti-inflammatory medication, and nerve block injections resulted in only transient relief of her pain.

Psychological evaluation revealed that during the past year the patient had become increasingly depressed and anxious, suffering from disturbances of sleep and appetite. In addition, she had nightmares about the accident, intrusive daytime images of the accident (especially while at work), and avoided the area of the file cabinets (which had been labeled with "Danger" signs). She described becoming increasingly confused during the past year, having difficulty with memory, concentration, balancing her checkbook, and remembering her two-digit computer account number. Based on this information, the patient was diagnosed as suffering from a Posttraumatic Stress Disorder (PTSD) accompanied by Major

Depression. The nature of the very disabling cognitive deficits that she reported was less clear, as was the possibility that her ongoing involvement in workmen's compensation litigation was playing a role in her presentation.

To further evaluate her cognitive deficits, the patient was referred for psychiatric, neurological, and neuropsychological evaluation. The results of all diagnostic studies were normal, and the impressions of the neurologist and psychiatrist were that her cognitive deficits were probably secondary to her depression. Her neuropsychological evaluation, however, suggested that her problems with attention and concentration were the result of a closed head injury, and that these deficits could be expected to last indefinitely given that the accident had happened over one year before. About this time, workmen's compensation required the patient to undergo an evaluation by a neurosurgeon, who concluded that there was no evidence of disability causally related to the accident.

Based on the above evaluations, the patient was prescribed the tricyclic antidepressant desipramine and weekly sessions of psychotherapy and relaxation training were initiated. After six sessions, hypnosis was begun, in which her relaxation training was augmented with deepening techniques and she was instructed to reexperience the accident. For the first several sessions of hypnosis, the portion of the trance devoted to reexperiencing the accident was about 5 minutes. Although the patient had been in treatment for about three months, she reported little amelioration of her presenting symptoms. During these initial hypnosis sessions, the therapist became aware that the "file cabinet" that fell on the patient was actually three large lateral file cabinets bolted together (each about 6 feet high by 4 feet wide); the fact that all of the patient's medical evaluations had assumed that the file cabinet in question was the narrow four-drawer kind might have contributed to the consistent impression that the patient's symptoms were excessive given the trauma she had experienced. At about this time, the psychotherapist read an account of PTSD which suggested that it may be necessary for the traumatic event to be reexperienced for 30 to 60 minutes for treatment of this disorder to be effective (Barlow, 1988). The sessions of hypnosis were modified

and the patient was made to recount her experience of the traumatic event in as much detail as possible for about 30 minutes. Each session, her reexperiencing of the accident was intensely vivid and accompanied by sobbing and great distress. It became clear during these sessions that, in addition to the severely traumatic accident, driving home afterward—alone, in pain, and confused and disoriented—had been terrifying for the patient (she had pulled off the road several times because she was afraid that she would get into a car accident and injure someone). These sessions were exhausting and emotionally draining for the patient (as well as for the therapist, who noticed that he was becoming anxious when opening large file cabinets), and at the end of each session she was instructed to go to the hospital cafeteria and spend some time composing herself before driving home.

After several of these sessions, the patient's symptoms began to improve. Not only did the symptoms of PTSD lessen, but her depression, pain, and cognitive problems improved. At this point in treatment, she was instructed to approach the file cabinets at work for gradually increasing amounts of time and to gradually decreasing distances (but not to open the drawers unless the Danger signs were removed and the cabinets bolted to the wall). Her improvement continued and eight months after treatment began she reported that the symptoms from which she had suffered for almost two years—especially her disabling cognitive deficits—were absent, and that she had resumed leading a normal life. At this point the frequency of her sessions and the dose of desipramine were tapered; treatment was terminated about five months later. Although the patient reported that she was completely recovered, she was encouraged to continue her litigation to obtain lost wages for time missed from work as a result of her doctor appointments.

We think that this case makes a number of important points about the treatment of chronic pain. We have already argued that multidisciplinary evaluation and treatment of the chronic pain patient is necessary; none of the numerous nonpsychiatric physicians who had evaluated the patient were aware of her PTSD. The psychological evaluation of the chronic pain patient must also be careful and ongoing, continually taking into account the patient's treatment response (or lack of it). In addition, the case makes the point that in working with chronic pain patients, the psychotherapist's knowledge of psychopathology and of treatment options should be as extensive as the range of mental and physical disorders, personalities, and coping styles that characterizes these patients; if the therapist had not happened to read Barlow's (1988) book, this patient might still be suffering from her symptoms. Therapeutic pessimism regarding this patient's prognosis—the neuropsychological evaluation predicted that her cognitive deficits would persist indefinitely—was never warranted, nor were attributions that her pain and other symptoms were the result of "secondary gain" or a "compensation neurosis" (Dworkin, 1990; Dworkin, Handlin, Richlin, Brand, & Vannucci, 1985).

Throughout the treatment, the therapist considered the possibility that the patient had developed PTSD as a result of some pre-existing psychosocial vulnerability, and he explored aspects of the patient's past and current life that might have contributed to her disorder. However, the only evidence of such factors was that the patient's former spouse had been physically and emotionally abusive, but exploration of possible links between the trauma of her accident and the abuse of her past was not productive. What may have contributed most to the development of her severe PTSD was the total absence of any validating social support of her experience; all of the physicians who evaluated her believed that her complaints were excessive given the physical trauma she had suffered. This lack of support from the social surround may have played a role in her PTSD, as it may have in the development of PTSD in Vietnam veterans (e.g., Keane, Scott, Chavoya, Lamparski, & Fairbank, 1985). Developmental experiences may make more of a contribution in other cases of PTSD and chronic pain. For example, a patient who had suffered a severe electric shock related that during hypnosis she had become aware that the "blackness and loneliness" of the shock were very similar to experiences she had as a child. These occurred when she would suddenly discover that her mother had gone to visit her father in another state and that she had been left with a grandmother for several months (the mother and grandmother apparently believed that the separation would be easier if it came as a complete surprise).

Chronic Pain in the Context of a Personality Disorder. By and large, the DSM-III-R Axis I disorders (American Psychiatric Association, 1987) that are most common in chronic pain patients (mood, anxiety, and somatoform disorders) have a better response to treatment—whether psychological or pharmacological—than Axis II disorders. When chronic pain occurs in the context of a long-standing personality disorder, for psychological intervention to have any beneficial effect at all it cannot be limited to the techniques of cognitive-behavior modification. Although most readers of this chapter probably think that this statement is self-evident, almost no attention has been paid in the literature on the psychological treatment of chronic pain to the complicating effects of personality disorders. The following case illustrates the necessity of such attention.

A 56-year-old married father of two developed left-sided arm and leg pain which remained undiagnosed for several years. At the time of referral, he had recently been given a diagnosis of rheumatoid arthritis and it was thought that this might account for much of his pain. Initial psychological evaluation found him to be moderately depressed, and psychotherapy and antidepressant medication were begun. After several weeks of relaxation training, instruction in hypnosis and self-hypnosis was started, and the patient reported that all of these techniques were moderately helpful in managing his chronic pain but that he remained depressed. His feelings about his rheumatoid arthritis were explored, as was his relationship with his wife, who had been diagnosed with "borderline schizophrenia" many years before and was maintained on a low dose of neuroleptic medication. After several months of weekly sessions of psychotherapy, the patient discovered that his son had become engaged to a woman of a different religion. He reported a dramatic worsening of his depression accompanied by prominent suicidal ideation and an effective suicide plan. His psychotherapy sessions were increased to twice weekly and a "contract" was initiated regarding mandatory telephone contact when he was feeling suicidal. The patient now revealed that he had been preoccupied with suicide since his childhood, had had a large amount of barbiturate medication readily available for this purpose for many years, and had suicidal ruminations on an almost daily basis.

The patient had been sexually and emotionally abused as a child and adolescent by both parents in a home where both his mother and his paternal grandmother had spent most of his childhood bedridden from ill-defined illnesses. He was considered an embarrassment to the family, and all aspects of his appearance and behavior were criticized and devalued (e.g., after receiving an award in high school, the only comment made by his mother and brother was that the way he walked down the auditorium aisle was "peculiar"). Perhaps not surprisingly, he had a very disturbed adolescence, with multiple suicide attempts, a course of electroconvulsive therapy, and one brief psychiatric hospitalization. The patient complained of feeling at least moderately depressed for much of his life, felt hopeless about the possibility of any change in a marriage that brought him no gratification, suffered from chronic insomnia, and reported life-long feelings of guilt, sinfulness, and low self-esteem. He was, and is, severely intropunitive, maintains an impressive array of depressogenic self-statements, and has marked fears of interpersonal closeness (which he experiences as "infantile dependency") and abandonment, within the therapy as well as in other relationships.

In psychotherapy, the patient has focused his attention on the traumas of his past and on his extremely poor self-image. In addition, much of the therapeutic work has consisted of exploration of the transference, in which the therapist has been experienced as the violent incestuous father, the intrusive yet neglecting mother, and the brutally critical brother. Although various antidepressant medications have been tried, neither therapist nor patient has seen much benefit with respect to pain or depression. After six years of twice-weekly therapy, his self-esteem has increased somewhat, his relationships with friends have become more numerous and deeper, and he is much more able to see connections between the way he experiences himself and the toxic relationships he had with his family (both parents were dead when the patient began treatment, and after about three years of therapy he essentially cur-

tailed contact with his abusive brother). However, he continues to suffer from intermittent episodes of severe dysphoria which have decreased in frequency but are still accompanied by suicidality and feelings of depersonalization and profound worthlessness.

After the onset of his chronic pain, the patient continued to work part-time as a graphic designer, but he has been unable to return to full-time employment because of his pain. He continues to find self-hypnosis effective in managing his pain, which fluctuates in intensity and varies in quality and location but which has not seemed closely linked to his psychological state. The patient has used self-hypnosis to retrieve memories of his childhood, which are then discussed in therapy, but he has become increasingly convinced that he has repressed the most traumatic events of his past. Given his understandable desire to remember his past as clearly as possible and in so doing achieve some mastery over it, the patient and therapist have begun to discuss whether to use hypnosis within the psychotherapy sessions for this purpose.

Some Psychodynamic Themes. We have argued that personality style, psychological conflict, and developmental experiences can play a large role in complicating the sensory aspects of chronic pain. On the surface, it may appear that we are suggesting that there is a psychodynamic explanation of pain. But to reiterate what we suggested above, because the role of psychological factors varies with each patient, sometimes this may be true and sometimes it will not be. It is therefore always necessary for the therapist to evaluate on an ongoing basis the multifactorial aspects of the experience of living with chronic pain. The following vignettes illustrate a small and select sample of the psychological processes that can complicate the patient's experience of chronic pain.

Pain and Conflict. A 36-year-old married male with back pain had been valedictorian of his graduating class at an Ivy League college but dropped out of a prestigious dental school after one semester and now works as a high school teacher. He reported the following dream: I was walking with my father, he was getting further and further in front of me, and I couldn't keep up. I said to myself: "I cannot even keep up with my father and my father is a cripple!" Further inquiry revealed that his father had a bad leg, ambulated with a marginally functional gait, and was constantly falling behind. This was the first that the psychotherapist had heard of the father's physical disability, and possible psychic meanings of the disability as it related to early identifications and introjects, including both fear of success and failure, were explored. Noteworthy is the fact that the patient appeared markedly ambivalent about outdistancing his father. A rehabilitation approach focusing on physical therapy and psychotherapy enabled him to return to his work as a high school teacher.

Both clinical observations and retrospective research have suggested that social modeling (Craig, 1978) and early identification with ill or disabled family members may play a role in the later development of a chronic pain syndrome. Such internalized objects are often not immediately accessible to conscious recall but, on occasion, the experience and behavior of a chronic pain patient can be associated with early experiences and exposure to the ways in which significant others have coped with pain or illness.

Learning How to Express Pain and Suffering. A 51-year-old divorced female was seen for psychotherapy as part of her multidisciplinary pain management program. She had had spinal surgery for a ruptured disc and during the postoperative period developed an infection in the area of the incision; the pain returned and never remitted. The psychotherapist initially focused on her depression, but from the perspective of the pain management team, she presented problems of compliance and appropriate use of prescribed medications, both analgesic and anti-inflammatory. In psychotherapy she reported the following memory: In early adolescence she had lived near a favorite aunt who had back pain. One day after school, the patient received a frantic telephone call from her aunt who implored her to come over immediately as her pain was severe and she had already summoned the family doctor. She raced around the corner to her aunt's house and was dumbfounded to be met by her aunt, all smiles and cheer. Before she could question her aunt, the

doorbell rang; the doctor had arrived. In a flash, the aunt transformed herself into a suffering person. Her face took on the expression of terrible pain, her gait became antalgic, and she limped into the bedroom where she then received her physician. The doctor inquired of her, provided reassurance, wrote a prescription for pain pills, and promised to visit the next day. Now, the patient was totally bewildered by what she had just seen and asked her aunt what this was all about. The aunt replied: "When you have a pain like mine, sometimes people don't believe you. You have to make them believe you to get help."

Patients may consciously or unconsciously exaggerate their symptomatology simply for the sake of credibility. They are not malingerers and they are not feigning illness. The processes that caused their symptoms were initially biological, take on psychological meaning because of idiosyncratic historical events and learning, and then become driven—in the absence of or in combination with continuing biological input—by psychological and social processes.

We have argued throughout this chapter that a chronic pain syndrome consists of both pain and suffering. Not surprisingly, many patients experience their pain and the suffering it causes as punishment for a past transgression. Some individuals can identify the event for which they believe they are being punished (e.g., the patient mentioned above who believed that her pain was punishment for an abortion); others cannot, but have a strong belief that such things as chronic pain and chronic illness only happen when people deserve them.

Pain and Punishment. A 32-year-old woman with chronic progressive multiple sclerosis was referred for psychotherapy and management of pain. Both of her parents had survived the Holocaust and her father had become a very successful businessman who was able to provide the best for his family. The patient's family was unable to comprehend that her illness was continuing to progress in spite of the expert medical evaluation and treatment she had received. In psychotherapy, the patient agonized over the limitations imposed by her disability and struggled to figure out the reason she had become ill. Her parents had been saved, but it seemed like she was being punished. Because she could not identify a wrong that warranted such punishment, the feeling of being punished alternated with a numbing despair that her illness (and the impact it had had on her) was senseless.

Unresolved Questions

In this section we will briefly identify some unresolved questions about treating chronic pain patients in the manner we have described. Although we have considered these questions at various points in conducting integrative psychotherapy with chronic pain patients, we have not been able to address them to our satisfaction. It is possible that more extensive experience with psychotherapy integration will provide answers, but we believe that it is more likely that these are issues that we will continue to struggle with in our work with chronic pain patients.

One issue that is relevant to all psychotherapy but which seems especially salient in integrative approaches is *timing*. By virtue of its nature, in an integrative psychotherapy the therapist is often choosing between two or more very different approaches to working with the patient. It is sometimes difficult to decide when to suggest changing approaches. This is equally true of changes from psychodynamic exploration to, for example, relaxation or hypnosis as it is of changes from a cognitive-behavioral approach to a psychodynamic one. To suggest such alterations in the course of therapy is a major intervention on the part of the therapist. Such suggestions by the therapist (or by the patient for that matter) must be discussed, and the patient's experience of them must be explored. Although such discussions can be very valuable, timing is still a central consideration in the art of integrative psychotherapy, one for which there are few guidelines for the practicing therapist.

Similarly, we can offer little practical advice about when to confront a patient's *denial*. Many chronic pain patients are suffering from chronic illnesses, and the psychotherapist may know more about the medical aspects of the patient's condition than the patient. As we suggested above, we believe that education of the patient plays an important role in integrative psychotherapy. However, it can be very difficult to decide whether to confront a patient's denial of an illness

or of its threatening consequences. It is often valuable for the patient to be knowledgeable about his or her medical situation, but in making this assessment the therapist must consider whether education serves the patient's best interests or whether the patient copes more effectively by avoiding threatening information. The therapist must also consider whether informing the patient about an illness reflects some need on the part of the therapist, or a tacit belief that knowledge is a valuable method of gaining a sense of control (even though the illness may in fact be uncontrollable).

We have briefly discussed occasions when the therapist has information that the patient appears not to. Another situation that arises in the multidisciplinary treatment of chronic pain patients is when the therapist has information, obtained during psychotherapy sessions, that the remainder of the treatment team does not. Often the patient gives the therapist permission to discuss some of the content of the sessions with other members of the team, but there are times when the therapist has information that is confidential but which could help the team to understand various aspects of the patient's behavior (for example, a female patient abruptly discontinues a series of nerve block injections administered by a male anesthesiologist because they revive feelings of vulnerability resulting from past sexual abuse). Although one of the arguments for a multidisciplinary treatment approach has been the value of coordinating different types of information, protecting the patient's confidentiality has priority. In these situations, therapists must address any perception by their colleagues that they are being withholding while at the same time remaining a part of the team and endorsing a team approach to treatment.

To the best of our knowledge, there are no empirical studies that have investigated the efficacy of an integrative psychotherapeutic approach in the treatment of chronic pain patients (but see Pilowsky & Barrow, 1990, for a study of psychodynamic psychotherapy with pain patients). Hopefully, this chapter has provided both a rationale and case material that provide support for the value of an integrative approach. Among our personal experiences that seem to speak to the value of such an approach are the not infrequent occasions when we have been asked to provide a behavioral intervention (most often, relaxation training or hypnosis) for a chronic pain patient who already has a psychotherapist. In these situations, both patient and psychotherapist are typically enthusiastic about such adjunctive treatment. However, we have found it very difficult to provide effective behavioral interventions when they are unaccompanied by psychotherapy. Indeed, given the absence of empirical research, our discomfort and lack of effectiveness when working in this nonintegrative fashion has made an integrative approach to psychotherapy with chronic pain patients seem all the more compelling to us.

CONCLUDING COMMENTS

The overwhelming majority of the chronic pain patients we have evaluated and treated have suffered from a very real physical illness or injury that has led to a chronic pain syndrome that has failed to respond to appropriate medical or surgical treatment. Although we do not believe that every case of chronic pain reflects a complex combination of biological, psychological, and social processes, we do believe that almost all chronic pain patients suffer from a disorder that can be characterized this way. There are some patients with short-term chronic pain (of, say, three to six months duration) with a purely physical etiology who do not yet suffer from psychosocial consequences of pain. Likewise, there are a few patients who do seem to suffer from pain of a purely psychological origin (e.g., "delusional pain" in a patient with schizophrenia; France & Krishnan, 1988). However, such unifactorial pain syndromes are rare, and we hope that the cases we have presented have illustrated that the etiology of chronic pain is complex but that the suffering that accompanies it is often more a function of psychosocial processes than of physical disorder.

In addition to advocating an integrative approach to psychotherapy with chronic pain patients, we would also like to stress the need for flexibility in intervention. Persons (1991), in a recent review of psychotherapy research, has noted that the fundamental nature of psychotherapy is betrayed by the methodologies used in outcome studies. She stated that psychotherapy has always been, and needs to remain, individualized and theory-driven. The most widely practiced psychological intervention for chronic pain—cognitive-behavioral modification—has failed to take into account the very great individual differences among chronic pain patients and the heterogeneity of their treatment needs.

Our title refers to the integration of mind and body. As we have argued throughout this chapter, we conceptualize the chronic pain experience as the result of a complex combination of factors, reflecting processes of both the body and the mind. But that is not the only meaning of integration we considered in choosing the title. As we reviewed our cases, we became aware that in the successful treatment of patients with pain and suffering the individual comes to accept his or her pain. By this we mean that pain and illness are accepted as an important but not self-defining part of the person's life, and as an unfortunate and only partially controllable aspect of the human condition. We cannot specify how the cognitive-behavioral and psychodynamic components of an integrative psychotherapy contribute to this process whereby the mind no longer disavows the body's pain and illness. However, we do know that when this process occurs, the chronic pain patient becomes an individual with persistent pain—one who is no longer disabled, but able to remove pain from the center of awareness and to replace suffering with meaning.

ACKNOWLEDGMENTS.   The authors wish to thank Sharon Gordon, Ph.D., for her critical comments on this chapter. An earlier version of some of this material was presented by the second author at the meeting of the Society of Behavioral Medicine, Washington, D.C., March, 1991.

REFERENCES

Adler, R. H., Zlot, S., Hurny, C., & Minder, C. (1989). Engel's "psychogenic pain and the pain-prone patient": A retrospective, controlled clinical study. *Psychosomatic Medicine, 51,* 87–101.

American Psychiatric Association. (1987). *Diagnostic and statistical manual of mental disorders* (3rd ed., revised). Washington, DC: Author.

Aronoff, G. M., & Rutrick, D. (1985). Psychodynamics and psychotherapy of the chronic pain syndrome. In G. M. Aronoff (Ed.), *Evaluation and treatment of chronic pain* (pp. 463–469). Baltimore: Urban & Schwarzenberg.

Atkinson, J. H., Jr. (1989). Psychopharmacologic agents in the treatment of pain syndromes. In C. D. Tollison (Ed.),

Handbook of chronic pain management (pp. 69–103). Baltimore: Williams & Wilkins.

Bakal, D. A. (1982). *The psychobiology of chronic headache.* New York: Springer.

Barber, J. (1982). Incorporating hypnosis in the management of chronic pain. In J. Barber & C. Adrian (Eds.), *Psychological approaches to the management of pain* (pp. 40–59). New York: Brunner/Mazel.

Barber, J. (1990). Hypnosis. In J. Bonica (Ed.), *The management of pain* (Vol. II, 2nd ed., pp. 1733–1741). Philadelphia: Lea & Febiger.

Barlow, D. H. (1988). *Anxiety and its disorders: The nature and treatment of anxiety and panic.* New York: Guilford.

Barsky, A. J., & Wyshak, G. (1990). Hypochondriasis and somatosensory amplification. *British Journal of Psychiatry, 157,* 404–409.

Basch, M. F. (1980). *Doing psychotherapy.* New York: Basic Books.

Basch, M. F. (1988). *Understanding psychotherapy: The science behind the art.* New York: Basic Books.

Bellissimo, A., & Tunks, E. (1984). *Chronic pain: The psychotherapeutic spectrum.* New York: Praeger.

Blumer, D., & Heilbronn, M. (1989). Dysthymic pain disorder: The treatment of chronic pain as a variant of depression. In C. D. Tollison (Ed.), *Handbook of chronic pain management* (pp. 197–209). Baltimore: Williams & Wilkins.

Bonica, J. J. (1990). General considerations of chronic pain. In J. J. Bonica (Ed.), *The management of pain* (Vol. I, 2nd ed., pp. 180–196). Philadelphia: Lea & Febiger.

Bradley, L. A., Prokop, C. K., Margolis, R., & Gentry, W. D. (1978). Multivariate analyses of the MMPI profiles of low back pain patients. *Journal of Behavioral Medicine, 1,* 253–272.

Chapman, C. R., & Turner, J. A. (1986). Psychological control of acute pain in medical settings. *Journal of Pain and Symptom Management, 1,* 9–20.

Chaturvedi, S. K. (1987). Family morbidity in chronic pain patients. *Pain, 30,* 159–168.

Ciccone, D. S., & Grzesiak, R. C. (1984). Cognitive dimensions of chronic pain. *Social Science and Medicine, 19,* 1339–1345.

Ciccone, D. S., & Grzesiak, R. C. (1988). Cognitive therapy: An overview of theory and practice. In N. T. Lynch & S. V. Vasudevan (Eds.), *Persistent pain: Psychosocial assessment and intervention* (pp. 133–161). Boston: Kluwer Academic Publishers.

Ciccone, D. S., & Grzesiak, R. C. (1990a). Chronic musculoskeletal pain: A cognitive approach to psychophysiologic assessment and intervention. In M. G. Eisenberg & R. C. Grzesiak (Eds.), *Advances in clinical rehabilitation* (Vol. 3, pp. 197–214). New York: Springer.

Ciccone, D. S., & Grzesiak, R. C. (1990b, October). *Psychological vulnerability to chronic pain.* Paper presented at the meeting of the American Pain Society, St. Louis, MO.

Craig, K. D. (1978). Social modeling influences on pain. In R. A. Sternbach (Ed.), *The psychology of pain* (pp. 73–109). New York: Raven Press.

Crue, B. L., Jr. (1986). Multidisciplinary pain treatment programs: Current status. *Clinical Journal of Pain, 1,* 31–38.

DeGood, D. E. (1983). Reducing medical patients' reluctance to participate in psychological therapies: The initial session. *Professional Psychology: Research and Practice, 14,* 570–579.

Dohrenwend, B. S., & Dohrenwend, B. P. (1981). Life stress

and illness: Formulation of the issues. In B. S. Dohrenwend & B. P. Dohrenwend (Eds.), *Stressful life events and their contexts* (pp. 1–27). New York: Prodist.

Dohrenwend, B. P., Shrout, P. E., Link, B. G., Martin, J. L., & Skodol, A. E. (1986). Overview and initial results from a risk-factor study of depression and schizophrenia. In J. E. Barrett & R. M. Rose (Eds.), *Mental disorders in the community: Progress and challenge* (pp. 184–212). New York: Guilford.

Dworkin, R. H. (1990). Compensation in chronic pain patients: Cause or consequence? *Pain, 43,* 387–388.

Dworkin, R. H. (1992). What do we really know about the psychological origins of chronic pain? *American Pain Society Bulletin, 1*(5), 7–11.

Dworkin, R. H., & Caligor, E. (1988). Psychiatric diagnosis and chronic pain: DSM-III-R and beyond. *Journal of Pain and Symptom Management, 3,* 87–98.

Dworkin, R. H., & Gitlin, M. J. (1991). Clinical aspects of depression in chronic pain patients. *Clinical Journal of Pain, 7,* 79–94.

Dworkin, R. H., Handlin, D. S., Richlin, D. M., Brand, L., & Vannucci, C. (1985). Unraveling the effects of compensation, litigation, and employment on treatment response in chronic pain. *Pain, 23,* 49–59.

Dworkin, R. H., Hartstein, G., Rosner, H. L., Walther, R. R., Sweeney, E. W., & Brand, L. (1992). A high-risk method for studying psychosocial antecedents of chronic pain: The prospective investigation of herpes zoster. *Journal of Abnormal Psychology, 101,* 200–205.

Eimer, B. N. (1989). Psychotherapy for chronic pain: A cognitive approach. In A. Freeman, K. Simon, L. E. Beutler, & H. Arkowitz (Eds.), *Comprehensive handbook of cognitive therapy* (pp. 449–465). New York: Plenum Press.

Engel, G. L. (1951). Primary atypical facial neuralgia: An hysterical conversion symptom. *Psychosomatic Medicine, 13,* 375–396.

Engel, G. L. (1959). "Psychogenic" pain and the pain-prone patient. *American Journal of Medicine, 26,* 899–918.

Feuerstein, M., Papciak, A. S., & Hoon, P. E. (1987). Biobehavioral mechanisms of chronic low back pain. *Clinical Psychology Review, 7,* 243–273.

Ford, C. V. (1983). *The somatizing disorders: Illness as a way of life.* New York: Elsevier Biomedical.

Fordyce, W. E. (1976). *Behavioral methods for chronic pain and illness.* St. Louis: C. V. Mosby.

France, R. D., & Krishnan, K. R. R. (1988). Pain in psychiatric disorders. In R. D. France and K. R. R. Krishnan (Eds.), *Chronic pain* (pp. 116–141). Washington, DC: American Psychiatric Press.

Frank, K. A. (1990). Action techniques in psychoanalysis. *Contemporary Psychoanalysis, 26,* 732–756.

French, A. P., & Tupin, J. P. (1974). Therapeutic application of a simple relaxation method. *American Journal of Psychotherapy, 28,* 282–287.

Gamsa, A. (1990). Is emotional disturbance a precipitator or a consequence of chronic pain? *Pain, 42,* 183–195.

Gamsa, A., & Vikis-Freibergs, V. (1991). Psychological events are both risk factors in, and consequences of, chronic pain. *Pain, 44,* 271–277.

Gitlin, M. J. (1990). *The psychotherapist's guide to psychopharmacology,* New York: Free Press.

Goldsmith, S. (1983-84). A strategy for evaluating "psychogenic" symptoms. *International Journal of Psychiatry in Medicine, 13,* 167–171.

Grzesiak, R. C. (1977). Relaxation techniques in treatment

of chronic pain. *Archives of Physical Medicine and Rehabilitation, 58,* 270–272.

Grzesiak, R. C. (1980). Chronic pain: A psychobehavioral perspective. In L. P. Ince (Ed.), *Behavioral psychology in rehabilitation medicine: Clinical applications* (pp. 248–300). Baltimore: Williams & Wilkins.

Grzesiak, R. C. (1989). Strategies for multidisciplinary pain management. *Compendium of Continuing Education in Dentistry, 10,* 444–448.

Grzesiak, R. C. (1991). Psychologic considerations in temporomandibular dysfunction: A biopsychosocial view of symptom formation. *Dental Clinics of North America, 35,* 209–226.

Grzesiak, R. C., & Ciccone, D. S. (1988). Relaxation, biofeedback and hypnosis in the management of pain. In N. T. Lynch & S. V. Vasudevan (Eds.), *Persistent pain: Psychosocial assessment and intervention* (pp. 163–188). Boston: Kluwer Academic Publishers.

Guidano, V. F., & Liotti, G. (1983). *Cognitive processes and emotional disorders.* New York: Guilford.

Harness, D. M., & Donlon, W. C. (1988). Cryptotrauma: The hidden wound. *Clinical Journal of Pain, 4,* 257–260.

Hartstein, G., & Dworkin, R. H. (in press). Psychological aspects of postoperative pain. In C. Weissman & E. Delphin (Eds.), *Acute postoperative pain management.* New York: Elsevier.

Hilgard, E. R., & Hilgard, J. R. (1983). *Hypnosis in the relief of pain.* Los Altos, CA: William Kaufmann.

Holzman, A. D., & Turk, D. C. (Eds.). (1986). *Pain management: A handbook of psychological treatment approaches.* New York: Pergamon Press.

Horowitz, M. J. (1988). *Introduction to psychodynamics: A new synthesis.* New York: Basic Books.

Horowitz, M. J., Marmar, C., Krupnick, J., Wilner, N., Kaltreider, N., & Wallerstein, R. (1984). *Personality styles and brief psychotherapy.* New York: Basic Books.

Katon, W., Egan, K., & Miller, D. (1985). Chronic pain: Lifetime psychiatric diagnoses and family history. *American Journal of Psychiatry, 142,* 1156–1160.

Keane, T. M., Scott, W. O., Chavoya, G. A., Lamparski, D. M., & Fairbank, J. A. (1985). Social support in Vietnam veterans with posttraumatic stress disorder. A comparative analysis. *Journal of Consulting and Clinical Psychology, 53,* 95–102.

Kellner, R. (1986). *Somatization and hypochondriasis.* New York: Praeger.

Kutz, I., Borysenko, J. Z., & Benson, H. (1985). Meditation and psychotherapy: A rationale for the integration of dynamic psychotherapy, the relaxation response, and mindfulness meditation. *American Journal of Psychiatry, 142,* 1–8.

Lichstein, K. L. (1988). *Clinical relaxation strategies.* New York: Wiley-Interscience.

Lipowsky, Z. J. (1988). Somatization: The concept and its clinical application. *American Journal of Psychiatry, 145,* 1358–1368.

Loeser, J. D. (1982). Concepts of pain. In M. Stanton-Hicks & R. Boas (Eds.), *Chronic low back pain* (pp. 145–148). New York: Raven Press.

Loeser, J. D., & Black, R. G. (1975). A taxonomy of pain. *Pain, 1,* 81–90.

Love, A. W., & Peck, C. L. (1987). The MMPI and psychological factors in chronic low back pain: A review. *Pain, 28,* 1–12.

Maruta, T., Vatterott, M. K., & McHardy, M. J. (1989). Pain management as an antidepressant: Long-term resolution of pain-associated depression. *Pain, 36,* 335–337.

Meehl, P. E. (1962). Schizotaxia, schizotypy, schizophrenia. *American Psychologist, 17,* 827–838.

Merskey, H. (Ed.). (1986). Classification of chronic pain: Descriptions of chronic pain syndromes and definitions of pain terms. *Pain,* Suppl. 3.

Monks, R. (1990). Psychotropic drugs. In J. Bonica (Ed.), *The management of pain* (Vol. II, 2nd ed., pp. 1676–1689). Philadelphia: Lea & Febiger.

Moss, E., & Garb, R. (1986). Integrated psychotherapeutic treatment of somatoform and other psychophysiological disorders. *Psychotherapy and Psychosomatics, 45,* 105–112.

Oxman, T. (1986). Psychotherapy. In R. P. Raj (Ed.), *Practical management of pain* (pp. 821–828). Chicago: Yearbook Medical Publishers.

Persons, J. B. (1991). Psychotherapy outcome studies do not accurately represent current models of psychotherapy: A proposed remedy. *American Psychologist, 46,* 99–106.

Pilowsky, I. (1978). Psychodynamic aspects of the pain experience. In R. A. Sternbach (Ed.), *The psychology of pain* (pp. 203–217). New York: Raven Press.

Pilowsky, I. (1988). Psychotherapy. In N. T. Lynch & S. V. Vasudevan (Eds.), *Persistent pain: Psychosocial assessment and intervention* (pp. 189–194). Boston: Kluwer Academic Publishers.

Pilowsky, I. (1989). Pain and illness behaviour: Assessment and management. In P. D. Wall & R. Melzack (Eds.), *Textbook of pain* (2nd ed., pp. 980–988). Edinburgh: Churchill Livingstone.

Pilowsky, I., & Barrow, C. G. (1990). A controlled study of psychotherapy and amitriptyline used individually and in combination in the treatment of chronic intractable, 'psychogenic' pain. *Pain, 40,* 3–19.

Pinsky, J. J. (1975). Psychodynamics and psychotherapy in the treatment of patients with chronic intractable pain. In B. L. Crue, Jr. (Ed.), *Pain research and treatment* (pp. 383–389). New York: Academic Press.

Pinsky, J. J., & Malyon, A. (1978). The eclectic nature of psychotherapy in the treatment of chronic pain syndromes. In B. L. Crue, Jr. (Ed.), *Chronic pain* (pp. 321–327). New York: Spectrum Publications.

Raphael, K. G., Dohrenwend, B. P., & Marbach, J. J. (1990). Illness and injury among children of temporomandibular pain and dysfunction syndrome (TMPDS) patients. *Pain, 40,* 61–64.

Roberts, A. H. (1987). Literature update: Biofeedback and chronic pain. *Journal of Pain and Symptom Management, 2,* 169–171.

Romano, J. M., & Turner, J. A. (1985). Chronic pain and depression: Does the evidence support a relationship: *Psychological Bulletin, 97,* 18–34.

Rudy, T. E., Turk, D. C., Zaki, H. S., & Curtin, H. D. (1989). An empirical taxometric alternative to traditional classification of temporomandibular disorders. *Pain, 36,* 311–320.

Shapiro, D. (1965). *Neurotic styles.* New York: Basic Books.

Sternbach, R. A. (1974). *Pain patients: Traits and treatment.* New York: Academic Press.

Sternbach, R. A. (1984). Acute versus chronic pain. In P. D. Wall & R. Melzack (Eds.), *Textbook of pain* (pp. 173–177). Edinburgh: Churchill Livingstone.

Sternbach, R. A., & Timmermans, G. (1975). Personality changes associated with reduction of pain. *Pain, 1,* 177–181.

Turk, D. C. (1990). Customizing treatment for chronic pain

patients: Who, what, and why? *Clinical Journal of Pain, 6,* 255–270.

Turk, D. C., & Flor, H. (1984). Etiological theories and treatments for chronic back pain: II. Psychological models and interventions. *Pain, 19,* 209–233.

Turk, D. C., & Rudy, T. E. (1987). Towards a comprehensive assessment of chronic pain patients. *Behaviour Research and Therapy, 25,* 237–249.

Turk, D. C., & Rudy, T. E. (1988). Toward an empirically derived taxonomy of chronic pain patients: Integration of psychological assessment data. *Journal of Consulting and Clinical Psychology, 56,* 233–238.

Turk, D. C., Meichenbaum, D., & Genest, M. (1983). *Pain and behavioral medicine: A cognitive-behavioral perspective.* New York: Guilford.

Turner, R. J., & Noh, S. (1988). Physical disability and depression: A longitudinal analysis. *Journal of Health and Social Behavior, 29,* 23–37.

Violon, A., & Giurgea, D. (1984). Familial models for chronic pain. *Pain, 18,* 199–203.

Von Korff, M. R., Le Resche, L. A., & Dworkin, S. F. (1990, March). *Depression and risk of onset of chronic pain: A 3 year follow-up of a pain-free population sample.* Paper presented at the meeting of the Society for Behavioral Medicine, Washington, DC.

Wachtel, P. L. (1977). *Psychoanalysis and behavior therapy: Toward an integration.* New York: Basic Books.

Watson, D. (1982). Neurotic tendencies among chronic pain patients: An MMPI item analysis. *Pain, 14,* 365–385.

CHAPTER 26

Severe Mental Disorders

David T. Hellkamp

INTRODUCTION

It is generally agreed that effective interventions with persons experiencing severe and persistent mental disorders are based upon a multidisciplinary, multilevel set of treatments which can occur in an inpatient or outpatient setting, ideally integrated via case management through a myriad of community support services. The philosophy of treatment is embedded in a rehabilitation framework. The effective interventions most frequently cited are psychoactive medications and psychiatric rehabilitation technologies. Examples of psychiatric rehabilitation technologies include developing psychosocial rehabilitation centers, teaching clients medication management skills, conducting family psychoeducational groups, teaching social skills to clients, developing supported employment programs, and teaching inservice and preservice personnel how to set overall rehabilitation goals, conduct functional assessments, and teach skills (Anthony, Cohen, & Kennard, 1990). These psychiatric rehabilitation technologies are clearly promising and consistent with the desires of many consumers and their

David T. Hellkamp • Department of Psychology, Xavier University, Cincinnati, Ohio 45207.

Comprehensive Handbook of Psychotherapy Integration, edited by George Stricker and Jerold R. Gold. Plenum Press, New York, 1993.

family members (Chamberlin & Rogers, 1990; Weisburd, 1990).

What is generally lacking in the psychiatric rehabilitation literature are references to the value of psychotherapy, especially individual psychotherapy, as an effective treatment for many persons with severe mental disorders (SMD). Clinicians who are reporting successful use of individual psychotherapy with the SMD population fall into the different theoretical orientations: psychoanalytic, behavioral, and humanistic-existential. In all instances, when one becomes acquainted with their psychotherapeutic methods, one finds modifications have been made in the therapeutic applications to fit the needs and experiences of the SMD patients. Although there are sometimes marked differences and even contradictions in the therapeutic applications (Cancro, 1983), one also becomes aware of the many similarities in the modifications that are being made. Unfortunately, references to the psychotherapeutic interventions that are showing great promise with persons experiencing SMD are generally scattered in the literature and, perhaps, as a result, do not have an "identity" that integrates them and identifies them as specifically appropriate for persons with SMD. The term *supportive psychotherapy* is many times considered "the therapy" for persons with SMD. It is my contention, however, that persons suffering from severe and persistent mental disabilities can benefit from a psychotherapy that is much broader in scope than supportive psychotherapy, if one defines supportive therapy in the usual manner (see Torrey, 1988, p. 259). I refer to these modifications of psychotherapy by the term *rehabilitative psychotherapy*.

Rehabilitative psychotherapy adopts what is "good therapy" for the SMD population while taking into account any existing biological, psychodynamic, and psychosocial issues in the patient's life, all of which are integrated in a rehabilitation philosophy. This is not to suggest that rehabilitative psychotherapy should be viewed as another type of psychotherapy to add to the more than 400 therapies. Rather, I consider rehabilitative psychotherapy as an integrative psychotherapy which identifies the wisdom gathered from the psychoanalytic schools, the practicality from the cognitive-behavioral approaches, and the humaneness from the humanistic-existential orientation.

This chapter will first describe the SMD population, then review some concepts regarding etiology and pathogenesis, particularly related to persons with one type of SMD, schizophrenia. I will then address some theoretical and clinical antecedents to be followed by a discussion of techniques and the process of rehabilitative psychotherapy, especially within an individual psychotherapy format. A case example will also be presented along with final comments about future developments for rehabilitative psychotherapy.

THEORETICAL AND CONCEPTUAL ISSUES

In this section I will focus on two questions: (1) Who are persons with SMD? and (2) What is the current thinking with regard to etiology of persons with SMD?

Description of the SMD Population

The term *severe* as a qualifier to mental disorders has been used historically as a reflection of "severity of symptoms" and "length of hospitalization." As social policy moved away from custodial treatment for these patients in a hospital environment to providing treatment in the patient's community, the definition of persons with SMD expanded to also include problems of disability, that is, problems in adapting to their own preferred environment. As a result, the term *severe* became broadened to include extent of role impairment (Bachrach, 1983).

From a DSM-III-R diagnostic perspective, individuals with SMD include categories of schizophrenia, delusional disorders, psychotic disorders not elsewhere classified, some mood disorders, and certain personality disorders, among others (Goldman, 1984). Such patients therefore represent a wide spectrum of diagnostic categories. The largest number of SMD patients carry a diagnosis of schizophrenia.

On a psychosocial level, Test and Stein (1978) identified five central characteristics of SMD patients, regardless of DSM categorization: (1) A high vulnerability to stress. They may develop severe psychopathology when experiencing only minimal to moderate stress situations, a dynamic sometimes referred to as "overstimulation." (2) Deficiencies in coping skills. Such persons frequently lack skills in daily living, such as budgeting money, using public transportation, doing laundry, preparing meals, and having and/or keeping housing clean and organized. (3) Extreme dependency. The patient frequently experiences feelings of extreme helplessness which requires massive support from families or institutions to adapt. When such support is threatened or cut-off, they frequently develop severe symptomatology. (4) Difficulty with working in the competitive job market. Vocational disability is a central feature in these persons. Employment histories usually reveal frequent job changes interspersed with long periods of unemployment. It is not infrequent that no employment history is found. Nevertheless, many of these patients can do quite well in sheltered workshop experiences where expectations are geared to the patient's capabilities, indicating the employment difficulties are probably related to stress factors. (5) Difficulty with interpersonal relationships. Considerable difficulties are found with such patients in developing and/or maintaining close relationships with others. Social support networks are therefore minimal and/or not frequently utilized.

Overall, it is necessary to consider the three "D's" (diagnosis, duration, and disability) as distinct criteria in any attempt to define SMD (Bachrach, 1988; Goldman, 1984). The person experiencing a SMD is frequently so disabled that without special support they cannot maintain a stable adjustment to community life. Proper assessment is considered to require not only a medical and psychodiagnostic workup, but also a rehabilitational, functional workup (Farkas & Anthony, 1989). For purposes of this chapter, I will limit most of my discussion on SMD patients to persons with a diagnosis of schizophrenia. Other writers have discussed promising developments with other DSM disorders, that is, bipolar disorders (Teixiera, 1990; Pollack, 1991), severe personality disorders (Masterson & Klein, 1989; Rowe & MacIsaac, 1989), to cite just a few.

Etiology

Any discussion of etiology of SMD, especially within schizophrenia, is likely strongly influenced by the primary assumptions the clinician makes about his or her understanding of the disorders. For example, if the assumption is made that schizophrenia is a disease, then biological (e.g., neurologic, neurochemical, genetic) theories are likely to be emphasized with psychological and social issues being considered secondary. On the other hand, if schizophrenia is conceptualized more as a dis-ease rather than a disease, phenomenological and life-experience theories (e.g., psychodynamic, behavioral, rehabilitative) are likely to be emphasized as primary with biologic ways of understanding perceived as secondary. Without addressing the pro's and con's of these assumptions, let us turn our attention to a discussion of some biological and psychological hypotheses regarding etiology.

Biological Hypotheses. It is beyond the scope of this chapter to thoroughly review the biological literature in schizophrenia. The interested reader is referred to articles by Buchsbaum and Haier (1987), Gottesman, McGuffin, and Farmer (1987), Holzman (1987), and Meltzer (1987). A few of the most salient developments will be discussed.

Current biological research on schizophrenia is attempting to find the best way for classifying and defining the characteristic symptoms in order to better search for the underlying mechanisms and causes. One such idea that is receiving much current attention is the notion of positive and negative symptoms in schizophrenia (Crow, 1982). Positive symptoms of schizophrenia in-

clude those that represent a distortion of some normal function, such as hallucinations, delusions, bizarre behavior, and positive formal thought disorders. Negative symptoms refer to symptoms that likely represent a loss of normal function, a "deficit," such as alogia (poverty of speech and of content of speech), affective flattening (blunting of emotional responsiveness), avolition-apathy (loss of will, energy, and drive), and anhedonia-asociality (loss of the ability to experience normal pleasure and relate intimately to others). Hypothesis building has been developed to relate positive symptoms of schizophrenia with neurochemical abnormalities, especially related to the neurotransmitters, such as excessive dopamine. In contrast, negative symptoms have been associated with certain types of brain lesions rather than to neurochemical disturbances of the brain. A number of structural brain abnormalities have been suggested: ventricular enlargement, a slight decrease in brain weight, a decrease in the volume of the basal ganglia, temporal lobe, or limbic regions, disorganization of the pyramidal cell layer of the hippocampus, and atrophy of particular cortical layers (Meltzer, 1987).

From a treatment standpoint, the formulation of a relationship between positive symptoms of schizophrenia and certain neurotransmitter dysfunctions provides a theoretical basis for psychopharmacologic interventions, such as the neuroleptics. Positive symptoms are considered responsive to antipsychotic medications. On the other hand, negative "deficit"symptoms are considered to be unresponsive to medications. Unfortunately, the association of negative symptoms of schizophrenia to structural brain abnormalities lends itself to a theoretical bias of therapeutic pessimism with clinicians, patients, and families feeling helpless and discouraged when confronting the severe negative disabling symptoms of the disorder.

Based on a review of data from a variety of biological studies coupled with basic facts of what is known about schizophrenia, Weinberger (1987) developed a hypothesis that "schizophrenia is a neurodevelopmental disorder in which a fixed brain lesion from early in life interacts with certain normal maturational events that occur much later" (p. 60). He speculated the lesion to be a congenital, static lesion in the prefrontal cortex, specifically within the dorso-lateral prefrontal area, which produces a disturbance in the functioning of the dopaminergic neurons. Such impairment is considered to produce a diathesis so that certain stressors might not only cause variable degrees of symptoms in different consequences, but may also account for differences in age of onset of schizophrenia. Weinberger discussed possible medical causes of the proposed lesion in the brain including the possibility, though remote in his mind, that "early developmental psychosocial experience could produce a structural brain lesion in plastic neural symptoms" (p. 666). Before Weinberger's hypothesis is interpreted as a panacea, it should be remembered that it is very speculative. Weinberger, himself, also reasons that it is possible there "may not be a true lesion at all, but simply a relative hypoplasia or dysplasia of the symptoms implicated, resulting in a quantitative physiological deficit" (p. 666).

Genetic studies typically report that schizophrenia runs in families. Risk tables for relatives of persons with schizophrenia usually include the considerably higher frequencies of family members being schizophrenic as compared to the general population when the patient is a parent, sibling, or twin (Gottesman et al., 1987).

Although the above ideas regarding biological hypotheses relating to schizophrenia have stimulated a new wave of biological research, the results are far from conclusive. For example, biochemical explanations such as the dopamine hypothesis may need to be tempered when one considers the reality that persons experiencing acute, florid, "positive" symptoms of schizophrenia can also be effectively treated psychologically without any medication. Numerous case studies, including my own experience, support this finding as do the results of a more systematic study (Karon & VandenBos, 1981). Similarly, the proposed brain lesions and identified differences in brain structures may be iatrogenic to the biochemical treatments themselves (Karon, 1991; Matthysse, 1987). Some evidence exists that the brain can target some of its own cells for destruction when under conditions of prolonged severe exposure to an impoverished external environment. With regard to the genetic studies, some of the evidence, including the twin studies most recently reported in Finland, are being interpreted in very contradictory ways by different researchers (i.e., see Nuechterlen & Haier, 1991 vs. Karon, 1991). At

least one researcher, following a reanalysis, has even questioned the integrity of some of the data (Karon, 1991).

Psychological Hypotheses. Psychological theories regarding the etiology of schizophrenia were developed principally from the psychoanalytic school of thought. The psychoanalytic theories and treatment procedures help illuminate the importance of early childhood experience in understanding later psychopathology. No other theory of psychopathology has articulated a detailed developmental perspective. Within a psychoanalytic context, schizophrenia is seen to evolve from problems that originate early in life, especially during the first year. This is true for any of the psychoanalytic theories, whether an id psychology (conflict theory), an ego psychology (object relations theory), or a self-psychology (deficit theory). What is not always clearly understood by nonpsychoanalytic clinicians and theoreticians is that a discussion of etiological factors in schizophrenia goes beyond solely psychodynamic concepts for developmental paradigms. On the basis of their research, Mahler and Furer (1960) described the symbiotic psychotic child as both constitutionally vulnerable and predisposed toward the development of a psychosis. Most psychoanalytic writers will refer to a "constitutional ego defect" in the child that lends itself to a vicious cycle in the pathogenetic mother/child relationship (Mahler & Gosliner, 1955). Both regression and fixation (developmental arrests) are important concepts in psychoanalysis and in the predicament of the person with schizophrenia. The preOedipal developmental arrest found in schizophrenia may not always be "caused" by poor parenting. Mahler found there was a "good enough mother" in terms of parenting style in half of the cases she studied of infantile psychosis. It was conjectured that the cause was probably related to some "intrinsic vulnerability" in the child. In contrast, in the other half a debilitating emotional unavailability on the part of the mother was found as the mother was usually depressed. Regardless, rather basic intrapsychic structures of the ego and self are theorized as having failed to develop. Consequently, distinct boundaries between the self and others in the environment are considered fragile, fluid, and undifferentiated. In addition, the self-experience of the person with schizophrenia includes an unstructured and under-developed self-identity along with feeling states of fright, confusion, loneliness, anger, and terror. Persons with schizophrenic disorders often realize that they are different from others in their environment as their friends and family members also understand. They frequently withdraw from others in their life and notice that others do not react favorably to them. Mistrust is usually central in their interactions with others. Karon and VandenBos (1981) theorized that all of the symptoms of schizophrenia can be understood as attempts to deal with chronic terror. Underlying themes and issues regarding annihilation and death are paramount in the transference issues found in the schizophrenic individual.

Many family members passionately object to faulty parenting as an etiological factor in schizophrenia. Such an explanation is perceived as "parent bashing." Although this has certainly occurred, it is important that a distinction be made between true parent bashing and the uncovering of stressors within a dysfunctional family system that may have pathogenetic influences on the family member with a schizophrenic disorder. Interventions with family members can be conducted in a sensitive, empathic manner in order to elicit the invaluable support and aid of the family in working with the patient with a schizophrenic disorder.

Rather than considering psychological factors as "causes" (etiology), it is perhaps more heuristic to consider psychological processes as critical in understanding the course and outcome (pathogenesis) of schizophrenia. In this way, family members can live with minimal guilt and other destructive feelings, while focusing their attention on those factors that can positively influence the course of their own lives, including that of the patient.

Along these lines, psychological and social factors, such as stressful life events (Day et al., 1987), family factors, for example, expressed emotion (Koenigsberg & Haddley, 1986), failures in support networks (Bennett & Morris, 1991), and the patients' own personal reaction to their condition (Selzer, Sullivan, Carsky, & Terkelsen, 1989) can be addressed by educating both patient and family members about the relevancy of these factors in precipitating acute symptoms.

In summary, research findings with regard to either biological or psychological factors of schizophrenia are inconclusive at this time with regard to "causes" of the disorder. Whatever the future portends in regard to etiology, it is apparent that clinicians and theoreticians should be very careful in their reasoning regarding "causality" factors in relation to schizophrenia and other severe mental disorders (Matthysse, 1987). Fortunately, more clinicians and researchers are adopting a theoretical position which promotes a biopsychosocial model for not only understanding SMD disorders such as schizophrenia, but also for providing a basis for both treatment planning and implementation. Examples of biopsychosocial models are found in works by Selzer et al. (1989) and Pollack (1991). Such approaches recognize the complexity of persons with schizophrenia and the likelihood that a large number of different processes are at work.

CLINICAL AND THEORETICAL ANTECEDENTS

Just as the biologic versus psychologic etiology controversy of schizophrenia can be reduced to an either/or discussion with one view or the other being considered "the winner," so, too, in my opinion, do we find a similar mentality being advocated by a segment of clinicians and theoreticians in the literature with regard to the efficacy of individual psychotherapy for this population. More specifically, tension has sometimes developed between the relative efficacies of individual psychodynamic psychotherapy versus behavioral and/or psychiatric rehabilitation technologies as appropriate intervention procedures with persons with schizophrenia. Some writers (Mueser & Berenbaum, 1990) are calling for a moratorium in the use of psychodynamic psychotherapies for schizophrenia, while others (Drake & Sederer, 1986) caution about "adverse effects" of intensive psychotherapy, and yet another (Torrey, 1988) goes so far to indicate that using psychoanalytic psychotherapy "is not only negligent, it is malpractice" (p. 223). In my opinion, it is extremely unfortunate and scientifically unconscionable that such dogmatic conclusions are being made by these writers. Neither the clinical nor the research data support such a conclusion at this time. The majority of these writers who call for the demise of psychodynamic psychotherapy are usually very selective in their literature reviews. At the minimum they are either unaware or ignore the recent upsurge in books and review articles that provide support for the efficacy of psychodynamic psychotherapy with persons experiencing schizophrenic disorders. Moreover, they frequently overgeneralize in their reasoning, treating psychodynamic psychotherapy in a very superficial and/or distorted manner. Mueser and Berenbaum (1990) are especially superficial in their analysis of the longitudinal psychotherapy studies that have been done. As one example, they interpret the results of the Boston Psychotherapy Study (Stanton, Gunderson, Knapp, Frank, Vannicelli, Schnitzer, & Rosenthal, 1984; Gunderson, Frank, Katz, Vannicelli, Frosch, & Knapp, 1984) in a manner that supposedly demonstrated that psychodynamic psychotherapy was clearly "inferior" to reality-adaptive supportive psychotherapy even though some of the same investigators who participated in the original Boston Psychotherapy Study have reported more recently (Glass, Katz, Schnitzer, Knapp, Frank, & Gunderson, 1989) in a further analysis of their data the importance of skilled dynamic exploration for predicting outcome in the domains of denial of illness, global psychopathology, and retardation-apathy in persons with a schizophrenic disorder. Since the Boston researchers found a relationship between dynamic exploratory activity and reductions in the so-called negative symptoms of schizophrenia, and since such negative symptoms are generally unresponsive to biochemical interventions, their results appear especially important insofar as the symptoms influenced may be core aspects of schizophrenic psychopathology. Mueser and Berenbaum (1990) did not report these later results from the Boston Study.

It is not my intent in this chapter to review the studies demonstrating the efficacy of individual psychodynamic psychotherapy in working with persons with SMD. Other writers have recently done so (Karon, 1991; Karon & VandenBos, 1981; Pollack, 1991; Teixeira, 1990). Suffice it to say, based on their reviews, it is fair to conclude that individual psychodynamic psychotherapy can be "good therapy" when it is modified appropriately to fit the needs of persons with SMD and conducted by skilled psychotherapists. "Good

therapy" for the patient may require a greater flexibility in the psychotherapist's manner of practicing. For example, the therapist might consider a missed appointment as a symptom to be actively resolved, rather than seeing it as a resistance and remaining passive. Also, the "place" of the therapy might not be rigidly perceived as always being the therapist's office, but, periodically, creatively conducted in places that are mutually considered to be safe and comfortable.

It appears the psychotherapist can play a central role in integrating rehabilitation technologies that are available to such patients and their families since the psychotherapist can provide a sense of continuity in care as compared to most other providers who intervene on behalf of the patient and the family. The integration of the relevant principles of psychotherapy within a rehabilitation framework comprises the work of the rehabilitative psychotherapist.

TECHNIQUE AND PROCESS OF REHABILITATIVE PSYCHOTHERAPY

I believe it is possible to synthesize what constitutes "good therapy" for the SMD patient with a schizophrenic disorder, thereby identifying the characteristics, qualities, and skills that are most likely to lead to success. Such an integrative approach in psychotherapy is not new. Recent integrative approaches can be found for the treatment of anorexia nervosa (Steinlin & Weber, 1989), bulimia nervosa (Johnson & Connors, 1989), cocaine addiction (Washington, 1989), borderline clients (Kroll, 1988), narcissistic disorder (Gold, 1990), and phobic disorders (Wolfe, 1989), to cite just a few. For psychotherapists committed to working with patients with SMD, it is my contention that the focus of the psychotherapy must not only be on a more traditional area of psychopathology and impairment, but also on themes related to the patient's disabilities. One of the major elements that has been shown to distinguish persons with schizophrenia (as well as most other forms of SMD) from virtually all other patients with various mental disorders is their difficulties in adapting and coping autonomously in their own preferred environments, especially between "psychotic episodes" when the acute symptoms subside (Summers, 1981).

Before discussing assessment and treatment techniques, I wish to address some of the characteristics of the rehabilitative psychotherapist who chooses to work with the SMD patient.

Characteristics of Therapists

Many psychotherapists currently perceive the major obstacle for providing their services to the SMD population as the failure of the health care system to provide insurance coverage for the treatment. Even if the financial incentive was there (which is not likely to occur in the private sector), I believe most providers of care would not be adequately trained to provide the necessary services. Discussions of specific training voids in the core mental health disciplines with regard to working with the SMD population have been detailed elsewhere (see Lefley, 1990). Succinctly, successful psychotherapy with persons with schizophrenic disorders occurs when the psychotherapist has not only been trained as a psychotherapist, but specifically to do psychotherapy with the population of persons with schizophrenic disorders. Among other traits, the psychotherapist must possess a comfort level for accepting, empathetically understanding, and communicating with a person who sometimes displays "crazy behavior." Not all psychotherapists can feel comfortable with the patients "crazy," bizarre behaviors. Additionally, SMD patients are not likely to provide much positive feedback to the psychotherapist about any progress. This lack of feedback can be very disconcerting for many therapists, activating countertransference feelings of insecurity, helplessness, frustration, anger, and projected resistance on the part of the patient.

Just as importantly, the psychotherapist who commits to work with the SMD population must also be trained in the area of psychiatric rehabilitation technology. Psychiatric rehabilitation is conceptualized as a comprehensive model that includes knowledge and skills about (1) appropriate psychoactive medications, (2) community support services, (3) collaboration in working with patients, family members, employees, the courts, landlords, agency personnel, and other treatment providers, (4) psychoeducational and psychosocial technologies, (5) case management, and (6) subcultural nuances of minorities and the socioeconomically impoverished groups. Finally, the rehabilitation psychotherapist should also be knowledgeable and skilled on a systems level about how to influence social policy through advocacy procedures. In my opinion, psychiatric rehabilitation technology must be perceived as a central aspect of the treatment for this population.

Once a commitment is made to do individual psychodynamic psychotherapy with an SMD patient, a number of issues need to be considered: assessment, the therapeutic alliance, the therapeutic procedures to be employed, and how to deal with the ending of the therapy. Before discussing these issues, it should be assumed that the rehabilitative psychotherapist will commit to involvement for the long-term so as to provide the necessary stability and continuity in the patient's life. Although specific temporal factors are hard to pinpoint with this population, a minimum of a commitment of a year to an ideal of three to five years is recommended. The rehabilitative psychotherapist is truly making a commitment at the outset. My comments are not directed at those psychotherapists who do only brief interventions with the SMD population. Although brief psychodynamic psychotherapy has been applied successfully to other populations (e.g., Budman & Gurman, 1986), more work needs to be done with the SMD population to determine its proper utility.

Assessment

Assessment is an important stage for the treatment and rehabilitation of the SMD population. The assessment will usually include an appraisal of any medical problems, including related somatic illnesses as well as an appraisal of medications. Psychiatric and psychological evaluations will be conducted for principally arriving at a good differential DSM diagnosis. These are standard medical, psychiatric, and psychological evaluation techniques which include the armamentarium of medical and psychological testing procedures that are a central part of diagnostics in psychology and psychiatry. In addition to these standard assessment techniques, a rehabilitation diagnosis also needs to be developed. Such an assessment would include setting the overall rehabilitation goal with the patient, conducting a functional assessment, and conducting a resource assessment (Farkas, O'Brien, & Nemec,

1988). Just as the skills for learning how to administer, score, analyze, and interpret, a psychological IQ test takes training and practice under supervision, so, too, are the skills and assessment procedures for good rehabilitation diagnosis (Cohen, Farkas, & Cohen, 1986; Cohen, Farkas, Cohen, & Unger, 1987). Finally, a good assessment must also integrate an analysis of the patient's self-functioning into the overall evaluation. This is a phenomenological analysis of the patient which is critical for developing an empathetic understanding of the unique psychological reality of the particular person. It is by getting into the patient's inner psychological world that the psychotherapist will be in a position to best collaborate with the patient for effective interventions on any level, medical (dental), psychological, rehabilitational (or habilitative). Compliance in treatment is a natural byproduct once the patient and the therapist learn how to collaborate; meaning that the therapist and patient are communicating effectively and the patient experiences himself as a critical part of the intervention process. In this way, the patient becomes educated about intervention techniques, while playing a critical role in helping develop the treatment goals.

Therapeutic Alliance

From the beginning, it is considered critical that the patient experience active participation in the therapeutic process. It is assumed that reasonable psychological readiness exists within the patient, meaning the patient possesses a nominal capacity for self-reflection and education. These characteristics are considered fundamental for working with the patient toward the initial goal of developing a therapeutic alliance. In my experience, many patients are mistakenly considered to lack psychological readiness, when, in fact, what is being observed within the patient is passivity and apathy (negative symptoms). A good assessment will usually shed light on the psychological readiness of the patient. It is my experience that such behavioral cues do not come from formal psychodiagnostic evaluations alone, but rather from analysis into the phenomenological world of the patient. Apart from feedback from the patient, I pay particular attention to descriptions about the patient from persons who spend considerable time with the patient, such as ward

personnel, case managers, and family members. Two other variables of readiness that have been hypothesized to predict successful therapeutic outcomes in these patients are: a patient's motivation to avoid acute psychotic episodes and the patient's desire to achieve social and vocational goals (White, 1989). I have found a majority of patients with schizophrenic disorders possessing a reasonable degree of psychological readiness.

Persons with schizophrenic disorders typically do not communicate clearly with the therapist. The neophyte rehabilitative psychotherapist is generally not prepared to work with such patients and receive little or no feedback from the patients that they are being helped or even being clearly understood. As implied before, training rehabilitative psychotherapists to deal with their own countertransferences and biases is critical. The prevailing attitude among mental health professionals is that working with the SMD population is unrewarding, nonprestigious, and hopeless. These attitudes, if present, need to be clearly understood and resolved.

The treatment alliance involves both the therapists' and the patients' capacity to work together and clearly understand the objectives of the psychotherapy. The therapeutic alliance assumes both the therapist and the patient have the capacity to observe each other as separate individuals who together can observe, clarify, and interpret the patient's psychodynamics and coping behaviors. Whereas the treatment alliance is generally the starting point in the psychotherapy process for most patients with mental disorders, it typically becomes a goal of the treatment for the patient with a schizophrenic disorder. The therapists' empathic style and associated attitudes of acceptance, sensitivity, and understanding are critical, but not sufficient, toward that end. Through the therapist's skilled interventions, the patient will slowly acquire a working alliance with a greater knowledge of the therapeutic method and the collaborative role.

Therapeutic Procedures

Specific strategies for facilitating a therapeutic alliance include searching for ways to involve the patient in an examination of his or her relationship with the therapist, while improving (frequently educating) his or her understanding of the treatment process. How the patient attempts to adapt in his or her own preferred environment will frequently provide clues for the therapist. Such clues can be related to the rehabilitation goals the patient has established, thereby providing the opportunity for examining intra- and interpsychic issues. Another avenue for the therapist is to accept a patient's symptoms (e.g., delusions), regardless of how bizarre or "crazy," in order to have the client reflect on the intrapsychic implications. Whatever is chosen, it must be something which both the therapist and patient agree reflects a fundamental orientation of the patient's experience which will be meaningful enough to remain useful as the therapeutic work moves in an increasingly interpretive direction (Selzer & Carsky, 1990). Segments of the patient's experiences from the rehabilitation diagnosis can be extremely useful toward that end. For example, the therapist might explore the patient's current rehabilitation goal setting in relation to a specific, preferred environment in which the client chooses to live, learn, socialize, or work throughout the next year. In this way, the psychotherapy becomes embedded in a psychiatric rehabilitation framework. Moreover, if the rehabilitation diagnosis was done properly, such a focus will have direct meaning for the patient. As the rehabilitative psychotherapy progresses, it permits the opportunity for the therapist to deal with the patient's strengths and resistances, including internal struggles in dealing with both the patient's growth and rehabilitation.

Although the specific rehabilitation interventions are usually carried out by others, I would suggest it would also be appropriate for the rehabilitative psychotherapist to assume a prime collaborative role in that endeavor. Consequently, both psychosocial and psychoeducational interventions could be facilitated by the rehabilitative psychotherapist. The guiding rule would be that the therapist does not continue to do for the patient what the patient can learn to do for himself or herself. Dynamically, the psychotherapist must allow the patient to test reality very gradually at the patient's own pace. The function of the psychotherapist is to ally with the patient at the symbiotic level of functioning so as to permit a strengthening of the patient's self functions, including self-identity. Just as the mother functions as an auxiliary ego for the child, that is, performing functions the child is not yet able to perform for himself, so too must the rehabilitative psychotherapist function frequently as an auxiliary ego for the patient. In that way, higher levels of adaptation can be either reclaimed or become newly established.

As the treatment alliance becomes more established, the technical procedures for rehabilitative psychotherapy become more pronounced. From a psychodynamic perspective, interpretation is the hub of the three other insight-furthering techniques: confrontation, clarification, and working through. They are the principle therapeutic techniques that provide an experiential base for psychodynamic rehabilitative psychotherapy.

Confrontation permits making a behavior or experience evident to the patient. This is accomplished by focusing on a phenomenon and bringing it into the patient's awareness. However, it must be done in a timely and empathetic manner so as not to put too much pressure on the patient. If done unskillfully, confrontation can create too much pressure and precipitate unnecessary regressive behavior in the patient. For example, confronting a patient who has delusions of persecution about a neighbor by trying to convince the patient the neighbor is not out to get him, could easily promote in a patient a greater suspiciousness about the therapist. In contrast, by accepting the patient's symptoms about the neighbor—and then confronting the patient about the discomfort that anyone experiences when they are suspicious about another—can help promote the patient's understanding of his intrapsychic experience. The occasional reactivations of acute psychotic symptoms when a patient is pressured unwittingly whether by medications, psychotherapy, family members, in a rehabilitation program, or premature hospital discharge, is now well known and has been observed in systematic research studies (Goldberg et al., 1977; Stevens, 1973; Stone & Eldred, 1959; Wing, 1991; Wing et al., 1964).

Clarification as a technique is frequently an extension of the phenomenon that has been confronted. The therapist will provide detail about the phenomenon by explaining and identifying patterns in its expression. For example, elaboration of the phenomenon of suspiciousness can help elucidate for the patient some of his or her own self-feelings and how they relate to functioning in his or her own specific daily activities. It is frequently necessary to continually check with the patient as to what the patient has heard from the therapist's confrontation and clarifications. Both confrontation and clarification can aid patients in better understanding their often confusing experiences.

Later in the psychotherapeutic process, more and more interpretations can be executed with success. It is through the interpretation that observable behavior and phenomena are given psychological meaning and experiential associations for the patient. It basically helps patients to organize and integrate their own intrapsychic experiences. Needless to say, interpretations must be empathic otherwise they are meaningless. More importantly, confrontations, clarifications, and interpretations are usually performed in rather concrete manners with a person suffering from a schizophrenic disorder. As mentioned above, as the client gets personally invested in rehabilitation interventions, an abundance of concrete experiences and phenomena usually become available as fertile material for the therapy. Simultaneously, patients' self-identity frequently begins changing from that of perceiving themselves as *patients* to perceiving themselves as persons who can become viable members of society. Such a change in their self identity is self-rewarding, opening up more and more possibilities in the evolution of patients' growth and rehabilitation. As the patient's insight becomes expanded, such a "working through" usually lends itself to intrapsychic structure building, while leading to symptomatic improvement. The patients' resistance to change becomes diminished as they experience more of their own developing strengths.

Ending the Psychotherapy

About two-thirds of persons with schizophrenic disorders improve by reaching a level of functional adaptability even though many will remain vulnerable to periodic regressions. We know that many persons with schizophrenic disorders usually require rather lengthy interventions, usually with periods of interruption, so as to promote, at the minimum, a functional adaptability. As a result, perceiving the ending of treatment as an interruption rather than a termination

seems to make most sense (Karon & VandenBos, 1981). I have found in my own clinical experience that interruptions in treatment will frequently occur with premature separation, or by mutually stopping the therapy. It has not been unusual to have patients recontact me at a later date as different life stressors periodically interfere with their adjustment. I might add, the later contacts are not always accompanied by acute psychotic symptoms. The presenting symptoms can be "more neurotic," including increased tensions, anxiety, and/or depression resulting from stressors in their current life.

CASE ILLUSTRATION

To illustrate aspects of rehabilitative psychotherapy, I would like to introduce you to Jack S., a then 22-year-old Caucasian male with a high school education who spent six months in the Navy and then received a medical discharge. At the time of the first session, Jack was hospitalized in a private psychiatric, acute care setting with a diagnosis of schizophrenia, paranoid-type. Medical assessment indicated Jack was in relatively good physical health with the exception of a disc problem which was the result of an injury in the service. He was limited to little lifting, although he was permitted to participate in light contact athletics. Psychiatric and psychological evaluation revealed loose associations in the thought process, some delusional thinking of a grandiose and persecutory nature, and dulled affect. His symptoms were developing over the previous year. Mental testing indicated a WAIS Verbal IQ of 122 and a Performance IQ of 99. No neurological symptoms were reported. An EEG, brain scan, and neuropsychological evaluation were normal. No significant history of alcohol or substance abuse existed. Patient presented a very complicated developmental history in which he was separated from his biological mother at the age of 4, with apparently little home stability during the first four years. He remembered living in 11 different homes and an orphanage at different points in his childhood and adolescent development. He reported the hospitalization to be his first psychiatric contact. He appeared to have no family support, although later it was learned adopted parents were in the picture, but Jack wanted no contact with them. An analysis of his self-functioning revealed deep feelings of rejection from the adoptive parents coupled with a rejection a year earlier from a young woman with whom he felt deeply in love. The content of talk in the first therapy session contained the following exchange.

After announcing myself as his therapist and asking him what he was going through, Jack replied that he "was evil, devil-man whose job it was to punish the good." I asked him if he would tell me what he saw he needed to do, and he began to recite, with rather loose associations, how "Satan demanded the punishment of the good." When I asked him whom Satan should punish, he replied "the Virgin Mary." When I confronted him with the notion that it must be difficult for even Satan to feel so angry that he must punish someone, the patient looked at me for the first time and said after a pause, "it hurts." For those few moments, an empathetic sense of understanding occurred. After about 10 seconds, Jack went back to staring at a wall, free associating to his delusional thinking, making little more direct contact with me.

Over the next week, Jack was medicated with Thorazine. I had several random contacts with him in the hospital halls. On the first contact, I asked him how he was doing, and he ignored me. I elaborated back to him that sometimes I don't feel like talking either. On the second random contact, I again asked him how he was doing and he did respond with brief eye contact, but nothing more. Over the next three months, I saw him twice a week in my office for therapy and would occasionally run into him in continued random manners. Apart from helping him focus on his own intrapsychic experiences, especially many of the confusing feelings underneath, I became aware that he had no real direction for himself when he was ready to leave the hospital. In collaboration with his psychiatrist, social worker, and rehab counselor, I explored with him his efforts to establish rehabilitation goals for himself. As I got to know the person behind the symptoms, I was impressed by his intelligence and growing interest in possibly attending college. This became one of the focal areas in the psychotherapy which provided the opportunity for him to examine his own attitudes, values, and anxieties about possibly attending college. The rehab counselor

and social worker educated him about the specifics of attending college, while in the therapy, I helped him explore the anxieties, fears, and, on occasion, the terror he experienced when considering college. As these destructive feelings were examined, he became aware how the numerous rejections he experienced in his life were being transferred to college. Simultaneously, he established specific rehabilitation goals with regard to college, including goals for a living environment. Following discharge from the hospital at a little over three months, he did apply and begin college on a full-time basis, deciding to major in philosophy. He was also able to find an apartment with two older students.

For the next seven months, he continued his psychotherapy on a bi-weekly basis. During that period of time, there were five different occasions when he missed his appointments. Regressions with some delusional thinking reappeared during four of the five missed appointment times. In each instance of a missed appointment, I took the initiative and contacted him, meeting him on three occasions in a quiet restaurant near his apartment. About one year later, he told me no one in his life came to him during times of confusion. At the time, however, while in the restaurant, he was usually distant, upset, and uncooperative. Among other things, I would merely relate to him that sometimes I can get distant, upset, and not feeling like I want to be cooperative. On two other occasions during that first year, he experienced major conflicts, one with his roommates, the other with a professor in one of his classes. After thoroughly exploring with him how other people sometimes have difficulties understanding persons with problems such as his, I told him I would be happy to contact the others, assuming he would be willing to help me with the process so that he would be in a position to learn from it for the future. Although he was at best ambivalent about the matter, he agreed. My intervention was essentially educational for both the professor and roommates. It provided the opportunity for Jack to develop greater social skills, to communicate with all of them on a more personal level which then allowed him to examine more direct problem-solving skills in the therapy for future interpersonal conflicts.

His grades during the first academic year were marginal, although he did obtain two A's in courses. Moreover, on a written paper, his professor provided a lot of positive feedback encouraging him to develop his writing skills. That experience had a great deal of meaning for Jack and permitted a great deal of self-examination with regard to not only his strengths, but also helping him identify some of the past self-deficits in his own experiences. It was during the latter part of the first year that interpretations became meaningful to him, a time when I believed a therapeutic alliance had been firmly established. A self-identity was developing as he reported experiencing himself as a "student, a budding philosopher," rather than as a patient.

During the second year of treatment, I saw Jack an average of once a week. There were several time periods when we increased the frequency of the sessions, but that was during times of stress related to ongoing crises in his life. Therapy was interrupted after the first 2½ years and I did not hear from him until 4 years later. At that time, he was beginning to become delusional again, but primarily tense and depressed. His call came early one evening and I saw him later on the same evening. He was mildly agitated and delusional and knew he could be rehospitalized. I told him I would see him the next day, providing assurance and encouragement that we could resolve the problems together. Therapy continued for eight months, averaging about once a week. His psychotic symptoms cleared up relatively quickly, although he remained somewhat apathetic and withdrawn for a period of several months. He was now in graduate school and was coping marginally with his studies. He spoke of having terrifying "dreams" of his early girlfriend and biological mother. From this point on his psychotherapy started becoming more traditional and less rehabilitative. His therapy was interrupted again by mutual agreement as he successfully won a scholarship for a doctoral program. He had also met a woman who was very self sufficient and was able to provide both emotional and financial support for Jack. Since that time, I have heard no more from Jack.

CONCLUDING COMMENTS

The rehabilitative psychotherapist is considered to be a core mental health provider who treats persons with psychiatric disabilities. Our discussion has been limited to persons experiencing SMD, especially schizophrenia. How rehabilitative psychotherapies might be extended to persons with other psychiatric disabilities could be explored in future treatises.

When it comes to providing rehabilitative psychotherapy to persons with SMD, at least two issues need to be confronted. One issue has to do with training, the other has to do with economics.

A small number of training programs exist or are being developed for training core mental health professionals in state-of-the art knowledge and skills in working with the SMD population and their families. Primarily through initiatives by the National Institute of Mental Health (NIMH) and a number of state departments of mental health, a significant number of core professionals will be trained to provide relevant treatment to the SMD population throughout the 1990s. The major barrier will focus on financing such treatment. In other words, increased resources will need to be obtained to support such comprehensive services, including rehabilitative psychotherapy. Currently, neither the private nor public sectors of service delivery are willing to reimburse extended psychotherapy services for SMD patients and their families. It is a paradox in our society that persons with the most severe forms of psychopathology are being treated primarily by persons with the least training, while, frequently, the SMD persons are isolated from receiving comprehensive treatment. Our current policies for working with SMD patients are frequently not effective. The percentage of SMD among the homeless is regrettably too high as is the frequency with which our headline news focuses on an SMD patient who experiences a tragedy following discharge into the community. No doubt, improved treatment services need to occur. It is my belief that the rehabilitative psychotherapist can play a vital role in that endeavor.

How would these services be funded? In my opinion, improved resources will come about through changes in priorities regarding how monies are spent. Advocacy groups such as the alliances for the mentally ill (AMI) will need to establish goals and lobby hard for such changes. Through such efforts, more comprehensive treatment by highly trained providers can be delivered to the SMD population and families.

REFERENCES

Anthony, W. A., Cohen, M., & Kennard, W. (1990). Understanding the current facts and principles of mental health systems planning. *American Psychologist, 45,* 1249–1252.

Bachrach, L. (1983). Planning services for chronically mentally ill patients. *Bulletin of the Menninger Clinic, 47,* 163–188.

Bachrach, L. L. (1988). Defining chronic mental illness: A concept paper. *Hospital and Community Psychiatry, 39,* 383–388.

Bennett, D., & Morris, I. (1991). Support and rehabilitation. In F. Watts & D. Bennett (Eds.), *Theory and practice of psychiatric rehabilitation* (pp. 189–211). New York: Wiley.

Buchsbaum, M., & Haier, R. (1987). Functional and anatomical brain imaging: Impact on schizophrenia research. In D. Shore (Ed.), *Special report: Schizophrenia 1987* (pp. 129–146). Rockville, MD: U.S. Department of Health and Human Services.

Budman, S., & Gurman, A. (1988). *Theory and practice of brief therapy.* New York: Guilford.

Cancro, R. (1983). Individual psychotherapy in the treatment of chronic schizophrenic patients. *American Journal of Psychotherapy, 37,* 493–501.

Chamberlin, J., & Rogers, J. (1990). Planning a community-based mental health system: Perspective of service recipients. *American Psychologist, 45,* 1241–1244.

Cohen, M., Farkas, M., & Cohen, B. (1986). *Psychiatric rehabilitation training package: Functional assessment.* Boston: Boston University, Center for Psychiatric Rehabilitation.

Cohen, M., Farkas, M., Cohen, B., & Unger, K. (1987). *Psychiatric rehabilitation training package: Setting an overall rehabilitation goal.* Boston: Boston University, Center for Psychiatric Rehabilitation.

Crow, T. (1982). Two syndromes in schizophrenia? *Trends in Neurosciences, 5,* 351–354.

Day, R., Nielsen, J. A., Korken, A., Ernberg, G., Dube, K. C., Gebhart, J., Jablensky, A., Leon, C., Marsella, A., Olatawura, M., Sartorius, N., Stromgren, E., Takahashi, R., Wig, N., & Wynne, L. C. (1987). Stressful life events preceding the acute onset of schizophrenia: A cross-national study from the world health organization. *Culture, Medicine and Psychiatry, 11,* 123–205.

Drake, R. E., & Sederer, L. (1986). The adverse effects of intensive treatment of chronic schizophrenia. *Comprehensive Psychiatry, 27,* 313–326.

Farkas, M., & Anthony, W. (1989). *Psychiatric rehabilitation programs: Putting theory into practice.* Baltimore: Johns Hopkins University Press.

Farkas, M., O'Brien, W., & Nemec, P. (1988). A graduate level curriculum in psychiatric rehabilitation: Filling a need. *Psychosocial Rehabilitation Journal, 12,* 53–66.

Glass, L., Katz, H., Schnitzer, R., Knapp, P., Frank, A., & Gunderson, J. (1989). Psychotherapy of schizophrenia: An empirical investigation of the relationship of process to outcome. *American Journal of Psychiatry, 146,* 603–608.

Gold, J. R. (1990). The integration of psychoanalytic, cognitive and interpersonal approaches in the psychotherapy of borderline and narcissistic disorders. *Journal of Integrative and Eclectic Psychotherapy, 9,* 49–68.

Goldberg, S., Schooler, N., Hogaty, G., & Roper, M. (1977). Prediction of relapse in schizophrenic outpatients treated by drug and sociotherapy. *Archives of General Psychiatry, 34,* 171–184.

Goldman, H. (1984). Epidemiology. In J. Talbott (Ed.), *The chronic mental patient: Five years later* (pp. 15–31). New York: Grune & Stratton.

Gottesman, I., McGuffin, P., & Farmer, A. (1987). Clinical genetics as clues to the "real" genetics of schizophrenia (A decade of modest gains while playing for time). In D. Shore (Ed.), *Special report: Schizophrenia 1987* (pp. 39–64). Rockville, MD: U.S. Department of Health and Human Services.

Gunderson, J., Frank, A., Katz, H., Vannicelli, M., Frosch, J., & Knapp, P. (1984). Effects of psychotherapy in Schizophrenia: II. Comparative outcome of two forms of treatment. *Schizophrenia Bulletin, 10,* 564–598.

Holzman, P. (1987). Recent studies of psychophysiology in schizophrenia. In D. Shore (Ed.), *Special report: Schizophrenia 1987* (pp. 65–92). Rockville, MD: U.S. Department of Health and Human Services.

Johnson, C., & Connors, M. E. (1989). *The etiology and treatment of bulimia nervosa: A biopsychosocial perspective.* New York: Basic Books.

Karon, B. (August, 1991). *Psychotherapy: Treatment of choice for schizophrenia.* Paper presented at the 99th Annual Convention of the American Psychological Association, San Francisco, California.

Karon, B. P., & VandenBos, G. R. (1981). *Psychotherapy of schizophrenia: The treatment of choice.* New York: Jason Aronson.

Koenigsberg, H., & Haddley, R. (1986). Expressed emotion: From predictive index to clinical construct. *American Journal of Psychiatry, 143,* 1361–1373.

Kroll, J. (1988). *The challenge of the borderline patient.* New York: Norton.

Lefley, H. P. (Ed.). (1990). *Clinical training in serious mental illness.* Rockville, MD: U.S. Department of Health and Human Services.

Mahler, M., & Furer, M. (1960). Observations on research regarding the "symbiotic syndrome" of infantile psychosis. *Selected Papers,* Vol. 1.

Mahler, M., & Gosliner, B. (1955). On symbiotic child psychosis: Genetic, dynamic and restitutive aspects. *Selected Papers,* Vol. 1.

Masterson, J., & Klein, R. (Eds.). (1989). *Psychology of the disorders of the self: The Masterson approach.* New York: Brunner/Mazel.

Matthysse, S. (1987). Schizophrenia 1987: A theoretician's perspective. In D. Shore (Ed.), *Special report: Schizophrenia 1987* (pp. 187–196). Rockville, MD: U.S. Department of Health and Human Services.

Meltzer, H. (1987). Biological studies in schizophrenia. In D. Shore (Ed.), *Special report: Schizophrenia 1987* (pp. 93–128). Rockville, MD: U.S. Department of Health and Human Services.

Mueser, K. T., & Berenbaum, H. (1990). Psychodynamic treatment of schizophrenia: Is there a future? *Psychological Medicine, 20,* 253–262.

Nuechterien, K., & Haier, R. (August, 1991). *Update on schizophrenia: Evidence for early cognitive abnormalities and brain dysfunction.* Paper presented at the 99th Annual Convention of the American Psychological Association, San Francisco, California.

Pollack, W. (August, 1991). *Is psychotherapy dead? The role of empathy and depth psychology in a treatment continuum for serious mental illness.* Paper presented at the 99th Annual

Convention of the American Psychological Association, San Francisco, California.

Rowe, C., & MacIsaac, D. (1989). *The technique of psychoanalytic self psychology.* New York: Jason Aronson.

Selzer, M., Sullivan, T., Carsky, M., & Terkelsen, K. (1989). *Working with the person with schizophrenia: The treatment alliance.* New York: New York University.

Selzer, M., & Carsky, M. (1990). Treatment alliance and the chronic schizophrenic. *American Journal of Psychotherapy, 44,* 506–515.

Stanton, A., Gunderson, J., Knapp, P., Frank, A., Vannicelli, M., Schnitzer, R., & Rosenthal, R. (1984). Effects of psychotherapy in schizophrenia: I. Design and implementation of a controlled study. *Schizophrenia Bulletin, 10,* 520–563.

Steinlin, H., & Weber, G. (1989). *Unlocking the family door: A systematic approach to the understanding and treatment of anorexia nervosa.* New York: Brunner/Mazel.

Stevens, B. (1973). Evaluation of rehabilitation for psychotic patients in the community. *Acta Psychiatrica Scandinavica, 49,* 169–180.

Stone, A., & Eldred, S. (1959). Delusion formation during the activation of chronic schizophrenic patients. *Archives of General Psychiatry, 1,* 177–179.

Summers, F. (1981). The post-acute functioning of the schizophrenic. *Journal of Clinical Psychology, 37*(4), 705–714.

Teixeira, M. (August, 1990). *Psychoanalytic theory and therapy in the treatment of manic-depressive disorders.* Paper presented at the 98th annual convention of the American Psychological Association, Boston, Massachusetts.

Test, M., & Stein, L. (1978). Community treatment of the chronic patient: Research overview. *Schizophrenia Bulletin, 4,* 350–364.

Torrey, E. (1988). *Surviving schizophrenia: A family manual.* New York: Harper.

Washington, A. M. (1989). *Cocaine addiction: Treatment, recovery, and relapse prevention.* New York: Norton.

Weinberger, D. (1987). Implications of normal brain development for the pathogenesis of schizophrenia. *Archives of General Psychiatry, 44,* 660–669.

Weisburd, D. (1990). Planning a community based mental health system: Perspective of a family member. *American Psychologist, 45,* 1245–1248.

White, R. (1989). Psychotherapy with schizophrenic patients. *American Journal of Psychiatry, 10,* 1352–1353.

Wing, J., Bennett, D., & Denham, J. (1964). *The industrial rehabilitation of long-stay schizophrenic patients.* Medical Research Council Memo. No. 42, HMSO, London.

Wing, J. (1991). Schizophrenia. In F. Watts & D. Bennett (Eds.), *Theory and practice of psychiatric rehabilitation.* New York: Wiley.

Wolfe, B. E. (1989). Phobias, panic, and psychotherapy integration. *Journal of Integrative and Eclectic Psychotherapy, 8,* 264–276.

PART V

Psychotherapy Integration with Specific Populations

CHAPTER 27

Couples and Families

Sam Kirschner and Diana Adile Kirschner

To see a world in a grain of sand
And a heaven in a wild flower,
Hold infinity in the palm of your hand,
And eternity in an hour

—William Blake (1946, p. 150)

INTRODUCTION

The family is a complex living organism with subsystems which include interpersonal relationships and individual emotions and cognitions all in dynamic exchange. Like Blake's "world in a grain of sand" each subcomponent of the family dynamic provides a reflection of the others embedded within. These two primary subsystems, the interpersonal and the individual, system and psyche, can be viewed as independent entities for the purpose of analysis. Yet mounting research and clinical evidence suggest that the two entities are very interdependent and that they shape and influence each other throughout the life cycle.

This chapter will describe comprehensive family therapy (Kirschner & Kirschner, 1986;

Stein, 1980), a theoretical framework in which system and psyche are integrated in the treatment of couples and families. Specific techniques which draw from both the systemic as well as the individual therapy literature will be discussed. We will then illustrate the approach with a brief description of a family which entered treatment with the first author around the problems of a child.

THEORETICAL AND CONCEPTUAL ORIENTATION

The marital, rearing, and independent (or career) transactions are the three most important interpersonal areas of the family. In family life, disharmony in any of these arenas will have repercussions of different strengths on all the members and their relationships with each other. Nowhere is this clearer than in the example of a distressed couple whose explosive marriage has impaired their ability to parent the children as a united team. The children in this family become

Sam Kirschner and Diana Adile Kirschner • Private Practice, Gwynedd Valley, Pennsylvania 19437.

Comprehensive Handbook of Psychotherapy Integration, edited by George Stricker and Jerold R. Gold. Plenum Press, New York, 1993.

so upset by the level of conflict in the home that their behavior in school becomes disruptive or shows signs of severe anxiety and depression.

This example also illustrates how critical the marriage is in family life. As many clinicians including Minuchin (1974) have noted, the marriage underlies the spouses' functioning as parents and shapes each spouse's interactions with the children. These parenting, or rearing transactions, in turn, greatly influence the children's independent functioning whether at home, at school, or with peers. The children's independent performance then, in turn, feeds back to affect the rearing and marital relationships. Thus, the three transactions form a multiloop feedback system in which changes in one impact on the others. This feedback system is largely regulated by the marriage, which we consider to be at the center of family life.

We define the marital relationship as the pattern of behavioral interactions between the spouses. These patterns consist of repetitive sequences of behaviors that control and shape intimacy, distance, sexuality, giving, taking, and power. These sequences are shaped and reshaped throughout the life cycle but tend to remain fairly stable for long periods of time.

Two examples will illustrate how these sequences work. In one couple, the husband who was a rather rigid attorney would cough or twitch during sexual relations when his wife became overly aroused. She would then become angry with him. The husband would then apologize and resume lovemaking, but in a way that was more toned down and not threatening to him. This pattern recurred over many years and was a source of great unhappiness to both spouses.

In another marriage, the wife had no idea of the family's finances, since the husband was in complete control. If the husband wanted to buy some new "toy" for himself, he would do so and tell his spouse afterward. Whenever the wife suggested that the couple go on a vacation or spend money on something she wanted, the husband would angrily retort that "she had no idea of how strapped they were financially and what a burden he already had to carry." The wife would then withdraw her suggestion. This sequence of behaviors had gone on for about 20 years.

Marital interactions are extremely powerful and set the emotional tone for family life. To a very large degree they can shape the psychosocial functioning of each and every family member. First of all, spouses empower each other to influence each other's behavior. From the time they first "fall in love" and throughout the life cycle, the mates lend the considerable authority they once gave their parents to each other. This authority is rooted in the drive to attachment, which as Bowlby (1973) and others have observed, is the predominant behavioral tendency in mankind.

Because attachment behavior is so powerful and the fear of loss so frightening, the spouses empower each other to become agents of reinforcement over their behavior. Spouses can then choreograph each other by positively reinforcing certain behaviors while negatively reinforcing others.

The spouses' ability to reinforce each other's behaviors is also based on the relative amount of power each one is assigned. In most relationships, each spouse is assigned power over particular domains of family life. In our second example the husband controlled the finances and the wife was in charge of the children. In these areas, the dominant spouse's perceptions or suggestions were given more authority.

Another way in which spouses exert great influence over each other is through personality or role allocation. As Sager (1976) has indicated, it is common for spouses to both assume and allocate roles to each other which are complementary in nature. Each spouse may program the other to enact aspects of the personality which are undeveloped or unacceptable. Role allocations include the hysterical wife and the rigid husband, the shy wife and the overly talkative husband, as well as the caretaker and the child. By enacting only delimited roles, the spouses inhibit their ability to have a flexible repertoire of behaviors and as a result tend to manifest equivalent degrees of immaturity or inadequacy (Bowen, 1961).

One explanation for how the spouses shape each other's behaviors and roles is through the process of projective identification (Zinner, 1976). Aspects of the self which are perceived as undesirable, unacceptable, or shameful are disowned and projected onto the other. Because the mates exert tremendous influence over each other, they will accept these projections as legitimate representations of who they really are. This process operates in much the say way that children's perceptions of themselves are formed—largely through the messages they receive from the parents.

As the projections become a congruent part of the spouse's self, behaviors or roles which reflect the projection are enacted. These behaviors/roles are then reinforced by the other spouse, who validates their appearance. Over time these behaviors and roles become routinized in ongoing cycles of interaction. The earliest family researchers used the term "homeostasis" (Jackson, 1957) to refer to the stability of these cycles and of the family's tendency toward the equilibrium of predictable interactions.

These homeostatic cycles eventually tend to include the children. For example, when marital tensions are high, the cycle may expand to include the children's becoming anxious or acting out in school as part of a repetitive sequence. This particular sequence of behaviors, marital conflict, followed by serious disagreements over dealing with a child, followed by the child misbehaving in school, could result in the parents' coming together finally in the interest of helping their child. The family's equilibrium is thus maintained, since the marital tensions do not escalate to the point of the couple's separating.

The marital transaction's strong influence on the spouses' individual functioning, in turn, shapes the children. The children look very carefully to model their parents' cognitions, emotions, and behaviors. In addition, the spouses will use projective identification with the children by assigning parts of their own or their parents' personalities to the children and treating them accordingly (Klein, 1975).

Thus, the marriage is the heart of power in the family dynamic. Domestic role allocation, personality scripting, choreographed behavioral sequences, and projective identificatory processes play out to strongly shape the spouses' and the children's self-percepts, attitudes, beliefs, and behavior.

The Intrapsychic or Self-System

The intrapsychic or self-system, as we term it, of each family member also impacts on the transactions to varying degrees. We conceive of the self-system as a tripartite system derived from object relations and psychodynamic models.

At the core of the self-system is the foundation of the ego (Guntrip, 1969), which is formed in infancy through the relationship with the parents. The infant must experience both acceptance/nurturance and limit-setting in relation to the parents. The symbiotic relationship with the parents confirms the infant's sense of belonging and lovableness. Their limit-setting or refusal to meet the child's needs at times helps him or her to experience a separate sense of self.

The foundation of the ego is formed through the introjection of aspects of the parents and the essential characteristics of the rearing relationship, which oscillates between symbiosis and separation/individuation (Mahler, Pine, & Bergman, 1975). When the parents create a "good enough" environment, the infant experiences fulfillment of physiological and safety needs, and a sense of the world as soothing, mirroring, attentive, filling, and prizing. The infant forms a core feeling of the good self and experiences self-love.

The introjection process profoundly shapes the ego's development, such that internalizing a good enough environment creates the basis for relatively conflict-free movement to later phases of maturation (Fairbairn, 1952; Winnicott, 1965). The good environment internalized gives the toddler enough selfhood to explore and learn about the world. On the other hand, times of autonomous exploration, or times when parents are frustrating or limit-setting with the child, help the latter to differentiate between himself or herself and the parents, thus setting the stage for the recognition and acceptance of a separate self. In these ways, then, the earliest paradigm of relating, that of parent and child, generates the foundation models for intimate relating.

Foundation issues revolve around basic trust and the ability to tolerate both intimacy/closeness/fusion and individuation/distance/separateness. Primitive terrors of engulfment, annihilation, and abandonment develop at the foundation level based on the earliest traumata with the parents.

As adults, spouses may unconsciously regulate the closeness and distance of the marital relationship based on their foundation issues. Many couples will present with choreographed conflict cycles in which engulfment issues surface in the face of "too much" intimacy, which then give rise to conflict and then to emotional distance. This is then followed by a coming together fueled by abandonment terrors triggered by "too much" distance. In this way, a kind of stability emerges in proximity and distance such that basic insecurities are not allowed to become overly disruptive.

The next level of the self-system is gender identification. This is a gender-based differentiation model of the self based on anatomical realities, parental expectations, perceptions and projective identifications, along with the child's identification with the same-sex parent and aspects of the opposite-sex parent. The father becomes the prototype of the child's own masculine potentials while the mother becomes the prototype of the feminine potentials. Various characteristics of each parent are incorporated into the blueprint that becomes the child's template for future behavior as a marital partner (Dicks, 1967).

The gender identifications of each spouse strongly shape domestic role allocations and personality assignments. Usually there is a "fit" in terms of gender identification, both at the outset and later in the relationship. As the relationship develops, spouses will reinforce behaviors and transactions which are congruent with their self-perceptions and self-concepts and extinguish or punish those that are not. For example, a client had identified with his weak, soft-spoken father, a man who had worked at a low level in a corporation all his life. He, in turn, was modeling his career life accordingly. His wife, on the other hand, had identified with her father who was chief executive officer of a bank. Although she was frustrated with her own career progress, she demanded that her husband be more assertive and angle for a higher level position. These confrontations would usually end with the man withdrawing in silence and the woman expressing regret over marrying him.

The third level of the self-system is the triangulation level. This is an internal model for relating in groups of three or more based on experiences generated in the various triangles of relationships with mother, father, and siblings. Competitive struggles for attention and loyalty, or alternatively cooperation and collaboration shape the triangulation model. This internal paradigm includes messages about parentally sanctioned behaviors with members of the same or opposite sex and programming regarding how to be a spouse and parent. Pathological variations of the triangulation model include: illicit coalitions and

enmeshments between a parent and child in which the other parent is left out or becomes the common and hated enemy; parents bonding together around a misbehaving child; the use of the child as a scapegoat to reduce marital tensions; or parental enmeshment with a favored sibling while other siblings are rejected or abandoned emotionally. These triangular relationships and gender-related models then become the blueprint upon which later marital and parenting behaviors are constructed.

For example, in one case, a family presented with a "spoiled" daughter who had been suspended from school. Any attempts on the mother's part to discipline the child were consistently undermined by the father. In conjoint family interviews, the therapist learned that the father had been exceedingly close with his mother while his younger sister had been his father's favorite. He told the therapist that he was always jealous of his sister for "taking his father away" and at the same time disclosed that he was his mother's confidant—a role he both enjoyed and resented.

The therapist hypothesized that the father had developed an internalized triangulation model in which the opposite sex parent and child collude in a closer relationship than the same-sex parent and child. In the father's family of origin, the collusion often resulted in the mother and him laughing at and deriding the other parent. Although this exact type of interaction did not occur in the family with the spoiled daughter, the father had undermined the mother's authority and was colluding with his daughter instead of teaming with his spouse.

In summary, then, the individual dynamics of each family member and most especially those of the spouses shape and influence the rearing, marital, and independent transactions. These transactions, in turn, reciprocally alter and shape the three levels of the self-system over the life cycle. We believe that the spouses' self-systems in ongoing interaction through the marital relationship set the tone for the quality of family life and for the maturational developmental of each family member.

Psychopathology

At the heart of most psychopathology lie failures in relationships with significant others (Fairbairn, 1952; Framo, 1970). From a systemic viewpoint, the spouses reenact and/or reexperience in rigid homeostatic fashion some of the original failures and disappointments they each had in relation to their own parental figures (Boszormenyi-Nagy, 1973; Dicks, 1967; Jackson, 1957). In troubled families, these reenactments take the form of marital interactions punctuated by verbal and even physical abuse and the lack of emotional support and nurturance. The couple becomes stuck in ongoing cycles of behavior in which they ultimately involve the children through the parenting function.

These enduring marital and rearing transactions powerfully shape each spouse's self-perceptions and identity. The more destructive the interactions, the more they solidify and even amplify core fears about attachment/separation and trust, shame about self-image, and guilt about power and competition.

We consider the interaction between marital dysfunction and the core fears, insecurities, and immaturities of each spouse to be the major factor in the development or maintenance of psychopathology in the family whether it manifests in a child, a spouse, or in one of the familial transactions. The marital dysfunction adversely affects the mates as parental partners, so they cannot team adequately, and as individuals in the outside world, so they cannot fully actualize themselves. In these families, children are raised by a divided leadership and are caught in the crossfire of unsatisfying and destructive marital interactions. The children's self-esteem and self-perceptions are then formed in the context of hostility, guilt, and blame. Their school performance, peer relationships, and normal socialization can then be adversely affected.

It must be noted, however, that, in our view, based on much clinical experience with children in treatment, the children's self-systems are extremely malleable and reactive to changes in parenting, and in the family system. Barring organicity, the children are quickly responsive to parental teaming and improved parenting up to the adolescent years.

For example, in the Moore family, 10-year-old Tom was a serious disciplinary problem both at school and at home. The parents were unable to team together in a consistent fashion to discipline the boy. At times, the mother would undermine the father's authority over Tom by rescinding various punishments, but at other times she would lose control and scream furiously at him. At those times, the father would step in to calm things down and end up defending Tom.

This type of parental disagreement coupled with confusion about the provision of discipline, nurturance, and guidance for a child is a symptom of dysfunction in the rearing transaction. Often, these "problem" children come to the attention of school guidance counselors who, in turn, refer them for treatment. When therapy aims at uniting the parents as a parenting team, behavioral problems in children usually stop quickly. In the Moore family, the confusion was settled in several family therapy sessions, in which the parents actually signed agreements with each other concerning how they would team to parent Tom. Tom's affect improved and he began to function more appropriately at home and at school. Ten weeks into treatment, Tom was asked to draw a picture of himself. The figure was smiling and unlike earlier drawings, Tom's self-portrait showed a more central placement on the paper.

In a situation like Tom's, however, further treatment was necessary. This is because the rearing dysfunction was symptomatic of a much larger and more serious issue—the Moores' marriage. The Moores had suffered through 18 years of a relationship devoid of emotional and sexual fulfillment, and lacking in mutual respect and reciprocity. As we will see in the case example, Tom Moore's presenting problem was merely the beginning of the family's therapeutic odyssey.

CLINICAL AND THEORETICAL ANTECEDENTS

The integrative approach we have described is built on the work of family theorists and therapists, object relations theorists, and cognitive/behavioral clinicians.

Our work with families and couples uses assessment procedures and interventions derived from the systemic literature. In particular, mapping family relationships, understanding boundaries and hierarchies in relation to existing psychopathology, and actively restructuring parental relationships are based on Minuchin's "structural family therapy approach" (1974). Understanding and intervening in families' and couples' homeostatic cycles are based on Hoffman (1976), whereas specific strategic techniques have been drawn from Haley (1976, 1984).

The model of the self-system we have described is based on object relations theory. In particular, we have built on the works of Guntrip, Fairbairn, and Winnicott, who paid careful attention to how their patients' earliest experiences shone through their adult lives.

Our thinking about projective identification and its use as a bridge concept from an individual to a systems viewpoint especially in couples and family work has been shaped by Melanie Klein's original formulations (1975) and by Zinner (1976).

Traditional psychodynamic techniques are also utilized in our clinical work although they have not played as central a role as other approaches. However, the role of the therapist as envisioned by Freud certainly matches our view. Freud wrote: "We serve the patient in various functions, as an authority and substitute for his parents, as a teacher and educator" (1923/1975, p. 181). We feel that these various roles require the therapist to be a more active agent of change (Kirschner & Kirschner, 1986; 1990a,b).

As such, we have borrowed heavily from those schools of thought which use active or directive techniques in therapy and especially from the cognitive/behavioral approach. We regularly use such interventions as behavioral rehearsal, homework assignments, relaxation, and desensitization in our couple and family work (Jacobson & Margolin, 1979; Lazarus, 1976; Stuart, 1980).

The indirect techniques which characterize our work include paradox, symptom prescription and prediction, and reframing. These interventions were developed initially by Haley (1963) and Watzlawick (1978) among others.

Comprehensive family therapy, which was originally developed by Arthur Stein (1980), has been refined and reshaped by us in light of new clinical research and findings. For example, data which indicate the advantages of short courses of antidepressives for certain patients has forced us to rethink how we view and treat a married person who is on medication. In the past, we would seek to shift attention away from a depressive lest they continue to be the "symptom bearer." Today,

we recognize the validity of using antidepressive medications and reframe this, for example, as "insulin for a diabetic" to provide support for the person.

We have also been strongly influenced by other theoreticians whose work has put psychotherapy integration in the forefront of psychology. They include Pinsof (1983) and Gurman (1981) who, like us, have advocated step-wise models of integration which combine family and individual work.

PROGRESSION OF TREATMENT

In the clinical practice of comprehensive family therapy, most presenting problems of children are viewed as merely the tip of the family iceberg. All contributory factors, whether in the rearing, marital, or independent transactions, or in the self-systems of the child or the parents are examined, and, if necessary, addressed in the treatment process. There are three distinct phases in the process: (1) remediating the presenting problem and bonding as a nurturant and authoritative figure; (2) working on the spouses' individual issues as they relate to the marriage and the children; and (3) furthering the collaborative teamwork in the couple so they can assist each other to grow. There may be considerable overlap at times among these foci.

Because of space limitations in this chapter, we will present the overview of our treatment process and a case example with a preadolescent child. The treatment of adolescents will not be discussed. Adolescent problems are often complex and sometimes severe and, therefore, require more intensive individual work with the adolescent in addition to conjoint family treatment. Nevertheless, we have found that an approach which integrates individual and family therapy has been shown to be effective with many adolescent problems, including the serious conduct disorders typical of juvenile delinquents. (See Kirschner & Kirschner, 1986, for a review of some findings.)

It should also be noted that, because of their special needs, the treatment of single-parent and step families require different interventions. The reader is referred to the same text for a more detailed description.

Phase 1

In Phase 1, the practitioner focuses on the presenting problem(s) of the child and bonds with each spouse or adult client as a nurturant authority figure. In initial sessions, the practitioner meets with all those members of the nuclear client family who are willing to participate in treatment. He or she joins with the family, adopting their language and style.

The practitioner assesses the marital, rearing, and independent transactions, and gains an initial understanding of how the child's symptomatology is maintained by the system and what role it serves in the family. Since the child's symptom is often part of a larger homeostatic cycle which includes his or her parents, the sequence of behaviors which make up the cycle must be understood by the therapist. Conjoint sessions create the opportunity to not only observe these cycles *in vivo*, but also to intervene and interrupt them as well. For example, interrupting these cycles during a session and getting the parents to agree on a reward or punishment can be the first step toward changing the child's behavior.

Based on the assessments gained in the first few sessions, the therapist may give tasks both in session and homework assignments outside the session to the family. These tasks are designed to counter tendencies toward overly distanced or enmeshed rearing relationships as well as to foster a united executive team. The assignments are followed up in the next sessions and resistance dealt with, either through interpretation, mild confrontation, or paradox.

The clinician also explores the rearing, marital, and independent transactions in each spouse's family of origin. This is because these transactions have not only influenced the spouses' individual development but also have become incorporated as the patterns for their behavior as parents and marital partners. The therapist can then interpret deficiencies in parenting, for example, to each spouse as a way of promoting insight into their behavior and, it is hoped, then facilitating changes.

Information about each spouse's family of origin is usually best obtained in conjoint sessions. This is because each spouse can add to or correct misperceptions, gaps in memory, or distortions that the other may have. Children often are useful sources of information about grandparents although their experiences may be different than their parents.

Sometimes, in Phase 1, the therapist will meet with the spouses alone without the children. In these sessions, the therapist can model or role play various types of behaviors and roles vis à vis the children or the spouse. For example, he or she can demonstrate a confrontational or disciplinary stance which a father could take with an acting out son. The therapist can also educate and model for the spouses the growth-promoting stances each child needs.

The therapist's interruption of the homeostatic cycle which supports the symptom, assignment of tasks which foster executive teamwork and good parenting skills, and interpretations about family or origin issues which are being replicated by the parents with their children will usually result in the abatement of symptoms in the children. Behavioral change and insight occur in tandem, with each reinforcing the other. This combination not only promotes change, but is also a catalyst for further growth of the children.

Phase 2

In our experience, positive changes in the children and in the rearing transaction lead to positive behavioral changes in the spouses as well. Yet, paradoxically, these alterations also tend to create disequilibrium in the family system. As symptoms and acting-out are reduced in the family, the spouses' inner conflicts and other dissatisfactions emerge. They will often then ask the practitioner for further assistance with either individual problems or, more commonly, the marriage.

The shift from working on the presenting problems to these other issues is best accomplished using a combination of session formats. In Phase 2 of treatment, the therapist flexibly alternates between conjoint sessions and individual concurrent sessions with each spouse as needed. The therapist will also continue to monitor the progress of the child/children and may call for additional family sessions.

During conjoint sessions the clinician can

track and observe the recurring interactional sequences in the marriage which maintain symptomatology. Cycles manifesting unresolved conflict, inadequate mutual support, and lack of tenderness are common examples of these sequences. As with problems in the rearing transaction, the therapist first indentifies and then interrupts the dysfunctional marital sequence(s) in the session. Alternative methods of relating to each other are then modeled, taught, or role played.

In these conjoint sessions the practitioner works to build health in the marriage. He or she promotes a context of mutual support and understanding by encouraging active listening, enhanced communication, as well as good negotiation skills. These skills can be practiced both *in vivo* and through homework assignments to be done at specific times of the day.

Couples' sessions also allow the practitioner to see how role allocations and projective identifications are used as part of the marital dance. These delimiting and destructive labels also can be interrupted through interpretation or more directly through paradoxical techniques like relabeling or reframing.

The therapist uses these sessions to observe how the marital transaction maintains or amplifies the individual self-systems of each spouse. As needed, the therapist will invite one or both spouses for individual sessions in which he or she can discuss and work on conflicts, anxieties, or other problems.

Individual sessions allow each spouse to process his or her own thoughts and feelings more freely, without familial role constraints. This also allows for abreaction of hostile feelings or other powerful emotions which have been suppressed over the years. The freeing of these emotions can be very therapeutic (Greenberg & Safran, 1987) and can create new vitality and purpose. In addition, the therapist can often overcome resistance to behavior change when certain emotions and attitudes are abreacted.

The individual sessions aim at cultivating a strong therapeutic alliance with each spouse in which each feels "held" by the nurturant-authoritative therapist. In this "good enough" environment, the therapist's direct and indirect interventions emanate from an empathic and benevolent attitude. In this way, he or she can co-create with each spouse corrective transactional experiences with the practitioner, each other, and their children. These healthier transactions facilitate individual growth in terms of self-esteem, self-perceptions, and increased behavioral competence.

Phase 3

The third and final phase of treatment begins when clients achieve enough ego strength and demonstrate that they have incorporated the therapeutic inputs sufficiently to use them creatively on their own. The focus changes to assisting the spouses to become more active growth agents for each other.

With intact or remarried families, the practitioner helps enhance the marital relationship so that it can fulfill some of the needs for understanding and nurturance that the therapeutic relationship was satisfying. The therapist again uses the conjoint session format to foster bonding between the spouses and to wean them away from individual sessions with him or her. The therapist may educate them as to each other's dynamics, emotional needs, or how to interact under stressful circumstances. Optimally, this process results in the formation of a collaborative relationship in which each spouse is dedicated to the growth of the other.

During this phase, each mate is encouraged to achieve a healthy degree of psychological separation from the other, so as to be able to function with greater autonomy and individuation. The spouses undertake independent and risk-taking activities in which they grow in self-appreciation and self-reliance and master their fear of separation and loss. As they develop as separate and more self-confident individuals, they relate with less conflict and experience greater mutual respect and appreciation. This furthers their ability to be more effective growth agents for each other.

The termination process begins when the couple and therapist agree that the major goals of treatment have been accomplished. Clients will then begin to attend sessions less frequently and work toward a firm termination date.

In sum, then, the treatment of couples and families proceeds in an orderly fashion from presenting problem to marital and individual treatment. In our view, the therapist must recognize that growth and maturation in therapy proceed in a biphasic fashion. As clients increase in competence behaviorally or attempt to break through personal ceiling barriers in functioning, a countervailing, regressive trend in emotions and cognitions emerges. These regressive phenomena of pain, anxiety, insecurities, and self-doubts must be dealt with and worked through in order for treatment to be successful (Kirschner & Kirschner, 1991).

Treatment, therefore, proceeds in a biphasic fashion with a progressive strategy and a regressive strategy. The progressive strategy targets changes in behavior and in the transactions and utilizes techniques from structural and strategic family therapy and cognitive-behavioral work. On the other hand, the regressive strategy is psychodynamically based and designed to handle the regressive reactions and cognitions that emerge in treatment.

In the progressive work, the therapist maps out the distance, conflict, and enmeshment and the hierarchical power structure in the various family relationships. He or she then assigns tasks and educates in a way that (1) promotes shared executive teamwork by the parents vis à vis the children; (2) develops positive reciprocal behaviors in the marriage; and (3) diminishes the homeostatically maintained dyadic and triadic distance, conflict, and enmeshment patterns of interactions.

The practitioner also utilizes behavioral rehearsal, desensitization, and relaxation techniques to deal with individual psychopathology. The progressive strategy additionally involves the use of indirect techniques when direct techniques fail. These include paradox, symptom prescription, and prediction and reframing, given either from a more confrontational or a more nurturant stance.

As clients relate to the nurturant-authoritative practitioner and develop behaviorally, natural regressive phenomena arise both in relation to the self and to the partner. The practitioner then utilizes client-centered and psychodynamically based techniques, which include reflective and empathic listening, unconditional positive regard, promotion of abreaction of emotion, and interpretation of family of origin issues and material related to the transference.

CASE STUDY

We will return to the Moore family which was briefly described above. The family consisted of Bob and Toni Moore ages 45 and 47, respectively, and their three children, Joanne, 15, Dina 13, and Tom, age 10. The school guidance counselor had referred Tom and his family to the first author because of continued disruptive behavior in class. The boy manifested a similar tendency at home but less so when his father was at home. Mr. Moore had taken a job as an outside sales representative in the past year which necessitated far greater travel requirements than his previous inside sales position had required.

The school psychologist had completed a full psychological battery with Tom and was almost certain that neither attention deficit disorder nor any organicity was involved. Tom's reading scores were at grade level and his IQ score in the bright, normal range. The test results along with the teachers' comments on his last report card were brought by Mrs. Moore to the first session at the therapist's request.

The parents' inability to agree, even as to what the problem was, characterized the first interview. In Toni Moore's view, the boy was less of a problem when her husband was home and, therefore, Bob's job was the issue. In Bob's view, Toni's screaming at Tom and/or undermining Bob's authority when he did discipline Tom, was the real problem. The therapist reframed the disagreement by saying; "Well, at least you agree on one thing—it's not Tom's fault, the problem is either father's or mother's." The humor allowed the couple to relax somewhat and be more open to the therapist's suggestions.

The therapist explored the cycle of rearing interactions around the crucial issue of discipline. He asked, "What happens at home when the assistant principal calls you with a report that Tom has been sent to her by the teacher for being disruptive yet again?"

"I call Bob. He's usually in some God-forsaken place. Then we have some kind of fight," replied Toni.

Bob retorted that he had tried to suggest some disciplinary actions, but that Toni did not follow through and "took it out on Tom," who would then phone Bob crying and complaining.

The next sequence of events was that Bob would protect Tom and also mollify Toni on the phone. He reported that "That's the way women are—overreactive, blowing things way out of proportion."

Thus, the therapist gained an understanding of the behavioral sequences in the rearing transaction, and some of the marital issues, along with initial understanding of the type of projective identificatory processes at work in the relationship between Toni and Bob.

The therapist worked to unify the parents and to disrupt the dysfunctional rearing cycle by having the parents write down a list of consequences upon which they agreed for Tom's problem behavior. In front of Tom, the therapist asked them to sign an agreement about following through on the disciplinary actions on the list and to post it on the refrigerator at home.

Over the next several months, Bob and Toni were able to follow through for the most part. Whenever they would come and report some breakdown in the contract, the therapist would mildly confront them and/or explore their resistance through the lens of their families of origin.

Bob reported that in growing up, he had felt somewhat engulfed by his histrionic mother and abandoned by a father he perceived to be passive and weak. He had vowed not to let this happen when he became a father. Toni, on the other hand, identified with Tom as the all-good and prized male child who was longed for in her patriarchal Italian family of origin, in which all of the children were female. She had become enmeshed with Tom and found it very difficult to set appropriate limits for the "golden boy." The therapist also hypothesized that Toni had projectively identified her own power into Tom so that she generally felt powerless. Nonetheless, over a few months time as the parents teamed, Tom improved both at school and at home.

Phase 2 began when the couple asked for help with their marriage. Toni complained that Bob was never there for her emotionally, while Bob said that all that ever happened when they were together was "more jobs, work, and things to do." Upon further exploration, the therapist learned that the couple rarely spent time alone and had sex infrequently.

The therapist began conjoint couples' sessions twice monthly, along with monthly individual sessions with Bob and Toni. During the conjoint sessions he helped to initiate a renewed courtship by asking the couple to go out on a date each week. He also disrupted the couples' distancing/closeness sequence which was played out through the rearing difficulties with Tom by asking Bob to phone Toni each day at a prescribed time whenever he was out of town.

In individual sessions, Toni began to explore her role as a housewife. She was encouraged to explore gender identification issues and began to examine how she felt like a devalued and incompetent woman. During this process, she decided to go back to school although she was terrified of the idea. As her gender issues surfaced, she expressed strong doubts about her academic abilities. The therapist used interpretation, relaxation, and visualization techniques to deal with these fears. He also asked Toni to share her dreams with Bob.

In conjoint sessions, the therapist prompted Bob to support Toni's return to school. At the same time, he suggested that Toni make herself available as a sounding board for Bob's problems at work.

The weekly dates helped bring the couple closer together and Toni overcame her reluctance to register for courses. As Toni became more involved in her schoolwork, her overinvolvement with her son, Tom, also lessened. Toni was becoming more independent and her self-esteem rose.

At the couple's request, the therapist then initiated a series of interventions aimed at enhancing their sexual life. First, he asked the couple to add some alone time at home once a week during which the couple would learn to pleasure each other. Because the two older children were busy teenagers and young Tom was more able to make friends, the couple found that an hour alone was usually available to them on the weekends.

The therapist prescribed sensate focus and other sensual exercises (Kaplan, 1974) to build the spouses' skills in becoming aware of their own and the other's sexual likes and dislikes. Sessions were used to discuss problems that arose or to overcome the inevitable resistances which occur when spouses deal with sexual dysfunction.

Bob reported, in his individual sessions, that he disliked the exercises and that occasionally he experienced a strange anxiety during them. The therapist then began to explore and interpret Bob's engulfment fears, which had developed in the relationship with his mother and were resurfacing as he allowed Toni to get closer. In a corrective transactional maneuver, the therapist also pressed Bob to use some relaxation exercises before doing sensate focus and also challenged him by saying that "a man works through his problems." In this manner, he modeled the strong father and targeted change at the level of Bob's weak male gender identification.

Over the course of 18 months, Toni was ultimately accepted at a social work graduate school. The couple's romantic and sexual relationship improved and Tom continued to do well. All family members seemed to have grown in basic trust at the foundation level—which was expressed in the closeness around the dinner table and on weekends. They had developed greater self-esteem and self-acceptance at the level of gender identification, which was expressed in more vibrancy, expressiveness and better appearance. The Moore's were also better able to collaborate with each other and avoid destructive collusions and coalitions.

Many couples choose to terminate treatment somewhere in the process we call Phase 3. The Moore's told the therapist that they had accomplished their personal and familial goals. Even though Toni did not consider Bob her best friend nor their sexual life more than "moderately satisfying," both spouses reported that their marital, family, and personal life was better than they could have ever hoped for.

The therapist suggested a 6-month vacation from treatment. He hoped that during the time, the spouses would achieve some degree of separation from him and in his absence would choose to become growth agents for each other. Bob and Toni did return for treatment, but after a hiatus of 2 years. At that time, the spouses were more ready to learn the skills needed to complete the third phase of the therapy.

CONCLUSION

In sum, then, comprehensive family therapy integrates models from the family therapy, cognitive-behavioral, and psychodynamic schools of thought. Each approach can generate useful and effective interventions when applied in a strategic and timely manner to the various problems of children, couples, and families. We continue to refine our understanding and application of various types of interventions to specific disorders.

Our continued involvement in the Society for the Exploration of Psychotherapy Integration reflects an ongoing commitment to understanding the various factors common to all successful psychotherapies. We realize that one approach cannot account for all the elements in normal individual and family development, psychopathology, or even the wide range of treatment interventions. We believe, therefore, that advances in life span theory, longitudinal research on childhood and family disorders and their impact on later adult development, and research which compares specific treatment approaches with specific disorders will all contribute to the building of more useful integrative models.

REFERENCES

Blake, W. (1946). *The portable Blake*. New York: Penguin Books.
Boszormenyi-Nagy, I. (1973). *Invisible loyalties*. New York: Harper & Row.
Bowen, M. (1961). Family psychotherapy. *American Journal of Orthopsychiatry*, 31, 40–60.
Bowlby, J. (1973). *Separation*. New York: Basic Books.
Dicks, H. V. (1967). *Marital tensions*. New York: Basic Books.
Fairbairn, W. R. D. (1952). *An object relations theory of the personality*. New York: Basic Books.
Framo, J. L. (1970). Symptoms from a family transactional viewpoint. In N. W. Ackerman (Ed.), *Family therapy in transition* (pp. 125–171). Boston: Little, Brown.
Freud, S. (1975). An outline of psychoanalysis. In J. Strachey (Ed. and Trans.) *The standard edition of the complete psychological works of Sigmund Freud*. (Vol. 23, pp. 141–208). London: Hogarth Press. (Original work published 1923.)
Greenberg, L. S., & Safran, J. D. (1987). *Emotion in psychotherapy*. New York: Guilford.
Guntrip, H. (1969). *Schizoid phenomena, object relations, and the self*. New York: International Universities Press.
Gurman, A. S. (1981). Integrative marital therapy. In S. Budman (Ed.), *Forms of brief therapy* (pp. 415–457). New York: Guilford.
Haley, J. (1963). *Strategies of psychotherapy*. New York: Grune & Stratton.
Haley, J. (1976). *Problem solving therapy*. San Francisco: Jossey-Bass.
Haley, J. (1984). *Ordeal therapy*. San Francisco: Jossey-Bass.
Hoffman, L. (1976). Breaking the homeostatic cycle. In P. Guerin (Ed.), *Family therapy: Theory and practice* (pp. 501–519). New York: Gardner Press.

Jackson, D. D. (1957). *The question of family homeostasis. Psychiatric Quarterly Supplement* (Part I), *31*, 79–90.

Jacobson, N. S., & Margolin, G. (1979). *Marital therapy*. New York: Brunner/Mazel.

Kaplan, H. S. (1974). *The new sex therapy*. New York: Brunner/Mazel.

Kirschner, D. A., & Kirschner, S. (1986). *Comprehensive family therapy*. New York: Brunner/Mazel.

Kirschner, D. A., & Kirschner, S. (1990a). Couples therapy: A new look. *Journal of Couples Therapy, 1*, 91–100.

Kirschner, D. A., & Kirschner, S. (1990b). Comprehensive family therapy. In F. W. Kaslow (Ed.), *Voices in family psychology*. (Vol. 2, pp. 231–243). Newbury Park, CA: Sage Publications.

Kirschner, S., & Kirschner, D. A. (1991). The two faces of change: Progression and regression. In R. C. Curtis & G. Stricker (Eds.), *How people change* (pp. 117–127). New York: Plenum Press.

Klein, M. (1975). *Envy and gratitude & other works*. New York: Dell Publishing. (Originally published 1946.)

Lazarus, A. A. (1976). *Multimodal behavior therapy*. New York: Springer.

Mahler, M. S., Pine, F., & Bergman, A. (1975). *The psychological birth of the human infant: Symbiosis and individuation*. New York: Basic Books.

Minuchin, S. (1974). *Families and family therapy*. Cambridge: Harvard University Press.

Pinsof, W. M. (1983). Integrative problem-centered therapy. *Journal of Marital and Family Therapy, 9*, 19–35.

Sager, C. (1976). *Marriage contracts and couple therapy*. New York: Brunner/Mazel.

Stein, A. (1980). Comprehensive family therapy. In R. Herink (Ed.), *The psychotherapy handbook* (pp. 204–207). New York: New American Library.

Stuart, R. B. (1980). *Helping couples change*. New York: Guilford.

Watzlawick, P. (1978). *The language of change*. New York: Basic Books.

Winnicott, D. W. (1965). *The maturational processes and the facilitating environment*. New York: International Universities Press.

Zinner, J. (1976). The implications of projective identification for marital interaction. In H. Grunebaum & J. Christ (Eds.), *Contemporary marriage: Structure, dynamics and therapy* (pp. 293–308). Boston: Little, Brown.

CHAPTER 28

Integrative Child Therapy

Sheila Coonerty

In many ways, integrative models of psychotherapy are well suited for the tasks of conceptualizing child psychopathology and child therapy. This chapter will attempt to outline the unique demands of child therapeutic work and to demonstrate the appropriateness of the integrative approach for such work. Specific types and sequences of intervention will be outlined and demonstrated through case examples. It is hoped that the adoption of an integrative approach to child psychotherapy will add a sense of cohesion to the many roles of a child therapist.

In contrast to adult therapy, successful child therapy usually demands that the therapist wear many hats, skillfully changing his or her stance to meet the changing needs of the child as well as those of the various members of the child's life. At one moment, the therapist is intensely involved in play, enacting the internal struggles of the child; at the next, he or she is discussing the latest problems with a parent or fielding calls from the school psychologist or classroom teacher. In addition to the necessity of responding to the various other players in a child's life, the therapist is also thrust into the role of limit setter, educator, or mediator with the same child that he or she involves in deeply evocative, often intensely conflictual, play therapy.

Often, such conflicting and rapidly changing roles result in the adoption of an eclectic style, in which therapeutic interventions are chosen and changed according to the most external demand. Such a style can leave all involved somewhat confused as to the purpose of, and their role in, the therapeutic process. Alternatively, the pressure to wear many hats may result in confusion as to what is "true" child therapy and vague feelings of malaise and guilt as the therapist departs from the expected path of treatment defined by the process of adult psychotherapy. Such demands to constantly alter the therapeutic sense of self threaten the clinician with emotional burnout; as a result, the clinician often narrows and redefines his or her role to fit a clearer, adult-based model, limiting himself or herself to play therapy, cognitive therapy, family therapy, or behavioral intervention alone. To do so at times demands altering or reinterpreting the perceived needs of the patient to fit one model.

To develop an integrative approach to treatment is to attempt to broaden the therapist's concept of what is appropriate to his or her theoretical point of view and to then give the therapist a wider array of tools. Rather than jump from one type of treatment to another, the therapist can

Sheila Coonerty • Doctoral Program in Clinical Psychology, Long Island University, Brooklyn, New York 11201.

Comprehensive Handbook of Psychotherapy Integration, edited by George Stricker and Jerold R. Gold. Plenum Press, New York, 1993.

conceive of all interventions as coming from an integrative sense of the needs of children and families in the midst of emotional crisis (see Gold, 1988). The integrative approach is by no means a set and well-defined entity, but one in the process of being formed. It would seem that the demands of child work particularly call for a more integrated and refined understanding of the overall role of therapy in the ongoing lives of children. At present, child therapists are often hampered by role confusion and a sense of being less legitimate than adult therapists, rather than seeing their many-hatted status as in itself a rational and cohesive approach to understanding children.

The child in treatment is still in the midst of psychological growth and development, only gradually establishing a separate sense of self from important others and acquiring the ego defenses and coping skills necessary to master impulses, desires, and conflicts adequately. Because of this, much of what will eventually become intrapsychic is still actively present in the child's reactions to parents, siblings, teachers, and to his own unintegrated experiences of his self.

The predominantly present-oriented nature of a child's psychological development changes the therapeutic task. Rather than searching for the past derivatives of present conflicts and interpreting them, the therapist must make sense of both the internalized and the "real" present experiences of the child while helping him or her develop coping skills and ego functions to allow for continued development. And the work does not stop there: the analyzing and educating functions must also be extended outward to those in the present who are actively forming a child's experience.

Early in this century, followers of child analyst Melanie Klein advocated a model of child treatment that utilized the basic techniques of psychoanalysis, focusing solely on the analysis of transference and resistances and assuming that children acted on internalized object relations, or patterns of experiencing the self and other. Anna Freud (1965) disagreed with this emphasis, asserting that to emphasize the unconscious was to ignore the developing ego of the child. She suggested that child therapy must include attention to ego development, including in her description of the roles of a child analyst those of educator and nurturing adult. In recent decades, both fam-

ily therapy advocates and behavioral-cognitive advocates went even further. They stated that, given the still-dependent, still-developing state of the child, analysis of the inner state of the child is of secondary importance. Instead, they advocated changing external circumstances, through family intervention or behavioral change. Cognitive therapists, in their focus on the development of cognitive processes, closely parallel Anna Freud's (1965) view of the importance of the development of the ego; however, they are minimally concerned with underlying conflicts and unconscious processes which still have a central place in Anna Freud's work. Instead, the development of maladaptive cognitive schemata are of central importance, as is helping the child to recognize and consciously alter such schemata. The field of child treatment today recognizes the importance of both the internalized representations as well as the crucial roles of cognition, developing ego functions, internal and interpersonal relatedness, family, and society.

Adopting an integrative model as basis for assessment and treatment of children allows for the consideration of all of the above aspects of child development. After careful assessment of the appropriate treatment goals, the relative weight of the unconscious dynamic, systemic, behavioral, and cognitive aspects of a child's psychopathology can be evaluated. The integrative approach offers a coherent therapeutic rationale as well as a conceptual system for the "many-hatted" child therapist. In this way, once a clear formulation of a child's psychological difficulties and overall development is made, a wealth of tools are made available to aide in appropriate growth-inducing interventions.

THE INTEGRATIVE APPROACH:
AN OVERVIEW

Integrative models of psychopathology and psychotherapy attempt to address the limitations of traditional theories. Traditional theories, whether psychoanalytic, behavioral, or cognitive, tend to see psychological disturbance as arising from a single source (or a closely related set of sources) in a direct causal progression. For instance, as noted by Gold (1992), the psychodynamic theories are based on the assumption that psychological disturbances derive from the interaction of biology and environmental events with the normal and predictable progression of intrapsychic development. A fixation or conflict at one point in development is seen as generating later emotional, cognitive-behavioral, and/or interpersonal disturbances. Similarly, cognitive theorists see psychopathology as arising out of early faulty cognitions developed in response to developmental crises. In all such theories, causation is seen as linear, and the resulting complex set of symptoms and disturbance can be seen as variations on the original theme.

In direct contrast to such linear models, integrative theories of psychopathology assume an interweaving of various aspects of experience. The theoretical groundwork for integrative models has been laid by clinicians of various backgrounds. Each attempt at integration originally intended to emphasize one school of thought while integrating another (see Fitzpatrick and Weber, 1989, for an excellent description of such integration). Fensterheim (1983), for instance, enlarges the behavioral model to include psychodynamic concepts; these concepts are seen as aids in the task of understanding a patient's personality organization or resistances to treatment. Wachtel's (1977) work on cyclical psychodynamics uses psychodynamic theory and technique as a base while attempting to enlarge the scope of technique to include the more active interventions of cognitive and behavioral treatment. Both Feldman (1989) and Wachtel and Wachtel (1987) address the task of integrating systemic therapy with the theory and techniques of individual work. Gold's (1992) recent extension of Wachtel's work offers a broader theoretical view in asserting that it is possible to conceptualize psychopathology from the viewpoint of multicausation, giving equal weight to the various aspects of personal functioning and seeing them as an interwoven and unified whole. Such interweaving implies circularity as well as multiple relationships between cognitive, dynamic, interpersonal, and behavioral aspects of the individual.

The model assumed in this chapter is based on the concept of cyclical psychodynamics put forth by Wachtel (1977, 1989) as well as the extension of this concept proposed by Gold (1992). A brief summary follows.

Wachtel (1977) questioned the assumed linearity of psychodynamic, behavioral, and cognitive models and challenged the belief that these models are incompatible. He advocated a directive, action-oriented psychodynamic approach which considers the importance of early experiences but has a strong present orientation. Rather than seeing the individual as run by early determined inner structures which persist through life and shape all of experience, Wachtel has asserted that the inner life of individuals is also influenced by their present encounters. Unconscious wishes, fantasies, and ideas representing early experience are not seen as in a one-way relationship with the person's present life, but also as interacting with present experiences.

Although existing psychological structures and internal representations are seen as strongly influencing our perceptions of the present, the resulting interactions and feedback in turn shape those structures. The reactions and feedback and chosen "actors" in our present life may act to maintain our internal belief system and unconscious fantasy, but they may also result in modifications and further distortion. Thus, according to Wachtel, "every neuroses requires accomplices" (1977, p. 17).

The model of cyclical psychodynamics, then, assumes that neurotic symptoms persist because of constant feedback. Neurotic belief systems create life circumstances, which maintain and continue to modify these same belief systems. Such a model would not only allow for, but demand, therapeutic action that encompasses both present and past. In later work, Wachtel, in collaboration with Ellen Wachtel (1987), extended this model to the consideration of the interaction of family systems with individual internal representations. Thus, it is assumed that the demands and stresses of the family system also act on, and are acted upon by, the internal needs, conflicts, and beliefs of the individual.

Gold (1992) summarized the importance of this circular, interacting model and expanded it to a model of multiple causation in which "individual, family and the socioeconomic and political context are construed as mutually influencing and influenced by each other in an interlocking system of feedback circles and loops" (p. 21). Such a model rejects the notion of a primary site of causation or influence; rather, initiation and reaction flows back and forth among the various components. The areas of disturbance which are causing and/or maintaining pathology, then, are multiple, and the therapist is free to, if not obliged to, work in whichever sphere is thought to lead to change.

With this cyclical, rather than linear, view of the development of psychopathology, the concept of change also ceases to be unidirectional. Rather, it is assumed that a pathological development in one sphere is likely to lead to difficulties in other spheres of experience, thus both reinforcing and exacerbating the original area of conflict. Although one may conceive of a problem as having a specific starting point, this does not by any means infer that the starting point is the essential source of the problem. Rather, the emotional illness or crisis has spread to other aspects of functioning while difficulties in other areas have, in turn, modified or increased emotional stress overall. As to the prospect of change, then, one can see intervention in any arena as potentially leading to broad reverberations and changes throughout all aspects of an individual's functioning.

The task, then, of the therapist is one of developing a comprehensive understanding of the relationship among the intrapsychic, cognitive, behavioral, and larger systemic aspects of a patient's psychopathology. In doing so, care must be given to avoid reverting to single causal, linear explanations. With such a complete assessment, a treatment plan can follow that allows for intervention in the arena where it will be most effective in laying groundwork for further change. Such a treatment plan is similar to Lazarus' (1981) BASIC ID model, with the addition of Gold's (1992) broader inclusion of political and socioeconomic factors as systemic influences.

INTEGRATIVE APPROACHES TO CHILD TREATMENT: RATIONALE

Turning now to the question of child therapy, integrative approaches seem particularly suited to working with children. Because children are still in the process of developing within the context of larger social systems, understanding and working with the interaction of those systems with a child's psychopathological symptoms would appear to be a necessity in developing a comprehensive treatment plan. Because of the child's pro-

pensity toward action under stress as well as society's demands for socialization, a consideration of behavior in treatment planning also would be of considerable importance. Since childhood is a crucial time for the development of lifelong cognitive styles and self-concepts, intervention in the cognitive arena may be seen as powerfully affecting the quality of later development. And, of course, no one who has worked intensively with children in treatment would doubt the intense fantasy life of children and the constant interplay between conscious and unconscious thoughts, feelings, needs, and conflicts. Thus, an understanding of the intrapsychic life of children must be combined with an analysis of behavioral, cognitive, and systemic aspects of their psychological experience.

For children, it is most important to focus oneself therapeutically on making possible their ongoing progress developmentally. The progress of development must in itself be taken into consideration, as we assess what roadblocks exist in the path of ongoing development in all spheres. Of utmost importance, however, is the vulnerability of the still-developing child to cross-over effects from one area of functioning to another. Thus, a conflict which arises in the internal fantasy life of a child can quickly generalize to the behavioral or cognitive spheres, leading to altered and negative behavioral habits or to the beginnings of maladaptive cognitive schemata. Similarly, a parental or school-based assumption of a negative trait in a child can soon become part of that child's active schematic representation of his or her self.

As we review the complicated arena of child assessment, we begin to see the reason for the many-hatted therapeutic role. In child treatment, the therapist is not simply an agent of change within a single relationship; his unique position requires that he intersect with all others responsible for the child's care. An integrative model allows for an even-handed assessment of all areas of a child's functioning and demands the consideration of interventions that extend well past the child himself. It is assumed that a child's fantasies, cognitions, and behavior are shaped by the influence of the family and the larger society, as well as by his inherent temperamental and genetic makeup. In addition, the child's particular ways of experiencing and acting upon his own self and his environment will affect and shape the environment's response to him. When we now consider the internalized pressure on child therapists to adhere to models limited to one sphere of functioning (models which assume a straight and simple linear progression), it is easy to understand the role conflict involved. How to make one hat fit when many are needed? And how, on top of this, do we learn to juggle all of these different hats without losing sight of our own heads? The problem becomes more manageable if all of the parts, or hats, are seen as connected, forming a more complete whole; considerable skill in juggling, however, is still needed. In the next section, assessment and treatment planning within an integrative model will be addressed, with the assumption that one's first task is to discover which hats are required.

Assessment and Treatment Planning

The basic task of assessment in the integrative model is similar to that of any model: data on the child's development, concerns, strengths and weaknesses, the circumstances of the present problems and the level of involvement of the family system must be obtained. The therapist must keep his or her ear tuned for important connections and signs of crises. While collecting the factual material, the therapist also watches and listens for what may be said outside of the arena of words. Gradually, like a skilled detective, the therapist begins to piece together a coherent picture. However, since the picture searched for is a multilayered, multiconnected one, the therapist must be aware that each piece of the puzzle represents only a single dimension, an incomplete picture until all connections are made and the problem can be viewed in a true multidimensional fashion. In addition, each traditional area of assessment is viewed from a slightly different vantage point within the integrative model, leading the therapist to notice and stress certain kinds of information and connections. The areas of assessment will be covered in greater detail below.

The Problem Leading to Treatment. Children are rarely brought to a mental health worker to aide in a self discovery process or to achieve maximum potential. Rather, a significant problem has been identified or suspected by someone close to the child: a family member, teacher, or other powerful adult. The usual assessment begins with ascertaining the nature of the problem as well as *for whom* it is a problem. For the integrative therapist, the task is to broaden and deepen the inquiry so as to view it in a multidimensional, multicausal way, as is illustrated by the example below:

A 5-year-old child, Andy, is brought to treatment for severe and persistent phobic reactions during all outside activities at school. The child explains this as a fear that there might be a thunderstorm. The parents say that the school reports being unable to soothe him or coax him to enter into play with other children. The problem is becoming increasingly crippling, as he is being teased by others. The school suggested a psychological consultation, and the parents reluctantly consented, feeling that they had been handling the problem well, and that the school was overreacting. Despite this, the parents are embarrassed and chagrined that their son is unable to conquer these irrational fears, and feel that they cannot identify the cause. Andy seems quite unperturbed about this problem. He describes himself as "just a little boy," "too little" to be brave. At that moment of the thunderstorm, however, he becomes panicked and inconsolable. The parents have resolved this by taking him to an inner room without windows each time a thunderstorm threatens, and cuddling with him among warm blankets, eating cookies, listening to his favorite music, and reading stories. But now that their child must interface with the outside world, this solution does not seem good enough.

To see the problem as one of a dynamic conflict over the expression of or experience of aggression may accurately portray the original source of the symptomatic behavior. Of course, should one work on such issues, one might eventually help the child. However, the problem had now become so much more complex, involving the child's concept of himself (cognitively as well as emotionally), the effect of that concept on the rest of his behavior, the family system, and the interaction of these with the outside world. It was quickly clear that, if one looked at this presenting problem from an integrative point of view, multidetermined, circular dilemmas were being created which were shaping the understanding and the actions of all involved.

The therapist attempted to engage first the parents and then Andy himself in recasting the problem in a multileveled light. The parents quickly understood the way in which they had contributed to Andy's symptom through gratifying it, and asked for help in changing their previous method of managing his fear. Working together with the therapist, they came up with a less regressive way to handle thunderstorms and spontaneously presented Andy with other alternative ways to get special attention. Although the parent's plan did not solve the whole problem, it led to a sense of competence and control for everyone involved. They were now much more available for and actively involved in, the work of therapy; even Andy wanted to know more about the ways to be less afraid.

This case example illustrates the value of reformulating a problem from its initial presentation, always remaining alert to the complex interactions between the underlying dynamic conflict and the active process of keeping the conflict alive and expanding on it to produce other difficult emotional knots. It also highlights the active, collaborative role of the therapist from the very beginning of the process. Rather than eliminate the dynamic work mentioned earlier, the process of reformulation and active involvement cleared the way for intensive play therapy in which Andy repeated and expended on his fantasies of aggression and his solution of helpless "littleness." The problem had truly "entered the room" rather than being created, recreated, and enlarged upon in the eternal world.

Development of a Treatment Plan. Once care has been taken to reformulate the presenting problem and develop a formulation for the emotional conflict and distortions apparent within that problem, the therapist must turn his or her efforts to a treatment plan. This is a crucial step in the integrative process, as the many connections and feedback loops between different levels of the problem must be clarified so as to decide where intervention must begin.

There are no definite rules to lead this process. The therapist must call on all of his or her clinical experience to differentiate symptoms which are primarily powerful expressions of internal conflict from those which indicate the active reshaping and reknotting of present experi-

ence. In the latter, a behavioral intervention may lead to the realignment of experience in a way that may bring further maladaptive connections to a halt. In the former, intensive dynamic work may be seen as being the first point of entry. Whatever direction the therapist takes, care must be taken to ascertain how change in one area may affect other areas of functioning. For instance, one must be alert to apprehend early what changes in a child's functioning may so threaten a systemic solution that the parents panic and end treatment. Also, one must take pains to try to identify the primary areas of resistance and the multiple levels of that resistance so as to evaluate the best direction and/or level of functioning at which to attempt resolution.

Throughout this process, the therapist must attempt to develop and refine a sense of this child, where the child is moving developmentally and where he or she may be stuck. In addition, it is important that the therapist bring to this task some knowledge of child development and age-appropriate achievements. In this way, the therapist will be able to evaluate what cognitive leap or behavioral advance may be possible and which ones may be beyond that child's reach.

It is a crucial component of the integrative model that the therapist involve both parents and child as active collaborators in treatment. Therefore, once the therapist has decided on a tentative treatment plan, essential aspects of that plan should be made known to the parents, with encouragement for them to establish some goals of their own. Even small children can actively participate in the formation of a treatment plan by consulting them as to what worries them and what might help. One caution here is that care be taken to avoid narrowing the scope of the problem while engaging the parents and child in the plan. It should be clear to all involved that problems in one area reflect changes and distortions in other areas, and that choosing the ground to being therapeutic work in no way implies that the starting point is the whole problem.

For many therapists, eliciting an active role in beginning dynamically oriented play therapy seems impossible. Play therapy's success often depends on neither child nor parents being too aware of the meaning of the play. However, few children or parents will disagree with the concept that the first thing to do is to let the child follow his own ideas and fantasies, letting them take shape in play. Parents' help can be elicited in encouraging the child's involvement in the play therapy sessions while reserving the concerns of external reality for phone calls, family sessions, or parental conferences. Children need little more than an invitation to come for help with problems and worries and spend the time engaged in play. The nature of the child's play is always an active choice and can be encouraged as such; your role in that play is also mostly determined by the child.

Setting the stage for active collaboration at the beginning allows for cooperative work in re-evaluation as change begins. As both parents and children learn to perceive the signs of change and gain a sense of perspective on themselves, they will be encouraged to identify and work toward undoing other knots in their functioning. The therapist, meanwhile, can gain valuable information as to the many layers of experience as child and parents learn how to view themselves with perspective and insight.

Child Development and the Major Aspects of Experience

When attempting to understand adults from an integrative viewpoint, we often speak about dynamic conflicts, behavioral habits, and cognitive self schemata embedded in early life experiences but actively kept alive and elaborated upon in the adult present. With children, the early life experiences are still forming their perceptions, and the nature of the child's critical experiences is enormously affected by the developmental process itself. Children's development proceeds along lines of increasing complexity in all areas of functioning. Early limitations in behavioral, affective, and cognitive spheres lend force and distortion to early internal conflict. Early conflicts themselves are heavily invested in fantasy and colored by the child's powerful experience of his or her physical self. As a result, the form and shape of later problems must be understood in the light of the limitations of a developing child.

The Behavioral Sphere of Development. Children experience the world first through their bodies. Due to their tendency to absorb and integrate experience physically, their bodily reac-

tions are intense. Because they only gradually learn to use cognition for expression, action and bodily experience are central modes of knowledge. Ironically, the child only gradually learns how to observe and control bodily expression, controlling the use of the body both constructively and destructively. A child learns to combat the enforced passivity of infancy and childhood by attempting to act, to take control. Although the propensity toward expression through the body and through action is strongest in early childhood, that propensity remains in somewhat diluted form throughout childhood and adolescence.

The clinician, then, must learn to evaluate a child's behavioral expressions in the light of development, so as to know what it is realistic to expect. Also, an understanding of the gradual process of synthesizing body behavior with verbal behavior should allow the clinician to have a realistic sense of what behavioral controls are within the reach of the child.

The Cognitive Sphere of Experience. As with behavioral control, children only gradually develop cognitive skills. Concepts are first only understood through action-oriented schemata. As the child develops the capacity for more complex schemata and for language, schemata become internalized as unconscious or subconscious thoughts, feelings, and behaviors. Through a gradual process of internalization, the child begins to develop cognitive maps for his experience of himself and of the world. It is precisely these maps which can limit the emotional vision in adult years. Since children are still developing, intervention can have a powerful effect. In addition, children gain cognitive skill through the development of gradually more refined capacities for cognitive maps.

In understanding the role of cognition in emotional disturbance, it is also important to remember the central and crucial role of egocentricity in the child's tendency to experience his or her self as the center and cause of all negative and conflictual experiences. Such early egocentricity plays a crucial role in the later power of early experiences, but also resurfaces in later distortions.

Another aspect of cognitive development which is of central importance to child therapy is the gradual differentiation of fantasy from reality, external from internal. Until middle childhood, the child has little ability to make clear distinctions between that which is fantasy and that which is reality. Even in middle childhood, stress is likely to cause the child to regress to a less reality-oriented state. The fantasy life of a child is at peak intensity between the ages of 3 and 6, and the coloring of all experiences with internal fantasy adds to the power of conflicts at that age. A child who continues to have a propensity for vivid fantasy after the age of 6 will often translate any problematic situation into one laden with internal meaning.

Finally, the internalization of patterns of relating and of experiences of the self and other is a cognitive achievement which grows in strength throughout early childhood. A child achieves a sense of object permanency and of the essential constancy of the aspects of an object, thus setting the stage for schematic representations of the world, the self, and relationships which may be the foundation for later action and experience.

The Interpersonal/Affective Sphere. Children only gradually learn to recognize and label their own affective states and those of others around them. Long before that, however, they react to life with experiences such as sadness, anger, shame, and gladness. Until they can recognize and label their experiences, there is little room for understanding and working through emotional experience. Therefore, very young children must be taught how to recognize, label, and express their internal affective experiences before they can be taught how to understand and make use of their reactions to such experiences. They must also be taught to understand and respond to the emotional reactions of others, gradually (by middle childhood) gaining the ability to take another's perspective and to truly empathize with another.

As to the interpersonal sphere, the primary source of learning is through the intense and at times exclusive relationship with the mothering figure. Mahler, Pine, and Bergmann (1976) referred to this central relationship as the source of the psychological birth of the infant, implying that it plays a key role in all cognitive and behavioral achievements as well as in the child's emotional life. It is through this relationship, from early infancy onward, that a child learns about the

intimate attachment to another and about the essential physical, cognitive, and emotional boundaries that exist between the self and all that is not the self. Mahler spoke of this process as that of gradually establishing a sense of separation-individuation, the end result of which is object constancy (i.e., a constant internalized and integrated sense of all aspects of the self as well as a constant sense of the other). Stern (1985) and others question whether separation is the essential task here, asserting that from early infancy it is relatedness that is learned and developed in the infant–mother relationship. What seems likely is that a child develops, through an essentially good relationship with the mother, a core sense of the individual self *as well as* a core experience of the self as related.

Because of the centrality of the progression of relatedness and separation-individuation in the mother–child relationship, the developmental progression in this area is important to our understanding of the child's relative emotional health and capacity relatedness. Thus, child clinicians must take care to evaluate the nature of the child's progression along this continuum.

Children, of course, also learn a great deal through relating to others. Although always actively seeking involvement and reciprocity, the child only gradually learns the skill of relating. A very young child relates through parallel play and moves to more and more complex abilities in interpersonal relating. Although the establishment of a best friend relationship can come about quite late in childhood, a clinician should be evaluating the ability of the child to progress toward that type of relationship.

The Dynamic Sphere: Conflicts in Childhood. The Freudian model of dynamic conflicts in childhood stresses intrapsychic conflict arising between aspects of the id, ego, and superego as the child progresses through the oral, anal, phallic, and Oedipal stages. The object relations models of dynamic conflict stress instead the conflictual nature of unintegrated internalized object relationships. Self-psychology models stress essential disruptions in the development of an integrated and benign sense of self. Whichever focus of childhood conflict you subscribe to, it is essential to child work that not only the area of dynamic conflict but the interweaving of that conflict with cognitive, behavioral, and interpersonal development be thoroughly understood. It is through the intersection of dynamic conflict with other areas of personality development that the first multilayered emotional disturbances begin. It is of little use of understand the dynamic conflicts of a child unless one understands how that conflict interplays with other areas of development.

Treatment Issues in Early Childhood (Ages 4–7)

As has been clear in our earlier discussion, very young children are egocentric, present-oriented, struggling to develop a constant sense of self and other, and dominated by internal, fantasy-oriented experience. One can see in their actions, thoughts, and moods the beginning of the kind of complex cognitive schemata that they will later use in understanding and acting upon their world. To intervene now may be to save a child from the painful effect of distorted cognitions and maladaptive behavioral and affective reactions. A few central considerations when treating a young child are listed below:

1. Due to their intense involvement with fantasy and a fuzzy sense of the fantasy/reality boundary, young children often relate well to play therapy. Helping a child to express his internal experience through play may allow the child to place that experience and the fantasies about it outside of himself. This leaves distortions and maladaptive reactions more subject to intervention without the child having to be too distressed by the meaning of his internal experience. Thus, traditional, dynamically oriented play therapy allows a child to develop and expand upon both his internal and external experience. Expression itself allows for some cathartic relief, but beyond that the therapists dynamic interventions may lead to the lessening of the conflict, allowing the child more energy to respond to the external world.

2. While viewing the play version of a child's internal world and conflicts, the integrative therapist will often see the early and essential cognitive schemata by which a child begins to make sense of experience. When a child appears to have developed a theme depicting his internal struggle as far as he can dynamically, the integrative therapist may look for opportunities to help a child understand and adjust such conscious and unconscious schemata. This is often most simply done through gentle questioning and discussion within play. Questions, such as "what would happen if . . . ?" or "I wonder why it always happens that . . ." may lead to answers which allow the clinician to engage the child in a simplified reformulation process *within* the play. Once that reformulation is introduced and gradually worked with, the replay may be altered to make room for new schemata of experience. If the clinician has moved too quickly or has broken off a necessary dynamic working through, such remarks will more than likely lead to the abrupt ending of the play itself, signifying that the clinician has moved too quickly or intrusively rather than following the lead of the child.

3. Once new schemata have been explored through play and appear to be of some compelling interest to the child, the therapist may also wish to look for opportunities to relate them to reality dilemmas. Thus, a child's mention of a problem at school, with friends, or at home may allow for a practice use of new schemata to see problems in new ways. At times, this can be best achieved through some form of play which allows for movement back and forth between fantasy and reality. Thus, one child's upsetting conflict with his grandmother was first talked about briefly, then acted out in play acting, and finally talked about with alternative understandings proposed in regard to the conflict itself and to his ability to perceive and act differently. It is important to remember that, as in all therapy work, timing is everything. If one is able to elicit the active involvement of the child and follow his or her lead, one can think of offering alternatives when the child clearly states his or her dead-end dilemma, or maladaptive cycles. The timing and effectiveness of the cognitive intervention can often be evaluated by the child's curiosity and interest in engaging in a new world view.

4. Directly addressing behavioral problems is often a necessity in child treatment. As in the example given earlier, parents must be helped to discover their reactions to behavioral problems and, if necessary, develop more adaptive ways to intervene. Thus, although care should be given to avoid isolation of behavioral symptoms as the entire problem, active educating of and collaboration with the parents may lead to behavioral solutions that decrease the cyclical effect of a child's

problems and give both parents and child back the sense of a controllable world.

It is also possible to address behavioral dilemmas with both the child and parents from an early age. By the age of 6 or so, children can contribute to a discussion as to what would help and what does not help in controlling their behavior. At an even younger age, children can be helped to understand the necessity of learning to control one's "hands and feet," a concrete description of the processes of frustration tolerance and impulse control. To allow a child an active voice in the process of controlling maladaptive behavior is in itself esteem-building and a greater insurance that the child will view the solution to his problems as his own.

5. Finally, in addition to the therapist's having extensive contact with the systems in which the child functions (contact with parents and teachers are a *must* in working with young children), systemic work can be done even within a predominantly individual model. Children can be asked if they would like to use the therapist to help talk to their parents about a concern; parents also can be encouraged to ask for such sessions as long as they understand that the decision to use the therapist in that way is in the end the child's. Within such sessions, the therapist tries to establish a collaborative relationship, aimed at engaging everyone in sharing his or her viewpoint and discussing possible solutions. After such sessions, the effect on the child and on the parent must be carefully monitored by the therapist. However, such systemic interventions often lead to breakthroughs in dynamic play.

Treatment Issues in Middle Childhood (Ages 8–13)

In middle childhood, a child becomes capable of more types of active involvement in treatment than that of fantasy play. In fact, in middle childhood, children become concerned with and fascinated by the rules and complexities of reality. In conflictual areas, though, a middle child may still work best indirectly through play. The kind of cognitive interventions described with young child can be used more frequently; however, care must be taken to notice whether a child's increasing self-awareness makes such indirect interventions uncomfortable. In addition to all of the techniques described for younger children, middle children may respond to the following:

1. More elaborate discussions of internal schemata through extension of play into the arena of play-acting. Thus, a piece of play that begins in the dollhouse may be encouraged to evolve into play in which the therapist and child take roles. Once this extension has been accomplished, discussions about cognitive dilemmas and assumptions and reformulations can take place as author/director/producer discussions of the issue at hand. Agreements as to characters and their dilemmas can also lead occasionally out of the play/fantasy realm and back into real life.

By this age, children are somewhat more conscious of the meaning of their play and will often make such connections themselves. For instance, a 8-year-old girl, Jamie, took puppet play further, with each of us staging and directing productions in which the other was advisor. When a familiar conflictual dilemma was introduced, Jamie would sit in front of the "stage" and direct the play. After a while, Jamie began to enter the play and shape it through her role as a character. The puppets would interact with each other and with her, leading to long discussions and tearful protests about what needed to be done. After several months of working with a theme in this way, Jamie would disrupt the play to enlighten the therapist as to how this same thing had happened in her life. At this point, dynamic interpretations and/or cognitive techniques could be directly offered and discussed as possible solutions to her internal dilemmas. Inevitably, this would lead back to the world of play and movement onward to other knots to untie.

2. A child's increasing ability to empathize with the other's viewpoint often clashes head-on with his or her need to assert increasing control and individuality. In such clashes, the therapist often needs to offer his or herself as consultant to the resultant conflict, verbalizing the dilemma in both the cognitive and the affective realm.

3. Children can be encouraged to make increasing use of systems work through sessions with parents or through discussions about therapists' contact with teachers (i.e., "What would you like me to address with your teacher?" "What might your teacher say?") In doing so, the therapist is assuring that the whole system is given attention so that change in the child does not

backfire and lead to parental or teacher treatment-destructive resistance.

4. In addition, as in the above example, children can be increasingly encouraged to look at therapy as a cooperative adventure with the therapist, in which together they explore the increasingly apparent individual experience of the child. From such a viewpoint, therapists can engage a child in the work of adjusting internal representations and facing the inevitable disappointments of life. If a therapist is always ready to reenter the world of indirect, fantasy-oriented communication, comfortable cycles of work can be developed which allow for the child to solve problems across many layers.

Case Example: Early Childhood

John, a 4-year-old boy, was brought for a therapy consultation by his parents. John's presenting problem was one of increasing aggression toward other children and teachers at his nursery school. The parents, who were extremely worried that "something" was wrong with their child, were asked to bring him for a consultation by the nursery school head teacher. John was reported to be hitting constantly and without apparent provocation; in addition, he became particularly out of control when others seemed to be looking at him. His father, who had some acquaintance with psychology and psychopathology, was afraid that his son was becoming aggressive and somewhat paranoid. Would he eventually turn into a sociopathic person? The mother was terrified that he would continue to have severe difficulties interpersonally. When closely questioned, most of the parents' data seemed to come from the school. At home, their son was prone to stubbornness and occasional temper tantrums but had only recently been out of control in any way.

In order to understand the system, the therapist visited the school before meeting the child. What she saw was a dreamy, solitary boy who liked to build and create. He tended to be suddenly and dramatically aggressive, but mostly in reaction to being surprised by another child's wish to share something he was using in his building. The teachers kept him constantly in their vision and called out his name every time it appeared that he might be getting upset. After hearing his name called in warning 15 times in

10 minutes, John became more active and violent, telling the teacher to "stop looking at me." After being sternly called aside and spoken to, John then climbed inside of a box and pulled another over his head, staying there for the remainder of the play period. Meanwhile, the head teacher told the therapist that she had taken John on as her "special project," sure that she could help save this child from his badness. However, despite her best efforts, she felt that he was beyond help in a normal setting. Thus, she now worked for total control.

Later meetings with the parents revealed that the father had been the good child in a family with an out-of-control sibling. As he began to hear that his son was out-of-control, he had begun to respond by informing his son that he could not be with other children if he was bad, and by withdrawing his love. The mother, a rather clear (and at times somewhat abrupt) limit setter, did not always use these skills since she had often been told that she was not nurturant enough as a mother, and did not want to harm her child.

A few play sessions with John revealed that he saw the world as divided into the dangerous and the safe, the good guys and the bad guys. The more divided and violent his play became, the more likely that he would suddenly need to stop. However, during the time of these sessions, his aggressive behavior elsewhere decreased.

The therapist also noted the same dreaminess in John that was seen at school. He seemed to ignore, or not hear, many of the comments made to him. His verbal description of the play was fairly simple.

Reformulation of Presenting Problem. The therapist, in both parent and teacher meetings, pointed out the assumption of a "bad, aggressive boy" hypothesis, and offered the evidence that she had seen to the contrary. She then invited the parents and teachers to work with her in developing a new way to conceptualize John's difficulties. The parents spontaneously wondered about hearing or language problems and offered to have John evaluated. In addition, the possibility that he was upset, experiencing failure at school and reacting aggressively was addressed by John's mother. John's father was able to begin to relate his fears to his own early experience.

With the teacher, the reformulation attempt

failed over several attempts. The teacher insisted that this boy was the most disturbed, most aggressive boy she had ever seen, and that without her constant attention and control, he would be uncontrollable. She recommended an intensive therapeutic nursery for disturbed children.

Until the problem was understood better, little attempt was made to reformulate with John himself. He became tense at any direct mention of nursery school and expressed his feelings through withdrawal from the therapist and increasingly disorganized play.

Treatment Planning. The parents returned for treatment planning with two new pieces of information: John had suffered a mild, chronic ear infection and his language evaluation indicated a mild to moderate disorder in reception of and integration of language. For the mother, this information was enough to confirm the reformulation, and she was ready to be actively involved in the solution. The father was hopeful but remained skeptical. All involved were unanimous that a change in nursery schools was in order, as well as extra language therapy as well as play therapy.

In developing a treatment plan, the parents requested help in handling their son's behavior in and outside of the home, as well as developing ways to explain the school change. On her part, the therapist recommended intensive play therapy in order to help John express and work through his extremely negative and angry feelings and conflicts in regards to aggression. In addition, the therapist hoped to use the play to help John develop alternative ways of understanding himself, his behavior, and others. In addition, she suggested that she and the father meet further to explore his intense and negative reactions to his son's behavior. The following treatment plan was made:

1. Several therapist–parent sessions were scheduled to develop and evaluate behavioral techniques to deal with aggressive and out-of-control behavior. These sessions followed the pattern of analysis, specific modifications, and evaluation of effectiveness.

2. John's mother took on the responsibility of finding a nursery school that would meet his needs. In addition, a language therapist was requested through the Board of Education.

3. Three sessions were agreed to by the fa-

ther to further understand his own reactions and explore ways of dealing with those reactions.

4. Twice a week play therapy was agreed to for a 6-month period, with a parent–therapist meeting monthly to discuss progress.

5. Privately, the therapist completed an analysis of John's difficulties from a multimodal point of view. She concluded that to intervene first through helping John's parents and teachers to develop behavioral approaches was crucial to stop the downward cycle now apparent. At the same time, it seemed important to begin helping John release his anger and begin to express his shame at being bad and his fear of retaliatory aggression through traditional play therapy. Opportunities to alter cognitive schema and interpersonal relationships could wait.

Progress of Treatment. Initial behavioral approaches, combined with school change, were gradually but dramatically successful on the part of the mother and new teachers. The father initially faltered in applying new approaches, but after his work with the therapist was able to develop and initiate creative new approaches of his own. The result was a steadily decreasing amount of aggression and out-of-control behavior at home and school. In addition, as they experienced success, the parents began to see ways to pick up early "signal" behavior and avert trouble.

Language therapy has significantly improved John's ability and willingness to use words to express his feelings. This has also led to a decrease in frustration and aggression.

Play therapy has flourished, with John deeply involved in scenarios of good guy/bad guy and accident/injury and rescue. Gradually, he has increasingly verbalized his concerns through discussing the play. As this has happened, the therapist offered some simple interpretive interventions within the context of play. Perhaps even more importantly, John and the therapist were able to discuss whether little kids can be bad guys, or if they are too little to be really bad. In addition, John has responded to the therapist's attempts at cognitive reformulation (through questions, comments, and active role playing) with an attempt to give the bad guys an occasional redeeming characteristic as well as making the good guys act up occasionally. As these changes have progressed, John's play has become less chaotic and more playful. The good guys are no longer beleaguered and alone, but have houses, furnitures, dogs and cats, and friends. They no longer spend all of their time fearing and fighting the bad guys. In addition, the good guys sometimes get in mean moods and hurt someone, but the bad guys sometimes become doctors and ambulance drivers. Evidence of altered cognitive schemas abound in John's external life, where he only occasionally refers to himself as a bad boy and where he has begun to enjoy play with other children. Recently, he has begun to enjoy nursery school.

Finally, an understanding of the integrative model demands constant reevaluation and reformulation as the balance of the different spheres of experience changes. As the 6 month point is reached, therapist, teacher, parents, and John himself will be involved in further reformulations and treatment planning, perhaps attempting to intervene in other areas of functioning.

SUMMARY

Due to the continuous interweaving of growth and development in intrapsychic, behavioral, cognitive, and interpersonal spheres, integrative approaches to treatment in childhood seem *essential* to the process of change. Due to the child's significant dependence on parents and teachers for the satisfaction of physical and affectional needs as well as for self-esteem, the involvement of outside systems in treatment is also crucial. The tools of child therapy, then, can be seen as ever-changing; the therapist, however, can use these tools much better if he works wearing only one conceptual "hat," that of integrative theory. It is hoped that the theoretical and clinical discussion presented here helps to elucidate some of the theory and techniques of the still-developing integrative model of child treatment.

REFERENCES

Feldman, L. B. (1989). Integrating individual and family therapy. *Journal of Integrative and Eclectic Psychotherapy, 8*(1), 41–52.

Fensterheim, H. (1983). Introduction to behavioral psychotherapy. In H. Fensterheim & H. I. Glazer (Eds.), *Behavioral psychotherapy: Basic principles and case studies in an integrative model.* New York: Brunner/Mazel.

Fitzpatrick, M. M., Weber, C. K. (1989). Integrative approaches in psychotherapy: Combining psychodynamic and behavioral treatments. *Journal of Integrative and Eclectic Psychotherapy, 8*(2), 102–117.

Freud, A. (1965). *Normality and pathology in childhood: Assessment of development.* Madison, CT: International Universities Press.

Gold, J. R. (1988). An integrative psychotherapeutic approach to psychological crises of children and families. *Journal of Integrative and Eclectic Psychotherapy, 7*, 135–151.

Gold, J. R. (1992). An integrative-systemic treatment approach to severe psychopathology of children and adolescents. *Journal of Integrative and Eclectic Psychotherapy, 2*, 58–63.

Lazarus, A. (1981). *The practice of multimodal therapy.* New York: McGraw-Hill.

Mahler, M., Pine, F., & Bergman, A. (1975). *The psychological birth of the human infant.* New York: Basic Books.

Stern, D. N. (1985). *The interpersonal world of the infant.* New York: Basic Books.

Wachtel, P. (1977). *Psychoanalysis and behavior therapy.* New York: Basic Books.

Wachtel, P. (1989). Cyclical psychodynamics: An amplification. *Journal of Integrative and Eclectic Psychotherapy, 8*(2), 118–124.

Wachtel, P., & Wachtel, E. (1987). *Family dynamics in individual psychotherapy.* New York: Basic Books.

CHAPTER 29

Adolescents

Mary FitzPatrick

Adolescence begins with the onset of puberty and can continue into the twenties with the accomplishment of a series of developmental tasks, including growing independence from parents, forging an enduring sense of identity, establishing satisfactory peer relationships, and developing a satisfactory set of life goals. Those who work with adolescents encounter a broad array of issues and problems which vary considerably based on developmental levels, family and environmental supports, and the nature of the presenting problem. Work with adolescents demands an integrative approach. In contrast to adult therapy, where the external world often remains outside the bounds of direct therapeutic intervention, the problems posed by adolescent patients often demand interaction with an array of adults including parents, school authorities, and, at times, others in the community. In addition to combining psychodynamic and behavioral approaches, the integrative therapist must decide when and how frequently to include family members in the therapy.

Although an interest in the integration of

psychodynamic and behavioral models began in the 1930s (French, 1933; Kubie, 1934), and continued to grow and flourish in the late 1970s and 1980s, there is little research on the use of integrated treatments with adolescents. A recent review of the literature yielded fewer than 15 articles which had any relevance to adolescent integrative therapy. Relevant articles discussed the integration of individual and family therapy (Dreman & Cohen, 1990; Feldman, 1989), reality integrative therapy (Weiner, 1986), humanistic and cognitive-behavioral therapy (Thompson & Spana, 1986), and multimodal therapy (Keat, 1990).

In this chapter, the integration of psychodynamic and behavioral perspectives in working with adolescents in individual and family therapy will be presented. Modifications of technique and specific problems encountered with this population will be discussed. Two models will be used to represent integrative approaches. Fensterheim's model of behavioral psychotherapy (Fensterheim & Glazer, 1983) blends behavioral and psychodynamic perspectives, while Feldman's (1989) multilevel perspective looks at interpersonal and intrapsychic problem-stimulation and problem-reinforcement processes with adolescents and their families. The use of both models provides the clinician with a broad base from which to assess, formulate a treatment plan, and treat the adolescent patient. In addition, since the adolescent is in a process of developmental change, a

Mary FitzPatrick • Department of Psychiatry, The New York Hospital–Cornell Medical Center, New York, New York 10021.

Comprehensive Handbook of Psychotherapy Integration, edited by George Stricker and Jerold R. Gold. Plenum Press, New York, 1993.

third developmental perspective will be added to the integrative model presented. Physical, cognitive, and social-emotional developmental levels will be considered. A brief summary of developmental shifts and adolescent psychopathology will precede the discussion and application of the models.

DEVELOPMENTAL ISSUES

Adolescent developmental literature (Hamburg & Wortman, 1990) describes three phases of adolescent development each with its own set of tasks which facilitates the change from childhood to adult status. During these periods, the child matures physically and gains the cognitive abilities and emotional independence to separate from the nuclear family, form new attachments and forge a stable identity with regard to vocational choice, values, and goals. Early adolescence spans the years from 11 to 15, middle adolescence continues from 15 to 17 years, and late adolescence extends into the early 20s with the final accomplishment of the developmental tasks.

Although numerous cognitive, physical, and emotional shifts occur, the shifts described by Piaget, Erikson and Blos will be singled out for discussion as changes which are particularly important to note in therapeutic work. Cognitive changes during adolescence include the transition from concrete to formal operational thinking, the final stage of cognitive development according to Piaget (1969; Inhelder & Piaget, 1958). The development of formal operational abilities allows the adolescent to go from concrete to abstract thinking, to leave the objective world and enter the world of ideas, and to think about possibilities versus reality. The ability to be able to consider the past, present, and future simultaneously, to understand systems of thought (ethical, political, and philosophical) which can guide life choices, and to be able to postulate a self are mental operations which enable the adolescent to become open to influences apart from the immediate family and to be able to identify and understand conflict and identity issues.

Identity issues are at the center of Erikson's (1950, 1968, 1975) psychosocial view of development. According to Erikson, development leads to increasing psychosocial differentiation seen

over eight stages which extend through the life cycle. Adolescence is the period where the individual must establish a sense of personal identity. This includes a sense of continuity and sameness over time, the formation of a personal philosophy, and a commitment to a system of values. Consolidation of the ego identity is the main characteristic of adolescence. Failure to achieve an identity results in self-doubt, role confusion, and role diffusion.

A second, psychoanalytically based view of adolescent development is offered by Blos (1967, 1975, 1979) who introduced the concept of adolescence as a second separation–individuation period. During this stage of development, the adolescent faces the task of disengaging from infantile internalized objects and finding a new extrafamilial love object in the outside world. This shift is fueled by an increase in drive as a result of puberty and ends with the organization of a stable self where drive and ego organization are harmonized, and where parents are evaluated in a more realistic manner. As part of the separation process, relationships outside of the family occupy a central role. The process of separation involves internal as well as external shifts in object choice, relationship with parents, and self-definition.

ADOLESCENT PSYCHOPATHOLOGY

In spite of the rapid changes and shifts occurring during adolescence, normative studies of adolescents (Hamburg & Wortman, 1990) not only report that there is not a significant increase in psychopathology during adolescence, but that parent–child relations remain stable and positive during this period. It is important to differentiate between pathology and so called adolescent turmoil and to note that certain disorders and behavioral problems are more prevalent during the adolescent years.

In their study of British 14 and 15 year olds, Rutter, Graham, Chadwick, and Yule (1976) found that adolescent turmoil differs from a mental disease in its scope and duration. The 10% of their population who reported feelings of "inner turmoil" described feelings of internal misery and self-depreciation at subclinical levels. These feelings, although quite painful to the adolescents, often went unnoticed by significant adults. Rutter's group concludes that psychiatric disorders are somewhat more common during adolescence than during middle childhood and that patterns of disorders shift to school refusal and depression. There appears to be a continuity in adolescent and adult psychopathology with prognosis more dependent on diagnosis than age of onset.

Table 1. Summary of DSM-III-R Diagnostic Categories in Adolescence

Developmental disorders
  Mental retardation
  Pervasive developmental disorders
    Autistic disorder
    Pervasive developmental disorder not otherwise specified
  Specific developmental disorder
    Academic skills disorder
    Motor skills disorder
Disruptive behavior disorder
  Attention-deficit hyperactivity disorder
  Oppositional defiant disorder
  Conduct disorder
Anxiety disorders of childhood or adolescence
  Separation anxiety disorder
  Avoidant disorder
  Overanxious disorder
Eating disorders
  Anorexia nervosa
  Bulimia nervosa
  Pica
Gender identity disorder
Tic disorder
Elimination disorders
Speech disorder
Other disorders of infancy, childhood or adolescence
  Elective mutism
  Identity disorder
  Stereotypy disorder
  Undifferentiated attention-deficit disorder
Adult disorders evident in adolescence
  Organic mental disorders
  Psychoactive substance use disorder
  Schizophrenia
  Mood disorder
  Schizophreniform disorder
  Somatoform disorder
  Sexual disorder
  Adjustment disorder
  Personality disorder
  Psychological factors affecting physical condition
Parent–child problem
Phase of life problem

Risk factors which predict psychopathology are not directly related to developmental issues and include socioeconomic status, history of antisocial behavior, marital discord, family size, sexual abuse, and family history of psychiatric disorders (Garmezy, 1985; Garmezy & Rutter, 1983).

What are the disorders which may occur during adolescence? Table 1 summarizes the diagnostic categories listed in the *Diagnostic and Statistical Manual of Mental Disorders* (DSM-III-R) published by the American Psychiatric Association. This system is most commonly used in classifying and identifying disorders in the United States. Many of the disorders first appear in childhood or are adult disorders which become evident during adolescence.

There is a steeply rising suicide rate and prevalence of adolescent depression according to Hamburg and Wortman (1990). Reported suicide rates have tripled in the past 20 years with 8% to 10% of all adolescents reporting suicidal feelings. Other issues reported by these authors include a significant rise in level of sexual activity, younger age of first sexual experience, and an increase in adolescent pregnancies (one quarter of all births). Rates of psychiatric adolescent inpatient admissions have risen in the past decade. In addition to psychiatric disorders, areas of concern with this population include violence and abuse, reaction to parental divorce and death, mood fluctuation, problems associated with sexual activity, drug abuse, and the impact of chronic illness. In determining what is normal and what is pathological, Kessler's (1966) guidelines remain valid: difference in the child's chronological age and behavioral age level, number of symptoms, frequency and duration of symptoms, degree of social disadvantage, intractability of the behavior, general level of adjustment, and degree of inner suffering.

INTEGRATIVE MODELS

Behavioral Psychotherapy

Behavioral psychotherapy is a model proposed by Fensterheim in 1983 which integrates behavioral and psychodynamic perspectives. It is a model designed to provide the therapist with a blueprint for organizing information about the patient and determining how and where to intervene. Fensterheim follows the law of parsimony in selecting the simplest explanation for a given phenomenon over a more complex explanation and following with a simple in contrast to a more complex treatment. With this model, an understanding of psychodynamic concepts aids in appreciating the processes which underlie a given behavior, as well as how a patient's personality organization can lead to a particular constellation of behaviors. When a more straightforward behavioral treatment approach is unsuccessful, this model can provide alternative treatment approaches as well as an understanding of why a particular treatment may be ineffective. While Fensterheim essentially uses a behavioral approach to asses and treat specific target behaviors using direct, systematic behavioral interventions, he relies on both behavioral and psychodynamic models to formulate hypotheses about relationships between behaviors and decide where to intervene to effect the greatest change. Treatment begins with a standard behavioral interview including a focus on the presenting problem with detailed, concrete illustrations, a history of the presenting problem, and a general history of the patient. The following broad areas are included in each assessment: (1) automatic emotional reactions or phobias defined as automatic conditioned responses of the central nervous system to a stimulus; (2) general disturbance which includes a variety of feeling states, including tension, anxiety, anger, or fatigue; (3) obsessions defined as unwanted intrusive thoughts which lead to a negative affective state; (4) assertive difficulties in close personal relations, social situations and at work; and (5) behavioral deficits and unwanted behaviors which include skills deficits and compulsive habits.

Before treatment strategies are selected, data is organized into a behavioral formulation in which core problems are identified and related issues represented in a flow chart. Such a formulation allows the therapist to effect change in personality organization as well as symptom reduction by hypothesizing how symptoms are interrelated. Thus, symptoms may be the consequence of a deeper conflict or simply an autonomous behavior. For example, an assertive problem may be viewed as a skills deficit or a problem with the expression of aggression having its roots in

early experiences with parental figures. Although each problem could be treated using behavioral techniques, the type of techniques used (desensitization to early memories or skills training) could vary considerably. If the initial selection of target behaviors is unsuccessful or leads to unexpected results, Fensterheim recommends reformulating the case and intervening in a different manner or at a different level.

An example of the use of a behavioral formulation in an adolescent treatment is presented by FitzPatrick (1983). The patient, Ann, was a 19-year-old girl who had first been seen at age 13 when she was referred for treatment to a day hospital and school. Her diagnosis was Schizophrenia, Paranoid Type, in Remission (DSM-III). During the initial two years of treatment, the patient received supportive therapy as well as a psychodynamically informed treatment. During the subsequent two years, a shift was made using Fensterheim's model. This shift occurred after the therapist received training in the use of the model and could incorporate it into the treatment.

Ann presented with a history of school avoidance beginning in the seventh grade, fear of aggressive outbursts both from self and others, obesity, auditory and visual hallucinations, and symptoms of both depression and anxiety. She was socially isolated and had become increasingly withdrawn. Over the course of treatment, Ann was prescribed a variety of antipsychotic and anti-anxiety medications. She had a history of two psychotic episodes, both involving serious aggressive outbursts and subsequent hospitalization. Developmental and family information showed normal pregnancy, delivery, and early development. Ann was the oldest in a large intact family who lived in a poor and violent neighborhood. There was a history of psychiatric disorders in the family, particularly with the mother who had been hospitalized for depression.

Initial treatment involved an expressive, supportive therapy where Ann discussed her fears, the nature of her emotional disorder, concerns about anger, daily interpersonal problems, and somatic complaints. The therapist served as a stable adult in an unstable internal and external world. Treatment focused on separating reality from fantasy as well as enhancing ego strengths which would allow her to function more effectively. Even though she improved considerably as a result of the combination of medication, therapy, and a structured daily program, Ann remained socially isolated, anxious, and fearful.

The addition of a behavioral treatment resulted in a more active therapy to treat fears, phobias, and assertiveness problems. In the behavioral formulation developed (see Fig. 1), problems were seen to center around two major components. One involved a biologically based psychotic process, the other a learned anxiety reaction resulting both from the trauma of the psychotic episodes and the severe psychosocial stressors in Ann's life. In addition, Ann was found to have a learning disability which further interfered with

her ability to keep up with her peers in school. Finally, Ann's family continued to make demands on her as the oldest child as well as to infantilize her. Far from separating emotionally from her family, she remained tied to them. Developmentally, she had not separated physically or emotionally, nor had she developed the skills needed to be successful away from home.

It was hypothesized that Ann's core fear was of losing control and becoming angry or "crazy." Her fear led to oversensitivity and overcontrol, increased vigilance to moods, and phobic avoidance of anxiety-provoking situations. As she became more isolated, she became more depressed

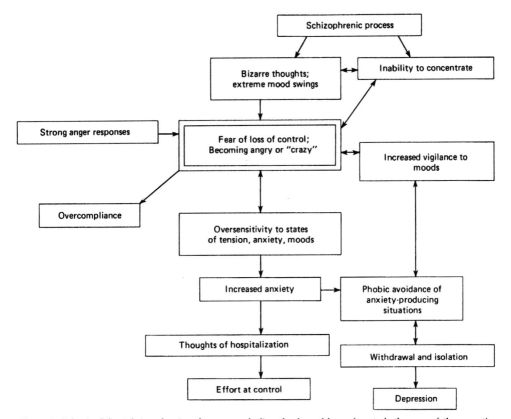

Figure 1. Behavioral formulation showing the process fueling the fear of loss of control, the core of the neurotic organization. From *Behavioral Psychotherapy: Basic Principles and Case Studies in an Integrative Clinical Model* (p. 117) by H. Fensterheim and H. I. Glazer (Eds.), 1983, New York: Brunner/Mazel. Copyright 1983 by Brunner/Mazel. Reprinted by permission.

and anxious. Her subsequent behavior maintained the core phobia. Treatment centered on reducing the core fear of losing control in the hopes of affecting all elements of the proposed formulation. A first step was to teach Ann to differentiate between psychotic and neurotic levels of disturbance. She had learned to manage psychotic symptoms by consulting with her psychiatrist and adjusting her medication. The second level involved her separating anxiety reactions from psychotic states and taking the appropriate actions. In the course of the behavioral treatment, Ann was taught training in anxiety management through a combination of relaxation and cognitive techniques, desensitization to anxiety-provoking situations and feelings, and practice in handling angry feelings by learning to be more appropriately assertive. As Ann became more able to accurately label feeling states, her fear of "going crazy" was reduced. She was encouraged to approach rather than avoid situations. As her level of fear diminished, she remembered details of her hospitalization experiences which had been particularly traumatic and was able to express appropriate reactions of fear and anger as well as put the experience in perspective. Reducing her fear of hospitalization allowed her to approach the staff psychiatrist for help more readily. Work with her phobias was accomplished through the use of desensitization procedures and graded exposure.

As Ann's anxiety reactions diminished, work focused on expanding her skills and moving out into the world. She began to discuss a number of age-appropriate topics in therapy including dating and finding a job so that she could be more independent. As Ann's social contacts and experiences increased, her anger responses diminished. It became apparent that her feelings of extreme anger were directed at family members. With less time spent at home, she was able to be more objective in dealing with others and to transfer this objectivity back home. Although it would have been advantageous to include family therapy as part of Ann's treatment, her family was unwilling to become engaged in therapy. In spite of their reluctance, Ann's changed behavior patterns had an expected effect on family dynamics, and family members were forced to shift their behaviors and reactions toward Ann as she changed and made different demands on them.

Integrating Individual and Family Therapy

Feldman (1988, 1989), described an integrative, multilevel perspective which looks at both interpersonal and intrapsychic problem-stimulation and problem-reinforcement processes. A clinical assessment of an adolescent using this approach would seek to clarify both the intrapsychic and interpersonal factors which stimulate and reinforce individual symptoms, and lead to dysfunctional family systems. Problems are stimulated at an intrapsychic level by feelings and cognitions, as well as at an interpersonal level by parental emotional response and behavior. Likewise, symptoms may be reinforced when followed by a reduction in anxiety level or by the gratification of an impulse, as well as by the attention paid to the child by other family members as a result of the symptom. Feldman used both conjoint and individual interviews to understand these dual factors. In the parental interview, Feldman assessed the presenting problem, the parents' views of the child's strengths and weaknesses, family developmental history, and strengths and weaknesses in the parental relationship. The adolescent interview leads to clarification of the adolescent's thoughts and feelings about the presenting problem as well as general impressions about the patient and his or her family. In the conjoint interview, there is an opportunity to observe functional and dysfunctional behavior patterns with particular attention given to problem identification and problem solution.

With the data gained from these interviews, it is possible to develop a formulation which includes an understanding of individual problems, how these problems are stimulated and reinforced, and what are the strengths present in both the adolescent and in the family which can be used to facilitate the therapeutic process. Subsequent therapeutic intervention is focused on promoting both intrapsychic and interpersonal change processes through a combination of conjoint and individual sessions. These may be integrated in either a symmetrical manner (alternating individual and family meetings) or in an asymmetrical manner where one format occurs more than the other. The structure of the process varies based on the types of resistances encountered as well as the relative degrees of pathology in either the adolescent or the family. This integration of both individual and family therapy broadens the scope of the assessment and provides an array of interventions which can be specifically geared to a particular child, family, and problem complex.

CASE ILLUSTRATIONS

The following cases illustrate the range of interventions available to the integrative therapist. Work with children may last over several years. Often, therapy may be terminated only to resume at another developmental point when new problems arise. The therapist must determine what therapy to use with what combination of family members. Work with children demands at least some contact with parents. As the child becomes older, frequently parental contact diminishes as the child becomes more emotionally separate. Long-term treatment is especially appropriate when working with children with developmental disabilities. These children and their families face new obstacles with each major developmental step. The following case describes such a treatment, one that is ongoing after 11 years of contact with the family.

Sarah, aged 12 years, was initially referred for a psychological evaluation to aid in designing a treatment plan which would include school placement as well as individual, group, or family therapy. At the time of the initial evaluation, Sarah was a student in a special school for learning disabled children which she had attended for seven years. Although she had received numerous types of therapy, including speech and language and occupational therapy, she had not been in psychotherapy. Presenting problems included a high degree of anxiety, general immaturity, thumbsucking, multiple fears, low frustration tolerance, and difficulty handling social situations with peers.

Developmental information indicated normal pregnancy and birth with immaturities present in all aspects of early development. Sarah walked at 2½ years and said single words at 3 years. Delays in expressive and receptive language as well as articulation problems were ap-

parent at an early age. At age 2, Sarah was seen for the first of many neurological evaluations and given a diagnosis of bilateral cerebral dysfunction with irritative features. She was described as a child with fine and gross motor incoordination, language disability, learning disability, and mild psychomotor delay. Over the years Dilantin, phenobarbital, and Depakene were prescribed to control for seizures.

In her initial assessment, Sarah was tense, anxious, and easily overwhelmed. She had little inner resources to deal with new situations and turned to her mother for support and aid, much like a very young child. Testing showed her to have poor problem-solving strategies. She relied on her good memory to respond to demands in a rote manner. In her response to Piagetian tasks, Sarah was clearly preoperational in her thinking. She could not reverse her thinking, nor could she consider two aspects of a situation simultaneously. Sarah was bound by what she saw and could not use the past to evaluate the present. She needed to rehearse responses to new demands to be able to respond appropriately without regressing or becoming overwhelmed. Perceptual-motor and language skills were deficient in spite of a good grasp of factual material. Sarah saw herself as fragile and physically damaged. She expressed a fear of physical injury and of death and was afraid to fall asleep for fear she would die. At an age when children are beginning to emotionally separate from their parents, Sarah remained dependent on her parents to help her to cope with a world that was becoming increasingly more complex as she became older and demands increased.

Sarah was the youngest of three children. Her older brother and sister were functioning well at home and in school. Sarah's parents were caring and supportive but confused by Sarah's uneven and atypical development. Alternately overprotective and encouraging, they were unsure of what they could realistically expect from Sarah and needed help in setting limits and realistic goals. The fights that erupted at home were fueled by Sarah's conflicting needs to move away from as well as cling to her parents. When overwhelmed, she had tantrums which elicited a considerable amount of parental attention. Her more adaptive, age appropriate behavior often went unnoticed in the busy household.

Sarah's problems were conceptualized as stemming from two sources. First, she was dealing with very real neurological problems and learning and language disabilities. Second, a response to her disabilities was to view herself as damaged and fragile. A core issue was a fear of growing up and separating from her parents which she associated with a threat to her survival. Her anxiety over emotional and physical separation intensified the degree to which she would cling to her parents and at the same time feel anger at them because of her dependence. Sarah's parents would respond to her clinging behavior in an inconsistent manner, a response which resulted in her being unable to separate.

Therapy began with individual weekly sessions with Sarah held in her house. Following the individual session, one or both parents were seen for conjoint sessions with Sarah. Parent meetings were held separately on a monthly basis to discuss the parents' feelings about their child's behavior and disabilities. The initial course of therapy lasted two years. Since Sarah was concrete and showed little motivation to either talk to the therapist or engage in any kind of open-ended play, a behavioral therapy was designed with the goals of helping her to manage anxiety, be able to become more emotionally separate from her parents, develop skills which would help her to become more independent, and confront rather than avoid her fears. Meeting in her home was very beneficial in working with this concrete child as it was possible to confront fears and perform tasks where they occurred. It was also possible to easily include the parents in the treatment. As she reached her goals, it was anticipated that the core fears of growing up and becoming separate would diminish.

Initial attempts to teach Sarah to physically relax through relaxation exercises involving diaphragmatic breathing and tensing and relaxing various muscle groups were unsuccessful. Because of her neurological problems, Sarah found it uncomfortable and frightening to change the level of physical tension in her body. However, she readily responded to a cognitive approach using cognitive restructuring and role playing to come up with alternative responses to situations which frightened or angered her. Sarah was able to list a number of fears including bad guys, faucet noises, strange noises at night, dark, staying

home by self, and going to bed by self. We designed a board game based on the rooms in her apartment, where she would have to act out alternative behaviors and responses to situations which frightened her. Next, a point system was designed where she received points for activities which involved separation, independent activities, and overcoming fears. Points could be converted into small presents and responses were put in a weekly chart. Tasks would change from week to week. Points were gained for such diverse behaviors as making her bed, cleaning up her room, cooking, staying home alone without becoming upset, trying new things without giving up, doing anything which scared her, and self-monitoring thumb sucking.

The behavioral chart was revised on a weekly basis in the family meeting. Sarah's parents became more adept at ignoring maladaptive responses and reinforcing positive ones. They were able to set more consistent goals and gradually became adept in negotiating the weekly charts with their daughter. After the first year, meetings moved out of the home and into the therapist's office. This allowed Sarah to function more independently and necessitated that she become more active in relating events of the past week without help from a parent. Family meetings were stopped at this point. The relationship between Sarah and her parents had improved, they were able to continue a point system with her, and it seemed important to focus on Sarah's life outside of her home. As part of the ongoing therapy, visits were made to Sarah's school and meetings were held with Sarah and her teacher to discuss problems dealing with peers, responsibility for challenging schoolwork, and hygiene. These themes would reappear in later years as she moved on to vocational training.

After two years of treatment, therapy was stopped both at Sarah's request and because the initial goals of treatment had been reached. Two years later, when Sarah was midway through high school, therapy began again at her parent's request. They were concerned that she had reached a plateau and related that issues of independence and responsibility were being discussed at school meetings. They planned that she would attend a two year vocational program in two years and wanted her to gain the necessary skills and emotional independence to make the move.

Although Sarah did not initiate therapy, she did not resist meeting once again. This time, it was decided to include another student at her special school to make a group of two. The goals of therapy were to encourage independence at a number of levels. Because the two girls were not able to talk without a structure guiding them, a version of the earlier behavioral plan was drawn up. Each week, each girl would select three tasks to perform over the week from a list of possible tasks. Points earned could be converted into popular tapes. Tasks involved social skills (talking to company, holding a 5-minute conversation with family members about one's feelings) or activities of daily living (cooking, cleaning, shopping). An important goal for both group members was to make them aware of and responsive to others as well as more independent. Again, the chart was very successful and resulted in a rapid rate of skill acquisition with two previously unmotivated girls. In addition to discussion of the chart, a 15-minute discussion period was made part of the weekly meetings. The girls were allowed to choose from a list of age-appropriate topics, such as allowance, dating, and getting along with friends. This treatment lasted until the girls graduated from high school.

Following her graduation from a vocational program, Sarah again returned to treatment. Again, she found it difficult to engage in an open-ended, expressive therapy and was more readily drawn into a small group of three young adults who met weekly to discuss problems encountered in moving out into the world. At this point, the feedback from group members served as a source of support and information which other group members could follow.

Developmentally disabled young adults continue to face the complications of separating from parents on whom they remain quite dependent. Because the separation process is extended, the therapist who stays involved over many years can play an important role as a consistent figure in the child's life who can facilitate the separation process by providing an alternative to the parents. For such a shift to be successful, it is essential that the therapist and the parents work as a team to help the child and that the approach be a flexible one.

Dan, aged 14, was referred with a presenting problem of depression following not achieving a

high enough grade on a citywide examination to be accepted into the top public high school in the city. Upon hearing this news in the spring of the eighth grade, Dan became tearful, expressed a wish to die, and a sense of hopelessness about his future.

When seen with his parents for an initial interview, Dan presented as an articulate, thoughtful, well-related adolescent who was very distressed and preoccupied with thoughts of failure. Dan related that he had been ill with mononucleosis for several weeks prior to taking the exam and that his fatigue had contributed to his poor performance. Both Dan and his parents were confident that when Dan took the test the following year, he would achieve a high enough score to enter the tenth grade in the school of his choice. His diagnosis was Adjustment Disorder with Depressed Mood (DSM-III-R 309.00).

Although Dan's parents supported his need to achieve, they felt that he was too concerned with academics and encouraged him to become more socially active. Dan's relationship with his parents was a positive one. He saw them as supportive and not intrusive, and felt that he was a valued member of the family. There seemed little need to meet as a family except to reassure his parents that their son, whose prior adjustment had been fine, would be able to overcome this disappointment. Short-term, individual therapy for Dan was recommended with the goals of restoring his sense of worth, reducing his level of depression, and helping him to make a plan for the following year which would capitalize on his strengths. Since the family did not present with problems, and since the parents were accepting of any choice Dan might make, this plan seemed to be the most efficacious one.

Dan had weekly therapy for a 3-month period. As we talked, it became apparent that Dan's sense of identity was solely defined by his level of scholarship. He had always been an excellent student and this blow affected not only his self-esteem but his core identity as a top student. In the course of a brief, supportive therapy, Dan was able to reexamine what gave meaning to his life. Although intent on remaining a top student, he struggled to put the failure into perspective and to search for a broader definition of himself. The opportunity to meet was sufficient to help Dan deal with the disappointment and focus on making the most of his immediate future, not on his failure. The selection of a treatment modality was based on ruling out rather than integrating various treatments which would complicate the treatment and possibly lead to less beneficial results.

SUMMARY

The use of integrative therapy with adolescents demands a knowledge of developmental processes as well as models of treatment. The integrative therapist must be comfortable working not only with families but with schools and other community members. In contrast to work with children, where parents are more frequently included in treatment, therapy with this population may be helped or hindered by actively including parents in the treatment process. Often adolescents will not enter treatment unless they are ensured total privacy. This age, more than any other, challenges the integrative therapist to tailor each treatment to the multiple developmental, intrapsychic, and interpersonal needs of the patient population.

REFERENCES

American Psychiatric Association. (1987). *Diagnostic and statistical manual of mental disorders* (3rd ed., rev.). Washington, DC: Author.

Blos, P. (1967). The second individuation process of adolescence. *The Psychoanalytic Study of the Child*, Vol. 22. New York: International Universities Press.

Blos, P. (1975). The second individuation process of adolescence. In A. H. Esman (Ed.), *The psychotherapy of adolescence* (pp. 156–176). New York: International Universities Press.

Blos, P. (1979). *The adolescent passage: developmental issues.* New York: International Universities Press.

Dreman, S., & Cohen, E. (1990). Children of victims of terrorism revisited: Integrating individual and family treatment approaches. *American Journal of Orthopsychiatry, 60,* 204–209.

Erikson, E. (1950). *Childhood and society.* New York: Norton.

Erikson, E. (1968). *Identity: Youth and crisis.* New York: Norton.

Erikson, E. (1975). The problem of ego identity. In Esman, A. H. (Ed.), *The psychotherapy of adolescence* (pp. 318–346). New York: International Universities Press.

Feldman, L. (1988). Integrating individual and family therapy in the treatment of symptomatic children and adolescents. *American Journal of Psychotherapy, 42,* 272–280.

Feldman, L. (1989). Integrating individual and family therapy. *Journal of Integrative and Eclectic Psychotherapy, 8,* 41–52.

Fensterheim, H., & Glazer, H. I. (1983). *Behavioral psychotherapy: Basic principles and case studies in an integrative clinical model.* New York: Brunner/Mazel.

FitzPatrick, M. (1983). Treatment of a schizophrenic adolescent. In H. Fensterheim & H. I. Glazer (Eds.), *Behavioral psychotherapy: Basic principles and case studies in an integrative clinical model.* New York: Brunner/Mazel.

FitzPatrick, M., & Weber, C. K. (1989). Integrative approaches in psychotherapy: Combining psychodynamic and behavioral treatments. *Journal of Integrative and Eclectic Psychotherapy, 8,* 102–117.

French, T. M. (1933). Interrelationships between psychoanalysis and the experimental work of Pavlov. *American Journal of Psychiatry, 89,* 1165–1203.

Garmezy, N. (1985). Stress resistant children: The search for protective factors. In J. E. Steverson (Ed.), *Recent research in developmental psychopathology.* Oxford: Pergamon Press.

Garmezy, N., & Rutter, M. (1983). *Stress, coping and development in children.* New York: McGraw-Hill.

Hamburg, B., & Wortman, R. (1990). Adolescent development and psychopathology. In R. Michels, A. Cooper, S. Guze, L. Judd, G. Klerman, A. Solnit, A. Stunkard, and P. Wilner (Eds.), *Psychiatry* (Vol. 2, pp. 1–15). New York: Basic Books.

Inhelder, B., & Piaget, J. (1958). *The growth of logical thinking.* New York: Basic Books.

Keat, D. (1990). *Child multimodal therapy.* Norwood, NJ: Ablex Publishing.

CHAPTER 30

An Integrative Approach to the Psychotherapy of the Elderly

Nicholas Papouchis and Vicki Passman

INTRODUCTION

The focus of this chapter will be to present an integrative approach to individual psychotherapy with the elderly patient. The theoretical basis for this approach is best understood from an object relational position which emphasizes the individual's relationships with significant figures in one's life as the basis for psychopathology. The approach relies heavily on attachment theory derived from John Bowlby's three volume work on Attachment and Loss (1973, 1980, 1982), and Mary Ainsworth's (1978) empirical strategies to studying this phenomena. From Bowlby's perspective, loss is a central factor in determining psychopathology. To the extent that aging involves the experience of loss in a number of arenas of psychic life, whether personal (physical), interpersonal (loss of spouse or family and friends), or social (occupational or financial), it is a crucial determinant of how the aging process is experienced. Bowlby's conceptualization that the indi-

vidual's needs are essentially relational and that attachment phenomena continue throughout the life cycle is also an important basis for this approach.

The therapeutic strategy suggested here accepts the assumption that developmental stages continue throughout the life cycle (Erikson, 1982; Haveren, 1986), and that any meaningful psychotherapeutic approach must take into consideration the psychological tasks of the developmental epoch with which the individual is dealing. Equally important to psychotherapeutic strategies with the elderly is the recognition that environmental factors play a critical role in an individual's ability to adapt to these developmental challenges (Blum & Tross, 1980; Kroetsch & Shamoian, 1986). From this perspective, the psychological tasks which the individual must face entering his or her mid-sixties, are more profoundly affected by physical and social factors than they were a decade earlier. Physical infirmities and changes in the social system in the elderly person often are critical factors (losses) impacting on the individual's ability to adapt effectively. The patient who has reached that stage in life which is defined as elderly must then reintegrate his or her sense of self based on changes in the psychological, physical and social spheres (Cath, 1975; Lazarus, 1988; Muslin, 1984).

Nicholas Papouchis and Vicki Passman • Doctoral Program in Clinical Psychology, Long Island University, Brooklyn, New York 11201.

Comprehensive Handbook of Psychotherapy Integration, edited by George Stricker and Jerold R. Gold. Plenum Press, New York, 1993.

The elderly patient, like the adolescent or child, is affected in a more significant fashion by environmental factors which are either impinging upon or facilitating his or her ability to negotiate the developmental tasks of this period (King, 1980; Sandler, 1982). This requires that the clinician be acutely aware of the complex interaction between the psychological issues of this phase of development and the physical and environmental factors which facilitate or impede successful negotiation of this developmental period.

The psychotherapeutic approach set forth in this chapter relies heavily on an appreciation and understanding of these multiple factors confronting the elderly, and the considerable individual variability within this cohort of patients. It emphasizes the diversity of therapeutic strategies which need to be employed, and argues that there can be no single integrative approach which can be specified which will meet the needs of all elderly patients. Instead, psychotherapy with this population must essentially be tailored to the specific patient, with a given biological integrity, living in a particular environmental context.

Although this integrative approach is fundamentally object relational, it also appreciates the relevance of cognitive-behavioral interventions which may be used to address more focal problems, and the significance of the systemic issues, familial or social, which the individual faces. The environmental context in which the individual lives is thus viewed as a critical factor in determining the appropriateness of the therapeutic strategies to be implemented.

THEORETICAL AND CONCEPTUAL ISSUES

The Elderly as a Heterogeneous Group

The reader should keep in mind the variability among people described as elderly. Clearly there are important differences between patients who are in their mid-sixties and those who are in their 80s. There is also considerable variability among the aging in their physical health, psychological resources, and the environments in which they live.

Berezin (1972, 1983, 1987) underscored the important distinctions within this population. He argued that this population is a heterogeneous cohort ranging from 65 to 90 years of age, with variable levels of adaptive functioning, psychological mindedness, family composition, social background, and history. Hansson (1986) differentiated between two groups of elderly: the young-old adults (ages 60–80) and the old-old adults (ages 80+). He concluded that the nature and meaning of social roles differed for these age groups and differentially affected life satisfaction and quality of life. Haveren (1986), arguing for an appreciation of the wide variety in individual differences, suggested that older people should be seen as individuals moving through their history with each person influenced by his or her unique early life experience.

There are important differences between those patients who are relatively healthy physically and those who are suffering from an illness which limits intellectual or physical functioning (Busse & Blazer, 1980). Blau and Berezin (1982) have described in detail the various myths and stereotypes about the elderly. These include stereotypes of increased rigidity and inflexibility and the assumption of underlying organic pathology. A therapeutic strategy which is directed toward treating the elderly, must take into account the considerable variability within this population, and the context within which each individual exists. For example, Berezin (1972) noted that prior to 1970, the largest number of studies investigating psychotherapy of the aged studied groups of institutionalized, and often chronically ill patients. Although it is understandable that these studies resulted in perceptions of the elderly as rigid, cognitively limited, and resistant to change, these conclusions were a direct result of the biased samples studied. It is important to underscore the fact that these conclusions are inaccurate (Caspi & Elder, 1986, Chodorkoff, 1982).

Cohen (1984) reviewed the question of cognitive capacity in the elderly and concluded that for the most part, those older persons who maintained their general health and remained intellectually alert and vital, showed no significant decline in capacity with aging. Similarly, Backman, Mantyla, and Erngrund (1984) found that while younger adults outperformed older adults on recall tasks in terms of speed of information processing, the overall effect of performance related to age did not show any differences in accuracy or patterns of processing information. Chodorkoff

(1982) cautioned that we should not equate old age with some of its characteristics, sickness, disability, and deterioration. Instead it seems that the healthy elderly person has the cognitive capacities to learn from new experiences, like those provided in the psychotherapy process (Blum & Tross, 1980; Kroetsch & Shamoian, 1986). Blau and Berezin (1982) concluded from their own clinical experience that the aged were as responsive to psychotherapy as any group with similar problems.

The literature regarding the psychological capacities of the aged and psychotherapeutic work with the elderly leads to the conclusion that each individual must be assessed according to a "case-specific" treatment approach. This approach has been advocated by others such as Lazarus (1988), and Silberschatz and Curtis (1980) who argued for a specific psychodynamic formulation for each patient with treatment strategies and goals specific for the case.

Similarly, Kroetsch and Shamoian (1986) developed a strategy for selecting treatment for the elderly individual based on upon the assessment of primary diagnosis, level of personality functioning, environmental stressors, and motivation for therapy. Depending upon the results of this assessment, one of three psychotherapeutic strategies were recommended: (1) environmental manipulation, (2) supportive psychotherapy, or (3) exploratory, insight-oriented psychotherapy. The present approach argues that a flexible approach which can move from one strategy to the other even within a single case may be called for in work with the elderly.

As Berezin (1972) noted earlier, it is important to assess each case in terms of age-specific changes and the timelessness of life-style. Age-specific changes include physical and physiological changes in the body, as well as extra-somatic changes such as occupational changes, retirement, loss of financial security, and loss of spouse, family members, and friends. The significance for the individual is not that such changes occur, but that such changes are inevitable (Cath, 1982). How each individual adapts in response to these changes is the critical factor. This is more a matter of individual variability than a general statement of how the elderly adapt. As Berezin (1982) pointed out "those who are rigid in youth are rigid in old age."

In fact, it would be unfortunate if any of the principles to be outlined later in this chapter were to be applied in a blanket fashion to all elderly patients, or were to be adhered to without constant review in the treatment of any individual case. The possibility for a dramatic change occurring at any point in time seems to have a high probability of occurrence in therapeutic work with the elderly. A debilitating physical illness or the trauma of losing a spouse may lead to a dramatic change in the patient's adaptive functioning. These stressors are likely to challenge the psychotherapist of the elderly patient to be prepared to be more adaptive than the therapist of the younger adult. The basis for the therapeutic approach articulated in this chapter depends upon a careful biopsychosocial assessment of each patient's functioning in all three domains, with an awareness that there may be dramatic changes in any of the areas at any point in time. Dogmatic adherence to a particular strategy is not only to be avoided, but is counterproductive. Instead, given the likelihood of considerable variability among the elderly, and the high probability that there will be significant change during an individual's lifetime, the therapist must remain open to modifying treatment strategies depending upon these changes. What is needed is a complex, integrated, eclectic approach which addresses the complexities of later life.

AN INTEGRATED PSYCHODYNAMIC PERSPECTIVE

The issue of individual variability and the ability to modify treatment strategies according to the integrative approach suggested in this chapter depends upon the therapist's ability to articulate a model of psychotherapeutic interventions appropriate to different areas of psychological difficulty. Pine's (1985, 1988, 1989) clinical theorizing provides a conceptual basis for just such an integrated model. He argues that psychoanalytic theory may be categorized into four psychologies, each distinctive but overlapping with the others. These psychologies of drive, ego, object relations, and self as they are called, each relate to a different domain of the individual's psychological functioning, and to different domains of development. Pine (1989) spells out in considerable detail the kinds of interventions appropriate to each domain and demonstrates convincingly how interpretative work is important in certain domains, while empathic or ego-building responses are appropriate in others.

Pine's (1988, 1989) major distinction seems to be between areas of conflict and areas of deficiency. When the patient's level of personality has developed sufficiently so that symptomatology reflects conflict in an otherwise basically integrated personality, interpretative work may be the primary mode of intervention. When there are severe deficiencies in the patient's level of ego functioning or sense of self, empathic responses and ego-building efforts may predominate. This distinction, although oversimplified, may provide a basis for understanding how the therapist can move from a position which is largely organized around the attainment of insight, to a more empathic one designed to communicate an attitude of support and understanding to the elderly patient.

Bromberg (1980), in a series of papers, described the distinction between empathic responses and interpretative interventions from an interpersonal point of view. He argued that it was clinically useful to think of an empathy/anxiety gradient in working with patients with a range of personality difficulties. For problems stemming from the preverbal phase of development, the appropriate therapeutic response would be one of empathy. The impact of this intervention was a reduction in the patient's anxiety, leading toward increased trust in the therapeutic relationship and an improvement in psychic integration. When the patient's difficulties suggested a problem in later developmental stages, and personality integration seemed largely intact, interpretative work which evoked anxiety could proceed.

From an integrative perspective, the work of Pine (1985) and Bromberg (1980) provides us with the beginning of a working model which enables us to do away with the artificial dichotomy between "supportive" and "insight-oriented" psychotherapy. To the extent that empathic responses and ego building interventions provide the patient with support, then this approach working within specific domains of difficulty will dominate the work. To the extent that interpretative work is possible, then that will be the focus of the therapeutic strategy. It should be obvious that either approach depends upon the development of a trusting therapeutic relationship, and that working in one mode of intervention does not

preclude the other. What is critical is that the therapist feel that he or she can move comfortably from one position to the other without violating his or her therapeutic integrity.

Similarly, it is critical for the therapist to modify his or her position on therapeutic neutrality when needed. It is common for practitioners working with patients who are suffering from psychosis or other severe pathology to serve as real objects for their patients in times of crisis. The rationale for this modification in technique is based on the assessment that the patient's resources are psychically inadequate. In psychotherapeutic work with the elderly, the psychotherapist must similarly be prepared to modify the psychotherapeutic relationship when the patient needs to be supported by the therapist. This is especially important in cases where withdrawal, alienation, and helplessness in relation to the external environment dominate the world of the aging individual, and internal resources are depleted. Blum and Tross (1980) have offered some examples of when such modifications in the therapeutic relationship are indicated. The therapist may function as an auxiliary ego to the older person who has declined physically and sustained numerous ego assaults from a rejecting and hostile environment. The therapist may then work exclusively to strengthen the adaptive capacities of the older person, without challenging them. The therapist may offer advice in the midst of confusion and disorientation, offer support in the face of intense anxiety, or reassure in the face of a profound sense of inadequacy or guilt. Although it is crucial that the therapist recognize when such modifications in technique are warranted, it is equally important that the therapist working with the older person recognize that these interventions are case-specific modifications in technique. Working with the elderly does not by definition require these modifications. When that is the case, the likelihood is that a significant countertransference problem exists, since many elderly patients may be treated without any significant modifications in technique.

BOWLBY'S ATTACHMENT THEORY

Bowlby's (1973, 1980, 1982) seminal contribution to developmental and clinical theory was to demonstrate convincingly the significance of attachment theory in human development. His theories were the basis for the work of Ainsworth (1964, 1969) and other developmental researchers who have studied attachment phenomena in young children (Sroufe & Waters, 1977).

Bowlby conceptualized attachment behavior as a primary motivating force in human behavior and argued that such behavior had evolved in a Darwinian sense to promote survival of the species. From this perspective, the absence of a secure attachment, and the loss of significant figures leads to psychopathology. For Bowlby, psychopathology is the end result when the individual deals with loss maladaptively, and the environment impedes the individual's ability to cope with such loss. On the other hand, healthy attachment to significant others promotes growth and development. Seen from this theoretical perspective, the individual is oriented toward attachment and relatedness, not isolation and loneliness as Cumming (1975) and Cumming and Henry (1961) suggested in their theory of the elderly's disengagement from the world. From an object relational perspective, the latter only occurs as the result of frustration and a hostile environment. There is no isolated independence, but rather healthy interdependence with the important people in one's life.

Although this theoretical perspective has not been applied directly in psychotherapeutic work with the elderly, it seems particularly relevant to do so. The life of the older person is filled with the potential for loss. Further, these losses are inevitable. Everyone ages, loses his or her youthful appearance, and experiences the loss of friends and family members. Many people give up their occupation and while retirement may have been planned, the potential for the experience of loss around status and meaningful activity is highly significant. The realignment of relationships with children is often an issue that represents significant stress for the older person. The task for the older person is to struggle with these losses and adapt to them. Often the central task is to reintegrate a different sense of self. When that is the problem, it becomes the focal point of the psychotherapeutic encounter (Lazarus, 1988; Muslin, 1984).

From the life-span developmental perspective followed in this integrative therapeutic strategy it is critical to carefully examine how the patient negotiates this period. King (1980) argued that the elderly face many of the same problems

that they did as adolescents, though in reverse order. These include sexual, biological, and self-image changes and conflicts regarding dependency and independence. Sandler (1982), in a similar vein, described the pressures on the elderly as resembling the tasks of childhood. She noted that especially in childhood and old age, internal and external psychological, social, and biological pressures impose demands for change and adaptation on the individual. She suggested that the goals of psychotherapy with the aging are much like the goals in child work. The task is to remove the impediments to further development.

Unlike the child or adolescent, the elderly's experience of change is colored by an awareness of their mortality. The process of change occurs in a reverse fashion, and the elderly person has to successfully negotiate a state in life without a long life ahead to look forward to. Here Erikson's (1982) conceptualization is helpful. For Erikson, when wisdom, defined as the informed and detached ability to live life in the face of death, prevails, this last stage may be negotiated successfully. Disdain, the alternative, results in a state of confusion and helplessness. From this perspective, the therapeutic relationship must provide the elderly patient with the additional resources to resolve this developmental conflict. In Bowlby's (1973, 1980, 1982) language, secure attachment to the therapist promotes the capacity to withstand anxiety. It is for this reason that Bowlby's (1973, 1980, 1982) conceptualizations of attachment and loss seem most fitting.

Like the adolescent, changes in physical appearance and body image are significant. There are also realignments in relation to family members and peers, and concerns with occupational status or career are often paramount.

CLINICAL AND THEORETICAL ANTECEDENTS

A number of authors have pointed out how the "elderly" have remained an underserved population (Cohen, 1984; Kastenbaum, 1964; Kroetsch & Shamoian, 1986; Rechtschaffen, 1959; and Steuer, 1982). The explanations for the paucity of psychotherapeutic services and substantive theoretical work dedicated to understanding the psychotherapeutic process have been attributed to factors such as stigmatization of the elderly (Small,

Fong, & Beck, 1988), the inability of the elderly to benefit from psychotherapy because of personality limitations (Fenichel, 1945; Gitelson, 1948; Hollender, 1952), and countertransference issues in the therapist dealing with this population (Blau & Berezin, 1982; Kastenbaum, 1964; Steuer, 1982; Small, Fong, & Beck, 1988; Wershow, 1981).

Compared to therapeutic approaches with other populations, relatively little has been written with regard to psychotherapy with this population (Small, Fong, & Beck, 1988; Steuer, 1982). In an early review of the literature, Rechtschaffen (1959) reported that psychotherapy with geriatric patients did not compare with the extensive work done with other adult populations. Later Kastenbaum (1964) confirmed the previous findings and described the lack of psychotherapeutic services for elderly individuals.

Berezin (1972) noted that many of the early conclusions about the prognosis of work with the elderly developed from studies done in nursing homes with a cohort of patients whose prognosis for change was highly unfavorable. In an earlier study (Papouchis, 1971), the senior author reviewed much of the early literature on institutionalization and concluded that many of those who studied the institutionalized elderly failed to appreciate the pernicious effects of life in such milieus. The study that followed indicated that even a group of chronically disabled elderly patients confined to a nursing home would demonstrate the capacity for adaptation, given some control over their environment (Papouchis, 1971). Thus, the assessment of psychological functioning in the elderly, even among the chronically disabled, should be examined in conjunction with the context in which the individual lives (Haveren, 1986). Looking at the elderly person in isolation is analogous to describing the child's ability to be attached without examining the child's behavior within the mother–infant dyad (Ainsworth, 1969).

Early arguments about the viability of the traditional Freudian approach to working with the elderly centered on the elderly patient's ability to benefit from more insight-oriented approaches. In recent years, however there appears to have been some increase in interest in working with the elderly, although this shift has not yet resulted in a significant improvement in mental health services for the elderly (Kastenbaum, 1964; Small,

Fong, & Beck, 1988; Steuer, 1982). This change seems to have come from several sources. One emphasis may be said to come from the shift in developmental psychology to a life-span developmental approach. Erikson (1982) for example, articulated the inherent difficulties of old age as an essential aspect of the developmental process. From a similar perspective, Haveren (1986) suggested that the primary focus of one's experience at any point along the life course continuum needed to be examined, lending further support for including old age as an important stage in adult development.

Changes in psychoanalytic theorizing have also contributed to the increase in interest and optimism to working with elderly. The contributions of ego psychology (A. Freud, 1936; Hartman, 1939), object relations theory (Bowlby, 1973, 1980, 1982; Fairbairn, 1952; Guntrip, 1961; Winnicott, 1965) and self psychology (Kohut, 1971, 1977), have all facilitated a shift from the drive/libido model of Freudian Theory to an interest in the nature of ego functioning and the significance of object relationships as significant determinants of personality development and the development of the self (Pine, 1985). With this shift an interest in modifications in parameters of technique, and the possibility of working with patients previously not amenable to psychodynamic psychotherapy developed. Several writers (Hildebrand, 1986; King, 1980; Sandler, 1982), in fact have credited these changes in psychoanalytic thinking with influencing psychoanalytic practitioners' approaches to working with the elderly. For example, Sandler (1982) noted that the shift in focus from an archaeological model to understanding the patient's mental processes in the here and now is more appropriate for the elderly whose longer histories make extensive analytic work not feasible. Similarly, King (1980) suggested that increased interest in ego functions and object relations encouraged some analysts to reconsider working with patients in the older age groups.

One final factor may have indirectly contributed to the increase in interest in the elderly, and that is the progressive demographic shift toward an increased elderly population. Kermis (1986) reported that in the United States, older persons made up 4% of the population in 1900, 11.4% in 1984, and are projected to represent approximately 25% of the population by the year 2050.

Put in other terms, there is a net increase of more than one-half million people aged 65 and older each year. This demographic shift and the increased demand for services for this segment of the population, cannot help but be stimulating interest in this group.

THE TECHNIQUE AND PROCESS OF PSYCHOTHERAPY

The therapist must remember that working with the aging person requires an awareness of the complex psychobiosocial system impacting on the elderly person. Difficulties in any area of this system may have profoundly affected any other area. Hartman's (1939) concept of an "average expectable environment" does not apply to the elderly. Initial assessments of the presenting problems must therefore be especially thorough and detailed. The technique and process of therapy outlined in this section is applicable to outpatient work. When the initial assessment results in a decision for hospitalization, alternative approaches may be more appropriate.

Psychotherapeutic work with an elderly patient must carefully assess the patient's adaptive capacities, and evaluate his or her physical status and the surrounding environment. The initial assessment must involve a detailed examination of these three spheres. Each of these areas has the potential to contribute in a significant fashion to the patient's presenting symptomatology.

As with all patients, the initial assessment should begin with a detailed description of the presenting problems and the factors contributing to their development. Following this, it is crucial to evaluate the patient's level of functioning, to determine if it has changed in certain areas. Here the clinician is looking for clues to the impact of the aging process on the problem, and attempting to rule out physical and environmental factors.

In this context, a careful assessment of the patient's capacity for object relationships is essential. Who are and have been the important figures in the patient's life? Are they still present? What is the composition of the patient's family? If the issue is related to important losses, what is the patient's history of dealing with loss? Which significant figures in the patient's life have been lost, and at what age? Next is the question of the patient's capacity for dealing with conflict. What are the patient's preferred modes of dealing with inner conflict? Have they changed recently or not? Here we may borrow from Kroetsch and Shamoian (1986) who suggested that it was essential to determine a primary diagnosis and the level of personality functioning before deciding on a therapeutic strategy.

It is essential to identify the stressors in the patient's life. Does the change in the patient's functioning respond to environmental stressors or does it continue older maladaptive ways of coping? Included among the stressors may be a host of physical and environmental factors.

A careful evaluation of physical problems is important. Does the presenting symptomatology suggest an incipient physical problem whose early manifestations are psychological? Has the change in psychological functioning, in terms of illness or injury, followed a physical assault? If so has there been a careful and thorough medical evaluation of the problems? If the psychological symptoms are temporally associated with the physical illness, the therapist can explore the impact of the physical problems on the patient's functioning, and determine whether they are the expected consequences of the illness or side effects of the medication used to treat it. Although not the subject matter of this chapter, the therapist working with the elderly should be familiar with the cognitive and psychological sequelae of the numerous physical illnesses to which the elderly are vulnerable. The skilled clinician will also note the way in which minor losses in physical functioning may impact negatively on the elderly patient's psychological equilibrium.

Finally, it is essential that the therapist inquire in a detailed manner about the nature of any environmental changes that may have occurred prior to the development of the presenting symptoms. A significant change in quality of life, such as that accompanying the loss of a job, a change in the home environment, changes in family composition, or the loss of a significant support system in the community may all contribute to the presenting symptomatology. For example, relocation to a retirement community, although planned for, may precipitate symptomatology if the change involves the loss of a significant support system. In a similar fashion, financial problems may be an important factor when unexpected expenses begin to appear. In all instances the therapist should be aware that the patient may have considerable difficulty admitting to problems in any of these areas, particularly when they are embarrassed by their reaction to what has happened.

When the patient's symptomatology involves difficulty with the family, it is important that the therapist involve the appropriate family members. Minuchin (1974) has described the pathological consequences which may follow significant alterations in family structure. Even when the family is not initially consulted, the therapist should remain open to involving members of the family when problems in that domain are the crux of the patient's psychopathology. Since disturbances in the attachment bond between parents and children can often lead to pathological consequences, a careful assessment of these interpersonal relationships is important.

THE PROCESS OF PSYCHOTHERAPY

Once a psychotherapeutic contract has been established, therapy with the elderly patient should proceed along a direction determined by the case-specific psychodynamic treatment plan. The beginning of psychotherapy with the elderly may not be very different than it is with younger adult populations except where it may be particularly helpful to devote extra time to socializing the older patient to treatment (Gallagher & Thompson, 1983). This involves an examination of the patient's expectations and a discussion of the limits of what therapy can and cannot accomplish. Glantz (1989) writing from a cognitive perspective, emphasized the importance of understanding the elderly patient's particular sociocultural and historical past, and stressed that therapists of the elderly should demonstrate empathy and positive regard to a greater degree than with other age groups. This suggestion is reminiscent of Greenson's (1981) emphasis on the real relationship between therapist and patient writing from his psychodynamic perspective. In the language of attachment theory, the establishment of a secure attachment bond can facilitate healthy functioning.

From the integrated perspective suggested here, the principal therapeutic task in the first few sessions is the initial development of an empathic bond between therapist and patient, where the elderly patient feels understood and respected. This bond, which underscores the relational nature of the therapeutic encounter, is facilitated when the therapist takes the time to know and understand the patient's sociocultural history (Glantz, 1989) and enables the patient to begin to trust the therapist's interest in knowing who they are as a person (Bromberg, 1980a,b). It is even more important for those patients whose social support system has deteriorated and who are in need of a trusting relationship, where the numerous assaults on their self-esteem can be addressed.

At the outset of therapy, it is important that the therapist concretely identify the patient's problems. To the extent that the ambiguity of a more open-ended examination of the symptomatology raises the elderly patient's anxiety, initial focus on the symptomatology should also be oriented more to the present than the past. This focus helps to build the therapeutic alliance and enables the therapist to assess the patient's typical ways of dealing with conflict and emotional experiences. The patient's life history may then be used as a means of clarifying and illuminating the present problem.

This problem-oriented focus gives the therapist the opportunity to investigate the patient's misconceptions about therapy. It may then help the therapist to dispel the impression some of the elderly have about therapy, namely that it is only for "crazy" people or that emotional problems are a sign of moral weakness (Chaisson-Stewart, 1985; Gallagher & Thompson, 1983; Glantz, 1982). This problem-oriented approach thus reduces the patient's anxiety while demonstrating to the patient that the therapist may be available to deal with "real" problems. At the same time, it gives the psychodynamically oriented therapist an opportunity to demonstrate to his sometimes skeptical patient, that emotional problems may contribute significantly to "real" problems. It is then possible over the course of later sessions to demonstrate the importance of reviewing the origin of these problems.

Following the initial development of the treatment contract, the psychodynamically oriented therapist may begin to demonstrate the relevance of earlier events to the present. All the while the therapist moves between engaging his patient on an empathic level with ego building interventions when they are called for, or interpreting the patient's problems when that is indicated (Bromberg, 1980b).

In psychodynamically oriented psychotherapy with younger adults, examination of the transference may be a central focus of the therapy (Greenson, 1967). In a series of articles Greenson (1981) argued that the ability to develop and work through the difficulties of transference phenomena depends to a large extent on the real relationship between therapist and patient. Similarly, Bromberg (1980a,b), Guntrip (1961) and Meissner (1986) have argued that the therapist or analyst provides the patient with the opportunity for a new interpersonal experience with old conflicts. Implied in these theoretical positions is the concept that the therapist becomes internalized as a new object in the patient's inner representational world. Here again we see an emphasis on encouraging the patient's attachment to the therapist as a major therapeutic agent.

With some elderly patients, the transference may be explored in much the same manner as it is with younger adults, while with others it may have to be lived in the same manner as it is with fragile patients (Arieti, 1974). In general, it seems that the older the patient, the more his or her inner resources and social system are depleted, the more likely the real relationship between therapist and patient will be significant. As with younger patients, especially adolescents, the emphasis on the relationship between therapist and patient becomes the foundation for the therapeutic work (Meeks, 1985; Papouchis, 1982). In this manner, resolution of transference issues becomes difficult, and interpretative efforts to examine the transference may leave the patient feeling alone and abandoned since they suggest that the nature of the therapeutic relationship is illusory. Meerloo (1954) seems to have had that in mind when he suggested that the transference assumed the primary mode of therapy with the elderly, and concluded that, unlike traditional psychoanalysis, no attempt at resolving the transference was indicated. He recommended that the most effective form of therapy was to remain in the transference and to use the relationship to substitute for the losses of social contact for the client. With the younger cohort of elderly patients in their 60s,

interpretative work may proceed as it does with younger adults.

The nature of transference relationships with the elderly is as varied as it is with younger adult populations. Blum and Tross (1980) in their review of the psychodynamic literature have summarized the four major types of transference which characterize the psychotherapy of the elderly: (1) the classical parental transference; (2) the therapist as child; (3) a sibling transference which may develop in patients who have experienced multiple losses of peers; (4) sexualized transference when patient experiences a limited and diminished need for intimacy. The implication of the above is that there is no unique form of transference relationship to be expected in work with the elderly, and that attachment phenomena assume many forms. The nature of the transference thus resembles the range of transference phenomena found in other adult populations.

The nature of the therapeutic relationship may be complicated when cognitive-behavioral interventions are introduced. These strategies often place the therapist in a didactic position in relation to the patient. When this occurs it is difficult for the therapist to move back into a position of therapeutic neutrality. Thus, the utilization of cognitive-behavioral techniques, however effective, should be used judiciously when the goal of the therapy is insight. Nonetheless, the therapist should always be aware when they have modified the treatment relationship, and the general rule should be to determine how little needs to be done to help the patient. The more directive and interactive the therapist becomes the more complicated the treatment relationship becomes.

COGNITIVE APPROACHES

Some cognitive approaches have been found to be effective interventions with the elderly (Glantz, 1989), particularly with regard to the treatment of depression and anxiety, two of the most commonly reported clinical pictures in the geriatric patient population. Although a discussion of the general principles of cognitive therapy is beyond the scope of this chapter, the basic premise is that disturbances in an individual's affect and behavior are largely determined by cognitive distortions (Gallagher & Thompson,

1983). Especially with regard to the genesis of depression, people are thought to maintain certain irrational and idiosyncratic beliefs about themselves, their environment, and the future, which produce depressive affect and behavior (Beck, 1967; Fry, 1986).

Although dynamic conceptualizations of psychological difficulties are at variance with this model, it is still possible and quite useful to integrate certain cognitive therapy strategies and foci into a dynamically driven treatment. In particular, with an elderly population, the modifications may be understood as enhancing and developing ego functioning.

UNIQUELY SUITED ASPECTS OF A COGNITIVE APPROACH

The elderly may not be accustomed to thinking of solving problems in terms of psychological solutions and may be resistant, at least initially, to therapeutic approaches that seem to be far removed from the problem at hand (Glantz, 1989). In addition, as has been mentioned earlier, because older adults face many real losses, some of these patients will present with immediate, practical problems for which traditional, longer term, exploratory techniques may not be the most efficacious.

For these reasons, it may be useful to integrate the generally active, directive, and interpersonally interactive aspects of a cognitive approach, at appropriate points, into a dynamic treatment. From the authors' psychodynamic perspective this may be conceptualized as working at improving the patient's ego functioning when it is needed. For instance, the present-oriented as well as the goal- and problem-oriented focus of cognitive techniques may facilitate the achievement of concrete success early on in treatment (Glantz, 1989), solidifying a therapeutic alliance, and then permitting dynamic work to be undertaken. In addition, some elderly patients may find the more overtly educational thrust of cognitive techniques to be less stigmatizing and more immediately empowering (Chaisson-Stewart, 1985).

Although dynamic treatments are educational, providing insight and understanding during the therapy, conveying information and developing skills is a less obvious and immediate emphasis of psychodynamic therapy than it is of cognitive therapy. For certain patients, and at various phases in a dynamically oriented treatment, focusing on these aspects of a cognitive approach in the work may be quite beneficial. For example, a recently widowed elderly woman, who finds herself alone and having to manage her own finances, will benefit most from an approach which focuses not only on the particular meanings, memories, affects, and so forth that are part of her experience of the loss and its consequences for her life, but also on an evaluation of the particular coping skills she may or may not possess.

Specific techniques with the elderly include identification and correction of maladaptive conceptualizations, beliefs, expectations, interpretations and attributions, cognitive monitoring and rehearsal procedures. Even though many of these problems are addressed by psychodynamic therapists, the added emphasis on cognitive distortions helps to focus the therapist's interventions on these distortions as preliminary approaches to dealing with them. After these distortions have been identified and pointed out to the patient, the therapist may begin to examine the underlying affects and object relationships which give them their power.

COMMON COGNITIVE DISTORTIONS AMONG OLDER ADULTS

Several common cognitive distortions exist among older patients. One is the idea that one is "too old to change" (Gallagher & Thompson, 1983). As Gallagher and Thompson point out, this is a particularly easy misinterpretation for the elderly, who often experience a series of negative life events (i.e., personal losses, physical illnesses, etc.). Similarly, the often heard concern of older patients, that their therapist is "too young" to be able to help or understand may be viewed as another cognitive error. Although the elderly almost always encounter therapists (and people generally) who are younger than themselves, this does not necessarily preclude a helping relationship, and an age differential is but one difference between themselves and their therapist with which patients of all ages often become concerned. Finally, it has been pointed out that the negative views of themselves, the world, and the future that frequently accompany depression in the elderly are compounded by widely held age stereotypes (Glantz, 1989). That is, the elderly themselves tend to internalize society's negative attitude toward aging and adopt the belief that "being old is being interior" (Fry, 1986). Even though this may be a "cognitive distortion," and is perhaps best conceived as a culturally embedded one, dynamically, one is always interested nonetheless in the idiosyncratic shaping of these "universal" beliefs. Therefore, a cognitive analysis and treatment of "dysfunctional" ideas, may, for some elderly patients, be a useful prelude to a dynamic understanding of the distortion.

This is especially true when the psychodynamically oriented therapist has succeeded in demonstrating to his elderly patient that he or she is genuinely concerned with their welfare. It is also helpful, if in the course of the first few therapy sessions, the therapist has an opportunity to demonstrate to his patient that he or she has the potential for change. This may happen when understanding the significance of a problem either in terms of its cognitive distortions or its emotional meaning leads to a reduction in the patient's symptomatology. For example, the patient who begins to sleep better when she understands the basis for her anxiety about sleeping can genuinely appreciate that change is possible.

OTHER SUGGESTED MODIFICATIONS

Gallagher and Thompson (1983), suggested that, particularly when using cognitive techniques, the therapist should take steps to enhance the elderly patient's learning capacities by presenting material multimodally (using visual as well as auditory input, including use of a therapy journal), using relevant, age-specific examples when explaining the influence of thought on feelings, and encouraging patients to practice these techniques outside of therapy sessions. When the psychodynamic therapist utilizes these cognitive techniques, he or she does so only after it is clear that he or she and the patient have determined which of these copying strategies is best suited to the patient's style of encoding information, and the patient has expressed the willingness to learn these new skills. It is essential in terms of the patient's autonomy and initiative that

these techniques develop organically out of the patient's needs.

In those instances where the patient's internal resources are depleted and the environmental supports are not sufficient to maintain his or her self-esteem, then environmental manipulation as suggested by Kroetsch and Shamoian (1986) may be more desirable. At such times, behavioral strategies which emphasize an approach to practical problems by intensifying the behavioral/environmental intervention are indicated (Glantz, 1989). Examples include helping the elderly person redevelop depleted external structures and supports, reorganizing the patient's living situation, or providing medication. In this regard, it is important for a therapist to discriminate between physiologically and psychologically based symptoms, and to be aware of the symptoms of medication side-effects and interactions that, in an age-group increasingly sensitive to chemical substances, can easily be mistaken for emotional and behavioral disturbances. Finally, it is important to note that cognitive ego-building treatment procedures with some elderly patients may involve a more lengthy process than with younger adults (Glantz, 1989).

ISSUES OF TERMINATION WITH THE ELDERLY PATIENT

Here again, the process of termination depends to a large extent on the initial assessment of the patient's functioning, and the case-specific treatment approach. However, since the world of the elderly often involves a great deal of loss, the planning of termination is especially important. In most cases a gradual termination with decreasing frequency of therapy sessions and increased time between sessions may be the optimal mode of termination.

It is especially important to allow the patient to set the pace for the termination, and to allow the possibility of telephone calls between sessions. Once the patient has stopped coming regularly to sessions, there may be some sporadic contact either by phone or by letter which allows the patient to stay in contact with the therapist. There may also be a need for the patient to resume sessions for a brief period of time if there is an upsurge in symptomatology. In all instances, it is our opinion that it is important to respect the patient's needs and to enable them to maintain the therapeutic relationship in whatever capacity they need to do this. Often the therapist has become a highly significant figure in the elderly patient's life and only a gradual termination which takes place over several years may be advised. For example, the patient may stop coming to regularly scheduled sessions and come intermittently or remain in contact by phone calls or letters every few months. Whenever possible it is essential that the therapist respond to the patient's efforts at maintaining contact with respect and warmth. Although this would seem to be the case in all good psychotherapeutic relationships, it seems especially important with elderly patients whose social network grows increasingly smaller. It is also important to underscore that the patient's continued attachment to the therapist is not a sign of dependency, but rather a continued indication of the basic human need for relatedness.

CASE EXAMPLE

Mrs. V., a 75-year-old woman, came to therapy, at the suggestion of her daughter because she had recently lost her right eye to cancer. She had trouble sleeping and blamed herself for not following the appropriate medical procedures.

In her first session, Mrs. V. described her difficulties and expressed the wish that something be done to help her sleep. She described waking up several times in the middle of the night and remembered dreams of being cut up in the hospital. She was quite anxious and concerned that her daughter had sent her to therapy to avoid taking care of her. At that time, Mrs. V. owned a flourishing business and was responsible for the welfare of a number of employees. She revealed that she previously learned not to make many demands on anyone. She also remarked casually that she often thought of herself as only 50 years of age, and that she exercised vigorously on a daily basis. By the end of the session, the therapist thought he understood something about her and offered the possibility that she was waking up because she was afraid of dying in her sleep. She responded by saying that she had refused to think about death, and that up until that moment she had blocked it from her mind. This was, she re-

vealed, a way she had learned to deal with things that troubled her. She also mentioned that she was reluctant to begin therapy since she had been in therapy several times earlier in her life and it had not been particularly useful.

The next session Mrs. V. reported that she had slept through the night for the first time in many weeks. The remainder of that session and the next several sessions were spent discussing her feelings of disfigurement and the horror she felt should anyone see her eye. The operation was so severe that the surgeons had not been able to save enough of the eye socket to make an artificial eye possible and Mrs. V. was deeply ashamed of her appearance. After some prolonged discussion of this issue during which the therapist empathized with her feelings about the assault of the cancer and then the operation, she decided to begin therapy on a twice weekly basis. Her goal was to deal with her feelings about this narcissistic assault on her body and the social apprehensions she felt about her appearance.

Much of the early focus in therapy was directed to her experience of the operation and to its impact on her life. She was deeply horrified by her appearance, and filled with self-recriminations about her failure to monitor her health care adequately, in spite of the fact that she seemed to have done a great deal to take care of herself. During these early sessions a significant amount of time was spent deciding on what kinds of eye patches to wear in order to help her feel better about her appearance. As the therapy progressed it was clear that Mrs. V. had begun to treat her therapist like a son, and that this filled an important void in her life. Her son was then living in South America, and she had little contact with her daughter who lived in a neighboring state.

As the concrete issue of her appearance began to recede into the background, and her depression began to lift, Mrs. V. began to report a tendency to ignore problems she had with those who were close to her. She reported that some of her most trusted employees were taking advantage of her. In one case, an employee had managed to get paid double for the same job and had hired members of her family to work for Mrs. V. As the issues involved in Mrs. V.'s reluctance to fire her employee became apparent, she began to report the difficulties in her relationship with her mother. Here the therapy moved into a more exploratory phase of work as Mrs. V. talked about her history and her relationship with her parents. During this phase, the work proceeded in much the same manner as it would with other adult patients.

During this next phase of the work, Mrs. V. began to report an image which appeared on the periphery of her consciousness. The image was of a man's genitals. After some encouragement to allow this image to emerge more fully, she began to report memories of her grandfather asking her to perform fellatio. This initial phase of exploration was followed by a long period of several years of exploratory work with resulted in the uncovering of memories of sexual abuse on the part of her grandfather and her mother's unwillingness or reluctance to listen to her complaints.

Interspersed with these deeply important and moving memories from over 60 and 70 years ago, were discussions from the present about problems with her business and her difficulties with both her children. The shift from present day topics to the early childhood memories was dramatic as though the therapy were moving at high speed through a time warp. Mrs. V. wanted to maintain her focus on these issues by using a diary to keep notes from her sessions, to jot down her dreams and thoughts she wanted to remember. The therapist strongly endorsed this idea rather than treat it as resistance. She reported that the diary was an aid against her sometimes failing memory. As the relationship between the past and the present began to be more integrated, Mrs. V.'s ability to withstand the traumas of her early life improved, and her relationships with current family and friends changed. Throughout this period the therapist's position shifted from an empathic one to a more interpretative one, depending upon Mrs. V.'s ability to tolerate the strain of her anxiety and guilt over betraying her mother's prohibitions that the story of her grandfather's sexual abuse not be told. At the same time Mrs. V. began to be able to express her anger at her mother for her failure to protect her.

During the course of therapy, when the weather was bad, and Mrs. V. could not drive, the therapy sessions were held on the telephone. Similarly, when Mrs. V. was bedridden for several months while recovering from a severe illness, the therapy sessions were continued on the telephone. Throughout this time, continuity in the therapeutic relationship was maintained whenever possible.

The case of Mrs. V. was presented in order to demonstrate selected aspects of the psychotherapeutic process with an elderly patient. Many of the interventions, particularly the challenging of many of Mrs. V.'s misconceptions, and the use of the journals could be called cognitive-behavioral interventions. In psychodynamic language they are conceptualized as ego building or ego enhancing. The transference relationship was not examined in detail except where the transference served as a resistance to the expression of a conflict, presented as an obstacle to treatment, or could be used as an example of how her way of avoiding conflict would get her into trouble. In many other ways, particularly with regard to the exploratory work done on her relationship with her parent and her grandfather, the work was very similar to the psychotherapy of younger adults. Similarly, except for the changes necessitated by Mrs. V.'s physical condition which required telephone sessions, the frequency and nature of therapy sessions have been similar to those of other adult patients. Moreover, work with Mrs. V. has been every bit as rewarding as with any other patient.

Mrs. V. is still in therapy. The principal focus is insight into the dynamics of her problems. She continues to work on the impact of her grandfather's sexual abuse, and on her anxiety about challenging her mother's admonitions. The gains she has made in therapy speak of her ability to grow from this experience. The therapeutic relationship has deepened and grown as the time working together has lengthened. In many respects, the work is not very different than it is with other bright and competent adults. In one respect it is. Mrs. V.'s age makes time a precious commodity. When she forgets her age momentarily, a friend dies or has a life-threatening illness. This is the environmental context in which she lives, no matter how healthy she feels, she is aware that her life is drawing to an end and she cannot take it for granted.

CONCLUSION

This chapter has presented an integrated psychotherapeutic approach to working with the elderly based largely on object relations theory and the attachment theory of John Bowlby. It has stressed the necessity for clinicians working with the elderly to keep an open mind regarding the aging person's capacities, and to treat each case according to a case-specific psychodynamic plan which emphasizes the patient's unique capacities and case-specific environmental context. From this perspective, there is no one psychotherapeutic approach which may be applied to the elderly. Instead insight and ego-building supportive approaches are applied to different kinds of problems in different contexts. Cognitive approaches were also suggested as useful additions to the therapist's repertoire of ego building interventions.

This approach also stresses the significance of the therapeutic relationship as a principal agent in the therapy process, in much the same way that the attachment bond articulated by John Bowlby (1973, 1980, 1982) functions to ally anxiety and promote psychic growth. From this theoretical perspective, attachment is a life-span developmental phenomenon which serves as a powerful force throughout the life cycle. There has been little if any empirical work on the meaning of attachment phenomena among the elderly and none relevant to psychotherapeutic work with an elderly population. This promises to be a fruitful area of future investigation, as empirical studies begin to examine the efficacy of different treatment interventions with different cohorts of that segment of the population known as the elderly.

REFERENCES

Ainsworth, M. D. S. (1964). Patterns of attachment behavior shown by the infant in interaction with his mother. *Merrill-Palmer Quarterly, 10,* 51–58.

Ainsworth, M. D. S. (1969). Object relations, dependency and attachment: A theoretical review of the mother-infant relationship. *Child Development, 40,* 969–1025.

Ainsworth, M. D. S., Blehar, M. C., Waters, E., & Wall, S. (1978). *Patterns of attachment: A psychological study of the strange situation.* Hillsdale, NJ: Lawrence Erlbaum.

Arieti, S. (1974). *Interpretation of schizophrenia.* New York: Basic Books.

Backman, L., Mantyla, T., & Erngrund (1984). Optimal recall in early and late adulthood. *Scandinavian Journal of Psychiatry, 25,* 306-314.

Beck, A. T. (1967). *Depression: Clinical and theoretical aspects.* New York: Harper & Row.

Berezin, M. A. (1972). Psychodynamic considerations of

aging and the aged: An overview. *American Journal of Psychiatry, 128*(12), 1483–1491.

Berezin, M. A. (1982). Psychoanalysis and psychoanalytic psychotherapy of the older patient. *Journal of Geriatric Psychiatry, 15*(1), 33–42.

Berezin, M. A. (1983). Psychotherapy of the elderly: Introduction. *Journal of Geriatric Psychiatry, 16*(1), 3–6.

Berezin, M. A. (1987). Reflections on psychotherapy with the elderly. In J. Sadavoy & M. Leszcz (Eds.), *Treating the elderly with psychotherapy* (pp. 45–63). Madison, WI: International Universities Press.

Blau, D., & Berezin, M. A. (1982). Neuroses and character disorders. *Journal of Geriatric Psychiatry, 15*(1), 55–97.

Blum, J., & Tross, S. (1980). Psychodynamic treatment of the elderly: A review of issues in theory and practice. In C. Eisdorfer (Ed.), *Annual review of gerontology and geriatrics* (pp. 204–234). New York: Springer.

Bowlby, J. (1973). *Attachment and loss: Vol. 2 Separation.* New York: Basic Books.

Bowlby, J. (1980). *Attachment and loss: Vol. 3 Loss, sadness and depression.* New York: Basic Books.

Bowlby, J. (1982). *Attachment and loss: Vol. 1 Attachment (2nd ed.).* New York: Basic Books. (Original work published 1969)

Bromberg, P. M. (1980a). Sullivan's concept of consensual validation. *Contemporary Psychoanalysis, 16*(3), 647–655.

Bromberg, P. M. (1980b). Empathy, anxiety and reality: A view from the bridge. *Contemporary Psychoanalysis, 16*(2), 223–237.

Busse, E. W., & Blazer, D. G. (1980). The theories and processes of aging. In E. W. Busse & D. G. Blazer (Eds.), *Handbook of geriatric psychiatry* (pp. 3–27). New York: Van Nostrand, Reinhold.

Butler, R. N., & Lewis, M. I. (1982). *Aging and mental health,* 3rd Edition. St. Louis: C. V. Mosby Co.

Caspi, A., & Edler, G. (1986). Life satisfaction in old age: Linking social psychology and history. *Journal of Psychology and Aging, 1*(1), 18–26.

Cath, S. (1975). The orchestration of disengagement. *Journal of Aging and Human Development, 6*(3), 199–213.

Cath, S. H. (1982) Psychoanalysis and psychoanalytic psychotherapy of the older patient: Discussion. *Journal of Geriatric Psychiatry, 15*(1), 43–53.

Chaisson-Stewart, G. M. (1985). Psychotherapy. In G. M. Chaisson Stewart (Ed.), *Depression in the elderly: An interdisciplinary approach* (pp. 269-287). New York: Wiley.

Chodorkoff, B. (1982). Psychoanalysis and psychoanalytic psychotherapy of the older patient: Prologue. *Journal of Geriatric Psychiatry, 15*(1), 7–10.

Cohen, G. (1984). Psychotherapy of the elderly. *Psychosomatics, 25*(6), 455–463.

Cumming, E. (1975). Engagement with an old theory. *International Journal of Aging and Human Development, 6*(3), 187–191.

Cumming, E., & Henry, W. (1961). *Growing old.* New York: Basic Books.

Erikson, E. (1982). *The life cycle completed,* New York: W. W. Norton.

Fairbairn, W. R. D. (1952). *An object-relations theory of the personality.* New York: Basic Books.

Fairbairn, W. R. D. (1952). *Psychoanalytic studies of the personality.* New York: Tanstock/Rutlege.

Fenichel, O. (1945). *The psychoanalytic theory of neuroses.* New York: W. W. Norton & Co.

Freud, A. (1936). The ego and the mechanisms of defense.

The writings of Anna Freud Vol. 2. New York: International Universities Press.

Freud, S. (1905). On psychotherapy. *Standard Edition, 7*, 257–268.

Fry, P.S. (1986). *Depression, stress, and adaptations in the elderly: Psychological assessment and intervention* (Ch.8). Gaithersberg, MD: Aspen.

Gallagher, D., & Thompson, L. W. (1983). Cognitive therapy for depression in the elderly: A promising model for treatment and research. In L. D. Breslau & R. Haug (Eds.), *Depression and aging: Causes, care and consequences* (pp. 168–192). New York: Springer.

Gitelson, M. (1948). The emotional problems of elderly people. In S. Steury & N. Blank (Eds.), *Readings in psychotherapy with older people* (pp. 8–17). Rockville: National Institute of Mental Health.

Glantz, M. D. (1989). Cognitive therapy with the elderly. In A. Freeman, K. M. Simon, L. E. Beutler, & H. Arkowitz (Eds.), *Comprehensive handbook of cognitive therapy* (pp. 467–489). New York: Plenum Press.

Greenson, R. R. (1967). *The technique and practice of psychoanalysis.* New York: International Universities Press.

Greenson, R. R. (1981). The "real" relationship between the patient and psychoanalyst. In R. Lamps (Ed.) *Classic in psychoanalytic technique* (pp. 87–96). New York: Jason Aronson.

Grotjahn, M. (1955). Analytic psychotherapy in the elderly. *Psychoanalytic Review, 42*, 419–427.

Guntrip, H. (1961). *Personality structure and human interaction.* London: Hogarth Press.

Hansson, R. (1986). Relational competence, relationships, and adjustment in old age. *Journal of Personality and Social Psychology, 50*(5), 1050–1058.

Hartman, H. (1939). *Ego psychology and the problem of adaptation.* New York: International Universities Press.

Haveren, T. (1986). Historical changes in the social construction of the life course. *Human Development, 29*, 171–180.

Hildebrand, P. (1986). Dynamic psychotherapy with the elderly. In F. Hanley & M. Gilhooly (Eds.), *Psychological therapies for the elderly* (pp. 22–40). New York: New York University Press.

Hollender, M. H. (1952). Individualizing the aged. *Social Casework, 33*, 331–342.

Kastenbaum, R. (1964). The reluctant therapist. In R. Kastenbaum (Ed.), *New thoughts on old age.* New York: Springer.

Kermis, M. D. (1986). *Mental health in late life: the adaptive process.* Boston: Jones and Bartlett.

King, P. (1980). The life cycle as indicated by the nature of the transference in the psychoanalysis of the middle-aged and elderly. *International Journal of Psychoanalysis, 61*, 153–160.

Kohut, H. (1971). *The analysis of the self.* New York: International Universities Press.

Kohut, H. (1977). *The restoration of the self.* New York: International Universities Press.

Kroetsch, P., & Shamoian, C. (1986). Psychotherapy for the elderly. *Psychiatry, 20*(3), 123–127.

Lazarus, L. W. (1988). Self psychology—its application to brief psychotherapy with the elderly. *Journal of Geriatric Psychiatry, 21*(2), 109–125.

Lewis, M. I., & Butler, R.N. (1974). Life-review therapy: Putting memories to work in individual and group psychotherapy. *Geriatrics, 29*(11), 165–173.

Meeks, J. (1985). *The fragile alliance.* (3rd ed.). Malabar, FL: Robert E. Krieger.

Meerloo, J. (1954). Transference and resistance in geriatric psychotherapy. *Psychoanalytic Review, 42*, 72-82.

Meissner, W. W. (1986). *Psychotherapy and the paranoid process.* Hillsdale, N.Y.: Jason Aronson.

Minuchin, S. (1974). *Families and family therapy.* Cambridge: Harvard University Press.

Muslin, H. L. (1984). Psychoanalysis in the elderly: A self-psychological approach. In L. Lazarus (Ed.), *Clinical approaches to psychotherapy with the elderly* (pp. 51–71). Washington: American Psychiatric Press.

Papouchis, N. (1971). *An evaluative study of the therapeutic community to treatment.* Unpublished doctoral dissertation. C.U.N.Y., New York.

Papouchis, N. (1982). Intimacy in the psychotherapy of adolescents. In M. Fisher & G. Stricker (Eds.), *Intimacy,* New York: Plenum Press.

Pine, F. (1985). *Developmental theory and clinical process.* New Haven: Yale University Press.

Pine, F. (1988). The four psychologies of psychoanalytic and their place in clinical work. *Journal of the American Psychoanalytic Association, 36*, 571–596.

Pine, F. (1989). Motivation, personality organization and the four psychologies of psychoanalysis. *Journal of the American Psychoanalytic Association, 37*, 31–64.

Rechtschaffen, A. (1959). Psychotherapy with geriatric patients: A review of the literature. In S. Steury & M. Blank (Eds.), *Readings in psychotherapy with older people* (pp. 45–61). Rockville: National Institute of Mental Health.

Sandler, A. (1982). Psychoanalysis and psychoanalytic psychotherapy of the older patient—a developmental crisis in an aging patient: comments on development and adaptation. *Journal of Geriatric Psychiatry, 15*(1), 11–32.

Silberschatz, G., & Curtis, J. T. (1989). Research on the psychodynamic process in the treatment of older persons. (unpublished manuscript).

Small, C., Fong, K., & Beck, J. (1988). Training in geriatric psychiatry: Will the supply meet the demand? *American Journal of Psychiatry, 145*(4), 476–478.

Sroufe, L. A., & Waters, E. (1977). Attachment as an organizational construct. *Child Development, 48*, 1184–1199.

Steuer, J. (1982). Psychotherapy with the elderly. *Psychiatric Clinics of North America, 5*(1), 199–213.

Wershow, H. (1981). The theory of disengagement. In H. Wershow (Ed.), *Controversial issues in gerontology* (pp. 77-92). New York: Springer.

Winnicott, D. W. (1965). *The maturational processes and facilitating environment.* Madison, WI: International Universities Press.

CHAPTER 31

Groups

Richard L. Wessler

PSYCHOTHERAPY INTEGRATION

Psychotherapy is inevitably an integrative activity when conducted with groups of persons. The presence of persons in addition to the practitioner and patient introduces certain variables associated with the social psychology of groups. The therapeutic efforts that ensue are a combination of psychotherapy and group process, whether or not the therapist explicitly attends to the process, or whether the therapist considers group dynamics to be a distraction to the therapeutic process or the very essence of it (Kissen, 1981).

The particular effects of additional persons depend upon patterns of group interaction. They may range from an audience effect upon the proceedings of a therapist working one-on-one with an individual in the presence of others, to the complex dynamics of face-to-face communications of participants (including one or more therapists). Psychotherapy in groups is already integrative even before therapists attempt to integrate two or more approaches or systems of psychotherapy.

What does it mean to integrate psychotherapy? When Goldfried (1980) sounded the clarion around which integration-minded people might rally, it was in the form of a question: What is it that psychotherapists do in common? Our methods might differ, our language and thinking might differ, our theories and assumptions about the nature of human nature certainly differ, but there could be something we do that is the same or similar. The call was to learn *about* each other as much as it was to learn *from* each other.

Goldfried's list of commonalities was a short one: therapist feedback about and to the patient, and corrective emotional experiences. Yalom (1985) has shown that a group setting provides an ideal opportunity for both to occur. Emotional experiences are an essential aspect of group interactions, and communications from group members (as well as from therapist or group leader) furnish additional feedback about and to the focal person.

Possibly the single greatest barrier to psychotherapy integration is the definition of the term *therapy*. What one school of thought considers therapy another deems merely palliative or worse: Our approach is therapy, yours might be helpful but it is not therapy. Or, the term psychotherapy is reserved for jingoistic purposes: we do *psychotherapy*, you do supportive therapy, auxiliary therapy, or treat such specific disrupted modalities as cognitions or behaviors. Another form of elitism is to claim that we do therapy, you do counseling.

Richard L. Wessler • Department of Psychology, Pace University, Pleasantville, New York 10570.

Comprehensive Handbook of Psychotherapy Integration, edited by George Stricker and Jerold R. Gold. Plenum Press, New York, 1993.

Perhaps the term *integration* does not serve us as well as it should. To some older ears, including those of this writer, the sound of the word evokes memories of school desegregation that began in the 1950s. The integration of public schools was not a merging of equals; in fact, because the schools were not equal integration was supposed to correct the inequalities. The integration of psychotherapy should not involve a blending of unequals in which an elite admits portions of the lesser-than approaches, with an attitude of superiors tolerating inferiors.

WHAT IS GROUP PSYCHOTHERAPY?

The difficulties in respecting each other's efforts as "true" psychotherapy extend into group psychotherapy. Here, too, we find a split between psychotherapy and other helping endeavors which, however well intended, are somehow lesser-thans. For example, Rosenbaum (1976), writing from a psychodynamic perspective, defined group psychotherapy as an intentional effort to strengthen weak defenses or to alter personality structures. Another approach, he wrote, could be classified as "directive-didactic," an intellectual approach that is directed at relief of symptoms and therefore not psychotherapy; but the directive-didactic approach is also seen as "repressive-inspirational," an approach that promotes a sense of identification with the group, and in which the group is strongly supportive (the best examples of these are the "anonymous" groups of alcoholics, drug addicts, gamblers, and overeaters, who share a common problem, and give and receive mutual acceptance and understanding).

If the question of what is "true" psychotherapy is one barrier to integration, the question of what is "true" group is another. What conditions must be met in order to consider an aggregate of people meeting in the presence of a psychotherapist a "true" group? The segregating accusation is that I do group therapy, you do therapy in groups. This is hardly surprising. Nearly every approach to psychotherapy has its form of group therapy. *The Psychotherapy Handbook* (Herink, 1980), for example, contains brief chapters on Adlerian, psychoanalytic, rational-emotive, transactional analysis along with chapters on

the group counterpart of each. There appears to be nothing distinctive about the group version except the number of persons simultaneously treated.

Rather than attempt a resolution of the controversy, we will simply present what someone (usually a practitioner of the approach) considers to be a valid example of group therapy.

VARIETIES OF GROUP THERAPY

Psychotherapy with an Individual and an Audience

In this situation, one therapist works with one person (patient or client) while other people watch and listen. In some instances onlookers are allowed or encouraged to ask questions, give advice, make interpretations, and share their own experiences.

There are two variants on this arrangement. One is when the onlookers are clearly identified as an *audience* and so labeled; the other is when the onlookers are persons identified as members of the same therapy group as the focal person and are called *group members*.

When the audience is specifically labeled as such, there is no doubt about the role of each participant. The therapist (who may not be called a therapist) is the person in charge. He or she creates structure for everyone's participation by specifying the rules of procedure, by dialoguing with the person (who is probably called a volunteer rather than a patient or client), and by setting time limits. The audience knows that it is to listen more-or-less silently until called upon to speak one at a time as called upon by the therapist. This format was used by Adler (Corsini, 1988) and by Ellis (Wessler & Hankin, 1988) for the purpose of helping the focal person with a specific issue and of educating the audience toward improved mental health. There is no expectation that the focal person will continue to see the therapist or become a patient of someone else.

This format is also an example of art imitating life, or perhaps of entertainment imitating psychotherapy. This same format may be seen each weekday on American television as the audience participation talkshow. Its leading practitioners are Phil Donahue, Oprah Winfrey, Geraldo Rivera, and Sally Jesse Raphaël. They and their audiences say what is wrong with the focal person (diagnosis), share experiences with emotionally expressive guests (self-disclosure), offer comments and observations (feedback), and make suggestions for change (corrective experiences). In the hands of a skilled host, the hour-long program becomes a sort of psychological town meeting where each comment is greeted with applause and for a brief moment at the microphone, each audience member is an expert.

Another version is when a therapist works with one member of a therapy group while others look and listen but do not interact with the therapeutic dyad. Because the audience consists of group members, each eventually gets an opportunity to assume the role of focal person with whom the therapist works. Perls used this version, and depending upon the therapist or upon his or her mood, the nonworking group members may be ignored, allowed to speak, or encouraged to speak (Harman, 1988). They may be recruited to give feedback or share experiences, or to participate in the enactment of exercises or the playing out of the fantasies of the focal member. The role of the therapist is that of expert who applies knowledge of psychotherapy with the focal person.

The communication pattern in this format may either center on the therapist or on the focal client. When the therapist is the center of attention, most of the group members' questions and comments are directed at him or her as they seek the wisdom of an expert. The therapist gives advice, makes interpretations, furnishes information, or might actively teach some theoretical or therapeutic points. In the other pattern, communications take place between group members and the focal person, often with the encouragement and guidance of the therapist-leader. There is usually an exchange of opinions and feelings between the focal person and the other group members. In both therapist-focused and client-focused communications, the pattern is that of hub-and-spokes (focal center and periphery), with little interaction among the "spokes" or nonworking group members. In this pattern, the focus is on an individual rather than on the group, and there is less attention given to the dynamics of the group and more to the individual problems and concerns as they are presented.

Psychoeducation and Skills Training Groups

In this model seldom are there focal persons nor are individual problems presented. Instead, the effort of the therapist is self-consciously educational. The activities of the group are structured around a core of mental health principles to be learned and applied. The group participants are not so much an audience as they are students and the therapist is their teacher. Homework may be utilized to reinforce the material of the lessons. Participants may learn how to help themselves by engaging in the monitoring and correcting of cognitions and behaviors. There is very little "group" in this approach to group therapy, just as there is little attention given to any individual.

Skills-training approaches are primarily educational endeavors and have been identified with behavioral and cognitive-behavioral approaches to group therapy. An educational model, as opposed to a psychopathological model, of therapy is assumed. Faulty learning is assumed to be the cause and training the way to eliminate poor performance. Examples of this type include parent-training groups, assertiveness-training groups, and social skills groups.

In a parent-training group, the therapist functions as a teacher and the main task is to present information that helps parents perform more effectively with their children. An individual problem can be used to illustrate a point the therapist tries to teach. Corsini (1988), for example, helped a mother who said that she had not been successful in influencing her child's undesirable behavior by teaching the use of "natural consequences" of the child's behavior. There was no interest in the causes of the problem, only in what to do to solve it.

Assertion training has been extensively used, usually in a time-limited, highly structured format (Lange & Jakubowski, 1976). Some didactic presentations teach differences between assertive and nonassertive behaviors, supplemented with in-group exercises and role-playing, and homework to be performed outside the group meetings. Although this approach is primarily training and not therapy, when the trainers work with the individual needs of participants the distinction is not so clear. Knowing how to do something is no guarantee that the person will do it, as the individual may have fears that inhibit the performance of a skill. Barriers that inhibit the implementation of skills taught may require a therapeutic rather than a training orientation. Such barriers represent an opportunity to integrate skills training with forms of therapy more suitable for removing them, such as tension- and anxiety-reducing exercises, the probing of individuals' dysfunctional schemata and cognitions, and in-depth exploration of self-attitudes.

Social skills training has been used for persons with deficits in interpersonal behavior. This training ordinarily relies upon the use of modeling and role-playing, with ample opportunities for feedback from both trainer and group members. Again, knowledge may not be sufficient to allow a person to function more effectively in a social environment, and therapy interventions that are more specifically aimed at removing barriers to implementation of skills may be needed (Wessler, 1984).

Among other applications of skills training are efforts to improve the self-management of behaviors. Meichenbaum (1977) identified components common to a variety of coping-skills training programs whose objective is to train a person to control behaviors that are troublesome. In simplest terms, persons are taught to identify negative self-statements about emotional distress and to replace these with these more adaptive self-statements that reduce behavioral excesses and promote effective behavior in one's environment. Likewise, Novaco (1978) presented a 10 session program for dealing with anger, featuring relaxation and desensitization techniques, and active rehearsal of covert coping strategies.

In such psychoeducation and social skills training, there is little emphasis on the treatment of either the individual or the group. The instruction could be done as an individual tutorial, although the advantage of time and cost efficiency would be lost if this were done. Since group members serve each other primarily as actors in role plays to rehearse new actions, they could be replaced by the therapist or by surrogates. Time-limited and limited to common problems or diagnoses (e.g., depression), these educational methods are considered to be an important form of group therapy by those who use an educational model of treatment, especially cognitive

and behaviorally oriented therapists (see, e.g., Hollon & Shaw, 1979; Sank & Shaffer, 1984).

Experiential Groups

At another extreme are groups in which leader activity is low and members interact with each other more than they do with the therapist. There is no designated focal member. This is an approach to therapy that emphasizes interpersonal relations. The focus is upon the group and upon how an individual relates with members of the group. Here-and-now experience and feelings are featured, rather than issues in any person's life outside the group.

The therapist is present to facilitate process, but otherwise provides little structure (Johnson, 1988). As a result, there are more opportunities for group dynamics to emerge and be recognized. Patterns of communication, what will be talked about, and how it will be talked about, and who finds their ways into what type of leadership roles are important dynamics that the leader fosters by remaining relatively passive. Because so little structure is imposed, group norms about acceptable communications and behaviors can be expected to develop, and the necessary internal feedback mechanisms that allow a group to be self-regulating will likewise emerge. Later, the leader can process (i.e., discuss) what happened, and how individuals felt and acted in response to what had occurred. The leader does not control the patterns of interaction but rather seeks to understand them and help the participants learn by experiencing.

Psychodynamic Groups

Rosenbaum (1976) seems typical of psychodynamic therapists in defining psychotherapy as an intentional effort to strengthen weak defenses or to alter personality structures. The group therapist promotes interaction among group members and their deep expression of emotion and offers interpretations. Transference is sought and worked through within the group. It is assumed that the presence of several group members creates more opportunities for transference to occur than would in the traditional therapist–patient dyad.

Other Varieties of Group Therapy

As noted at the beginning of this chapter, there are nearly as many varieties of group therapy as there are varieties of psychotherapy. They can be differentiated on the basis of theory, by noting the assumptions about psychopathology and/or treatment that underpin them. Theory largely dictates whether the primary modality of interest is affect, behavior, cognition, unconscious processes, or interpersonal patterns. The jargon employed by therapists is that of their theoretical orientation; their words will become the words group members use as well. Some are distinctive enough to permit instant classification, for example, "games and scripts" identifies the therapist's orientation as transactional analysis (Grimes, 1988). Similarly, the frequent mention of schemata and cognitions identifies a cognitive therapist, defenses and motives identifies a psychodynamic therapist, homework a behavior therapist, and so on.

It is possible to differentiate group therapies on the basis of therapists' styles of conducting a group, but this too is largely a matter of theoretical orientation. Whether a therapist is more active than passive, promotes interactions or requires listening, introduces exercises and simulations or invites presentation of personal problems, owes more to orientation than to personality variables of the therapist.

GROUP PROCESSES

If we restrict the meaning of group psychotherapy to include only instances wherein individuals have a relatively high probability of interaction and engage in a fair amount of face-to-face contact, certain important considerations emerge that cut across specific schools of thought about psychotherapy.

One of these is how to get the group to work together. This is a problem of group cohesion. Plutchik (1981) presents evidence to support the contention that group cohesion and emotions are very closely related. Here is Plutchik's position: Basic survival, in an evolutionary sense, requires organisms to deal with four general problems:

(1) hierarchy, (2) territoriality, (3) identity, and (4) temporality.

Hierarchy pertains to dominance within a group. It has been noted that all groups are stratified; even those that are the most democratic in spirit have leaders and persons in positions of power. One either fights to ascend the leadership ladder or submits to those who hold higher rank. Fighting requires anger and attack, while submitting is based on fear and retreat. Hence, *anger* and *fear* are emotions involved in sorting out one's position in a hierarchy.

Territoriality refers to those aspects of the environment to which the organism belongs, and the boundaries are wherein it is safe and nurtured. The emotional response to having one's territory invaded is surprise. This issue is raised in open-ended therapy groups when new members are introduced. Identity, or to what group do I belong, is associated with feelings of *acceptance* and *rejection*—to be allowed into or expelled from territory.

The third of Plutchik's concepts concerns *temporality* or the limited duration of an individual's life. Loss and separation are inevitable due to the inevitability of death, as are the emotions associated with loss and separation, sadness or distress. When a distress signal succeeds it produces *joy*, when it fails it can lead to *depression*. Since one is not expected to spend a lifetime in a therapy group, the temporality is a latent issue.

Finally, it is *sharing* that promotes group cohesion. Sharing proximate positions in a hierarchy, sharing space and identity contribute to the feeling of belonging. Significantly, feelings do the same:

the sharing of any emotion, pleasant or unpleasant, tends to increase group cohesion. . . . This is also true in the group therapy experience, where a group of strangers become tied together—become cohesive—as a result of sharing emotions. That the crucial element is the sharing of emotions and not the exchange of information is evident from the fact that people who simply attend a lecture do not thereby become cohesive. (Plutchik, 1981, pp. 141–142, italics in the original)

When applied to group therapy, Plutchik's analysis suggests that most of the learning that takes place is a result of experiences within the group rather than intentional lessons taught by the therapist. Members learn about themselves as persons and about interpersonal skills. The goal is to function more effectively outside the group and not simply to be better group members. The key that makes group therapy possible is the sharing of emotional experiences, or self-disclosure.

Self-disclosure is a requisite in group psychotherapy as it is in individual therapy. The same psychological factors that inhibit free expression of information about oneself, one's personal life and felt emotions in individual treatment are present in groups. Although many people can open up to a therapist in a one-on-one situation, they find it difficult to speak as freely and openly in a group. Shame and embarrassment cause them to defend by remaining quiet or closed about themselves. A measure of progress within a newly formed group is the degree to which persons disclose about themselves.

Therapists encourage specific types of disclosure, depending upon their theoretical orientation. Some approaches emphasize disclosure of past events, and may even try to help people recover memories about events long past, such as sexual abuse. Other approaches eschew the past and focus on the here-and-now experiences within the group. These here-and-now experiences require that persons not only know what they experience as feelings but also express these in the presence of other group members. Strong feelings about oneself and about one or more group members are less likely to be readily expressed.

The term *feelings*, as used here, include affective experiences (subjective emotional experiences) as well as less visceral and more cerebral mental products such as opinions and appraisals. More specifically, the group member is expected to discuss positive and negative feelings about self and other members of the group, to talk about conflicts and anger about other group members and the therapist, and to express confusions and sexual feelings.

SHAME AND SELF-DISCLOSURE

Within a therapy group one is expected to put into words what one would normally only discuss with persons very close to oneself—friends, relatives—or perhaps with no one at all. Although there are cultural and generational differences in regard to what is considered appropriate for disclosure, to whom and when, the key

emotional correlate is shame: I do not want you to know about me because I consider the information to be shameful. It is probably correct to assume that the way a person characteristically handles shame in everyday life is the way that person will handle it in a therapy group, at least initially. Nathanson (1987) identifies four characteristic defenses against shame that have relevance for group therapy.

A common method for concealing shame is to avoid and withdraw. The silent members of a group take no risks and reveal little or nothing about themselves or their feelings. Such persons must be encouraged to participate, and confronted if they do not.

Another typical defense against shame is to deny one's feelings by being active in the group, but always keeping the focus on others and their problems and feelings rather than on oneself. Such persons may appear helpful, give advice and attention to others, and seem to be highly involved with the group. In fact, because group cohesion depends on the expression of emotions, such a group member is sooner or later seen as on the periphery, as perhaps trying to function as the therapist's assistant or replacement. The group and its therapist have the task of confronting the overtly helpful but covertly concealing member to deal with shame and to become self-disclosing.

A third way to handle shame is through humor. Even though some good humor is beneficial by not taking oneself too seriously, excessive reliance on humor is not because it conceals shame and other emotions. By making oneself the butt of one's jokes, a person preempts confrontations by others. The person discloses what he or she considers safe rather than exploring and revealing more risky feelings. The joker may be amusing at first, but unless the humor is accompanied by serious self-disclosure the person will not integrate into the group, and will likely not benefit from psychotherapy.

Finally, the experience of anger may be a person's characteristic defense against shame. Rage is often what surfaces when shame has been provoked underneath. Shame-defended rage presents two problems for group therapy. First, unbridled rage is disruptive and inappropriate. Although the expressing of anger is desirable, it must be done according to social rules and conventions, and the leader must be ready to set limits if the group fails to enforce norms about the expressing of feelings. In general, feelings should be put into words and not acted out. Second, fear (and shame) about expressing anger or other negative affects may produce evasiveness or silence or passive-aggressive comments as anger is leaked out in relative safety. Whether shame-related anger is hotly expressed or hidden under ice, neither group cohesiveness nor personal therapeutic benefit is likely to result because true feelings are concealed.

A goal of therapy that cuts across psychotherapy orientations is to enable the individual to deal with feelings—his or her own and those of others. To some extent, therapy may be considered successful when the person fits cohesively into the group; it is a sign that feelings are being dealt with and lessons of interpersonal skills are being learned through experience, even if the problems in everyday life outside the group that led one to seek treatment have not been affected.

For group therapy to be effective, the group has to be perceived as "safe," which means that the group has to be a shame-free environment. If one is to surrender defenses against shame, one should expect to reveal shameful secrets in the safety of a noncritical setting. One way to do this is to give feedback with especial care.

FEEDBACK

Goldfried (1980) and Yalom (1985) have identified feedback as a hallmark of good therapy and commonality in various approaches. Feedback consists of comments made to a focal person, comments that might pertain to what the person has said or done. The term *feedback* did not originate in group therapy or even within the parent discipline of psychology. Feedback is a term taken from cybernetics, and refers to the information needed for self-regulation. In its original meaning, feedback was information about the output of a system that was used to control input and thereby allow the system to maintain a steady state of operation. If output exceeds a specified limit, the signal says "less input" in order to return output to the limit, and vice versa when output falls below the limit. Biofeedback retains part of this meaning; biological processes are detected, amplified, and presented in the form of

visual or auditory display to enable the person to accomplish self-regulation, although improvement rather than consistency (steady state) is the usual goal. Such feedback is neutral in that information is merely presented, without comment or criticism.

When used in an interpersonal sense, feedback consists of observations and opinions other people have and express about a focal person's statements and actions. The information feedback to the person is not so much about his or her behaviors as about observers' reactions to those behaviors. Because humans rather than gauges give the information, neutrality is hard to achieve. In therapy groups, members are admonished to give feedback neutrally, but since feedback consists of expressing feelings, these admonitions seem impossible to enact. Yet accurate, useful, but noncritical feedback is necessary for therapy to occur in a shame-free environment.

Group members are instructed to give feedback about statements and actions, and not about the person. Feedback should be about specifics and not about abstractions or generalizations; it should be useful to the focal person and not catharsis for the speaker (Johnson, 1988). The model sentence is, "I feel this way about what you just said or did." Such feedback is clearly an expression of feelings for which the speaker takes responsibility, expressed directly about a specific here-and-now behavior. The comment is designed to help the listener, not condemn him or her. Because the listeners are humans and not machines, even feedback that is optimally given may be taken as criticism. A result is further shame and a conclusion that the group is not a safe place to express intimate thoughts and feelings.

Feedback, because it consists of impressions, opinions, and feelings, promotes group cohesion, but because it can stimulate shame even when well-done, it can threaten group cohesion. Without feedback there can be no therapy. Feedback provides opportunities for reality testing when exploring transference; it provides opportunities for reality testing when exploring the accuracy of one's cognitive inference and predictions. Feedback serves as positive reinforcers for desirable behaviors, and aversive consequences for undesirable ones. Feedback helps clarify one's social impact, and allows the modifying of the self-image by hearing about impressions one makes on others. Feedback allows the person to learn to label feelings more accurately and to discover aspects of the self that are apparent to others but of which the individual is unaware. Without feedback there is no therapy.

Group therapy offers opportunities for multiple sources of feedback. This provides, on the one hand, a variety of perspectives, and on the other, heightened impact when feedback is univocal. An individual therapist's feedback can be minimized by thinking it is the opinion of a lone person (or by attributing it countertransference, if the patient is sophisticated). It is much less easy to disregard the comments of several group members.

CORRECTIVE EMOTIONAL EXPERIENCES

The sharing of emotional experiences promotes the group cohesion thought to be important in most approaches to group therapy, and it permits the individual to work through shameful feelings. The former creates conditions for therapy to occur, and the latter is an important aspect of psychotherapy, individual or group. However, the sharing of emotional experiences allows for another vital element in psychotherapy, corrective emotional experiences. Yalom (1985) declared that

the group setting offers far more opportunities for the generation of corrective emotional experiences . . . (because) the group contains a host of inbuilt tensions: for example, sibling rivalry, competition for the leader's attention, competition for the group's attention, the struggle for dominance and status, sexual tensions, parataxic distortions, differences in background and values among the members. (p. 26)

His research indicated that patients who have completed group therapy often recall a turning point in therapy, and that it is almost always an emotionally laden event involving some other group member and not the therapist. Turning points are typified by the patient's uncharacteristic expression of strong emotion (usually anger or affection), which to the patient's surprise is greeted with support rather than criticism or rejection by the group, and ensuing reality testing that allows examination of the experience and greater subsequent freedom of expression. The therapist's job, as Yalom sees it, is to keep the group directed at the self-reflective aspect of the

experiential process so that cognitive learning can take place. The intellectual part of the change process is essential, and the acquisition of information and/or generation of personal insight necessary in order to benefit from the emotional experiences a group provides. However, the process is both cognitive and affective in that insight strongly correlates with amount of affect: "The more real and the more emotional an experience, the more potent its impact; the more objectified and intellectualized the experience, the less effective is the learning" (Yalom, 1985, p. 44).

INTEGRATED GROUP PSYCHOTHERAPY

It is possible now to abstract a definition of group psychotherapy from the point of view of psychotherapy integration. Personal change results from experiences of interacting with other people, experiences that are both emotional and result in cognitive understanding of self, other people, and interpersonal relations. Personal change includes shifts in thinking and acting, and relief from emotional distress. When emotional distress cannot be relieved because it is associated with some aspect of the person he or she is unwilling or unable to change (such as the emotional distress associated with remaining in a marriage one's values prohibit one from leaving), the person at least is more accepting of this reality.

Various therapists will express the preceeding statement in different terminologies depending upon their primary orientation. They will also emphasize different modalities of disturbance and change, but not exclude any of them. What is unique about group psychotherapy is the attachments formed among group members and the importance they have in each other's lives, albeit only temporarily.

It is tempting but incorrect to say, in a spirit of integration, that all therapists do pretty much the same things. However eclectic or integration-minded therapists are, they can be differentiated by the way they conduct group therapy. Their dominant school of therapeutic thought will be revealed in how active they are in a group and, most particularly, by the type of comments they make in their attempts to be helpful. Are most of the comments about group process, interpersonal conflicts, intrapsychic events, cognitions, empathy, or what? Is the focus on here-and-now feelings, individual problems, symptoms, events inside or outside the group?

The best part of psychotherapy integration for this writer is that he can focus on all of the above and more at one time or another, and still return to his principal orientation of cognitive psychotherapy (Raimy, 1975; Wessler, 1990) and self-confirmation theory (Andrews, 1991). One can move across modalities rather than neglect significant issues that one's theory may not cover. One can learn about relationships in therapy by exploring object relations theory, without subscribing to its account of the development of the self (Cashdan, 1988), or understand a cognitive account of depression without neglecting its origins in the personality patterns (Millon, 1981). The concluding section of this chapter illustrates how the writer, in collaboration with Sheenah Hankin, combines these several foci in group psychotherapy (Wessler & Hankin-Wessler, 1989).

COGNITIVE APPRAISAL THERAPY IN GROUPS

Cognitive Appraisal Therapy or CAT contains some distinctive features as an approach to psychotherapy, and when applied in groups it gives nearly equal emphasis to the content of patients' personal and psychological problems, and to the process of interaction that unfolds among the group members. First, the distinguishing features of CAT.

CAT began as a cognitively oriented therapy, the work of Beck (1976), Ellis (1962), and Raimy (1975) forming its initial foundations. As it developed, greater importance was given to affect and to the affective aspects of the self. Thus, its basic concept, called personal rules of living, is the cognitive core around which much of the rest of the approach revolves, but it does not exclude other concepts. Personal rules are algorithms and cognitions pertaining to what a person knows and how that person thinks he or she and others should act. Knowledge and personal values combine to provide a guidebook for the appraisal of events, and of self and others. One of the important rules, which is largely unconscious, concerns how the individual should feel.

We postulate an emotional setpoint that prescribes, in effect, how one should feel. Deviations from this setpoint start a self-correcting process to return the individual's feelings to their customary state. A person who typically feels anxious, for example, when faced with success or affection, will engage in behaviors and/or perceptual and conceptual distortions that replace any good feelings with the more usual anxiety. Behaviors that result in a return to "normal" are called *security seeking maneuvers*, to acknowledge their mission of restoring the sense of security that familiar feelings bring. Distorted cognitions have the same effect; the person tends to regard them as truthful all the while knowing that they are not factual. These distortions, known as justifying cognitions, are particularly troublesome in a cognitive psychotherapy because they cannot be challenged on factual grounds—the person already knows and admits that they are not factual and do not make sense, but continues to act and feel as though they are truthful.

Affect serves as motivation to restore the setpoint, neither to feel too much better or too much worse than what is prescribed. Such familiarity of feeling provides a sense of security even when the felt affect is negative. The strong tendency to preserve the familiar works against change in therapy, as the person experiences gains only to face setbacks to progress due to need to have familiarity and security. These feelings provide confirmation about the self, by furnishing information about who we are. By behaving in ways that pull predictable responses from others, thereby stimulating certain affects, the individual engages in an unwitting set of interpersonal maneuvers that bring the security of both predictable responses from the environment and emotional feelings that confirm one's sense of self.

Further rationale and justification for CAT as an individual therapy is presented elsewhere (Wessler, 1993, in press). It is enough to say that the approach goes beyond cognitive psychotherapy, and explicitly integrates a focus on affect, interpersonal behavior, and self-confirmation notions, with more than a passing allusion to object relations principles.

The ultimate goal of CAT is the same as most other approaches to treatment. To help the individual reach self-defined goals, or correct maladaptive behavioral patterns, or to relate better to other people, or to feel less anxiety, depression, and so forth. In a phrase, the goal of almost any psychotherapy is to improve the individual's quality of life.

CAT does this by identifying less-than-functional rules, typical affects, and characteristic behavioral and cognitive maneuvers that provide a sense of security while preserving a lesser quality of life. Insights into one's patterns of thinking, emoting, and interacting are sought and repeatedly discussed with the patient. Therapist and patient together attempt to devise ways to work against these well-entrenched patterns, to recognize setbacks as motivated by a need for security, and to try again to attempt the unfamiliar. A solid therapeutic relationship is essential, cognitive insight is a goal, affect is regarded as something to learn about and from, not something to control, and a strong sense of personal responsibility (such as living up to one's consciously held rules) is encouraged.

What follows is an illustration of how these notions work in group psychotherapy, using an 8 member, 10 one and one-half hour session closed-end example. Longer closed-end groups are just as feasible as are open-ended groups. In an open-ended group there is less use of formal feedback periods, and more attention to personal issues presented by group members. There are planned themes for each group meeting in the 10-session format. These are:

1. Introduction and initial presentation of self
2. Feedback about first impressions
3. and 4. Current issues in each member's life.
5. and 6. In-depth understanding of past and present relationships
7. and 8. Open—to be used as needed by group members
9. Member-to-member feedback
10. Feedback to and from the therapist

Session 1

The emphasis in this first session is on content. Group members are asked to introduce themselves and to say something about their goals for therapy. Each of the 8 members uses about 10 minutes. It is not a monologue, as the therapist encourages members to ask the type of questions that promote getting acquainted with each other. The therapist also sets the tone for this in subsequent sessions, urging openness, dealing with issues of trust and confidentiality, and other rules for the group.

Session 2

In this session process is the focus. Each member is asked to give feedback to each other member about his or her initial impressions. In particular, group members are asked to describe their feelings about each person. (These will be compared to feedback given during Sessions 9 and 10.) The purpose of this procedure is to give each member an opportunity to learn about the impression he or she makes, and the impressions he or she gives off, and what feelings he or she inspires in others—in short, to discover the impact of one's self-presentation on other people and how one pulls responses from other people (projective identifications, in object relations terms). This is also a time when members can learn about the expectations about other people they bring to a new situation (transferences), and they can compare their biases against reality as defined by each person (who can protest, "I'm not like that") and consensually by the group ("We don't see the person that way").

Sessions 3 and 4

There is time during each session for four persons to present problems on which they wish to work in therapy. These are here-and-now issues which the therapist will work on with the assistance of group members. Interventions featured are characteristic of CAT, and of behavior therapy (such as the assigning of homework), of problem-solving therapy (Rose, 1989), and Rogerian counseling (the feeling of empathy and its communication). Group members are told to be empathetic and to share similar experiences, provided they have had any, but not to give advice or tell the focal person what he or she is thinking, feeling, or what his or her motivations are. The therapist stops an offending group member, and uses the occasion to illustrate and model more appropriate responses, and to encourage compliance with the sharing of experiences rule.

Sessions 5 and 6

Four persons per session explore in depth their present and particularly their past relationships. Each is led to review his or her personal developmental history of interpersonal relationships, and the interpersonal schemata that have resulted. For the focal person, the connections between past and present are sought, with the gaining of insights into present attitudes and relationships. For other group members, this is a time of discovering similarities between self and others. The therapist encourages empathetic relating by requiring each person to comment or question the focal person. Comments may be in the form of feedback or of shared experiences ("Something like that happened to me, too"). Questions are the least one can do to participate in the life of the focal person; even if one has no similar experiences one can seek to know more about someone else. By requiring full group participation, the therapist can work against the evasiveness that sometimes develops as an informal group norm; that is, group members sometimes handle shame by tacitly agreeing not to confront one another about anything that might produce shame. Since a tactic in CAT is to confront one's shame rather than avoid it, it is important to counteract this common tendency to "respect" another's privacy and not commit the social error of stimulating shame. Group therapy, however, is not an ordinary social situation, but a time to penetrate both individual and group defenses.

Sessions 7 and 8

These sessions provide a break in therapist-imposed structure and allow participants to return to a presentation of individual issues. Everything that has been developed within the group during the previous sessions can be used here. By now most group members can confront one another and give feedback by speaking about their feelings. Issues within the group are less likely to be dealt with here than issues outside the group. However, since patients have had some opportunity to work on their problems during the prior several weeks, noncompliance, procrastination, oppositionality, and other forms of avoidance come up frequently. Group members are urged to express their feelings about persons' failure to work on their problems, but not to condemn them for it. Empathy and sharing are stressed, advice and scolding not permitted.

Session 9

As in the second session, feedback from each person to each person is formally sought. Comparisons between initial and subsequent impressions are made, and the focal person can learn about his or her interpersonal style and about any attempts he or she made to modify it. The focus of this session is on changes (or lack) each person has made. The individual can compare what he or she perceives about himself or herself with what others notice. During this session in particular, strong feelings, either positive or negative, are expressed about others.

Session 10

Although this is nominally time for feedback to and from the therapist, in practice the first portion of the session is used to finish comments from Session 9. The therapist has probably given continuous feedback to each member during their weeks together, but this is a chance to do so more formally, and to hear what group members' feelings are about the therapist. It is also a time for deciding on the future course of treatment for each person and/or the continuation of the group for additional sessions.

In summary, this version of group therapy quite intentionally incorporates aspects of the other approaches mentioned above. It does so because CAT is not only concerned with surface issues (a criticism, not altogether unfair, leveled at behavior and cognitive therapies) but with broader aspects of personality and of genetic explanation as well. However, CAT is also concerned with current events in people's lives, and so includes problem-solving and behavioral homework. In addition, should lack of emotional expression be a problem in a specific group, tactics to promote emotional expression, such as those associated with psychodrama and gestalt therapy, can be integrated into the procedures. The use of guided imagery, for example, is explicitly included in the early sessions of some groups where members have difficulty opening up about themselves (Wessler & Hankin, 1988).

This version of group psychotherapy is hardly the last word on the subject. It is presented only as an example of integration and of what is possible when one is willing to cross therapeutic boundaries. It is a more-or-less technical integration around a core of theoretical assumptions that are themselves more-or-less integrated as CAT.

If I may close on a personal note, I once was asked at a Society for Exploration of Psychotherapy Integration meeting why a cognitive psychotherapist (as I was identified by the questioner) would be interested in his approach to therapy, as though the lines between his approach and another could not be crossed. I did not answer very well, but mumbled something about my not being a conventional cognitive psychotherapist. But the question stuck in my mind, as though there was something suspect with wanting to expand one's view of human nature and find additional ideas about helping patients. (Incidentally, I respect my questioner's views, and some of his ideas are included in this chapter.) May more boundaries be crossed as we learn about and from each other.

REFERENCES

Andrews, J. D. W. (1991). *The active self in psychotherapy.* Boston: Allyn & Bacon.

Beck, A. T. (1976). *Cognitive therapy and the emotional disorders.* New York: International Universities Press.

Cashdan, S. (1988). *Object relations therapy.* New York: Norton.

Corsini, R. J. (1988). Adlerian groups. In S. Long (Ed.), *Six group therapies* (pp. 1–48). New York: Plenum Press.

Ellis, A. (1962). *Reason and emotion in psychotherapy.* New York: Lyle Stuart.

Goldfried, M. R. (1980). Towards the delineation of therapeutic change principles. *American Psychologist, 35,* 991–999.

Grimes, J. (1988). Transactional analysis in group work. In S. Long (Ed.), *Six group therapies* (pp. 49–114). New York: Plenum Press.

Harman, R. L. (1988). Gestalt group therapy. In S. Long (Ed.), *Six group therapies* (pp. 217–256). New York: Plenum Press.

Herink, R. (Ed.). (1980). *The psychotherapy handbook.* New York: New American Library.

Hollon, S. D., & Shaw, B. F. (1979). Group cognitive therapy for depressed patients. In A. T. Beck, A. J. Rush, B. F. Shaw, & G. Emery (Eds.), *Cognitive therapy of depression* (pp. 328–353). New York: Guilford.

Johnson, F. (1988). Encounter group therapy. In S. Long (Ed.), *Six group therapies* (pp. 115–158). New York: Plenum Press.

Kissen, M. (1981). Exploring general systems processes in group settings. *Psychotherapy, 18,* 424–430.

Lange, A. J., & Jakubowski, P. (1976). *Responsible assertive behavior.* Champaign, IL: Research Press.

Meichenbaum, D. H. (1977). *Cognitive-behavior modification.* New York: Plenum Press.

Millon, T. (1981). *Disorders of personality.* New York: Wiley.

Nathanson, D. L. (1987). The shame-pride axis. In H. B. Lewis (Ed.), *The role of shame in symptom formation* (pp. 183–206). Hillsdale, NJ: Lawrence Erlbaum.

Novaco, R. W. (1978). Anger and coping with stress. In J. Foreyt & D. Rathjen (Eds.), *Cognitive behavior therapy: Therapy, research, and practice* (pp. 135–162). New York: Plenum Press.

Plutchik, R. (1981). Group cohesion in psychoevolutionary context. In H. Kellerman (Ed.), *Group cohesion* (pp. 133–140). Baltimore: Grune & Stratton.

Raimy, V. (1975). *Misconceptions of the self.* San Francisco: Jossey-Bass.

Rose, S. D. (1989). *Working with adults in groups.* San Francisco: Jossey-Bass.

Rosenbaum, M. (1976). Group psychotherapies. In B. B. Wolman (Ed.), *The therapist's handbook: Treatment methods of mental disorders* (pp. 163–183). New York: Van Nostrand.

Sank, L. I., & Shaffer, C. S. (1984). *A therapist's manual for cognitive behavior therapy in groups.* New York: Plenum Press.

Wessler, R. L. (1984). Cognitive-social psychological theories and social skills: A review. In P. Trower (Ed.), *Radical approaches to social skills training* (pp. 111–141). London: Croom-Helm.

Wessler, R. L. (1990). Cognitive appraisal therapy. In J. K. Zeig, & W. M. Munion (Eds.), *What is psychotherapy?* (pp. 155–159). San Francisco: Jossey-Bass.

Wessler, R. L. (1993, in press). Cognitive appraisal therapy and disorders of personality. In K. T. Kvehlwein & H. Rosen (Eds.), *Cognitive therapy in action: Evolving innovative practice.* San Francisco: Jossey-Bass.

Wessler, R. L., & Hankin, S. (1988). Rational-emotive therapy and related cognitively oriented psychotherapies. In S. Long (Ed.), *Six group therapies* (pp. 159–216). New York: Plenum Press.

Wessler, R. L., & Hankin-Wessler, S. (1989). Cognitive group therapy. In A. Freeman, H. Arkowtiz, L. E. Beutler, & K. E. Simon (Eds.), *Comprehensive handbook of cognitive therapy* (pp. 559–581). New York: Plenum Press.

Yalom, I. D. (1985). *The theory and practice of group psychotherapy.* New York: Basic Books.

CHAPTER 32

An Integrative Approach to Psychotherapy with Black/African Americans

THE RELEVANCE OF RACE AND CULTURE

Anderson J. Franklin, Robert T. Carter, and Cynthia Grace

This chapter is written for the purpose of bringing together a somewhat disparate body of knowledge about treatment with Black/African American patients.[1] We attempt to offer a view consistent with the goals of the handbook, in that we try to integrate the more recent theoretical concepts, research findings, and clinical thinking about psychotherapy with Blacks using knowledge about multisystems and racial identity development. Our particular perspective can be used in treating Blacks because it offers a unique and meaningful framework to conceptualizing a dynamic context for patients and therapist's behavior both in and out of therapy.

THE NEED FOR THEORETICAL INTEGRATION

During the training of many psychotherapists, one theoretical orientation is taught and many trainees and professionals are strongly encouraged to adopt a specific therapy framework. During our training we often heard the question, "What is your theoretical orientation?" This type of query often represented the direct and often not-so-subtle message that one needed to be identified with a particular theoretical orientation almost to the exclusion of initially understanding the individual in his or her psychological world and social context. In our training, there is virtually no emphasis on evolving a theoretical orientation from first an insight about the patient's

---

[1] We will use *African American* and *Black* interchangeably to refer and reflect the diversity of people with African heritage.

Anderson J. Franklin • Doctoral Program in Clinical Psychology, City College of the City University of New York, New York, New York 10031.   **Robert T. Carter** • Doctoral Program in Counseling Psychology, Teachers College, Columbia University, New York, New York 10031. **Cynthia Grace** • Department of Psychology, City College of the City University of New York, New York, New York 10031.

Comprehensive Handbook of Psychotherapy Integration, edited by George Stricker and Jerold R. Gold. Plenum Press, New York, 1993.

human condition, social ecology, or "psycho-ethno-history"; this, in spite of the fact, that our theory building comes from our knowledge of, and interaction with, a patient population having distinct personal legacies.

As a consequence, must psychotherapists become proponents of a primary theoretical orientation, psychoanalytic, behavioral, cognitive-behavioral, humanistic, psychodynamic and so forth? Although these approaches to understanding human behavior and motivation offer a unique view and often have associated with them a particular treatment approach, they all are grounded in the assumptions of Euro-American culture to the exclusion of other operative diverse factors and influences which may shape an individual's psychological world.

When other influences that shape one's identity are not included in the therapeutic process, a number of things may occur that prevent the therapy from being effective. Therapists can have difficulty in their assessment of the client or in conceptualization of the problem presented, they may have problems in forming a therapeutic alliance or relationship, they may not see the patient as a person, or as a Black person who is healthy but different from what the theoretical orientation dictates.

We believe that in order to understand the influences which affect the lives and intrapsychic dynamics of Blacks, it is essential to conceptualize the forces and influences which affect their life and psychological make-up in terms of a systems model. A multisystems/racial identity model will be used as a way to represent the various influences which affect Black people's psychological development. We believe it is essential for therapists to have this macro perspective in their efforts to address treatment issues with Black Americans. However, we should note that our approach will focus primarily on how the various macro influences manifest themselves in the person's intrapsychic system and as a consequence have relevance for their psychological functioning and ultimately strategies for psychotherapeutic intervention.

In this manner we conceptualize the elements and components associated with Black/African Americans' psychological functioning as a system. Thus, the sociocultural system which influences Blacks' lives is seen as having inter-dependent, interconnected, and interactive elements or units. In addition, participants (i.e., therapists and patients) in the system have a history together and relate to one another in relatively stable and consistent ways. We will not talk about sociocultural forces that influence the therapist–patient system as much as note that each are products of experiences which help form attitudes, assumptions, and beliefs about each other as people and representatives of their respective racial/ethnic groups.

For our purposes the whole system is American society and is characterized by its dominant cultural patterns (Carter, 1990a; Stewart & Bennett, 1991). And each racial/cultural group—Blacks, Whites, and members of other racial and cultural groups—also contains separate subsystems within the larger dominant culture. Therefore, in considering the treatment of African Americans, one must take into account the total pattern of intrapsychic dynamics, family system, sociocultural influences, economic resources, and community that has evolved over time and which regulates the interactions of the various sociocultural groups with the dominant culture. The behavior of each individual as a member of a racial/cultural group is therefore seen in the context of the whole system.

The life and psychological patterns of Blacks are a manifestation of the structure of the general society and how the society has regulated their role in American life and within their own communities and families. Boundaries within the system may be communicated to racial/cultural groups in many forms. For instance, ideas and beliefs about Black Americans may serve as one type of feedback (e.g., stereotypes); institutional inclusion or exclusion may be another way the dominant society communicates to Blacks their status and importance in the society. Socioeconomic resource distribution or labor force participation or the lack of it may also serve as a feedback mechanism that communicates the relative worth of some members of the society. Blacks have been excluded and minimized from participating in American society for much of their history in the United States. This type of message can have various psychological implications for individual African Americans.

Given this context, therapists who treat Black patients, utilizing our multisystems/racial identity perspective can develop formulations about Black/African Americans with a clear sense of how the forces of the environment affect an individual's psychological functioning. In addition, they can begin to understand how these social system factors and their own personal and group legacy affect their psychological framework and clinical perspective.

We argue that the systems perspective is more appropriate for treating Black people because the "systems" conceptual frame is the best vehicle for thinking about and developing effective interventions for the multiple problems that impinge on the psychological functioning of many blacks. The systems perspective is useful because it provides an orientation to problems and intervention strategies that allows for easier integration, and it gives coherence to complex issues. However, it is essential that therapists first work to understand their own cultural perspectives and the manner in which their racial and cultural perspectives of Blacks affects their treatment approaches and clinical conceptualizations.

We will briefly discuss the specific system influences upon the individual African American patient who presents himself or herself for treatment. Each individual black person must develop a sense of self or personal identity, within the context of his or her blackness or racial identity. One's identity must develop within a family system, the family must operate within a community, and the community functions within a society. Each African American's personality develops and integrates, in unique dynamic ways, responses to his or her race and skin color as well as myriads of other interacting personal experiences. Race is such a profound and salient life motif for African Americans (as well as whites and immigrants) that it must be incorporated into a theoretical and clinical framework. For example, skin color, facial features and hair texture, while relatively unimportant to members of some other ethnic groups, have played a significant role in the lives of African Americans (R. Jones, 1991). The "survivor's achievement guilt" that some economically successful African Americans experience when the majority of the Black community, including family members, remain impoverished or marginal puts a unique cast on entitlement conflicts. The multisystems/racial identity perspective provides

a framework for understanding these issues in psychotherapy with African Americans. It represents sociocultural realities in a fashion that assists therapists to comprehend better the psychodynamic organization and multiple problem focus of African American individuals and families. Moreover, the many issues brought to therapy by African Americans are emotionally loaded and infused with the messages and assumptions which specifically underlie being Black in America. The task of therapists working with African American patients is differentiating the mediating racial themes, from common developmental life stresses, and from fundamental pathology.

THE CONCEPTUAL FRAMEWORK: SYSTEMS ORIENTATION

Many social scientists and practitioners have struggled with the structure and condition of the Black family, comprehending its functioning and dynamics beyond the simplicity of nuclear family structure to a more complex extended family structure (Billingsley, 1968; Boyd-Franklin, 1989; McAdoo, 1988; McAdoo & McAdoo, 1985). It does not matter which *income group* of African Americans you treat—the extended family in Black life is profound, with extended family members playing an influential role in their lives. This family structure includes blood and fictive, or nonblood, kin. The powerful person in the family system may or may not be the most obvious, such as the father or mother. On the contrary, grandparents, aunts or uncles may be pivotal figures in the black family system, and the influence could be felt irrespective of residential location. Moreover, traditional labels may be misleading, since it is common for children to attach labels of aunt, uncle or cousin out of respect to friends considered as family. There is no "*the* Black family." Noting the empirical assumption that there is more diversity within than between groups, this holds true within the Black community. Black families are diversified by ethnic background such as African American, delineating descendants of African slaves in America, Afro-Caribbean, which reflects immigrant generations from the West Indies, African Latino, which includes descendants of Africans from Central and South America, and African immigrants. Of course, intermarriage between each of these groups brings the merger of values and practices to family life from each ethnic group orientation. Moreover, regional differences distinguish the Black families with distinct northern versus southern families as well as differences in generations of blacks in the Midwest and West. This is not to dismiss strong sharing of a Black experience, and certain values, traditions and practices which form group identity. Although there are differences among Black families, there is a cultural bond, particularly one which is shaped by experiences of disenfranchisement, discrimination, and racism. The similarities and differences of Black families present the challenge to psychotherapy. They also underscore the importance of utilizing a variety of knowledge bases and skills to maximize treatment interventions in individual, group, family and other forms of psychotherapy with Blacks.

To view the extended family as a primary organizing structure for the Black family is important. For example, the values and strengths of the Black family as presented by Hill (1972, 1977) are illustrative of how both structure and process operate within the Black family system. In characterizing the strengths of Black families, Hill talks about adaptability of roles, strong kinship bonds, strong work orientation, high achievement orientation, and strong religious orientation. Within these strengths represented by Hill are essential features of the structure and process of Black life. It is also illustrative of multisystems at work. For example, children are often shared among extended family members for child rearing. This is often done to relieve parents of child care while working and/or further educational achievement is being pursued. Therefore, sending a child South to family, for example, is quite common. A child could be sent because extended family members in the South may be more effective at controlling a behavior problem or providing another context to reduce the odds of a child getting into trouble. An aunt assuming a parental role for a sister's child or the more common grandmother taking care of her daughter's child is an illustration not only of the manner in which the family system can be utilized but also the strength through adaptability of roles.

Adaptability of roles in Black families presents a unique challenge to clinical assumptions and hypotheses generated by therapists. It also is a good context for utilizing the integrative approach to psychotherapy. Within this one family domain are both structure and value at work. To maximize family functioning, the extended family network is engaged as well as prized for role flexibility. It also adds to the complexity of family dynamics. A common example is determining who is the more influential parental figure, mother or grandmother, and how this impacts the therapeutic process. Often school problems of children potentially expose the degree of influence family members have. Parental influence can often be obscured by school authorities assuming nuclear family members (such as the biological mother) are the power brokers, when it could be matriarchical grandaunt.

Likewise, when considering the socialization of racial identity (i.e., the extent to which individuals identify with their racial group membership), family influences may also be equally differential. For example, many children during their pilgrimages to the South get a southern Black orientation to the history and experiences of racism, frequently framed by grandparents, or grand aunts and uncles. Consequently, children who move about the extended family network will be influenced by the values and orientation determined by the time spent in certain circumstances over others. This flexibility in child care, as well as occasions of informal adoption (i.e., nonparental family members assuming primary care of the child) can create a rich foundation of experiences affecting personal development (Hill, 1977; Stack, 1975). It can also account for differences in value orientation as well as value clashes within a family system. Unraveling the influences of the Black family is identifying parts of a system and determining its interrelationships. Even when one has few current direct ties to extended family, this circumstance can often have clinical significance, particularly in childhood experiences.

Understanding the influences and dynamics within a family system is also comprehending the multitude of external factors impacting the family as a unit. This constitutes the community, a system of structural and dynamic forces which come from the social institutions within the community, such as church, school, health, and human services. Each one of these entities forms a system within its own right affecting the family system. Of course, within that family system is the individual whom we consider is integrating these forces into a psychodynamic constellation of structure and process which forms character and style of relating to the world. We also strongly emphasize that all of these forces be considered within the special circumstance of racism and African American psychohistory (R. Jones, 1991; Kovel, 1970; Levine, 1977; White & Parham, 1990). This cannot be ignored, for the pervasiveness of racial and cultural themes is consistently present in our professional work with Black patients. Moreover, we state this position with the clear recognition of the pitfalls of the "color blind" and the "color myopic" orientation to the affectively loaded issue of race and psychotherapy (Thomas & Sillen, 1972). The former position attributes nothing to racial influence, and the latter attributes all factors to racial influence. Conceptualizing the individual in a world of interacting systems, therefore, is the fundamental basis and framework underlying an integrative psychotherapeutic strategy for African Americans. It involves distilling the dynamic transmissions between macro and micro systems. Such an approach, we believe, leads toward the development of a model of therapy which is better grounded and suited for the type of circumstances forming African American life. Perhaps an appropriate characterization is that it is more ecologically grounded.

This task is difficult for at least two reasons. First, it is theory building from the interactions of macro and micro systems within a social and cultural framework, and second, it subsequently requires demonstrating appropriate psychotherapy applications for individuals we consider as products of unique group psychosocial experiences. Clearly, it is no easy task, but we believe the strategy is correct. To further the possibilities of this approach, let us examine how developing racial identity interacts with and/or is a product of multisystems impacting the individual. We take racial identity as an example because it illustrates many of the features characterizing our approach to psychotherapy integration. Acknowledging the Black family as the socializing system and nurturer of racial identity, we will use this knowledge of the Black family to incorporate the larger social community systems. Social and community systems through the family form the theoretical and empirical basis of racial identity developments and the multilevel dimensions which determine some of the psychodynamic issues for psychotherapy with African Americans.

RACIAL IDENTITY DEVELOPMENT

In this section, we will present the relationship between racial and personal identity preceded by a discussion of how racial identity is a byproduct of the interaction of various social, family, and intrapsychic systems.

Personal identity is presumed to be made up of the dynamic interaction between one's self image, one's attitudes, beliefs, and feelings, which occur within an intrapsychic domain. That is, a person's "identity" is a complex integration of each person's sociocultural context, physical characteristics, personality attributes, unique experiences, and personal choices (Badad, Birnbaum, & Benne, 1983). Thus, within the context of one's family, each individual is believed to develop a constellation of characteristics which make up his or her personal identity. It is also true that our personalities are also "products" of various social identities. Some of our social identities are chosen, like religion and our political perspective, while others we are born with, such as race, gender, and ethnicity. There are various potential social identifies, and many are salient; however, we will focus on racial identity, in part because it has not received as much attention as other social identities, nor has it been given the same amount of attention as personal identity.

Racial group membership based on race *per se* is not a sufficient criterion for cultural group membership. That is, it is not appropriate to assume that all Blacks (or Whites) are the same psychologically because of their racial category, or that they share a common culture because they share a common racial category. It is possible for individuals to respond differently to their sociocultural environment and particular socialization experiences.

Furthermore, the legacy of racial attitudes of Blacks and Whites and their consequent behavior has affected individuals' psychosocial and cultural development (Helms, 1990; Kovel, 1970). Although many Blacks (and Whites) in America are subject to similar social norms and racial attitudes, Blacks (and Whites) might vary with respect to their psychological response to racial inequality. Therefore, to consider Blacks or Whites as a homogeneous group is probably as erroneous as the application of most Anglo-Saxon paradigms to racial/ethnic groups. The most promising models for examining psychological differences within racial groups are the Racial Identity Models (cf. Cross, 1978; Helms, 1990). Racial identity attitudes or stages are composed of attitudes, thoughts, feelings, and behaviors toward both oneself as a black or white person and Blacks and Whites as members of groups.

Cross (1978) hypothesizes a five-stage process of racial identity development for Black Americans that begins at a stage called *preencounter*, which is characterized by dependency on white society for definition and approval. Racial identity attitudes toward one's blackness are negative, and one views white culture and society as the ideal. The next stage is called *encounter*, and it is entered when one has a personal and challenging experience with Black or White society. The encounter stage is marked by feelings of confusion about the meaning and significance of race and an increasing desire to become more aligned with one's Black identity. The *immersion-emersion* stage follows the encounter experience, and it is characterized by a period of idealization of Black culture and intense negative feelings toward Whites and White culture. One is absorbed in the Black experience and completely rejects the White world. Immersion is followed by *internalization*; during the internalization stage, one has grasped the fact that both Blacks and Whites have strengths and weaknesses. In addition, one's Black identity is experienced as positive and an important and valued aspect of self. Therefore, one's world view is Afrocentric. One's attitude toward Whites is one of tolerance and respect for differences. *Internalization-commitment* is the last stage and reflects active involvement in promoting the welfare of black people (Goss, 1991). Empirical studies (Cross, 1991) involving racial identity have found it to be associated differentially with cultural value preferences (Carter & Helms, 1987), psychological functioning (Carter, 1991), self-esteem (Parham & Helms, 1985a), emotional states (Parham & Helms, 1985b), cognitive styles (Helms & Parham, 1990), psychotherapy process (Carter, 1990c; Pomales, Claiborn, & LaFromboise, 1986), and preference for race, gender, and social class of therapists (Helms & Carter, 1992;

Parham & Helms, 1981). What has been missing from the psychological literature is a consideration of how racial identity for Whites might influence their perceptions of Blacks and other racial/ethnic group people.

Whites may as a result of their dominant status in this country choose to develop or not develop racial identity. Whites, according to Helms (1984, 1990), can potentially move through a five-stage process. The first or lowest level of white racial identity development is *contact*. During this stage, the person is not aware of himself or herself or others in racial terms; in other words, the person at this level of development denies the importance of race and racial issues. Contact is followed by *disintegration*, which is entered as the person becomes aware of social norms and pressures associated with cross-racial interactions, either through confusing experiences with Blacks or negative reactions by Whites to interracial association. During this stage, the person is forced to acknowledge that he or she is White. The individual at this stage, according to Helms's (1984, 1990) theory, is "caught between internal standards of human decency and external cultural expectations" (p. 10). In order to cope with or resolve these negative feelings, the person may interact with Blacks or avoid contact with them altogether. The person who chooses to move forward toward Blacks may experience rejection by them. The rejection leads to feelings of helplessness and triggers movement to the reintegration stage of racial identity. During the *reintegration* stage, the person exhibits feelings of fear, anger, and hostility toward Blacks. The individual develops anti-Black and pro-White attitudes and sees Blacks stereotypically. However, "if the individual uses these feelings to become more aware of their whiteness and attempts to understand the sociopolitical implications of being White in a racist society, then it is possible that feelings of anger and fear will dissipate" (Helms, 1984, p. 148), which then leads to the final stages of white racial identity. The final stages, *pseudoindependence* and *autonomy*, are characterized by an acceptance of both Black and White cultures. Racially bound differences and similarities between the two groups are realized. The differences between the two stages are that the pseudoindependence person views similarities and differences with intellectual interest and is able to maintain emotional distance between herself or himself and racial issues, whereas the autonomous person values and actively seeks out interracial interactions and understands the personal implications of racial issues.

Empirical studies have found White racial identity attitudes were differentially associated with preference for counselor's race and respondents' gender and social class (Helms & Carter, 1991), cultural values (Carter & Helms, 1990), psychotherapy process (Carter, 1988, 1990c; Carter & Helms, 1992), self-actualization (Tokar & Swanson, 1991), and Whites' racist attitudes (Carter, 1990b). Taken together, these studies provide evidence that White racial identity attitudes influence a number of psychological and cultural variables and highlight the importance of the usefulness of this within group psychological variable. White racial identity attitudes can be used to help explain and understand the appropriate developmental tasks White therapists should undertake in their efforts to be effective in treatment with Black patients. Clearly their effectiveness will be determined in part by their own level of racial identity development and that of their patients, particularly since one's racial identity seems to guide one's thoughts, feelings, and behaviors.

Racial identity evolves as an aspect of one's personal identity and is influenced by several factors. Most children in American society are aware of racial differences from the age of 3 or 4 (Clark, 1988). Therefore, one's racial identity may begin to develop at these early ages and may be affected in many ways. As noted above, trips to visit extended family may have an effect, as would one's skin color as well as that of other family members, family composition, and their racial attitudes. Racial identity development is affected by the manner in which race is denied, avoided, or discussed in the family system or other systems interacting with the family, the racial make-up of one's community, and whether the school discusses, avoids, or denies racial issues. All of these factors can influence the individual's racial identity development process.

For example, a Black person who is light skinned and comes from a family that denies the importance and significance of race may grow up holding similar beliefs and thus may develop preencounter attitudes. Suppose though that this person grew up in a predominantly Black community; he or she might be the object of envy and hostility because of their physical features and consequently may have a harder time denying the significance of race and thus may develop encounter or Immersion-Emersion attitudes.

Personal and racial identity components can operate independently of one another, for example, a Black or White person might feel good about himself or herself, may believe the experiences of racial group members as of little significance to his or her life experience, and feel a commitment to no particular group. Personal and racial identities, nevertheless, interact with each other. As Helms (1990) notes,

To the extent that society stereotypes one racial group as "dirty," "shiftless," and "ignorant" and another as "clean," "industrious," and "intelligent" and can enforce such stereotypes, then it is likely that the individual will find it easier to use the second rather than the first as a reference group. It is apparent that under these circumstances identifying with the group which is seen in more positive terms will tend to feeling more positively about oneself than if one does not. However, this type of identification may become problematic if it requires denial and distortions of oneself and/or the racial group(s) from which one descends. (p. 21)

Just as individual experiences shape personal development, so does racial identity. Since these individuals can come to be therapists or patients, their individual developmental process can influence their therapeutic interaction. For instance, therapists at the preencounter or contact stages of development who are working with a Black client that stirs up these issues may avoid racial issues and may reject the client either by referral or by providing impersonal treatment (i.e., medication), or the therapist may deny his or her own feelings regarding racial issues and, consequently, deny his or her client's feelings also. It is also possible for therapists who are at low levels of racial identity development to deny the client's color and strive to react to the client as though he or she were not Black. They might take a color blind approach (Sager, Brayboy, & Waxenberg, 1972). In such cases, the therapist may wish simply to exercise power and dominate the relationship (i.e., have the client accommodate to the therapist). The dominating and powerful therapist, who denies the client's role and input into the relationship, typically behaves in a paternalistic, patronizing fashion (Jackson, 1973; Jones & Seagull, 1977; Seward, 1972; Vontress, 1971b).

Therapists at low levels of racial identity development (e.g., reintegration, disintegration, encounter or immersion-emersion) may view the Black client as emotionally and cognitively damaged by racism and oppression (Thomas & Sillen, 1972). For example, the therapist may view the Black client as a victim of racism and consequently may feel guilty. The therapist's guilt feelings might lead him or her to overindulge the client (Adams, 1950; Cooper, 1973; Gardner, 1971; Turner & Armstrong, 1981; Vontress, 1971a). The therapist's guilt feelings might also lead him or her to become defensive or to misperceive the Black client's emotional expressions (Grier & Cobbs, 1968). Therapists who engage in psychotherapy with Blacks who have ignored their own developmental process are likely to be confronted with a myriad of difficulties which stem from their own attitudes, motives, and knowledge of and experience with their own culture (e.g., Parker & McDavis, 1983; Vontress, 1971b). However, therapists at higher levels of racial identity (e.g., internalization or autonomy) would be more facile at using a multisystems approach because of the learning that occurred during their own racial identity developmental process. Through their development they have come to know and understand the various forces that affect the minds and lives of many Black (and White) people (Carter & Helms, 1992).

THE PSYCHOTHERAPY PROCESS

We do not believe that psychotherapists need to abandon their favored theoretical models; rather, what we advocate is that therapists integrate various models in their efforts to treat Black patients. We argue that it is not possible to be effective in treating Blacks when one uses a single orientation. We contend that the forces which operate to shape the intrapsychic life of individual Blacks are multidimensional and multifaceted and as such *cannot* be fully grasped through the lens of one theoretical model. One orientation does not help therapists learn how the Black person comes to terms with himself or herself as an individual, family member, racial/cultural person, a member of a community, and a member of the larger society.

Our intent has been to show how utilizing the multisystems/racial identity orientation and approach can form a strategy for integrating several perspectives toward the aim of providing effective psychotherapy with Blacks. The multisystems/racial identity approach integrates both sociological and psychological constructs, as well as the empirical and theoretical work from these disciplines. The fundamental steps of therapy are still essential in the process. That is, in meeting a patient some assessment of history and background takes place, as well as a referral process, joining and bonding, treatment, and termination. What governs the psychotherapy process is our model of behavior, psychodynamics, and intervention. There is no model of therapy, much less personality development, that incorporates the Black experience in the formation of its constructs or applications. Efforts in this regard, such as the racial identity models, are only in their infancy, and are often derided as too ethnocentric rather than universal. Our approach has been to use the process of racial identity development to show the utility of a systems orientation to this process in particular as well as conceptualizing treatment for Blacks in general. The following discussion about some aspects of the psychotherapy process with our orientation will further elucidate this position.

Assessing and interpreting history and background information is a critical aspect of the therapeutic process. It provides information, boundaries, dynamics, and framework for a therapist about the patient. If diagnostic assessment instruments are used, the manner in which they are interpreted can be extremely critical to a personal profile. For the assessment area alone, the proper conceptualization of the individual in a multisystem context becomes essential. Black families have too many factors—many of which are the product of race—that determine individual members' personal and socioemotional development. These are not adequately considered in the development, much less interpretation, of assessment instruments. There have been efforts by Black psychologists to address the exclusion of the Black experience in assessment tools by devising their own tests (Williams, 1971). This has become true for other ethnic psychologists who believe there are distinct ethnic sociocultural life experiences which need to be considered in all forms of assessment (Jones, 1988).

An example is taking information about social and/or developmental history of a Black patient. Certainly asking questions about family structure and relationships is important if the client's current functioning is to be fully comprehended. Genograms can assist in this regard; however, they are not encouraged to solicit until joining and bonding has occurred, since many Black people consider asking detailed questions about family intrusive (Boyd-Franklin, 1989). However, questions about significant others who might have played an important role provide information about lines of influence within the life of the individual. What it also conveys is something about the role multisystems play in the process. For example, knowledge about developmental milestones may be with several family members reflecting different times of shared child care. Recall of family history and dynamics may also be influenced by racial identity development. For instance, members in the family from different generations may have ongoing conflicts about how to live and survive in the United States as a Black person. Family elders may opt for the path of least resistance where race is underplayed or denied, reflecting preencounter or encounter attitudes, while family members who do not share the elders' experience with a more racially segregated society may be more aggressive in their behavior, believing in the achievements of Blacks and Africans. Their behavior may reflect internalization attitudes.

Also one of the common areas of misinterpretation is in the use of language, either in responses to formal assessment procedures or interview phases. Language style reflects the multisystem socialization process at its best and can form barriers to communication (Smitherman, 1977). For example, therapists often use first names as a way of reducing formality and aiding the joining process. Such informality is frequently not acceptable by Blacks at an initial meeting with a professional and stranger. In fact, to formally address a Black person by mister or misses is an extension of respect, particularly for elders, and informality should not be assumed until mutually agreed upon (Boyd-Franklin, 1989). The authors all have had Black patients who insisted upon calling us doctor throughout their treatment, and we in turn address them formally, in spite of mutually expressed intent to drop formality.

How a person is addressed in the Black community is an ethnic style fashioned by cultural and social experiences. In African society, elders are held with considerable respect and approached with humility. This legacy continues as an expected code of behavior in some Black families and communities. Further shaping the significance of how a person is addressed is the legacy of slavery, where stature was lessened and a Black person was "kept in place" by using only first names in superficial informality or by using humiliating labels such as calling an adult Black male "boy" or an adult Black female "gal." Consequently, what is used and how you address a person is a form of acknowledgement. For many Blacks, assessing respect and trust begins at introductions. Racism and discrimination psychodynamically can undermine self-esteem; therefore, seeking respectful behavior in initial meetings is one effort to counterbalance these destructive forces.

Another example of multisystems and racial identity interface for African Americans is around the experience of success. Success has many personal definitions and criteria; however, there is still a collective ethnocultural understanding of when you have made it and what are the acceptable indicators of success. For many people, the common indicators are position and money. However, each ethnic group, influenced by its history, creates different feelings about entitlement and how its members are to embrace it, whether with arrogance, guilt, or humility. The following case of a couple is illustrative of how the experience of success is influenced by multisystems socialization and racial identity.

One of the issues between a Black couple in marital therapy was the display of their wealth. He was very understating to manifest his money, dressing casual, frequently "bummy," driving an aged Volkswagen, and often indistinguishable from the average person in manner and appearance. He frequently stated being uncomfortable with his wealth and did not want to draw too much attention to it. His wife, on the other hand, was ostentatious with their money in manner, appearance, and display to the public. Their clashes about the house were related to costs and how much in location and decoration it advertised their wealth. Although both were aware their business and professional entertaining and networking required these accoutrements of wealth, both embraced them differently. Part of the open conflict between the two was determining what was appropriate for African Americans in their positions given their own personal/family history and their professed racial identity, which was expressed in their concern about not getting too far from the life-style of the Black community.

Several systems were behind this conflict for the couple—economically working poor childhoods, family values and expectations about managing success, the church's messages about success, the business/professional community's expectations about success, and society's attitude toward successful African Americans. Mediating their response to these forces were also their respectful levels of racial identity, which for both were at the Immersion-Emersion stage. Though they were in the latter phase of this stage, that is, they were emerging from Immersion and were in the Emersion phase and beginning to enter the Internalization stage, they experienced themselves as African Americans, identified with the psychohistory of the Black experience, particularly through personal experiences of community and family life plus the pain of discrimination and prejudice. Although their daily business and professional life, plus residence, distanced them from the typical Black community life, they maintained a network of African American friends and engaged in ethnic social and cultural activities as much as possible.

Their working poor childhoods were in an environment where few role models had achieved, socially or economically, much beyond their family status. Family values about education as a vehicle for upward mobility often meant becoming a teacher, minister and, if exceptional, a doctor or lawyer, working within the Black community. These were the traditional career options and paths for African Americans. In the church, humility was valued; talents and success were God given (Lincoln & Mamiya, 1990). No one was to become so successful that they would forget their family and community roots. Those who do, bring their racial identity into question and become subject to group sanctions. In contrast business and professional stature pulls for display of success, which competes with African American community values, particularly those which encourage severing ties with ethnic traditions and

practices. This is very often embodied in society's subtle expectation that successful African Americans will be more Euro-American than African American in behavior and values. Messages from the business/professional sector and the African American community form a multisystem with distinct values for internalization. They are forces which influence psychodynamic structure. This couple responded to these forces differently and individually.

Relationship building or joining and bonding is another domain within the psychotherapy process where the multisystems/racial identity knowledge base is useful. Early termination of Blacks in treatment is common, and for Black males it is difficult to get them to therapy at all (Franklin, 1992). Therefore, the initial process of joining and subsequently bonding with the patient for treatment to occur is critical. The development of a therapeutic alliance is heavily dependent upon trust between client and therapist, and the client's ability to tolerate the dependence demands inherent in the relationship. The complicated racial socialization of Black/African Americans and European Americans, as reflected in their respective levels of racial identity, can be an important variable in the process of relationship building. For example, it is helpful in understanding when and whether Blacks will self-disclose. Although client self-disclosure is generally considered essential for maximizing therapeutic outcomes, complex intrapersonal, interpersonal, and social factors often affect the Black client's willingness to self-disclose (Ridley, 1984).

Grier and Cobbs (1968) have suggested that the tendency for African Americans who are culturally identified (i.e., Immersion-Emersion and Internalization stages) not to trust white Americans is a healthy and expected response to the history of White oppression. They refer to this phenomenon as "healthy cultural paranoia." To the extent that the White or Black therapist exhibits racial identity attitudes that are comparable or more advanced than those of the client, then the establishment of a therapeutic alliance can proceed provided that the other factors that enhance the relationship are in place (see Helms, 1990). In addition, many other systems may influence why and how a Black person seeks and enters treatment. All of these factors may affect relationship building.

Many Black families and individuals enter treatment because they were referred by agencies and/or a host of significant others coaxing them into the process, such as traditional community service providers like their ministers, doctors, neighbors, or friends. They have already experienced several systems, some operating on their behalf and for their welfare and some not. It is rare that Blacks approach therapy in the orthodox manner of self-exploration common to the private practice model.

One way that multiple systems operate in the referral process is the frequent distrust of conventional therapy among Blacks. Herein is another area where our explanatory model may be useful. This distrust can be understood within the framework of multisystems which shaped an attitude toward social and mental health services—you know the experience of friends and family, which is often alienating and unrewarding—plus the sense of self, which comes from racial identity development, that forms personal beliefs about whether you can be helped or should entrust yourself to the considerations of psychotherapists. As part of the process for building trust, those blacks who are identified with their Blackness frequently must be able to differentiate racist behavior from other behavior. This is in part determined by their level of racial identity development. As victims of innumerable subtle acts of discrimination, trusting others is problematic; for persons immersed and identified with the personal legacy of African American life, this can be difficult at best, which is why some who suspect the motives of whites are judged to be exhibiting "healthy cultural paranoia" (Grier & Cobbs, 1968).

Therefore, trust in therapy for Blacks has an added meaning when considering extending this virtue. It is not only determined by the multiple systems that nurture the experience and understanding of trust, but also those experiences most central to the level of one's racial identity that determine how trust is manifested as a psychodynamic issue. Cultural bias and misunderstanding stemming from low levels of racial identity development on the part of the patient or therapist can lead to misunderstanding that results in empathic failure and, consequently, is a threat to the therapeutic alliance.

A case in point that illustrates the trust and distrust issue is that of an African American male who upon admission to an emergency medical room at a local hospital had an acute paranoid episode which led him to forbid any White doctor to touch or examine him in spite of symptoms of a heart attack.

Mr. M., a successful professional and long-time resident in the community, well known by even hospital personnel, was hysterical with fear that a loss of consciousness would put him at the mercy of White hospital personnel. He could not trust what they would do to his body. Although quickly treated by hospital staff and informed his symptoms were stress related with no serious cardiological involvement, Mr. M. was certain what medical interventions that had occurred compromised his health and safety, leading him to manifest greater paranoia. Moreover, every minute he remained under their care increased his risk for being done in—if not killed, then disabled.

Mr. M. thought his work and outspoken thoughts were too well known, too Black, and too threatening to the White community for them to allow him to remain alive. Being very secretive and noncommunicative, he resisted and rejected working with White psychiatrists. It was only upon securing a consultation with a Black psychiatrist friend that the episode began to subside, although one recurring thought was the old adage that "a good nigger is a dead nigger," which drove his demands for immediate hospital release. Needless to say, that hospital staff were perplexed by his behavior and saw the fear as common among persons with a possible cardiac emergency. The racial undertone to his outbursts during the episode was ignored or dismissed.

This is an example of a person whose racial identity was at an immersion-emersion stage, where Mr. M. publicly manifested his identification with African American and African history and legacy. He saw his personal and professional efforts as "bettering the conditions of his people." However Mr. M.'s heightened sensitivity to racism moved what Grier and Cobbs (1968) described as "healthy cultural paranoia" past the bounds of ethnic group normality when in life-threatening and helpless state, dependent upon those whose behavior and motives he constantly screened for discrimination and racism. In contrast, much of the interactions with him by the White hospital staff showed an insensitivity or lack of acknowledgement that racial issues were triggering his paranoid episode. Staff could appropriately be characterized as at the contact stage of White identity development (i.e., believing that racial issues are unimportant), thus setting the stage for a clash in orientation to the problem and reducing the effectiveness of intervention.

Within the personal legacy of Mr. M., there are several systems which contributed to his reaction and orientation to this problem that he could rely upon his psychologist friend to know, comprehend, and utilize in restoring his emotional balance. His family, friends, and professional networks were key in this regard for understanding what happened to him and devising a plan for his recovery. Upon his release to outpatient medical and psychiatric care, Mr. M. was brought home by his friend, where relatives and other friends visited him in a creation of a supportive environment which affirmed and validated his experiences but grounded the episode as a warning that his emotional condition was fragile and in need of treatment.

Choosing the appropriate intervention necessitates a clear definition and understanding of the problem. Lack of familiarity with cultural symbols, language styles, and the dynamics of racism interferes with problem definition and treatment. We will show the role of cultural knowledge through the following example:

A Black client of Jamaican descent told her white therapist that she had no friends because "Black people hated light skinned people." The client believed that her difficulties at work, her failure to maintain a relationship, and her extreme isolation were due to her skin color. She reported that in situations where there were significant numbers of darker skinned Black people, she feared for her safety.

In a case conference, the client was lauded for ability to cope with "such unbearable stress" and was reported to have an adjustment disorder. Upon the insistence of a few participants present at the conference, the woman's therapist reluctantly explored the possibility of a paranoid process as an alternative diagnosis.

The racial identity status of the therapist prevented him from identifying the distortions in this client's presentation. Her assertions, apart from revealing paranoid trends signaled signifi-

cant racial identity conflicts and were consistent with preencounter attitudes. Her paranoia reflected the externalization of her own negative and uncomfortable feelings about being Black. In the absence of any true understanding of the Black experience, the therapist's *Contact* attitudes prevented him from going beyond the surface of what was being communicated and identifying the patient's psychopathology. Typically, when this happens, the distortions are reinforced and the client becomes more deeply entrenched in the conflict. Clarity with respect to this client's dynamics would have come from an understanding of the position of the social system as regards skin color, the values and preferences of the smaller racial community, the contributions of the family system, and the client's own racial identity development.

Race, racial identity, or multisystems are not always such obvious factors in the psychotherapy process. They may very subtly and insidiously influence the course of therapy, however. It is important to deal with the racial and systems material presented in therapy as well as the racial themes that emerge outside of therapy (Adams, 1970). When this is not done, clients often terminate their treatment feeling that the therapist did not understand them (Brantley, 1983).

It has been observed that Black and White therapists frequently differ in their conceptualizations of clients' problems. In a study conducted by Jones and Gray (1985), White therapists rated a majority of problems in the stages of the treatment process as occurring more frequently than did Black therapists.

One myth that prevents African Americans from receiving suitable treatment is the notion that survival issues prevent the poor from exploring their inner world (Thompson, 1989). Another myth is that only emotionally inadequate and immature people succumb to environmental trauma as suggested by the following definition of psychotherapy.

In essence, psychotherapy is aimed at the alleviation of emotional problems that are reflected in symptoms, disturbed affects, and behavior problems . . . These are the outcome of unresolved intrapsychic conflicts, ego dysfunctions and failures in adaptation . . . Psychotherapy endeavors to produce these alterations primarily through structural changes in the patient, that is, the alleviation of systems through strengthening and maturing of the ego, modification of pathological ego mechanisms, constructive changes in superego and modifications of pathological instinctual drives. Essentially, the patient's intrapsychic conflicts and his methods of resolving them must be discovered and defined with special attention given to the ways in which the methods have failed. (Lange, 1981, p. 38)

Therapists clearly vary in their ability to understand the roots and foundations of clients' problems. Therapists who have not developed advanced levels of racial identity may tend to see Blacks solely in terms of their individual psychological structure without consideration for the interplay of other systems. Moreover, the type of relationship they eventually form will also be a function of the therapists' and clients' levels of racial identity development (see Helms, 1984, 1990).

The factors identified previously as hindering the psychotherapy process would be eliminated by concepts and approaches to treatment that take into account the multiple systems that impact the lives of African Americans. Ruiz (1990) offers the following counsel to therapists in cross-cultural dyads.

Mental health professionals would do well to be aware of racist feelings in themselves and to work through them when they arise. Furthermore, they must be open to perceiving and understanding the influences of racist forces on the problems of their Black clients . . . Therapists must become aware of their ethnicity and cultural heritage and come to value and respect racial differences. (p. 17)

The case which follows demonstrates the importance of flexibility in thinking, awareness, and approach.

A Black graduate student, one year into a doctoral program in sociology, sought treatment of severe work inhibition. At the end of his first semester in graduate school, he had only completed half of his course load and obtained incompletes in the other half. He attended a state-funded undergraduate school with a significant number of African American and Latino students and subsequently, a prestigious and predominantly White graduate school. This information was revealed only after some of the client's statements prompted an exploration of racial identity attitudes. When asked about the racial characteristics of the two schools, he responded that he "didn't see how that was important."

Racial identity attitudes were central to the client's approach to his work and in his comfort in taking his rightful place as a professional. The unhealthy racial identity attitudes that he held were related to the peculiar manner in which his family dealt with racism and became his rationale for the abuse he experienced. Subtle institutional racism precipitated the crisis but was denied by the client and consequently not immediately available for exploration. Success in treating this client was heavily dependent upon the therapist's understanding of systems, the dynamics of racism and racial identity issues, as well as the therapist's comfort with these issues.

Exploration revealed that the courses with which he experienced the most difficulty dealt with multiculturalism, racism, and other social themes. The course that engendered the greatest amount of anxiety was taught by a Black professor. His anxiety appeared related to a fear that his ideas about race and culture not being significant or important would not be accepted.

The client responded well to a multimodal/integrative approach. Cognitive-behavioral techniques were used initially to prevent further damage to his record. The treatment subsequently relied more heavily on cognitive restructuring, and then moved to psychoanalytic psychotherapy to address some long-standing characterological issues that interfered with healthy functioning.

Social forces are more likely to play a role in Black clients' motivation to seek treatment. In the case just described, the person was probably operating at the initial phase of the encounter stage. His racial identity was very likely a factor in his desire to work with a Black therapist. Multiple systems created racial identity conflicts and perpetuated them, and the interplay between them precipitated the current crisis. The larger society provided opportunities for this person to develop negative racial identity attitudes. The university system provided him with numerous reminders of his devalued status in society, thus highlighting his anxiety and calling into question some of his assumptions regarding how the world is ordered. Because racial issues were not discussed at home, the family system left him poorly prepared to deal with assaults to his racial self-concept.

In such a case, the racial identity status of the therapist had important implications for what was addressed. A therapist operating at low levels of racial identity would be more likely than a therapist at a higher level of racial identity to refer this person, or if not, to downplay, minimize, or ignore the significance of race and racial identity issues. A therapist operating at higher levels of racial identity would identify and experience less discomfort with the racial and cultural issues and would approach the treatment with greater clarity regarding the contributions of race, racial identity, and racism to the current problem. For example, the fear, anger, and hostility that a therapist in the reintegration stage feels toward Black people might lead the therapist to attribute the client's difficulties primarily to personal deficits. A therapist at the autonomy stage of White racial identity would be more likely to actively inquire about racial themes, make the appropriate connections, and demonstrate and assist the client in understanding the personal implications of racial issues.

In the case just illustrated, it would be easy to deny the significance of race. The denial of race represents an attempt to keep discomfort and conflict out of the client–therapist relationship. Often, however, this has the opposite effect. At the other end of the spectrum is a tendency to focus exclusively on the issue of race to the neglect of other issues. This might be the orientation of the White therapist at the pseudoindependence level of racial identity who has an intense intellectual interest in racial themes. It might also be the orientation of a Black therapist in the Immersion-Emersion stage of racial identity who is absorbed in the Black experience and rejects the White world.

CONCLUSION

This chapter presents the argument for psychotherapy integration to include ethnocultural considerations in the theory, research, and practice of our discipline. It specifically discusses how racial identity development, family, community, and the overall social context form multisystems that shape the psychodynamic world of African Americans in a unique fashion, which therapists must learn, and understand to maximize effective and empathic interventions. Our thoughts about treatment of African Americans lead us to suggest a paradigmatic shift in psychotherapy away from the conventional private practice model to a model and curriculum which teach the therapist how to include, utilize, and participate in a strategic multisystems intervention model that views the individual within a social context, with profound ethnocultural dimensions. Moreover, we suggest that introspective self-exploration that therapists should do to understand themselves in the therapeutic process needs to include awareness and knowledge of their own racial identity development. Expanding the models of psychotherapy practice and explorations of personal development to be more inclusive and innovative is, in our opinion, the future direction for effective treatment of African Americans, in a growing multicultural society.

REFERENCES

Adams, P. L. (1970). Dealing with racism in biracial psychiatry. *Journal of the American Academy of Child Psychiatry, 9*, 33–43.

Badad, E. Y., Birnbaum, M., & Benne, K.D. (1983). *The social self.* Beverly Hills: Sage.

Billingsley, A. (1968). *Black families in white America.* Englewood Cliffs, NJ: Prentice-Hall.

Boyd-Franklin, N. (1989). *Black families in therapy: A multisystems approach.* New York: Guilford.

Brantley, T. (1983). Racism and its impact on psychotherapy. *American Journal of Psychiatry, 140*(12), 1605–1608.

Carter, R. T. (1988). An empirical test of a theory on the influence of racial identity attitudes on the counseling process within a workshop setting. *Dissertation Abstracts International, 49*(3), 431-A.

Carter, R. T. (1990a). Cultural value differences between African Americans and White Americans. *Journal of College Student Development, 31*, 71–79.

Carter, R. T. (1990b). The relationship between racism and racial identity among white Americans: An exploratory investigation. *Journal of Counseling and Development, 69*, 46–50.

Carter, R. T. (1990c). Does race or racial identity attitudes influence the counseling process in Black/White dyads? In J.E. Helms (Ed.), *Black and White racial identity attitudes: Theory, research, and practice* (pp. 145–164). Westport, CT: Greenwood Press.

Carter, R. T. (1991). Racial identity attitudes and psychological functioning. *Journal of Multicultural Counseling and Development, 19*, 105–114.

Carter, R. T., & Helms, J. E. (1987). The relationship of Black value orientations to racial identity attitudes. *Measurement and Evaluation in Counseling and Development, 19*, 185–195.

Carter, R. T., & Helms, J. E. (1990). White racial identity attitudes and cultural values. In J.E. Helms (Ed.), *Black and White racial identity attitudes: Theory, research, and practice* (pp. 105–118). Westport, CT: Greenwood Press.

Carter, R. T., & Helms, J. E. (1992). Counseling process defined as relationship types: A test of Helms's interactional model. *Journal of Multicultural Counseling and Development, 20*(4), 181–201.

Clark, K. B. (1988). *Prejudice and your child.* Middletown, CT: Wesleyan University Press.

Cooper, S. (1973). A look at the effects of racism on clinical casework. *Social Casework, 54,* 78–54.

Cross, W. E. (1978). The Thomas and Cross models of psychological nigrescence: A review. *Journal of Black Psychology, 5*(1), 13–31.

Cross, W. E. (1991). *Shades of black.* Philadelphia: Temple University Press.

Franklin, A. J. (1992). Therapy with African American Men. *Families in Society: The Journal of Contemporary Human Services,* June, 350–355.

Gardner, L. H. (1971). The therapeutic relationship under varying conditions of race. *Psychotherapy: Theory, Research, and Practice, 8,* 78–87.

Grier, W. H., & Cobbs, P. M. (1968). *Black rage.* New York: Basic Books.

Helms, J. E. (1984). Toward a theoretical explanation of the effects of race on counseling: A Black/White interactional model. *The Counseling Psychologist, 12*(4), 153–165.

Helms, J. E. (Ed.) (1990). *Black and White racial identity attitudes: Theory, research, and practice.* Westport, CT: Greenwood Press.

Helms, J. E., & Carter, R. T. (1991). Relationship of White and Black racial identity attitudes and demographic similarity to counselor preferences. *Journal of Counseling Psychology, 38*(4), 446–459.

Helms, J. E., & Parham, T. A. (1990). The relationship between Black racial identity attitudes and cognitive styles. In J. E. Helms (Ed.), *Black and White racial identity attitudes: Theory, research, and practice* (pp. 119–131). Westport, CT: Greenwood Press.

Hill, R. (1972). *The strengths of Black families.* New York: Emerson Hall.

Hill, R. (1977). *Informal adoption among Black families.* Washington, DC: National Urban League Research Department.

Jackson, A. M. (1973). Psychotherapy: Factors associated with the race of the therapist. *Psychotherapy: Theory, Research, and Practice, 10,* 273–277.

Jones, A., & Seagull, A. A. (1977). Dimensions of the relationship between the Black client and White therapist. *American Psychologist, 32,* 850–855.

Jones, B. E., & Gray, B. A. (1985). Black and White psychiatrists: Therapy with Blacks. *Journal of the National Medical Association, 77*(1), 19–25.

Jones, R. (Ed.). (1988). *Psychoeducational assessment of minority group children: A casebook.* Berkeley, CA: Cobb & Henry.

Jones, R. (Ed.). (1991). *Black psychology* (3rd Ed.). Berkeley, CA: Cobb & Henry.

Kohut, H. (1983). *Restoration of the self.* New York: International Universities Press.

Kovel, J. (1970). *White racism.* New York; Pantheon.

Lange, R. (1981). *The technique of psychoanalytic psychotherapy.* New York: Jason Aronson.

Levine, L. W. (1977). *Black culture and Black consciousness.* New York: Oxford University Press.

Lincoln, C. E., & Mamiya, L. H. (1990). *The Black church in the African American experience.* Durham, NC: Duke University Press.

McAdoo, H. P. (Ed.). (1988). *Black families.* Newbury Park, CA: Sage.

McAdoo, H. P., & McAdoo, J. L. (1985). *Black children: Social, educational, and parental environments.* Newbury Park, CA: Sage.

Parham, T. A., & Helms, J. E. (1981). The influence of Black students' racial identity attitudes on preference for counselor race. *Journal of Counseling Psychology, 28,* 250–257.

Parham, T. A., & Helms, J. E. (1985a). Attitudes of racial identity and self-esteem in Black students: An exploratory investigation. *Journal of College Student Personnel, 26*(2), 143–146.

Parham, T. A., & Helms, J. E. (1985b). Relationship of racial identity attitudes to self-actualization and affective states of Black students. *Journal of Counseling Psychology, 32*(3), 431–440.

Parker, W. M., & McDavis, R. J. (1983). Attitudes of Blacks toward mental health agencies and counselors. *Journal of Non-White Concerns,* 89–99.

Pomales, J., Claiborn, C. D., & LaFromboise, T. D. (1986). Effects of Black students' racial identity on perceptions of White counselors varying in cultural sensitivity. *Journal of Counseling Psychology, 33*(1), 55–61.

Ridley, C. R. (1984). Clinical treatment of the nondisclosing Black client: A therapeutic paradox. *American Psychologist, 39*(11), 1234–1244.

Ruiz, D. S. (1990). *Handbook of mental health and mental disorder among Black Americans.* New York: Greenwood Press.

Sager, C. J., Brayboy, T. L., & Waxenberg, B. R. (1972). Black patient-White therapist. *American Journal of Orthopsychiatry, 42,* 415–432.

Seward, G. H. (1972). *Psychotherapy and culture conflict in community mental health* (2nd Ed.). New York: Ronald Press.

Smitherman, G. (1977). *Talkin' and testifyin': The language of Black American.* Boston: Houghton Mifflin.

Stack, C. (1975). *All our kin: Strategies for survival in a Black community.* New York: Harper & Row.

Stewart, E. C., & Bennett, M. S. (1991). *American cultural patterns: A cross-cultural perspective.* Yarmouth, ME: Intercultural Press.

Thomas, A., & Sillen, S. (1972). *Racism and psychiatry.* Secaucus, NJ: Citadel Press.

Tokar, D. M., & Swanson, J. L. (1991). An investigation of the validity of Helms's (1984) model of white racial identity development. *Journal of Counseling Psychology, 38,* 296–301.

Turner, S., & Armstrong, S. (1981). Cross-racial psychotherapy: What the therapists say. *Psychotherapy: Theory, Research, and Practice, 18,* 375–378.

Thompson, C. L. (1989). Psychoanalytic psychotherapy with inner city patients. *Journal of Contemporary Psychotherapy, 19*(2), 137–148.

Vontress, C. E. (1971a). *Counseling Negroes.* Boston: Houghton Mifflin.

Vontress, C. E. (1971b). Racial differences: Impediments to rapport. *Journal of Counseling Psychology, 18,* 7–13.

White, J., & Parham, T. (1990). *The psychology of Blacks* (2nd Ed.). Englewood Cliffs, NJ: Prentice-Hall.

Williams, R. L. (1971). Abuses and misuses in testing Black children. *Counseling Psychologist, 2,* 62–77.

PART VI

Teaching Psychotherapy Integration

CHAPTER 33

Supervision and Instruction in Doctoral Psychotherapy Integration

Conrad Lecomte, Louis Georges Castonguay, Mireille Cyr, and Stéphane Sabourin

INTRODUCTION

The movement of rapprochement and integration between different theoretical schools is currently one of the most active and dynamic areas of interest in the field of counseling and psychotherapy (Arkowitz & Messer, 1984; Lecomte & Castonguay, 1987; Marmor & Woods, 1980; Norcross, 1986). In fact, the sheer number of publications dealing with eclecticism, integration, or rapprochement has reached proportions that could have hardly been predicted 15 years ago (Goldfried & Newman, 1986). It can even be argued that the influence of this movement has reached the training boards of major professional associations (American Psychological Association, Canadian

Conrad Lecomte, Mireille Cyr, and Stéphane Sabourin • Department of Psychology, University of Montreal, Montreal, Quebec, Canada H3C 3J7. Louis Georges Castonguay • Department of Psychology, State University of New York at Stony Brook, Stony Brook, New York 11794-2500.

Comprehensive Handbook of Psychotherapy Integration, edited by George Stricker and Jerold R. Gold. Plenum Press, New York, 1993.

Psychological Association), which now expect future clinicians to become familiar with a wide range of assessment and intervention procedures, rather than being restricted to a single modality (APA, 1979; CPA, 1983).

Although clinical flexibility, conceptual pluralism, and professional versatility are highly valued goals, there is unfortunately scant empirical data to inform us concerning how students should be trained to attain these goals. Moreover, many arguments can lead us to believe that participation in a multitheoretical supervision program could have adverse effects on trainees' performance. Thus, some clinicians and researchers maintain that theoretical systems so highly different as humanism, behaviorism, and psychoanalysis are mostly irreconcilable (Franks, 1984; Messer & Winokur, 1980, 1984). The only result of a multitheoretical training supervision program would be to heighten the confusion level of trainees. Other clinicians believe that even if these theoretical systems can be partly integrated, at some level it necessitates a degree of cognitive complexity so high that the vast majority of students could not absorb the clinical teaching of supervisors of different theoretical orientations (Wright & Sabourin, 1987). Finally, a last group of thinkers objects that while a rapprochement is conceptually feasible, it is not practically feasible. Indeed, for them, the supervisor–supervisee relationship is conceived as an interpersonal influence process (Heppner & Clairborn, 1989). Accordingly, the supervisor's interventions represent compliance gaining tactics to model the behavior of the trainee. The efficacy of these strategies rests on the supervisor's perceived level of expertise, attractiveness, and trustworthiness. These variables are particularly determinant in the context of an integrated training program because the potential for marked divergence between supervisors and supervisees in their theoretical and clinical conceptions is very high. For example, it could be hypothesized that trainees of a humanistic orientation will emit compliance-resisting behaviors vis-à-vis the social influence strategies used by psychodynamic supervisors and vice-versa.

Notwithstanding these impediments, integrative supervision will, in most likelihood, grow into a major model of training over the next years. Even though we still do not have solid conceptual and empirical foundation to integrative psychotherapy and supervision, it will continue to attract a large number of practitioners. As underlined by Murray (1986), the majority of psychotherapists are not purists but use and will continue to use a diversity of combination or integration of different approaches in order to offer valuable and meaningful services to their clients. In addition, the conclusions of the Grand Prix study (Luborsky, Singer, & Luborsky, 1975) comparing different orientations are not only well known, they seem to have promoted a pervasive pattern based on relativism and pluralism. There is a growing number of clinicians who, while maintaining their own theoretical orientation, are viewing rival systems not as an adversity, but as a healthy diversity (Landsman, 1974). Finally, most of the psychotherapists seem to be looking for the best possible ways to help their clients while at the same time sensing the complexity and the uncertainty of human change processes. Integrative psychotherapy and supervision approaches may, in fact, be tentative efforts to explore and account for the multidimensionality and the complexity of psychotherapeutic change.

In fact, several attempts to delineate guidelines for integrative supervision have already been proposed. The first part of this chapter will provide a brief overview of existing multitheoretical training programs. A description of varied issues raised by these programs will then follow. The final sections of the chapter will be devoted to the presentation of the integrative model that guides our own program, and an attempt to illustrate how some of the issues related to eclectic training can be addressed at conceptual, clinical, and personal levels.

THEORETICAL AND CONCEPTUAL ISSUES

Integrative Training Programs

In recent issues of the International Journal of Eclectic Psychotherapy, and the Journal of Integrative and Eclectic Psychotherapy several major figures were invited to present their views on the training of integrative/eclectic psychotherapists (Beutler, Mahoney, Norcross, Prochaska, Sollod, & Robertson, 1987). Among the issues addressed by the authors were the ingredients and sequences of an ideal training program. For Beutler (in Beutler et al., 1987 and in Norcross (section ed.), 1986) such a program would first involve in-depth exploration of major models defining normal human functioning as well as psychopathology. The student would then be trained in basic skills that are used in most approaches to induce a positive therapeutic relationship. The trainees would also be expected to master theories of psychotherapy and the technological skills associated with each major orientation (i.e., behavioral, psychodynamic, experiential, cognitive, and group/interpersonal therapies). For Beutler, it would be only after students developed theoretical and clinical competencies in various individual orientations that they would explore models of integration. One such model is the one put forward by Beutler himself (Beutler, 1983, 1986) in which therapists are encouraged to apply diverse techniques that serve one of five therapeutic purposes (i.e., insight enhancement, emotional awareness, emotional escalation, emotion reduction, behavioral control or perceptual change) according to the client's symptoms, coping style, and interpersonal sensitivity. The ideal training model suggested by Beutler reflects similarities with the model proposed by DiClemente and Prochaska (in Norcross *et al.*, 1986; see also Prochaska in Beutler *et al.*, 1987). Like Beutler, DiClemente and Prochaska maintain that students should begin their training by learning major systems of therapy as part of the basic course work of the graduate studies, and by developing skills in the establishment of helping relationships. Also similar to Beutler's model, the exploration of integration is the last training step in DiClemente and Prochaska's program. The students are first exposed to different orientations by working gradually with more and more complex cases. Although they acknowledge the existence of other integrative models, they also recognize their biases toward their own transtheoretical approach (Prochaska & DiClemente, 1984, 1986). This approach consists of facilitating differential change processes (e.g., consciousness raising, self-evaluation) at different stages of therapy (e.g., precontemplation, contemplation) for different levels of problems (e.g., symptoms, maladaptive cognitions).

Both Halgin and Robertson's ideal models for an eclectic training (see Norcross *et al.*, 1986) differ from the two preceding ones by not requiring prior competence in one or more therapeutic approaches. For Halgin, integration must be presented at the outset of training, and the blending of major orientations should be attempted in basic courses and in the clinical curriculum. Supervision in this program is based on a model developed by Halgin (1986) which pragmatically blends psychodynamic, interpersonal, person-centered, and behavioral approaches. The basic postulate underlying pragmatic blending is that supervision should involve an individualized response to the particular needs of each trainee. Thus, through an exploration of transference/countertransference problems in the supervisory process, trainees probe issues of developmental significance which interfere with treatment effectiveness. Emotional issues emerging within the supervisor–supervisee relationship are also explored using the interpersonal theory as a guiding framework. In addition, applying supportive and empathic techniques, the supervisor facilitates the growth of the supervisee. Finally, didactic work, role modeling, and cognitive restructuring are some behavioral techniques employed to transmit specific knowledge and skills to the trainee. As for Robertson (in Norcross *et al.*, 1986), training should first focus on the similarities and differences between approaches that represent the three major orientations in psychotherapy: psychodynamic, phenomenological/humanist and behavioral/cognitive. In Robertson's model, a theoretical framework should then be taught to help students derive assessment and intervention strategies from an integrative perspective. During their clinical training, students should learn how to implement this integrative framework and should also acquire skills to develop a therapeutic relationship with a wide range of clients.

Clarkin and Frances (in Norcross, 1986) presented yet another model of ideal training. The goal of this program, called "differential therapeutic," is not to train a therapist to be always eclectic (i.e., to combine procedures from divergent orientations with all clients), but to train the supervisee in matching the therapeutic intervention (e.g., pure behavioral method; combination of pharmacotherapy and psychodynamic intervention) to the client's needs. Such training involves didactic seminars concerning the strengths and weaknesses of different approaches, as well as a clinical practicum covering the recommendations and execution of simple or combined treatment packages. A biomedical/sociobehavioral training model was also proposed by Suedfeld in Norcross *et al.* (1986). In this program, students would ideally be exposed to knowledge related to all dimensions of human organisms: biological, neurological, psychological, social, cultural, and environmental.

Other authors have described more or less explicitly, the training and supervision guidelines of their eclectic approach. Garfield (1980, 1986) has taught for more than 35 years an eclectic approach which rests heavily on factors that are common to different orientations. Although he considers it important to introduce students to the essential contributions of the major approaches, the supervisees are not expected to become competent in any specific school before becoming eclectic therapists. Lazarus's students, on the other hand, are required to be familiar with a large number of therapeutic approaches (Lazarus, 1976, 1986), giving priority to therapeutic procedures which have accumulated empirical support. Students learn to become "technical collectors." They are also taught that in order to effectively intervene in each basic modality of human functioning (e.g., behavior, affect, sensation), "useful techniques may be gathered from any sources and, if necessary, totally divorced from their origins" (Lazarus, 1986, p. 90).

In learning the eclectic time-limited therapy developed by Fuhriman, Paul, and Burlingame (1986), trainees are not exposed to the theoretical model and techniques of specific systems. What they learn are basic helping skills (e.g., empathy, self-disclosure, confrontation) relevant to different stages of therapy drawn from Egan's model (e.g., rapport building, enhancing self-understanding, active coping). In another eclectic approach to the teaching of psychotherapy, Watters, Rubenstein, and Bellissimo (1980) borrow theoretical concepts and technical skills from communication theory, psychodynamic theory, ego psychology, learning theory, and transactional theory. The integration of these models allows for the consideration of both intrapsychic and interpersonal phenomena. Concerned with the evaluation of student progress in their training, Watters *et al.* (1980) developed a set of learning objectives (e.g., "demonstrate a therapeutic stance characterized by genuine interest," "demonstrate the capacity to allow the patient to share powerful emotions"), which cover three classes of therapeutic skills: perceptual, conceptual, and executive.

Norcross (1988) also described several "consistencies" in his supervision approach. Relying on some of the eclectic models previously mentioned (Beutler, 1983; Lazarus, 1976; Prochaska & DiClemente, 1984), he focuses the students' attention on clients' characteristics that may indicate the use of specific treatments. Guided by an interpersonal perspective, he also trains his students to assess their clients' maladaptive patterns of relationship. Furthermore, consistent with an existential premise, he attempts to make his trainees aware that they will invariably have to make therapeutic choices (Messer, 1986). He emphasizes that, as an integrationist, his students' decisions at such therapeutic choice points should "embrace a continuum of indicated strategies based on the individuality of the client and the singulants of the situation" (Norcross, 1986, p. 160). Finally, other eclectic programs of training and supervision have been formulated for more specialized types of interventions like family therapy (Grebstein, 1986), marital/sexual therapy (Prochaska and Sollod in Beutler *et al.*, 1987), group therapy (Robertson in Beutler *et al.*, 1987), and social casework (Fischer, 1986).

Issues Related to Integrative Training

Although attempts to delineate and apply an integrative training program have been fairly recent, trainers and supervisors have already been confronted with a considerable number of issues. These issues are theoretical, clinical and concern personal characteristics of trainers and trainees. At the present time, there exists no definitive view on how to deal with these issues, and little empirical data has been generated to aid in the formation of firm guidelines on how to conduct an eclectic training. For the most part, eclectic therapists have relied on their experience and conceptual biases to determine what to teach, how to teach it, and who should be involved in this type of learning experience. In this section, we will introduce the most prevalent issues related to integrative training and then describe how we attempted to cope with them in the application of our own model of training. As one might expect, many of the issues concern the tasks of training and supervision in general, but we will focus our discussion on the characteristics and challenges that are specific to eclectic training.

The first issue raised by an integrative program of training is both a conceptual and a clinical one. The question is whether students should acquire a solid basis in one (or more) specific orientation(s) prior to learning an eclectic approach, or whether they should assimilate an eclectic perspective as early as possible. The issue has been aptly referred to by Norcross (1988) as a choice between depth and breadth. For some authors, a deep understanding of a model (or several of them) of human change and functioning, and minimal competence in the use of specific clinical skills should precede the acquisition of an integrative framework (see Beutler; Clarkin & Frances; DiClemente & Prochaska in Norcross *et al.*, 1986). The view is best summarized by Beutler (in Norcross *et al.*, 1988) when he argued that "one can usually integrate . . . only those things with which one is familiar, skilled or comfortable" (p.

84). For others, an optimal curriculum should be guided, from the beginning to the end, by an eclectic/integrative agenda (Fuhriman *et al.*, 1986; Halgin in Norcross *et al.*, 1986). Exposure to different conceptual models and methods of change is believed to foster an attitude of open mindedness, as well as encourages students to be guided by their clients' needs rather than by their conceptual biases (Halgin, 1986). What seems to be a growing consensus, however, is that trainees have to be provided with some conceptual framework (Norcross *et al.*, 1986). Whether it is first restricted to a unique orientation or whether involving the integration of divergent approaches, a model provides the beginning therapist with a cognitive structure to guide assessment, case formulation, and treatment selection (Norcross, 1988). Moreover, such a cognitive map may prevent mindless application of divergent procedures (Grebstein, 1986). As noted by Norcross (1988), there is some research evidence showing that students' appraisal of good supervision is based on the supervisor's ability to ground clinical interventions within a coherent conceptual framework. Even a proponent of technical eclecticism like Lazarus (1986) recognizes the inexorability of a theoretical position. His multimodal therapy is indeed based on a blending of several theoretical systems (i.e., social learning theory, general system theory, group and communications theory).

Another issue is related to the focus of supervision. The concern here is to what extent the relationship between the supervisor and supervisee represents the main vehicle for learning, and to what degree should training involve the teaching of techniques and therapeutic strategies. For several authors, no element of the supervisory process provides as much personal and clinical learning as the supervisee–supervisor relationship (e.g., Halgin, 1985; Lambert & Arnold, 1987). On the other hand, without negating the pedagogical power of the relationship, others have emphasized the importance of varied strategies to ensure the acquisition of skills and procedures (e.g., observation of expert therapists, co-therapy) (e.g., Lazarus, 1986). According to Robertson (1986), the general consensus is that eclectic programs should focus on both relational and technical skills. Norcross (1988) presented a similar position, arguing that the emphasis on techniques and the relationships need not be seen as a dichot-

omy, but rather as two different foci of a training sequence. Describing supervision from a developmental perspective, Norcross (1988) suggests that students have different needs depending on their level of training: techniques reduce the anxiety for the beginning therapists by providing concretely applicable tools; theory is needed later in the training to dissipate some of the confusion that gradually accumulates with involvement in more complex cases; and a focus on the relationship is finally indicated for more advanced students who are ready to address more directly their personal reactions (e.g., countertransference) that affect therapy.

A related issue is how strong is, or should be, the parallel between therapy and supervision. Several therapists have suggested that supervision is most beneficial for the trainee when it mirrors the focus and method used with the clients (Frances & Clarkin, 1981; Halgin, 1988). It is assumed, for example, that interpretive techniques are best learned and applied in therapy when the supervisor explores the therapist's countertransferential issues, and that behavioral procedures are more easily grasped in a supervision process that is directive and practice-oriented in context. Stricker (1988), however, cautioned that complete mirroring of the therapeutic situation may limit the learning potential of supervision. He argued, for instance, that interpretation of countertransference would not be only relevant for students learning psychodynamic techniques. It could also be very appropriate for students applying a behavioral technique without being aware of personal reaction toward the client that may prevent therapeutic improvement.

Other issues relevant to the training of eclectic therapists have been consensually identified. For instance, most authors agreed that an eclectic program required certain characteristics from their students: an ability to cope with stress, confusion, and uncertainties created by a relativistic and pluralist view of human functioning; a capacity to develop skills, knowledge, and personal confidence without the support of a distinct reference group; and the ability to achieve a professional identity without an allegiance to a unique and well-established theoretical model (Beutler *et al.*, 1987; Halgin, 1986; Norcross, 1988). It is also commonly believed that integrative supervisors should display a high degree of flexibility, and yet be fairly organized in their teaching of divergent perspectives (Clarkin & Frances in Norcross *et al.*, 1986). All integrative trainers are also confronted with the difficult task of presenting their conceptual model as only one possible integrative approach (Andrews, 1989; Norcross, 1988). This is an important issue, since failing to do so would defeat the purpose of the integrative movement (Goldfried & Castonguay, 1992). Hence, if future generations of students are exposed to a single eclectic system, we may soon witness a competition between opposing eclectic schools. It is essential for trainers to be aware that, as models, they can teach the merit of clinical diversity and inspire in their students a respect for conceptual complexity. As noted by Mahoney (in Beutler *et al.*, 1987), if open-mindedness is the essence of *what* integrative therapists teach, it should also dictate *how* they teach and supervise. Although such an attitude can increase the intrinsic difficulty of training, it makes it more rewarding. In Mahoney's words "I cannot imagine a more valuable or professionally relevant skill than that involved in nurturing and modeling critical, open inquiry" (p. 315).

Finally, most authors indicted that formal training in research is not a formal requirement to become an eclectic therapist (Robertson, 1986). The consensus seems to be that although such training can be useful, it is not necessary and certainly not sufficient (see Grebstein, 1986; Norcross, 1986; and Hart, 1986), for different views on that issue.

Pragmatic Blending of Self-Psychology Approaches: Rogers, Kohut, and Bandura

For more than 16 years, our training program in counseling psychology at the Université de Montréal consisted of a pragmatic integration of humanistic, interpersonal, and cognitive-behavioral approaches (Carkhuff, 1969; Egan, 1981; Mahoney & Lyddon, 1988). Students were first exposed to a generic model of psychotherapy based on research findings (Orlinsky & Howard, 1978, 1986). Using Carkhuff (1969) and Egan's (1981) therapeutic paradigm of self-exploration, self-understanding and action, a pragmatic blending of person-centered, psychodynamic, interpersonal influence and cognitive-behavioral techniques was achieved. The result was a form of systematic eclecticism (Lazarus, 1981; Norcross, 1986). Integration among various treatment modalities was achieved using specific guidelines and took place mainly at the level of intermediate principles and strategies (Goldfried, 1982) rather than at the level of theory or specific procedures. Training in fundamental relationship and communication skills, such as active listening skills, nonverbal communication, empathy, and modeling respect for client problems, was based on empirically demonstrated significant training procedures. The acquisition of facilitative psychotherapy skills and attitudes was systematically structured. The standard sequence involved instruction, modeling, practice, formative and summative evaluation, feedback, and more practice (Lecomte, 1990). With such training procedures, students did seem to acquire increasing levels of competence and flexibility (e.g., Tracey, Hays, Malone, & Herman, 1988).

During the practicums, students needed to demonstrate concretely, process and outcome competencies. Process competencies included therapeutic contract, establishment of an appropriate therapeutic relationship, formulation of relevant and valid dynamic hypotheses, choice of relevant and appropriate interventions, and indications of client progress. Psychotherapeutic efficacy referred both to micro and macro outcomes (Orlinsky & Howard, 1986). In our program, students were requested to achieve at least some therapeutic objectives with their clients, such as self-exploration, insight, resolution of conflicts or learning of new cognitive and interpersonal skills during therapy sessions.

In this program, students were offered limited exploration of various models of psychotherapy. Theoretical paradigms were introduced as tentative explanatory notions varying in level of analysis. Emphasis was put on the equivalence and relative efficacy of various models and the need to better understand therapeutic change.

At the same time, trainees were invited to consider personal issues related to difficulties or reactions to clients. This is how transference and countertransference issues were often dealt with. Using feelings and thoughts within therapists provoked by client expression of feeling, supervisors help trainees develop insight and affective sensitivity to clients.

Finally, supervisors tried to help trainees move to the integration of skills and personal issues and the supervisory relationship and therapeutic relationship were often examined as parallel processes. This process is conceptualized as one in which we ascertain in supervision specific vestiges of the relationship between the supervisee and his or her client (Stoltenberg & Delworth, 1987).

Evaluating the impact of our clinical training program on trainees in terms of professional development and degree of theoretical flexibility, a number of concerns and limitations were underlined (Girard, 1988). Most students emphasized that our systematic training program had helped them gain initial therapeutic competence, clinical flexibility, and professional versatility. On the other hand, a majority of them felt the need to have a coherent theoretical framework of human behavior and psychopathology. Instead, they were trained within a multitheory comparison suggesting that no truth exists. The result was flexible practitioners who possessed a confused professional identity. It seems that integration was for some, poorly or superficially achieved.

In order to correct, at least partially, the limits of our training model, we kept our commitment to a basic systematic and integrative eclecticism, but decided to identify and adopt a specific theoretical perspective that was harmonious with our clinical preferences. We decided that a rigorous mastery of the person-centered approach would provide a solid theoretical foundation for the learning of facilitative and generic interpersonal skills. In addition, this approach provides a phenomenological perspective and underscores the primacy of subjective experience, which provides a framework within which cognitive-behavioral methods could be initiated.

Our repeated confrontation with the complexity of certain clinical realities, led us gradually to question the adequacy of the Rogerian model for suppressing all types of psychological suffering. Without rejecting the heuristic qualities of the person-centered therapy, in the self psychology of Kohut (1977) and in the social cognitive approach of Bandura (1986), we found numerous contributions that seem to complement

and to harmoniously enhance the theoretical and clinical validity of our training model. Instead of juxtaposing contradictory theoretical approaches, we looked for a natural and complementary blending using the self as a central and unifying dimension. Finally, we brought nuance and temporal modalities to these notions by blending them into a developmental perspective.

Integrating Rogers, Kohut, and Bandura

Rogers' and Kohut's theories are well suited to provide this quiet blending. These theories share numerous similarities and their differences are in many respects complementary (Kahn, 1985, 1989).

Rogers (1951) developed a theory which primarily focuses on change and on conditions that bring about change. Self-concept is influenced by a need for positive regard, conceptualized by Rogers as a universal, pervasive, and persistent need in human beings. This need can only be satisfied by others. Empathy, positive regard, and genuineness are the catalytic agents of the therapeutic relationship that allow the client to experience his or her self in a wide range of ways, in a meaningful relationship with the therapist. Therapists have the responsibility to provide a climate which furthers the self-directed change of the client (Rychlack, 1981).

Kohut (1971, 1977) has focused on self psychology, and has studied the self in greater depth and complexity as compared to Rogers. He defined the self as a psychological structure which depends on the continual presence of an evoking-sustaining-responding matrix of selfobject experiences (Wolf, 1988). Selfobjects are neither selves nor objects, they are the subjective aspect of a function performed by a relationship. Disruption in the continuity of the sustaining selfobject experience results in disruptions in the continuity of the self. The structuration of the self is acquired by a process called *transmuting internalization* which is possible only when a consistent empathic intuneness is present between the self and its selfobject (Kahn, 1985).

If the selfobjects are not sufficiently empathic during childhood, the self may lose its inherent cohesion and may become fragmented (Kohut &

Wolf, 1978). Fragmentation means regression of the self, which is experienced as a loss of self-esteem or as feelings of emptiness, depression, worthlessness, or anxiety. Fragmentation occurs in varying degrees.

Throughout the course of life, the self is vulnerable to the absence, insufficiency, or inappropriateness of selfobject experience, which leads to selfobject relation disorders (Kohut & Wolf, 1978).

Kohut and Rogers have both stressed the importance of the subjective life. Psychotherapists should try to understand the inner world of the person, an objective which is achieved mostly through empathy. In both theories, the self is conceptualized as a perceiving, experiencing entity that is able to make choices and control its destiny. Consequently, during the therapeutic process, the therapist will help the person to attain self-enhancement. For Kohut, the aim is to bring the constituents of the self to maturity, whereas for Rogers, the self should attempt a greater congruence. Both authors have emphasized the importance of an empathic response from the environment throughout life as a major factor contributing to self-growth and optimal use of talents. The person is also viewed as motivated by future goals and as having free will.

Differences between Kohut's and Rogers' theories concern their understanding of the difficulties of the self, their goals, and their tools of treatment (Kahn, 1989). In Rogers' conception, a person feels maladjustment when he or she experiences incongruence between the organism and the self. The goal of therapy is to restore congruence, defined as the awareness of all organismic experiences, by offering unconditional positive regard, empathy, and genuineness to the client. Prizing the client and low-level inferences are used in a here and now context. For Kohut (Kohut & Wolf, 1978), the goal of therapy is the structuration of the self. As outlined earlier, psychopathology, for Kohut, consists of arrested development, characterized by significant failures to achieve cohesion, vigor, or harmony, which results in chronic distress and the lack of a purposive, satisfying, goal-directed life-style. By empathic understanding, therapists are able to establish and maintain the self-object bond between the patient and the therapist and later to offer some interpretations of the disruptions of the selfobject bond and its reestablishment, which inevitably occurs in therapy.

As mentioned by Kahn (1989), these two approaches are complementary in many aspects. Rogers stresses the importance of the qualities of the therapist as a person. Genuinely prizing and valuing the client will enhance self-esteem. Kohut asserts that optimal empathic attunement will restore to the self its coherence, vigor, and harmony. Kohut describes these attitudes within a developmental comprehension of the client's difficulties, an exploration and interpretation of the past into the present, and a discovery of the selfobject transferences. Integrating the insights of Rogers and Kohut provides a new and useful perspective of clinical relationships.

In recent years, some limited contact between object relations (for reviews, see Blatt & Lerner, 1983; Stricker & Healey, 1990) and social cognitive approaches has begun to occur (Tomkins, 1979; Westen, 1991). Within personality and social psychology, research spanning the two domains has begun to appear (e.g., Singer, 1984, 1985).

Cantor (Cantor & Zirkel, 1990) and Markus (Markus & Wurf, 1987) have noted the possible relevance of object relations theories for research on social cognition and the self. Westen (1991) is suggesting ways in which object relations theory and research can enrich, and be enriched by current research in social cognition.

Within this framework, the integration of the self perspectives of Kohut and Rogers with Bandura appears a relevant proposition. Bandura's (1986) social cognitive theory embraces an interactional model of causation in which environmental events, personal factors and behaviors operate as interacting determinants of each other, providing an interesting extension to the perspectives of Rogers and Kohut. Reciprocal causation provides people with opportunities to exercise some control over their destinies as well as set the limits of self-direction. Personal determinants of psychosocial functioning accords a central role to cognitive, vicarious, self-regulatory, and self-reflective processes. In particular, Bandura (1977a,b, 1982) postulates that all psychotherapy interactions effect change through their ability to alter the efficacy expectations that one can execute behaviors required to produce desired outcomes. This is an interesting extension and specification of Kohut's efficacy needs in the selfobject experiences (Wolf, 1988). For Bandura (1982), anxiety is viewed as the expectation that an individual lacks the necessary skills for coping with the demands of a threat situation. Teaching client skills that are needed to actually perform successfully will help the client to cope effectively with situational demands.

The integration of Rogers, Kohut, and Bandura appears as a harmonious blending that goes beyond simple juxtaposition or translation from one language to another by real complementary contributions that use the self as a unifying concept.

TECHNICAL ISSUES AND IMPLICATIONS FOR SUPERVISION AND TRAINING

We have proposed an integrative supervision and training model. Next we will look more closely at some basic issues and implications to the specific domain and process of supervision.

Integrative Approach to Supervising Trainees

The acquisition of theoretical and practical competencies are planned according to hierarchical sequences (Bernstein & Lecomte, 1976). The curriculum is articulated to ensure compatibility with pre-practicum and practicum activities. For example, students are simultaneously exposed to diagnostic activities, related concepts of psychopathology and psychotherapy while learning how to conduct intake and evaluation interviews. At each learning stage, there is a joint effort by faculty members and university supervisors to ensure the coordination of theory and practice. It takes substantial support among faculty and supervisors to adopt integrative approaches when various systems are stressing ideological uniqueness and zealotry. Specialized seminars and meetings are held each week, for example, to ensure the coordination and cohesiveness of faculty and supervisors, or to offer in-service training in some needed aspects of the program, and so forth.

Flexibility and Rigor

Trainees need to acquire a solid conceptual framework to guide their assessment, case formulation, and intervention process. The more difficult question is how to train rigorous yet flexible practitioners. Is it possible to have relevance and rigor (Cronbach, 1957)? The dilemma is between the single-theory suggesting one and only one truth and the multitheory suggesting that no truth exists. Are we condemned to produce either narrow adherents to rigid orthodoxy or "flexible" practitioners who possess a confused hodgepodge of half facts (Frances, Clarkin, & Perry, 1984).

We feel there is an intermediate position for a rigorous open-minded psychotherapist. To promote such a stance, students are first introduced to the relative equivalence of psychotherapy models in terms of efficacy. The exploration of various models is put into a pluralistic perspective underlining the complexity and multidimensionality of human behavior and therapeutic change. A pragmatic understanding that any theoretical system is a tentative and partial explanation of the person is provided. In addition, through an exploration of the complex reciprocal interpersonal influence and the multiple inferential errors and biases guiding human interactions, students are initiated to a flexible and pluralistic outlook on psychotherapy.

Within this framework, the self psychology perspectives of Rogers, Kohut, and Bandura are presented in a systematic manner. Students are required to demonstrate theoretical and practical proficiency. Even though students need to show a rigorous understanding and application of this orientation, they have to acknowledge the limitations of this approach and to remain guided by their clients' needs in a coherent and relevant manner.

In striving for rigor and flexibility, we also postulate that a clear conceptual and flexible framework provides the trainee with a sense of direction and coherence. Directionality and coherence are probably two basic ingredients of any psychotherapeutic enterprise. Integration and eclecticism, as long as they promote flexibility and the adoption of a pluralistic perspective, are commandable goals; if absolute truth is pursued through integration, then we are back to square one. Finally, perhaps what we should be aiming at is a flexible and open-minded trainee working in a coherent and rigorous fashion, aware of the relative contribution of any model but also conscious of his or her unique and meaningful interaction with his or her client, at each specific moment (Lecomte & Dumont, 1989).

The Crucial Variables in the Supervisory Process: A Quiet Blending of Self-Psychology Perspectives

It is our view that the processes that trainees undergo as they learn their craft and develop a sense of professional identity conforms to the developmental sequence which leads to individuation and identity formation in the human being.

Part of the process of becoming a psychotherapist involves developing a sense of professional identity. Once this has been attained with some degree of coherence, the professional identity serves as a stable frame of reference from which trainees make sense of their work. Ekstein and Wallerstein (1972) point out that professional identity is an extension of the self-concept.

Many authors have described developmental models of clinical supervision (Loganbill, Hardy, & Delworth, 1982; Littrell, Lee-Borden, & Lorenz, 1979; Stoltenberg & Delworth, 1987). These models serve as guidelines to chart the progress of supervisees in terms of the acquisition of knowledge, skills, personal growth, and integration. In addition, various consecutive types of supervisory relationships have been depicted (Loganbill et al., 1982).

Within these developmental models of clinical supervision, we are exploring the implications and the integration of Rogers, Kohut, and Bandura works with Stoltenberg and Delworth (1987) focusing on constructs such as self- and other-awareness, motivation, and autonomy.

When a supervisee begins his or her clinical training he or she is nominally a student trying to learn how to do psychotherapy. To start with, every trainee must define an initial role for himself or herself in the supervisory relationship. Some authors have identified this stage in terms of dependency and identification (Stoltenberg & Delworth, 1987; Loganbill et al., 1982) or imitation (Fleming, 1953). Supervisees are anxious initially and concerned about their apparent lack of skills, so they imitate their supervisor requesting suggestions. As supervisee confidence increases, the supervisor helps the trainee move into a corrective stage through various interpretations and techniques. Finally, a creative learning stage emerges when the supervises has found his or her style and identity and is working on meaningful and appropriate issues with his or her client.

In this process, the most fundamental role of the supervisor seems to be one of helping the trainee gain a cohesive and stable professional self. Rogers (1957) and Kohut (1977) bring a fundamental contribution to this process. A supervisor who conveys respect, genuineness, and empathy is likely to establish a relationship of trust in which personal and professional growth and clinical development are facilitated. Communicating a sense of acceptance contributes to heightening self-esteem and the manifestation of personal styles.

Describing the self as the structure of inner experience, Kohut (1977) introduces the notion of selfobjects referring neither to other persons nor to their behaviors, but to a dimension of one's experience of the behavior of others, namely, the subjective experience of others as serving certain functions for maintaining, restoring, or consolidating the organization of the self-experience. Fundamental human transaction is appreciating what something or somebody means to a person. These concepts provide meaningful insights into the process of the supervisory relationship. In order to develop a sense of a cohesive and stable self, Kohut suggests that supervisees need (1) to be recognized as unique and valuable; (2) to idealize a strong and soothing model; (3) to be accepted and recognized by professional peers; (4) to be able to impact and influence the supervisor or model in terms of self-efficacy; and (5) to feel accepted by the supervisor even when holding a different or adversarial position. The process through which a supervisee develops a cohesive and creative self implies the importance for the supervisor to provide an acceptable holding environment (Winnicott, 1965). Trainee's professional identity development is related to the supervisor's ability to adapt to the changing needs and capacities of the supervisee. Kohut (1968) seemed to view a critical part of the supervision as involving optimal empathic failures leading to disappointment. A supervisee who experiences disappointment of the wish to be perfectly understood, in small manageable portions, may move gradually toward individuation, professional identity, and creativity. This process needs to be embedded into a basic empathic understanding so that the empathic bond can be reestablished at a different level through optimal frustration (Winnicott, 1965).

The need for personal affirmation and creativity can be enhanced and enriched with the contribution of cognitive and behavioral theorists like Bandura (1986), Mahoney and Lyddon (1988), Beck (1976), and Meichenbaum (1985). Bandura's theory of self-efficacy, causal reciprocity, and social cognitive processes has numerous implications for training and supervision: (1) it is important to identify and treat a trainee's skill deficits in areas required for successful performance and for coping with situational demands; (2) procedures such as modeling that emphasize actual performance accomplishment represent potent procedures; (3) coping skills seem associated in correlated networks based on self-efficacy (Bandura, 1977) such that increasing one's coping repertoire may increase the probability of other types of coping skills; and (4) among the various cognitive-behavioral approaches (e.g., systematic desensitization, anxiety management, cognitive restructuring, stress inoculation), stress inoculation training (Meichenbaum, 1985) appears to be the one putting the greatest emphasis on coping as recommended by Bandura (1977) and offers the widest selection of coping strategies. As we do not know which techniques are effective for which problems, or the mechanisms by which they effect change for that matter (Lecomte & Castonguay, 1987), stress inoculation seems to offer better learning conditions than the other cognitive-behavioral techniques. Self-observation and internal dialogue procedures can also be meaningful techniques for consolidating self-perceptions.

Process and Outcome in Supervision

It is impossible to predict exactly what it takes and how long it will take a given trainee to achieve a professional identity. Our general assumption is that the process works not in linear fashion but in dynamic, multidimensional, and circular patterns (Lecomte & Castonguay, 1987). Within such a framework, we have found it useful and effective to conceptualize that at each developmental stage, the trainee needs to self-explore, self-understand, and also to act. The supervisor's tasks are to be able to assess the professional developmental level of the trainee and to provide learning conditions appropriate to that stage.

The ideal supervisor as depicted by Lambert (1986) seems to embody the same personal characteristics as the ideal psychotherapist. This notion should not be surprising insofar as many investigators have likened the client–therapist relationship to the supervisor relationship (Storm & Heath, 1985). It is relevant to consider the supervisory situation in terms of parallel processes. Rogers (1957) hypothesized that supervision must be a model of the psychotherapy process. Abroms (1977) described supervision as a "metatherapy," a therapy of therapy. There are components of the supervisory relationship which are analogous to the psychotherapeutic relationship. Within a Rogerian-Kohutian-Bandurian perspective, transference, countertransference therapeutic alliance, and real relationship (Gelso & Carter, 1985) can be utilized with some specific and relevant meanings and purposes. Using Marshall and Marshall's (1989) differentiated matrix of the supervisory relationship and Tansey and Burke's (1989) unique understanding of countertransference and transference, the therapeutic relationship components can be assessed and distinguished through three basic criteria: level of awareness, source specification, and degree of differentiation. Within this framework, notions of selfobject transferences like the need to be mirrored, to idealize, to be recognized, and to impact upon a significant other become relevant and useful for a better understanding of a trainee's professional identity development.

There are sound, objective reasons to believe that the supervisory relationship is the central vehicle for change and learning (Orlinsky & Howard, 1986). Our model suggests that it is within this evolving relationship that specific interventions and supervisory strategies have to be elaborated and integrated (Lecomte & Castonguay, 1987).

Strategies and Techniques

Within the process of helping a trainee become a psychotherapist with a cohesive and stable professional self, a number of techniques and strategies have been elaborated.

In the dependency or imitative stage, a skill-oriented model seems highly effective for the acquisition of generic and fundamental psychotherapy skills (Hart, 1982). Making therapy more objective reduces the anxiety of supervisees because they are evaluated in terms of what they do with clients, not who they are as people. Reducing anxiety to a moderate level helps supervisees learn more efficiently. If the supervisor provides an optimal climate of security and empathy, the trainee can risk exploring and gradually trust his or her own experience (Davis, 1987).

At this stage of skill development, coaching, modeling, rehearsing, feedback, and audio and videotaping are frequently used. Multiple sources of observation are used, for example, peers, clients, supervisors, and supervisees (Lecomte, 1990). Interpersonal process recall (Kagan, 1980) and microcounseling (Ivey, 1971) are structured approaches to supervision that work well with beginning trainees.

When the supervisee moves to some taking charge of himself or herself, intrinsic to this realization is the awareness that he or she is responsible for the treatment cures which he or she effects. Supervision will focus here more on transference and countertransference issues resulting in a corrective process. The supportive style has become insufficient. The process of solidifying one's professional identity will evolve through optimal frustration interactions with the supervisor (Kohut, 1968; Winnicott, 1965).

Videotaping and audiotaping remain basic procedures. At this stage, the supervisor may make some meaningful utilization of the parallel process of supervision and therapy. Rogerian and Kohutian strategies can serve as the bases for the supervisor/trainee relationship. Hart (1982) refers to this stage as the personal growth model when the goals are to increase insight and affective sensitivity about interpersonal relationships with the use of multiple techniques (e.g., audio, video, role playing, co-therapy, self-observation).

Finally, at the stage of creativity, affirmed professional identity, and integration, the supervisee has now acquired a cohesive and stable professional self (Fleming, 1953; Stoltenberg & Delworth, 1987). This sense is so firmly established that risk-taking has become an integral part of the therapeutic style. He or she knows how to use himself or herself in therapy. The supervisory strategies are then related to self-supervision, self-observation, and maintenance (Lecomte & Bernstein, 1978).

Although these stages of supervision seem sequential and linear, it should not be assumed that each stage has been fully mastered before moving to another. Learning, most of the time, is circular and dynamic. However, the supervisee who has completed these stages is often able to appreciate the complex interactions between clients, problems, relationship, techniques, and therapist.

PERSONAL ISSUES

Our model of integrative supervision evokes in trainees a constellation of affective, cognitive, and behavioral reactions. Over the first weeks, students are usually overwhelmed by the complexity of the task they are faced with: learning psychotherapeutic skills requires the integration of several abilities. Likewise, in a context of possible cognitive overload, self-exploration and disclosure of inner experiences can be an intimidating challenge. Thus, early personal reactions are generally tainted by anxiety, confusion, or anger. Such reactions can be intensified when supervisees feel particularly inadequate, vulnerable, or woundable.

Underlying these affective processes, supervisors frequently observe that there is a conflict between the emerging professional identity developed during undergraduate studies, and the theoretical requirements associated with a rapprochement between Kohut, Rogers, and Bandura. Indeed, during undergraduate training, trainees frequently adopt unidimensional or monolithic perspectives toward counseling and psychotherapy. Cognitively, at this stage, humanism, behaviorism, and psychoanalysis are perceived as antinomic approaches and students harbor, at best, ambivalent attitudes toward rapprochement. Spontaneously, they will invoke negative arguments frequently mentioned in the literature: "I do not think that anything goes with anybody in psychotherapy," "I do not even master a single model of intervention, how can you expect me to develop therapeutic skills in three very different intellectual traditions?" "It is naive to believe that Rogers, Kohut and Bandura have that much in common." Even if at first, such reactions are not overtly voiced, trainees comments often implicitly allude to such criticisms. Supervisors listening skills' will allow students to articulate their concerns more directly. After having explored in a sensitive way trainees' attitudes toward our general approach to integrative supervision and depending on the rigidity of cognitive schema students have developed, supervisors describe and illustrate, using theoretical presentations, case examples and modeling, how such apparently divergent viewpoints can be theoretically and clinically compatible.

It is important at this stage that supervisors explore these issues in the context of a positive therapeutic alliance. Integrative supervision is not a theoretical battlefield, diversity is not seen as an adversity, but as complementary. Integration adds fullness and richness to supervision by allowing the therapist to move easily from one domain to the other. As was said earlier, we do not attempt to simply juxtapose the principles of these schools of thought. Our approach to integrative supervision is based on the hypothesis that there exists commonalities and complementaries between these treatment methods. In this context, trainees are encouraged to identify strengths and weaknesses of main schools of psychotherapy. Reading recent reviews of the outcome literature (e.g., Orlinsky & Howard, 1986; Lambert, Shapiro, & Bergin, 1986) is a good method to foster openness to rapprochement and underline the potency of certain common factors to different conceptual approaches to psychotherapy.

Over time, and through concrete observation of trainees' therapeutic skills and behaviors in supervision, we have come to the conclusion that self-structure is a crucial parameter determining trainees' attitudes toward the supervisory environment. Trainees that initially present conscious or unconscious expectations of self-perfection pointing to an infantile grandiose self will per-

ceive supervisors as hostile or unresponsive. These grandiose beliefs of perfect control over the environment are tamed, optimally in a gradual way, by continuous performance and process feedback while supervisors maintain an empathic stance. The supervisor acts as a mirroring figure and shows nonjudgmental patience; supervisees need the supervisor's active approval. Upon admittance to a graduate study program in counseling or clinical psychology, students often feel that they have been accepted because they are special or because they have a special aptitude to become a psychotherapist. The development of these fleeting grandiose fantasies serves an appropriate psychological function; reducing anxiety over being an apprentice and decreasing feelings of inadequacy. Eventually, reality tempers these fantasies and students will often comfort themselves by idealizing their supervisor; this is another psychological coping strategy which helps supervisees to see supervision as a safe and controllable environment. The supervisor becomes someone to please. However, excessive idealizing will quickly prove ineffective. Trainees may feel that they have to prove themselves as worthy of attention from such an idealized parent imago; consequently, students can apply too concretely supervisors' suggestions. Cases of paralyzing embarrassment are also not infrequent. Supervisees will refrain from exposing their weak spots, discussing their learning needs, and asserting their clinical hypotheses. The supportive behaviors of supervisors can be rejected or interpreted as criticisms. At these critical points, supervisors often are perceived as self-objects for their students; i.e., someone who can help maintain coherence, continuity, and self-esteem (Norcross, Saltzman, & Gienta, 1990). Sustained empathic inquiry and support will help trainees work through difficulties they experience in supervision and with their clients. However, accomplishing these functions is not a simple endeavor, especially when supervisors have dual roles: encouraging self-exploration and assessing clinical competencies. This dual role may pose problems and provoke ruptures in the learning alliance.

In closing, it must be underscored that this description of personal issues in supervision is not exclusive and unique to integrative supervision. In a sense, every supervision program will evoke similar issues. However, we believe that in integrative supervision, such reactions are intensified by the multitheoretical nature of the program. This necessitates a good deal of tolerance of ambiguity in students and a low need for premature closure.

CONCLUDING COMMENTS

This chapter has presented a model of clinical training and supervision which is a pragmatic and harmonious blending using the "self" as a unifying concept. In this supervisory and training model, the supervisor and trainees take a multitheoretical approach to clinical supervision, whereby components of Rogers, Kohut, and Bandura are blended.

In recommending such an approach, attention must be given to numerous factors inherent to the complexity of the therapeutic reality. Among the most important are the personality of the supervisee, the stage of training and the needs of clients. For example, a trainee who is confused with fluctuating motivation and a dependency-autonomy conflict, would be a bad match for a supervisor who is anxious and stressing mechanistic performance. Trainers also have to remain aware that supervisees differ in the amount of support, direction, or interpretation they need. Their needs often change over time. Moreover, the client's needs must be appraised so as to ensure that supervision is being carried out in such a way that therapeutic gains will be maximized. Considerable amounts of knowledge, skills, and flexibility are thus required from supervisors. Most importantly, the effectiveness of our approach, as for any type of integrative training, rely on an ability to discern the clients' and trainee's requirements, and the capacity to teach various personal and technical skills in a coherent, articulated, and open-minded way.

ACKNOWLEDGMENTS. This chapter was written while the second author was receiving a fellowship from the Social Sciences and Humanities Research Council of Canada. Stéphane Sabourin was supported by the Social Sciences and Humanities Research Council of Canada through a Canada Research Fellowship. The authors wish to thank Susan Wiser and Marc-Simon Drouin for their editorial assistance.

REFERENCES

Abroms, G. M. (1977). Supervision as metatherapy. In F. W. Kaslow & Associates (Eds.), *Supervision, consultation and staff training in the helping professions* (pp. 81–89). Washington, DC: Jossey-Bass.

Andrews, J. D. W. (1989). Integrative languages in therapeutic practice and training: Promises and pitfalls. *Journal of Integrative and Eclectic Psychotherapy, 8,* 291–302.

APA. (1979). Criteria for accreditation of doctoral training programs and internships in professional psychology. *American Psychological Association.* Washington, DC.

Arkowitz, H., & Messer, S. B. (Eds.). (1984). *Psychoanalytic and behavior therapy: Is integration possible?* New York: Plenum Press.

Bandura, A. (1977a). Self efficacy: Toward a unifying theory of behavior change. *Psychological Review, 84,* 191–215.

Bandura, A. (1977b). *Social learning theory.* Englewood Cliffs, NJ: Prentice-Hall.

Bandura, A. (1982). Self-efficacy mechanism in human agency. *American Psychologist, 37,* 122–147.

Bandura, A. (1986). *Social foundations of thought and action: A social cognitive theory.* Englewood Cliffs, NJ: Prentice-Hall.

Beck, A. T. (1976). *Cognitive therapy and emotional disorders.* New York: International Universities Press.

Bernstein, B. L., & Lecomte, C. (1976). An integrative competence-based counselor education model. *Counselor Education and Supervision, 16,* 26–36.

Beutler, L. E. (1983). *Eclectic psychotherapy: A systematic approach.* New York: Pergamon.

Beutler, L. E. (1986). Systematic eclectic psychotherapy. In J. C. Norcross (Ed.), *Handbook of eclectic psychotherapy.* New York: Brunner/Mazel.

Beutler, L. E., Mahoney, M. J., Norcross, J. C., Prochaska, J.O., Sollod, R. M., & Robertson, M. (1987). Training integrative/eclectic psychotherapist II. *Journal of Integrative and Eclectic Psychotherapy, 6,* 296–332.

Blatt, S. J., & Lerner, H. (1983). Investigations in the psychoanalytic theory of object relations and object representations. In J. Masling (Ed.), *Empirical studies of psychoanalytic theories* (Vol. 1, pp. 189–249). Hillsdale, NJ: Lawrence Erlbaum.

Cantor, N., & Zirkel, S. (1990). Personality, cognition and purposive behavior. In L. Pervin (Ed.), *Handbook of personality* (pp. 135–164). New York: Guilford.

Carkhuff, R. R. (1969). *Helping and human relations.* New York: Holt, Rinehart & Winston.

CPA (1983). Accreditation criteria for clinical psychology programs and internships. *Canadian Psychological Association,* Old Chelsea.

Cronbach, J. L. (1957). The two disciplines of scientific psychology. *American Psychologist, 12,* 671–684.

Davis, W. N. (1987). The learning problem of the student in psychotherapy supervision. *Journal of College Student Psychotherapy, 1*(3), 69–89.

Egan, G. (1981). *The skilled helper* (2nd ed.). Monterey, CA: Brooks/Cole.

Ekstein, R., & Wallerstein, R. S. (1972). *The teaching and learning of psychotherapy* (2nd ed.). New York: International Universities Press.

Fischer, J. (1986). Eclectic casework. In J. C. Norcross (Ed.), *Handbook of eclectic psychotherapy* (pp. 320–352). New York: Brunner/Mazel.

Fleming, J. (1953). The role of supervision in psychiatric training. *Bulletin of the Menninger Clinic, 17,* 157–159.

Frances, A., & Clarkin, J. F. (1981). No treatment as the prescription of choice. *Archives of General Psychiatry, 38,* 542–545.

Frances, A., Clarkin, J., & Perry, S. (1984). *Differential therapeutics in psychiatry.* New York: Brunner/Mazel.

Franks, C. M. (1984). On conceptual integrity in psychoanalysis and behavior therapy: Two fundamentally incompatible systems. In H. Arkowitz & S. B. Messer (Eds.), *Psychoanalytic therapy and behavior therapy: Is integration possible?* (pp. 233–247). New York: Plenum Press.

Fuhriman, A., Paul, S. C., & Burlingame, G. N. (1986). Eclectic time-limited therapy. In J. C. Norcross (Ed.), *Handbook of eclectic psychotherapy* (pp. 226–259). New York: Brunner/Mazel.

Garfield, S. L. (1980). *Psychotherapy: An eclectic approach.* New York: Wiley.

Garfield, S. L. (1986). Research on client variables in psychotherapy. In S. L. Garfield & A. E. Bergin (Eds.), *Handbook of psychotherapy and behavior change* (3rd ed.). New York: Wiley.

Gelso, C. J., & Carter, J. A. (1985). The relationship in counseling and psychotherapy: Component, consequences and theoretical antecedents. *Counseling Psychologist, 13,* 155–243.

Girard, A. G. (1988). *Le développement professionnel et les préférences théoriques du psychologues débutant recevant une formation multithéorique.* Unpublished doctoral dissertation, Université de Montréal.

Goldfried, M. R. (Ed.). (1982). *Converging themes in the practice of psychotherapy.* New York: Springer.

Goldfried, M.R., & Castonguay, L. G. (1992). The future of psychotherapy integration. *Psychotherapy, 29,* 4–10.

Goldfried, M. R., & Newman, C. (1986). Psychotherapy integration: An historical perspective. In J. C. Norcross (Ed.), *Handbook of eclectic psychotherapy* (pp. 25–64). New York: Brunner/Mazel.

Grebstein, L. C. (1986). An eclectic family therapy. In J. C. Norcross (Ed.), *Handbook of eclectic psychotherapy,* (pp. 282–319). New York: Brunner/Mazel.

Halgin, R. P. (1985). Teaching integration of psychotherapy models to beginning therapists. *Psychotherapy, 22,* 555–563.

Halgin, R. P. (1986). Pragmatic blending of clinical models in the supervisory relationship. *Clinical Supervisor, 3,* 23–46.

Halgin, R. P. (Ed.). (1988). Special section: Issues in the supervision of integrative psychotherapy. *Journal of Integrative and Eclectic Psychotherapy, 7,* 152–180.

Hart, G. (1982). *The process of clinical supervision.* Baltimore: University Park Press.

Hart, J. T. (1986). Functional eclectic therapy. In J. C. Norcross (Ed.), *Handbook of eclectic psychotherapy* (pp. 201–225). New York: Brunner/Mazel.

Heppner, P. P., & Clairborn, C. D. (1989). Social influence research in counseling: A review and critique. *Journal of Counseling Psychology, 36,* 365–385.

Ivey, A. E. (1971). *Microcounseling: Innovation in interviewing training.* Springfield, IL: Thomas.

Kagan, N. (1980). Influencing human interaction: Eighteen years with IPR. In A. K. Hess (Ed.), *Psychotherapy supervision* (pp. 262–286). New York: Wiley.

Kahn, E. (1985). Heinz Kohut and Carl Rogers: A timely comparison. *American Psychologist, 40,* 893–904.

Kahn, E. (1989). Heinz Kohut and Carl Rogers: Toward a constructive collaboration. *Psychotherapy, 4,* 555–563.

Kohut, H. (1968). The psychoanalytic treatment of narcissistic personality disorders: Outline of a systematic approach. *Psychoanalytic Study of the Child, 23,* 86–113.

Kohut, H. (1971). *The analysis of the self.* New York: International Universities Press.

Kohut, H. (1977). *The restoration of the self.* New York: International Universities Press.

Kohut, H., & Wolf, E. S. (1978). The disorders of the self and their treatment: An outline. *International Journal of Psychoanalysis, 59,* 413–425.

Lambert, M. J. (1986). Implications of psychotherapy outcome research for eclectic psychotherapy. In J. C. Norcross (Ed.), *Handbook of eclectic psychotherapy* (pp. 436–462). New York: Brunner/Mazel.

Lambert, M. J., & Arnold, R. C. (1987). Research and supervisory process. *Professional Psychology: Research and Practice, 18,* 217–224.

Lambert, M. J., Shapiro, D. A., & Bergin, A. E. (1986). The effectiveness of psychotherapy. In S. L. Garfield & A. E. Bergin, *Handbook of psychotherapy and behavior change* (3rd ed., pp. 157–211). New York: Wiley.

Landsman, T. (1982). Not an adversity but a welcome diversity. In M. R. Goldfried (Ed.), *Converging themes in psychotherapy: Trends in psychodynamic and behavioral practice.* New York: Springer.

Lazarus, A. A. (1976). *Multimodal behavior therapy.* New York: Springer.

Lazarus, A. A. (1981). *The practice of multimodal therapy.* New York: McGraw-Hill.

Lazarus, A. A. (1986). Multimodal Therapy. In J. C. Norcross (Ed.), *Handbook of eclectic psychotherapy* (pp. 65–93). New York: Brunner/Mazel.

Lecomte, C. (1990). *Cahier de stages de M.Ps. en counseling.* Unpublished manuscript. Université de Montréal.

Lecomte, C., & Bernstein, B. L. (1978). *Development of self-supervision skills.* Paper presented at the annual meeting of the American Personnel and Guidance Association, Washington, DC.

Lecomte, C., & Castonguay, L. G. (1987). *Rapprochement et intégration en psychothérapie: Psychanalyse, behaviorisme et humanisme.* Montréal: Gaëtan Morin.

Lecomte, C., & Dumont, F. (1989). Erreurs, intuition et jugement en counseling et en psychothérapie. *Orientation, 3,* 1–18.

Littrel, J. M., Lee-Borden, N., & Lorenz, J. A. (1979). A developmental framework for counseling supervision. *Counselor Education and Supervision, 19,* 129–136.

Loganbill, C. Hardy, E., & Delworth, U. (1982). Supervision: A conceptual model *Counseling Psychologist, 10,* 3–42.

Luborsky, L., Singer, B., & Luborsky, L. (1975). Comparative studies of psychotherapies: Is it true that "Everyone has won and all must have prizes"? *Archives of General Psychiatry, 32,* 995–1008.

Mahoney, M. J., & Lyddon, W. J. (1988). Recent developments in cognitive approaches to counseling and psychotherapy. *Counseling Psychologist, 16,* 190–234.

Markus, H., & Wurf, E. (1987). The dynamic self-concept: A social psychological perspective. *Annual Review of Psychology, 38,* 299–337.

Marmor, J., & Woods, S. M. (1980). *The interface between the psychodynamic and behavioral analysis.* New York: Plenum Press.

Marshall, R. U., & Marshall S. V. (1989). *The transference-countertransference matrix: The emotional-cognitive dialogue in psychotherapy, psychoanalysis and supervision.* New York: Columbia University Press.

Meichenbaum, D. (1977). *Cognitive behavior modification: An integrative approach.* New York: Plenum Press.

Meichenbaum, D. H. (1985). *Stress inoculation training.* New York: Pergamon.

Messer, S. B. (1986). Behavior and psychoanalytic perspectives at therapeutic choice points. *American Psychologist, 41,* 1261–1272.

Messer, S. B., & Winokur, M. (1980). Some limits to the integration of psychoanalytic and behavior therapy. *American Psychologist, 35,* 818–827.

Messer, S. B., & Winokur, M. (1984). Ways of knowing and visions of reality in psychoanalytic therapy and behavior therapy. In H. Arkowitz & S. B. Messer (Eds.), *Psychoanalytic therapy and behavior therapy: Is integration possible?* (pp. 63–100). New York: Plenum Press.

Murray, E. J. (1986). Possibilities and promises of eclecticism. In J. C. Norcross (Ed.), *Handbook of eclectic psychotherapy* (pp. 398–415). New York: Brunner/Mazel.

Norcross, J. C. (Ed.). (1986). *Handbook of eclectic psychotherapy.* New York: Brunner/Mazel.

Norcross, J. C. (Section Ed.). (1986). Training integrative/eclectic psychotherapists. *International Journal of Eclectic Psychotherapy, 5,* 71–94.

Norcross, J. S. (1988). Supervision of integrative psychotherapy. *Journal of Integrative and Eclectic Psychotherapy, 7,* 157–166.

Norcross, J. C., Saltzman, N., & Gienta, L. C. (1990). Contention and convergence in the psychotherapies. In N. Saltzman & J. C. Norcross (Eds.), *Therapy wars: Contention and convergence in differing clinical approaches* (pp. 242–260). San Francisco: Jossey-Bass.

Orlinsky, D. E., & Howard, D. I. (1978). The relation of process to outcome in psychotherapy. In S. L. Garfield & A. E. Bergin (Eds.), *Handbook of psychotherapy and behavior change* (2nd ed., pp. 283–330). New York: Wiley.

Orlinsky, D. E., & Howard, K. I. (1986). Process and outcome in psychotherapy. In S. L. Garfield & A. E. Bergin (Eds.), *Handbook of psychotherapy and behavior change* (3rd ed., pp. 311–381). New York: Wiley.

Prochaska, J. O., & DiClemente, C. C. (1984). *The transtheoretical approach: Crossing the traditional boundaries of therapy.* Homewood, IL: Dow-Jones-Irwin.

Prochaska, J. O., & DiClemente, C. C. (1986). The transtheoretical approach. In J. C. Norcross (Ed.), *Handbook of eclectic psychotherapy* (pp. 163–200). New York: Brunner/Mazel.

Robertson, M. (1986). Training eclectic psychotherapists.

In J. C. Norcross (Ed.), *Handbook of eclectic psychotherapy* (pp. 416–435). New York: Brunner/Mazel.

Rogers, C. R. (1951). *Client-centered therapy.* Boston: Houghton Mifflin.

Rogers, C. R. (1957). Training individuals to engage in the therapeutic process. In C. R. Strother (Ed.), *Psychology and mental health* (pp. 76–92). Washington, DC: American Psychological Association.

Rogers, C. R. (1986). Rogers, Kohut, and Erickson: A personal perspective on some similarities and differences. *Person-Centered Review, 1,* 125–140.

Rychlack, J. F. (1981). *Introduction to personality and psychotherapy* (2nd ed.). Boston: Houghton Mifflin.

Singer, J. (1985). Transference and the human condition: A cognitive and affective perspective. *Psychoanalytic Psychology, 2,* 189–219.

Singer, J. (1984). The private personality. *Personality and Social Psychology Bulletin, 10,* 7–30.

Stoltenberg, C. (1981). Approaching supervision from a developmental perspective: The counselor complexity model. *Journal of Counseling Psychology, 28,* 59–65.

Stoltenberg, C. D., Delworth, V. (1987). *Supervising counselors and therapists: A developmental approach.* San Francisco: Jossey-Bass.

Stricker, G. (1988). Supervision of integrative psychotherapy: A discussion. *Journal of Integrative and Eclectic Psychotherapy, 7,* 176–180.

Stricker, G., & Healey, B. D. (1990). Projective assessment of object relations: A review of the empirical literature. *Psychological Assessment: A Journal of Consulting and Clinical Psychology, 2,* 219–230.

Storm, C. L., & Heath, A. W. (1985). Models of supervision: Using therapy theory as a guide. *Clinical Supervisor, 3,* 87–96.

Tansey, M. J., & Burke, W. F. (1989). *Understanding countertransference: From projection to empathy.* Hillsdale, NJ: The Analytic Press.

Tomkins, S. (1979). Script theory: Differential magnification of affects. In H. E. Howe Jr., & R. A. Dienstbier (Eds.), *Nebraska Symposium on Motivation* (Vol. 26, pp. 201–236). Lincoln: University of Nebraska Press.

Tracey, T. J., Hays, K. A., Malone, J., & Herman, B. (1988). Changes in counselor response as a function of experience. *Journal of Counseling Psychology, 35,* 119–126.

Watters, W. W., Rubenstein, J. S., & Bellissimo, A. (1980). Teaching psychotherapy: Learning objectives in individual psychotherapy. *Canadian Journal of Psychology, 25,* 111–117.

Westen, D. (1991). Social cognition and object relations. *Psychological Bulletin, 109,* 429–455.

Winnicott, D. (1965). *The maturational process and the facilitating environment.* New York: Basic Books.

Wolf, E. S. (1988). *Treating the self: Elements of clinical self psychology.* New York: Guilford.

Wright, J., & Sabourin, S. (1987). Les contributions du modèle behavioral à la problématique du rapprochement en psychothérapie. In C. Lecomte & L. G. Castonguay (Eds.), *Rapprochement et intégration en psychothérapie: Psychanalyse, béhaviorisme et humanisme* (pp. 81–100). Montréal: Gaëtan Morin.

CHAPTER 34

Supervision and Instruction in Postgraduate Psychotherapy Integration

Eugene H. Walder

I accepted the invitation to prepare this chapter in September of 1990. At the time of the charge by the editors, the launch of the Institute for Integrated Training in Psychotherapy (IITP) was still a week away.

In general, I am not inclined to procrastinate. Yet, as the weeks and months passed, I engaged in suppression or thought stopping (depending on whether one's orientation is psychoanalytic or behavioral). Sometime in March of 1991, I awoke from an anxiety or examination dream. In this dream, I was enrolled in a course and because I had forgotten to attend classes was suddenly faced with a final examination for which I was totally unprepared. It did not take any great feat of self-analysis to interpret this dream. Its meaning was clear—the deadline for this chapter was only 3 months away, however, I had not thought about it, let alone had I written a single word.

I took some comfort in the realization that heretofore I had not acquired the experience necessary to complete this chapter. Nor, for that matter, had anyone else—at least, not at the level of an in-depth training institute in psychotherapy integration, which was the main topic to be addressed.

Before this undertaking, training in an integrative or eclectic approach to psychotherapy had been confined to year-long integrative/eclectic graduate courses and seminars, and even these were few and far between; the reasons advanced for this scarcity of integrative training efforts have included the lack of sophisticated models of integration, the failure to achieve a consensus as to definitions of eclecticism, the level and method of integration, and the complexity of ensuring competence and skill in several theoretical orientations (Beutler, Mahony, Norcross, Prochaska, Robertson, & Sollod, 1987). So, besides these difficulties endemic to any integrative training effort, the undertaking of a postgraduate training institute in psychotherapy integration was bound to pose unforeseen and unpredictable issues. Until the latter took shape around just about every aspect of the program—involving the curriculum, faculty, and students—the topic of this chapter could not be developed fully.

Eugene H. Walder • Institute for Integrated Training in Psychotherapy, New York, New York 10019.

Comprehensive Handbook of Psychotherapy Integration, edited by George Stricker and Jerold R. Gold. Plenum Press, New York, 1993.

Unlike my dream, however, in which I engaged in motivated forgetting, the year during which the material for this chapter was gathered proved to be most fruitful, involving as it did the development, implementation, and evaluation of the program. This chapter is based on observations garnered from my experiences during the 1990–1991 academic year. They are offered as hypotheses and speculations in relation to what is at this point in time essentially an experiment in supervision and instruction in psychotherapy integration conducted by a postgraduate training institute.

THEORETICAL AND CONCEPTUAL ISSUES

Now it stands to reason that if you are going to provide integrated training in psychotherapy, you had better know just what it is that you mean by integration. The lack of a consensus of what constitutes a practical definition of eclecticism, the level at which integration is best conceptualized and the most effective method by which integration can be implemented, have been advanced as major stumbling blocks to the "paucity" of systematic training in integration (Beutler et al., 1987, p. 297).

Should we stay on the high ground and include only those approaches that involve a synthesis? Wachtel (1987, p. 126) eloquently characterized what such a synthesis would involve:

As I conceive it, an integration is not just a hodgepodge of eclecticism, a salad with a little of this and a little of that tossed in. The goal, rather, is the development of a new coherent structure, an internally consistent approach both to technical intervention and to the construction of theory.

As I understand it, this statement represents, at the present state of our knowledge, an ideal to strive for rather than actual accomplishment.

The cyclical model appears to come closest to realizing Wachtel's quest for a synthesis. What characterizes this model is a theoretical framework positing cyclical interactions that maintain and perpetuate psychopathology, and interventions from alternative approaches that are employed to break the vicious circles the patient is trapped in. To meet the criteria for a cyclical model, the interventions must be internally consistent with the theory. For example, in Wachtel's

(1987) cyclical psychodynamic model, the concept of transference as defined by classical psychoanalysis had to be revised to permit the utilization of action-oriented behavioral techniques by the therapist.

At the present time, there are only a handful of cyclical integrative models. Beutler et al. (1987, p. 297) maintained that the absence of "compelling" models of integration has impeded the advance of systematic integrative training. However, the difference between integrative training and training in integrative psychotherapy should be kept clearly in mind, because although we have some integrative models, we may be light years away from a comprehensive approach that could bear the designation, "integrative psychotherapy." However, that does not mean that we have to suspend scientific advance until we invent a single integrative approach. An analogous situation is the field of physics, where the universe is described in terms of theories that are inconsistent with each other—the general theory of relativity and quantum mechanics—yet the search continues for a complete unified theory that will be a combination of these two basic partial theories (Hawking, 1988).

The cyclical model appears to be the most promising development to date in the direction of an integrative psychotherapy. Wachtel's groundbreaking "cyclical psychodynamic" model (1987), involving the integration of psychodynamic and behavioral approaches, has influenced the development of other cyclical models (Frank, 1990; Safran, 1990). But what of other approaches that fall under the rubric of "integration"? Schacht (1984) described what he terms, "varieties of integrative experience" all of which he characterized as integrative models, including the following: the translation model; the complementary model; the synergistic model; the emergent model; and the synthetic model.

With the exception of the cyclical theories which represent a theoretical synthesis, are these truly integrative approaches or are they, to turn Freud's famous dream analogy around, beggars dressed in princely robes—eclectic approaches disguised in the noble garb of "integration"?

All of this leads to a related issue—is the line of demarcation between eclecticism and integration that well defined? I think not. To go back to Wachtel's culinary analogy, a Caesar's salad, for example, is more than just "a hodgepodge . . . with a little of this and a little of that tossed in" (1987, p. 128), but rather is a skillfully blended combination of ingredients. Our Caesar's salad might not meet the criteria for integration proposed by Wachtel, but it does correspond to Schact's synergistic model (1984). Our hypothetical Caesar's salad would also meet Wachtel's test of internal consistency: "The major constraint is that the elements must not be incompatible in the context of the new structure" (Wachtel, 1987, p. 128), since substituting sardines for anchovies would destroy the integrity of our salad and would be grounds for immediate dismissal of the salad chef committing such an atrocity. And furthermore, since the ingredients are combined according to a time-honored recipe, a Caesar's salad worthy of its name would certainly be more than just a "hodgepodge" of this and that but could well qualify as a "new coherent structure" (Wachtel, 1987, p. 126), another of Wachtel's criteria for integration. Now, I do not want to stretch Wachtel's analogy any further, but the point I want to make is that integration and eclecticism are not, at least at this time, entirely separate entities.

Since integrative theories at their best can accommodate only selected elements of theory and techniques, there is always a danger of ending up with a hodgepodge of *theories*, each contributing a little of this and a little of that. In order to forestall that possibility, elevating an imaginative and unruly eclecticism to the high ground might enable us to keep our powder dry, and in the end, might further the cause of developing a unified integrative theory.

Of late, the distinction between integration and eclecticism has been dealt another blow by the work of Messer and Winokur (1984). In their earlier work (1980), integration between psychoanalytic and behavior therapies was considered to be impossible, because at a metatheoretical level, contradictory "visions of reality" characterized the roles of the practitioners of these approaches. In their recent writing, however, Messer and Winokur (1984), have tempered their position, allowing for behavior therapists working analytically to shift from a comic to a tragic vision and psychoanalytic therapists working behaviorally to shift from a tragic vision to a comic vision.

Once Messer and Winokur admit to the possibility that therapists from different approaches can shift from one vision of reality to another, the question can then be raised—are we dealing with integration or with eclecticism? How does this shift in visions of reality differ from an eclectic approach in which the therapist borrows whatever meets the patient's or client's needs at that time, except in this instance, the therapist borrows a different vision of reality, rather than a theory or technique? Even at this rather lofty metatheoretical level, the differences between eclecticism and integration are ill-defined.

And then there is the matter of determining from whose perspective we define integration—the therapist's or the patient's. For example, let us take the hypothetical example of an analytic therapist employing cognitive restructuring with an analytic patient to identify negative thoughts, logical errors and negative schema, in an attempt to improve the patient's low self-esteem. I would doubt that Wachtel would consider that to be integration, since it would not satisfy his criteria for a synthesis from a theoretical standpoint, lacking as it is "a new coherent structure" (Wachtel, 1987, p. 126). However, I would suspect that from the patient's naive perspective, the effect is probably the same, with or without a coherent, internally consistent theory, because both approaches contribute to what the patient needs. It could be argued that the therapist might be more effective, with than without, an integrated theory. But we also know that patients improve, or do not improve, with or without our theories.

In anticipating the challenge of a burgeoning integration movement, Wachtel (1987, pp. 130–131) sounded a note of caution which bears on training in the field of psychotherapy integration. He said,

> But there are dangers as well. It would be unfortunate if integrative psychotherapy were to become a new "school" with gradually encrusting borders. It's strength lies precisely in its continued openness to the work of others.

In retrospect, I am glad that I settled on the name that I did, "Institute for Integrated Training in Psychotherapy." The alternative name under consideration, "Institute for Training in Integrated Psychotherapy" would have been a misnomer. Although at the present time we have a few integrated models, we are far from a comprehensive approach that could be characterized as "integrative psychotherapy."

In the foreseeable future, we need not be concerned about Wachtel's warning. The best that the field of psychotherapy integration has at its disposal is a sparse offering of integrative models, representing partial theories. So, in fact, there is no imminent danger of a new school of integrative psychotherapy coming on the scene. However, human nature being what it is, it can be predicted with a reasonable degree of certainty that there will eventually be such a threat from the extremes.

The most effective safeguard against Wachtel's warning becoming prophetic is to grant separate but equal status to integration and eclecticism, recognizing that even the best theories are necessarily selective. Theory building should be encouraged, to be sure, but so should an imaginative and unruly eclecticism that will act as a gadfly against orthodoxy.

I am, reminded of the Biblical story of the wise King Solomon who, when faced with a judgment about which of two women was a child's mother, requested a sword and said, "Now divide the living child in two and give half to one woman and half to the other." The real mother said, "Give her the living child and do not kill it" while the other woman said, "Let it be neither mine nor yours. Let it be divided." Now, of course, Solomon had no intention of carrying out his threat but it had been a test to discover who the real mother was.

Can we divide integration and eclecticism into two halves without seriously harming the cause of psychotherapy integration. I think not. Each can contribute something of value to the other: integrative theories—innovative and disciplined; eclectic approaches—imaginative and unruly; both striving toward a unified approach.

TECHNICAL ISSUES

The development of an integrative curriculum, involving as it does not only multiple approaches, but also integrative and eclectic models, poses an unparalleled challenge in therapist training (Beutler et al., 1987; Wolfe & Goldfried, 1988). The essence of the conundrum can be simply stated as "What to teach?" and "When should it be taught?" The ancillary issues concerning "Who

should teach it?" and "To whom it should be taught?" have to be addressed as well.

Moreover, what should be excluded from the curriculum is as much an issue as what should be included. It may be begging the question, but if an integrative program is to be manageable, it must concentrate on essentials; of necessity, providing training in multiple approaches, but in so doing, sacrificing breadth for depth. Any training program, regardless of orientation, must be selective with respect to subject matter (Beutler et al., 1987); an integrative training program must be more so. A curriculum that teaches everything, in effect, teaches nothing.

Unfortunately, logic alone does not provide a definitive basis for the design of an integrative curriculum. In designing our integrated curriculum, it appeared to be most sensible to follow the historical path along which the different theoretical orientations have developed—to provide a foundation in psychoanalytic theory, the cornerstone of psychotherapeutic intervention since the turn of the century; to exclude humanistic approaches that have branched off into an evolutionary dead end, leaving traces which have been assimilated by the larger therapeutic community; to behavioral and cognitive approaches that have evolved along separate lines from psychoanalysis, at a much later date but are now serious competitors in the psychotherapy marketplace; and to integration, that may someday achieve dominance over pure-strain approaches and result in their extinction.

Consequently, a three-track, sequential model was developed: psychodynamic, behavioral, and integrated. (See Tables 1 and 2.)

Each track was to be a year long. Aside from courses and modules, each track required 40 hours of group supervision and 40 hours of didactic group therapy, the latter representing a combination of instruction and treatment. In addition, 12 Integrative Case Seminars were held during the academic year. The integrative seminar was the centerpiece of the training program, involving dialogue between students and faculty representing divergent orientations. Through the vehicle of these seminars, students were exposed to the integrative process.

Although it appears to be sensible on the face of it, the sequential model proved to have

Table 1. Summary of Requirements for Serial Curriculum

First year	Second year	Third year
Psychodynamic track Fall semester	Behavioral track Fall semester	Integrated track Fall semester
Courses Theory and techniques I (15 sessions)	Courses Theory and techniques I (15 sessions)	Courses Theory and techniques I (15 sessions)
Modules Key concepts in psychodynamic therapy I (4 sessions) Transference and counter- transference	Modules Methods and procedures in behavior therapy I (4 sessions) Assessment	Modules Paradigms of integration I (4 sessions)
Key concepts in psychodynamic therapy II (4 sessions) Resistance	Methods and procedures in behav- ioral therapy II (4 sessions) Systematic desensitization	Paradigms of integration II (4 ses- sions)
Key concepts in psychodynamic therapy III (4 sessions) Dream interpretation	Methods and procedures in behavior therapy III (4 sessions) Cognitive restructuring	Paradigms of integration III (4 ses- sions)
Seminars Integrative case seminars: I–VI	Seminars Integrative case seminars: XIII–XVIII	Seminars Integrative case seminars: XXV–XXX
Supervision (see Spring)	Supervision (see Spring)	Supervision (see Spring)
Therapy (see Spring)	Therapy (see Spring)	Therapy (see Spring)
		Project Integrative case study

several serious drawbacks which became glaringly obvious during the first year of the program, including:

1. Integration requires a knowledge of the approaches to be integrated. Students could not derive optimum benefit from the integrative case seminars, during the first year of the program, because they lacked the most basic knowledge of behavioral, cognitive, and integrative approaches.

2. Consequently, integrative efforts were bogged down by this lack of basics. During the integrative seminars, time had to be taken to explain what the students should already have known, but had not been taught. Even so, only rudimentary knowledge could be imparted within this format.

3. Students were frustrated by having to delay gratification in relation to doing what they had set out to do; that is, acquire knowledge and skills in psychotherapy integration.

4. Even in these times of multinational conglomerates exercising a panoply of control over any number of diverse corporations, it is recognized as important for each company to maintain a separate identity, for the consumers, to be sure, but for the employees as well. In this vein, the sequential model did not provide the focus necessary to give students a sense of identity and loyalty to the program. It was as though our hypothetical employees worked for three separate organizations, each with a different identity, and what is more, identities that were often in sharp conflict with each other.

For the above stated reasons, a sequential curriculum proved to be an ineffective and inefficient method of going about the task of teaching

Table 2. **Summary of Requirements for Serial Curriculum**

First year	Second year	Third year
Psychodynamic track Spring semester	Behavioral track Spring semester	Integrated track Spring semester
Courses Theory and techniques II (15 sessions)	Courses Theory and techniques II (15 sessions)	Courses Theory and techniques II (15 sessions)
Modules Techniques in psychodynamic therapy I (4 sessions) Transference and counter- transference	Modules Clinical treatment strategies in behavior therapy I (4 sessions) Cognitive and behavioral treatment of anxiety and panic disorders	Modules Integrated treatment modalities I (4 sessions) Marital and sex therapy
Techniques in psychodynamic therapy II (4 sessions) Resistance	Clinical treatment strategies in behavioral therapy II (4 sessions) Cognitive and behavioral treatment of depressive disorders	Integrated treatment modalities II (4 sessions) Short-term psychotherapy
Techniques in psychodynamic therapy III (4 sessions) Dream interpretation	Clinical treatment strategies in behavior therapy III (4 sessions) Assertiveness and social skills training	Integrated treatment modalities III (4 sessions) Group therapy
Seminars Integrative case seminars: VII– XII	Seminars Integrative case seminars: XIX–XXIV	Seminars Integrative case seminars: XXXI– XXXVI
Supervision (total 40 sessions)	Supervision (total 40 sessions)	Supervision (total 40 sessions)
Therapy (total 40 sessions plus 80 ses- sions individual therapy)	Therapy (total 40 sessions)	Therapy (total 40 sessions)
		Project Integrative case study

psychotherapy integration. In an attempt to remedy the defects inherent in the sequential model, and to provide a curriculum that was integrative in every sense of the term, the curriculum was redesigned along the lines of a "concurrent" model.

Rather than exposing students to a logical series of approaches, as in the sequential model, the concurrent model exposes students to multiple orientations, including integrative approaches, simultaneously, as shown in Tables 3, 4, and 5.

Unlike the sequential model, in which integrative issues were postponed until the third year (with the exception of the integrative case seminars), the concurrent model will very quickly establish a "beachhead" in integrationist territory. The plan is to present an overview of integrative/eclectic models, to provide students with a conceptual framework around which to understand and organize subsequent learning. Simultaneously, the raw basics of psychodynamic and cognitive-behavioral theory and techniques will be presented, along with didactic group therapy and supervision, both on a rotational basis. Didactic group therapy will provide an opportunity for students to experience each of the orientations as a "patient," while at the same time will enable them to acquire knowledge and skills as a clinician.

Integrative Models 1, Approaches to Integration, will provide an overview of the field, introducing students to concepts and controversy in psychotherapy integration.

Safran's (1990) cognitive-interpersonal model will expose students to a cyclical model of inte-

Table 3. Summary of Requirements for Concurrent Curriculum (First Year)

Fall semester	Spring semester
Courses	Modules
Theory and techniques I (13 sessions) Interpersonal	Key concepts in psychodynamic therapy I (4 sessions) Transference, counter-transference, and resistance
Theory and techniques II (13 sessions) Cognitive-behavioral	Key concepts in psychodynamic therapy II (4 sessions) Dream interpretation
Modules Integrative models I (4 sessions) Approaches to integration	Methods and procedures in behavior therapy I (4 sessions) Systematic desensitization
	Methods and procedures in behavior therapy II (4 sessions) Cognitive restructuring
	Integrative models II (4 sessions) Cognitive-interpersonal
Seminars Integrative case seminars: I–IV	Seminars Integrative case seminars: V–VIII

Supervision Psychodynamic (14 sessions	Supervision Cognitive-behavioral (13 sessions)	Supervision Integrated (13 sessions)
Therapy Cognitive-behavioral (14 sessions)	Therapy Psychodynamic (13 sessions)	Therapy Integrated (13 sessions)

Table 4. Summary of Requirements for Concurrent Curriculum (Second Year)

Fall semester	Spring semester
Courses	Courses
Theory and techniques III (13 sessions) Cognitive-behavioral	Theory and techniques IV (13 sessions) Freudian
Modules	Modules
Techniques in psychodynamic therapy I (4 sessions) Transference, counter-transference, and resistance	Clinical treatment strategies in cognitive-behavioral therapy I (4 sessions) Cognitive and behavioral treatment of anxiety and panic disorders
Techniques in psychodynamic therapy II (4 sessions) Dream interpretation	Clinical treatment strategies in cognitive-behavioral therapy II (4 sessions) Cognitive and behavioral treatment of depressive disorders
Integrative models III (4 sessions) Behavioral psychotherapy	Integrative models IV (4 sessions) Cyclical psychodynamic
Seminars Integrative case seminars: IX–XII	Seminars Integrative case seminars: XIII–XVI

Supervision Cognitive-behavioral (14 sessions	Supervision Psychodynamic (13 sessions)	Supervision Integrated (13 sessions)
Therapy Psychodynamic (14 sessions)	Therapy Cognitive-behavioral (13 sessions)	Therapy Integrated (13 sessions)

gration. In synthesizing cognitive and interpersonal processes, Safran demonstrates the power of the cyclical model to reconcile disparate approaches.

The second year will see the introduction of Fensterheim's (1983) behavioral psychotherapy model and Wachtel's (1977, 1987) cyclical psychodynamic model, deriving from behavioral and psychodynamic frameworks, respectively. The behavioral psychotherapy model is a levels approach, proceeding from simpler behavioral explanations to more complex psychodynamic formulations, providing students with an approach that combines the respective strengths of psychoanalytic and behavioral approaches. By contrast, the cyclical psychodynamic model involves a theoretical synthesis of psychodynamic and behavioral approaches and represents the seminal contribution at this level of integration at the abstract level.

As an aside, the introduction of Freudian theory and techniques will be postponed deliber-

Table 5.   Summary of Requirements for Concurrent Curriculum (Third Year)

Fall semester		Spring semester
Courses		Courses
Theory and techniques V (13 sessions) Object relations		Theory and techniques VI (13 sessions) Self-psychology
Modules		Modules
Integrated treatment approaches I (4 sessions) Anxiety and panic disorders		Integrated treatment approaches III (4 sessions) Borderline personality disorders
Integrated treatment approaches II (4 sessions) Depressive disorders		Integrated treatment approaches IV (4 sessions) Sexual dysfunctions
Integrative models V (4 sessions) Relational-behavioral		Integrative models VI (4 sessions) Therapeutic choice-points
Seminars		Seminars
Integrative case seminars: XVII–XX		Integrative case seminars: XXI–XXIV
Supervision	Supervision	Supervision
Cognitive-behavioral (13 sessions	Psychodynamic (13 sessions)	Integrated (14 sessions)
Therapy	Therapy	Therapy
Cognitive-behavioral (13 sessions)	Psychodynamic (13 sessions)	Integrated (13 sessions)

ately until the second year, and will be preceded by Interpersonal Theory and Techniques. Wachtel (1977, 1987) examined the irreconcilable differences between classical Freudian psychoanalysis and behavior therapy and proposed an interpersonal psychodynamic position as a bridge between psychoanalysis and behavior therapy. Therefore, although Freudian theory is the foundation from which other schools of psychoanalytic thought have derived, it was decided to proceed counter-intuitively (K. A. Frank, personal communication, May 8, 1991), rather than historically. It is still deemed to be of substantial value for students to have knowledge of the contributions of classical psychoanalysis from a historical perspective; and who knows, perhaps to stimulate an inquiring mind to seek out an integrative solution in a heretofore unknown direction.

The emphasis of the third year will be on integrated treatment approaches with a focus on the most recent developments in theory and practice. Undoubtedly, these offerings will be the most susceptible to revision as the integration movement continues to undergo a rapid, even dizzying expansion.

In the third year, Frank's (1990) relational-behavioral model and Messer's (1986) therapeutic choice points will round out the presentation of integrative models. Frank integrates object relations and self-psychology, with cognitive-behavioral techniques—an application of the cyclical model to relational approaches. Although failing to meet Wachtel's (1987) criteria for an integrative model, Messer's concept of therapeutic choice points is worthy of inclusion, generating as it does, a number of exciting hypotheses related to the integrative process.

A word about our experience with the Integrative Case Seminars is in order. These seminars were considered to be the heart of the training program, involving the participation of students and two senior faculty members representing divergent theoretical approaches, including some of the foremost clinician/theorists in the integration movement. I hoped that this mix of faculty would catalyze discussion of case material in ways that would promote integration by increasing our understanding of the interface between psychodynamic and cognitive-behavioral approaches.

Unfortunately, these seminars, on the whole, proved to be disappointing. I suspect that the reason for this insufficiency—and I use that term rather than failure, because the seminars were not failures as judged by conventional standards—but my sense was that the discussants did not sufficiently address integrative issues as applied to the material at hand.

I am more than willing to accept the lion's share of the blame, since as moderator it was my responsibility to channel the discussion along the right path. In retrospect, I had the naive expectation that all that was required was to bring the discussants together and nature would take its course. Frankly, I was at a loss as to how to make integration "happen."

In the future, I plan to submit the case material to the discussants well in advance with the following list of questions to stimulate the integrative process:

1. How would you approach this patient from your dominant pure-form theoretical orientation, for example, psychoanalytic, cognitive-behavioral, and so forth?
2. Do you see this patient benefiting from integrating/eclectic approaches? Explain.
3. What integrative/eclectic theories and/or techniques are applicable to this patient? Elaborate.
4. What theoretical or technical problems might be anticipated from the utilization of integrative/eclectic interventions.

I would like to return briefly to a comparison of the sequential versus the concurrent model of integration. The sequential model requires that students become fluent in one language before learning another, with the risk of introducing a bias which might make subsequent learning difficult (K. A. Frank, personal communication, May 8, 1991; Wolfe & Goldfried, 1988) and even susceptible to deterioration under the stress of doing therapy, just as persons with a foreign background may revert to their mother tongue in stressful situations.

By contrast, the concurrent model requires students to learn several different theoretical orientations at the same time, in effect, asking them to become conversant in several different languages simultaneously. Besides slowing down the learning process (Norcross, 1988; Wolfe & Goldfried, 1988), it would be reasonable to anticipate a considerable amount of confusion (K. A. Frank, personal communication, May 8, 1991), at least in the early stages of the training process. Norcross (1988) likened the acquisition of competence in multiple theoretical orientations to the difficulties experienced by bilingual children.

However, a saving grace may be that psychodynamic and cognitive-behavioral theories, deriving from diverse origins, employ different root languages, resulting in basic vocabularies that are essentially unrelated to each other. Because they are so dissimilar, there should be less confusion in learning them than if they had arisen from one "mother tongue." Ultimately, these "protolanguages," I am speculating, will combine to form a modern linguistic branch that will define the basic vocabulary of integrative processes. In the meantime, students will have to learn these "ancestral" languages separately and in whatever

combinations are reflected in existing integrative models.

As was discussed earlier, the sequential curriculum essentially postponed the acquisition of integrative skills until the third year of the program. To be sure, some incidental learning took place as a consequence of the integrative case seminars. However, in a very real sense, a sequential model effectively postpones the inevitable. In contrast, the concurrent model forces the issue right from the start. Integrative issues have to be addressed at the outset. There is no pretense that the promised land is off in the distance; our ignorance and confusion are right there for all to see.

Integration, by its very nature, plays havoc with the orderliness of the student's universe and introduces institutionalized havoc. The student is faced with several divergent points of view which in some way have to be made peace with.

One could argue that students in psychoanalytic training are faced with a similar dilemma, with courses in several schools, including Freudian, ego psychology, object relations, and self-psychology. Yet, all of these share a common root language. Not so with psychoanalysis and behavior therapy, that have very different historical foundations, and from which, unrelated languages and concepts have evolved.

It requires a special kind of student to subsist in an integrationist environment; not necessarily a superior kind, but one who is willing to tolerate a high degree of ambiguity (Norcross, 1988), not found in more conventional training programs. In addition, the student has to be willing to forego a more traditional identity, as a psychoanalyst or a behavior therapist. Not that an integrationist lacks an identity, but to be a true integrationist requires a willingness to find oneself in a constant state of flux.

How one selects faculty for an integrated training institute is an even more complex issue than that of selecting students, since the latter more or less select themselves. Faculty are recruited, for the most part, because they have something to offer as an instructor or supervisor; that something may be an integrative or pure-strain approach.

Integrationists bring a particular "brand" of integration to teaching or supervision, especially when these faculty are selected because of their having made distinctive contributions to the integration movement. Undoubtedly, the unique way in which they view the integrative process will influence the content of the material they present in the classroom when teaching anything to do with integration. Even in those instances where the content is pure-form, their integrationist bent will influence the selection of material to be presented.

How do pure-strain faculty fare in an integrated training program? Not too well. Those who for one reason or another are really not that committed to the cause of integration tend to "hunker down" and entrench their positions. From this vantage point, they are secure in their professional identity, but are too well defended to make any significant contribution to the integrative process. Those pure-form instructors and supervisors who are truly intrigued with integration are in danger of being changed by observing the integrative process (a reversal of Heisenberg's uncertainty principle) and are, ipso facto, no longer pure-anything, having evolved into integrationists of a sort.

So, what we are left with is a bunch of integrationists, albeit representing many different approaches to integration. At this time, *glasnost* between pure-form and integrationist theorist/ clinicians is more an ideal than a reality.

The supervisory process is of equal, if not of greater importance than instruction, in the acquisition of integrative knowledge and skills. To this end, Messer's (1986) concept of "therapeutic choice points" has provided the most promising approach to integrative supervision from a pragmatic/clinical point of view.

Briefly, therapeutic choice-points represent crossroads at which decisions are made concerning psychoanalytic versus behavioral interventions— goal setting: client or therapist determined; promoting action versus exploring mental content; challenging versus understanding irrational cognitions; dissipating versus releasing emotions; and the therapeutic relationship—actual or projected. And we can add other polarities to this list, such as reducing anxiety versus increasing anxiety, supporting defenses versus attacking defenses, focusing on the present versus exploring the past, and so forth. As they stand, these divergent approaches are not easily reconciled and may not be reconcilable without some modifications in each of the orientations.

A problem inherent in Messer's therapeutic choice-points is the matter of internal consistency. From an orthodox theoretical perspective, you cannot have it both ways, for example, challenging the client's irrational cognitions, on the one hand, and helping the client or patient to understand their roots in childhood experiences, on the other. And once having made a choice, internal consistency would dictate all subsequent choices, which are theoretically consistent with the route originally decided upon. In the example provided by Messer to illustrate his concept, the behavior therapist he was supervising was counseled to take the analytic route, while discussing the rationale for going in one direction rather than the other. In that way, Messer's supervisee was internally consistent within a psychoanalytic framework.

But what would have happened if the therapist were really free to have made a choice at each therapeutic juncture, selecting a behavioral approach at one choice-point and an analytic approach at another? Here, one has to abandon orthodoxy. Given that flexibility, the principle of internal consistency could still be maintained at each therapeutic choice-point. Rarely does therapy address a single problem. It seems conceivable that depending on the problem being dealt with at that particular point in the therapeutic process, the therapist could proceed either analytically or behaviorally, in full regalia, so to speak, whereas in relation to another problem, the therapist could proceed in an entirely different fashion. Thus, depending on the problem or issue being addressed, the therapist could shift from one approach to another, and back again, as the situation required.

And the case material provided by Messer is consistent with this point of view. In one case vignette, the client Bill, in his layman's ignorance of the principle of internal consistency, would not accept an either–or approach to therapeutic choice-points, but rather proceeded to go his own way. For example, in one session Bill said that he wanted to see his therapist as a therapist only, not as a person, but in a later session he expressed what appeared to be a transferential distortion, referring to the therapist as a controlling "bitch."

The lesson to be learned from this case illustration is that regardless of the therapist's theoretical orientation, the patient's needs will out, calling for the therapist to shift from one approach to another; much as a driver will shift to a different gear, depending on prevailing road conditions.

Much as Messer emphasizes the differences between the orientations, he does call for a softening of positions of each of the therapies to permit a healthy infusion of attitudes, values, and interventions; for example, he urges behavior therapists to pay closer attention to the expression, rather than the control, of negative emotions, and analytic therapists to give more emphasis to the inhibition and control of affects.

However, Messer does not go far enough in advocating that therapists be willing to shift from one approach to another, as the situation or patient requires it. In the actual therapeutic situation, there is no reason not to shift from one approach to another; from challenging irrational cognitions, on the one hand, to exploring the roots of these beliefs in childhood experiences, on the other. And there is a pretty good chance that if the therapist will not, the patient will.

Not surprisingly, it has been proposed that parallel processes may exist between supervision and therapy (Halgin, 1986; Norcross, 1988).

A similar parallelism can be said to exist between the content and method of therapeutic choice-points (Messer, 1986) as applied to supervision and to therapy, both in relation to the best route to follow and the means by which a decision is made to go that route. Basically, the work of supervisor with supervisee is indistinguishable from the work of supervisee with patient. Alternative conceptualizations and interventions must be considered, along with the rationale for proceeding in one direction rather than another.

In this instance of parallel process, the ultimate focus, whether in the supervisory or therapeutic relationship, is clearly on the patient's needs; the latter being understood in a context broad enough to encompass unconscious processes.

It is axiomatic that in any supervisory relationship, the supervisee will be instructed in the particular approach espoused by that supervisor. Since the growth factor in the field of psychotherapy integration appears to be approaching exponential proportions, supervisees may be in the confusing position of being trained in as many models as they have supervisors. Coupled with having to acquire skills in a multiplicity of pure-form approaches, the lot of these supervisees will not be an easy one. But then, if they opted for the old order, they would not be in the vanguard of change.

PERSONAL ISSUES

Much of the foregoing, especially with respect to the section on Theoretical and Conceptual Issues, represents *post factum* developments occurring subsequent to the founding of IITP. Had I followed conventional wisdom about not putting the cart before the horse, to mix metaphors, we would not have been able to get off the ground as quickly as we did. In a very real sense, I moved into this project "ass backwards."

It would take me too far afield to chronicle the history of how I ended up, or more correctly, started in this rather awkward position. Briefly, however, the saga began in 1977 with the founding of Psychotherapies Selection Service (PSS), which was a response to the proliferation of therapies in the mid 1960s and early 1970s, which was an earlier instance of a changing climate creating an evolutionary niche for a new form.

What characterized PSS as being different from existing referral services was its eclectic nature. The goal of the service was to provide clients with whatever they needed to choose from a bewildering array of therapeutic approaches. To that end, I recruited therapists of different orientations—psychoanalytic, to be sure, but also Gestalt, bio-energetic, and even primal. Behavior therapy was represented by Masters and Johnson's sex therapy and rational-emotive therapy.

At that time, I regarded any therapist who was eclectic as a problem, since I believed that it was only with a "pure-strain" approach that the client could make a clear-cut decision. However, since even in those days, a majority of therapists tended to be eclectic, if only within a particular framework, I had to let go of that notion.

In order to familiarize clients with the different therapeutic approaches, I ran what I called orientation groups consisting of 16mm sound films and lecture materials. Several years ago, I discontinued the orientation program to reduce the lag time required to move clients into therapy. Some of the film images that remain with me are Janov, the father of primal therapy, riding a white stallion on a Pacific beach, saying something profound that has stuck with me ever since, to the effect that no sick system willingly gives itself up; it has to be fought with, struggled with, and finally overcome (as I complete the final edit of this material, those prophetic words ring in my ears as the headlines proclaim the deposing of Mikhail S. Gorbachev by the KGB and the military); I recall some erotic sex therapy sequences demonstrating sensate focusing; and a patient complaining to his analyst that he did not seem to have the money to do things anymore.

After an initial consultation, clients had the opportunity to "shop around"—to see three therapists, often representing different therapeutic approaches, before making a final decision. In retrospect, it was no accident that psychoanalytic therapy was the therapy of choice in the majority of cases; the film clips of primal therapy depicted emotionally wrenching experiences that most clients elected to steer clear of; the Gestalt exercises were gimicky; and I described psychoanalysis as the most powerful tool we have at our disposal to bring about deep-seated personality change—no wonder it ranked number one.

But beyond my bias, patients did appear to be turning away from the humanistic approaches of the 1960s toward the "old time religion" of psychoanalysis. The closing of hundreds of growth centers modeled after Esalen proved to be a manifestation of the decline of the humanistic movement.

In the mid 1980s, I added several cognitive-behavior therapists to our roster, but I did not really have a good enough understanding of how the approach worked to give it a fair shake (by this time I had replaced the film orientation with a verbal description of the approaches and how each was applicable to that client's symptoms and problems). And it was not until I undertook formal training in behavior therapy, that the balance between analytic and behavioral approaches equalized; and for our purposes here, clients began to ask about a "blend," "mix," or "integration" of these mainstream therapeutic approaches.

To move ahead in my story, after being a practicing analyst for almost three decades, I undertook formal training in cognitive-behavior therapy. I was like a kid in a candy store. I began to apply what I was taught, willy nilly, into my practice and to my surprise and delight found that behavioral interventions worked.

During relaxation training, a patient relived feelings of hatred, repressed since childhood, toward an alcoholic father, breaking through a previously impenetrable array of defenses. And I even had a bizarre success with an analytic patient with a flying phobia, who I suspect may have avoided my threat to desensitize her by curing herself before I had the opportunity to use her as a guinea pig to practice my newfound magic. Parenthetically, behavior therapists might call her "cure" a negative reinforcement, defined as any act that is successful in removing an aversive stimulus; in this case—me. By contrast, an analyst might call her cure "a flight into health." No pun intended. One can see that I am a true integrationist.

The lesson I learned was that there were indeed sorcerers who had spells and magic as potent as psychoanalytic therapists.

The germ of the idea for a training institute in psychotherapy integration was conceived during my training experience in behavior therapy. It seemed to be so simple. All one had to do was to train therapists in psychoanalytic and behavioral approaches and nature would take its course. Little did I know at that time the many complexities that would be involved in this effort.

Nor did I realize that being trained in more than one approach raises as many problems as it solves. It involves more than simply acquiring a "new bag of tricks" as one prospective student described her interest in the program.

I would like to think that in undertaking this project, I was a prime example of one of Bandura's "so called normals who are distorters of reality, but . . . exhibit self-enhancing biases that distort appraisals in the positive direction . . . if not unrealistically exaggerated, such beliefs foster the perseverant effort needed . . . to override the numerous dissuading impediments to significant accomplishments" (Bandura, 1989, p. 1177).

However, in order to distort reality one has to be aware of it. Yet, I must confess that at the time, I was ignorant of the existence of the Society for the Exploration of Psychotherapy Integration (SEPI). I was ignorant of the burgeoning literature in psychotherapy integration. And I was blissfully ignorant of the complex issues that had to be addressed in this chapter. So you see, I did put the proverbial cart before the horse.

Fortunately, the climate was right for an integrative training institute. SEPI preceded IITP by 6 years. However, the same conditions that were favorable for the development of SEPI provided the evolutionary niche for the Institute, the latter proving to be a parallel, rather than a linear development, by virtue of my lack of knowledge of what had gone before.

I was also lucky enough to be in the right place at the right time. New York City boasts some of the foremost clinician/researchers in the psychotherapy integration movement. In point of fact, as I was to learn later on, the concept of just such an institute had been discussed before I came on the scene. So, understandably, my proposal for this project was met with an initial reserve. After all, I was a virtual unknown, with no track record of having established a training program on this or any other level.

Nevertheless, so eager was the professional community for such a training institute that, one after another, faculty members assented, until we had "cornered the market" on the foremost integrationists in the area. The objections of one skeptic were successfully overcome and that person has since become an enthusiastic booster of our program. In retrospect, all things considered, the degree of cooperation, support, and encouragement tendered for this undertaking by the faculty was nothing short of amazing, attesting, as it does, to a sincere dedication and commitment, on their part, to the cause of integration.

CONCLUDING COMMENTS

It is important to bear in mind that integrative models are only as good as the schools they derive from. If that is the case, then, ironically, integrative efforts should proceed in tandem with the latest developments in psychoanalytic and cognitive and behavioral orientations.

In the middle ages, university-trained physicians wore long robes and barber-surgeons wore short gowns (surgery was considered a lower calling that could be performed by anyone who could wield a knife skillfully, including the barber and executioner who could shop off an arm or leg with the same alacrity that he could chop off the heads of the condemned). Neither had any knowledge of modern medicine, and if their patients survived it was by sheer luck, rather than any ministrations on their part. It is easy to see from this perspective that a third school, based on an "integrative" approach, whose practitioners wore midi gowns, would not in any likelihood be any more or less efficacious in treating patients than the other two. Integration can only be as good as the theories and techniques we integrate from.

In accord with the philosophy stated above, a curriculum in psychotherapy integration should encompass not only the latest developments in integration and eclecticism, but also a basic foundation in the theories and techniques form which they have derived. In this view, it is premature, and probably will always be so, to maintain an allegiance to a particular theory of integration, or even to Messer's "creative diversity" (Lazarus & Messer, 1991, p. 150) of integrative theories, without at least paying homage to the significant contributions of pure-strain orientations.

In this regard, I am reminded of the ancient Indian fable, *The Blind Men and the Elephant* which tells of:

> . . . six men of Hindostan,
> To learning much inclined,
> Who went to see the elephant,
> (Though all of them were blind)
> That each by observation
> Might satisfy his mind.

The poem goes on to relate how each of these learned men described the elephant according to which part of the beast's anatomy he happened to touch: the broad side, a wall; the tusk, a spear; the trunk, a snake; the leg, a tree; the ear, a fan; and the tail, a rope.

Apropos our fable, if we continue to be blind to alternative conceptualizations (Goldfried & Padawer, 1982), whatever their ilk, we will be like our learned men of Hindostan, who in describing the elephant,

> Disputed loud and long,
> Each in his own opinion
> Exceeding stiff and strong,
> Though each was partly in the right
> And all were in the wrong.

REFERENCES

Bandura, A. (1989). Human agency in social cognitive theory. *American Psychologist, 44*, 1175–1184.

Beutler, L. E., Mahoney, M. J., Norcross, J. C., Prochaska, J. A., Robertson, M. H., & Sollod, R. N. (1987). Training integrative/eclectic therapists. *Journal of Integrative and Eclectic Psychotherapy, 6*, 296–332.

Fensterheim, H. (1983). Basic paradigms and behavioral formulation. In H. Fensterheim & H. I. Glazer (Eds.), *Basic principles and case studies in an integrative clinical model.* New York: Brunner/Mazel.

Frank, K. A. (1990). Action techniques in psychoanalysis. *Contemporary Psychoanalysis, 26*, 732–756.

Goldfried, M. R., & Padawer, W. (1982). Current status and future directions in psychotherapy. In M. R. Goldfried (Ed.), *Converging themes in psychotherapy* (pp. 3–49). New York: Springer.

Halgin, R. P. (1986). Pragmatic blending of clinical models in the supervisory relationship. *Clinical Supervisor, 22*(4), 23–44.

Hawking, S. W. (1988). *A brief history of time.* New York: Bantam Books.

Lazarus, A. A., & Messer, S. B. (1991). Does chaos prevail? An exchange on technical eclecticism and assimilative integration. *Journal of Psychotherapy Integration, 1*, 143–158.

Messer, S. B. (1986). Behavioral and psychoanalytic perspectives at therapeutic choice points. *American Psychologist, 41*, 1261–1272.

Messer, S. B., & Winokur, M. (1980). Some limits to the integration of psychoanalytic and behavior therapy. *American Psychologist, 35*, 818–827.

Messer, S. B., & Winokur, M. (1984). Ways of knowing and visions of reality in psychoanalytic therapy and behavior therapy. In H. Arkowitz & S. B. Messer (Eds.), *Psychoanalytic therapy and behavior therapy: Is integration possible?* (pp. 63–100). New York: Plenum Press.

Norcross, J. C. (1988). Supervision of integrative psychotherapy. *Journal of Integrative and Eclectic Psychotherapy, 7*, 157–166.

Safran, J. D. (1990). Towards a refinement of cognitive therapy in light of interpersonal theory: II. Practice. *Clinical Psychology Review, 10*, 107–121.

Schacht, T. E. (1984). The varieties of integrative experience. In H. Arkowitz & S. B. Messer (Eds.), *Psychoanalytic therapy and behavior therapy: Is integration possible?* (pp. 107–131). New York: Plenum Press.

Wachtel, P. L. (1977). *Psychoanalysis and behavior therapy.* New York: Basic Books.

Wachtel, P. L. (1987). *Action and insight.* New York: Guilford.

Wolfe, B. E., & Goldfried, M. L. (1988). Research on psychotherapy integration: Recommendations and conclusions from an NIMH workshop. *Journal of Consulting and Clinical Psychology, 56*, 448–451.

CHAPTER 35

Countertransference Issues in Integrative Psychotherapy

Richard P. Halgin and Derek J. McEntee

Integrative psychotherapists encounter some interesting and confusing phenomena in their work due in great part to shifts in the techniques and models which they employ. At times, the confusion is in the mind of the client who may be perplexed by considerably different styles of therapeutic intervention over the course of the therapy, or even within a single session. At other times, the perplexity is in the mind of the therapist moving from one technique to another with a given client, or from one model to another across clients. In this chapter, we will discuss the impact of technical and theoretical shifts on clients and the therapists who are conducting integrative therapies. The issues discussed in this chapter are pertinent both to clinicians conducting multi-theoretical therapies and to advanced clinicians supervising such work.

THEORETICAL AND CONCEPTUAL ISSUES

Integrative Psychotherapy

During the past decade many clinicians have gone public with the acknowledgment that they are integrative or eclectic psychotherapists. Several writers (Beitman, Goldfried, & Norcross, 1989; Lazarus, Beutler, & Norcross, 1992) have pointed out that within the field of psychotherapy integration there are clearly different routes to be taken, and they call particular attention to the difference between technical eclecticism and theoretical integrationism. Beitman *et al.* (1989) differentiate between integration and eclecticism by noting that "integration" denotes a more conceptual synthesis of divergent theoretical systems, whereas "eclecticism" involves the pragmatic application of existing methods. Lazarus and his colleagues (1992) are critical of theoretical integrationism which they see as being comprised of flawed attempts to meld disparate ideas and conflicting theories into unworkable frameworks for therapy. In contrast, in technical eclecticism, procedures from different sources are tapped without necessarily adhering to the theories from which the techniques emerged.

Richard P. Halgin and Derek J. McEntee • Department of Psychology, University of Massachusetts, Amherst, Massachusetts 01003.

Comprehensive Handbook of Psychotherapy Integration, edited by George Stricker and Jerold R. Gold. Plenum Press, New York, 1993.

The distinction between technical eclecticism and theoretical integrationism is useful, yet our preference is to lean toward a middle point between the two camps seeing neither as necessarily excluding the other. Although our clinical work involves the careful choosing from an array of divergent techniques, our work also involves transtheoretical melding of the commonalities among different models. As Wachtel (1991) noted, "eclecticism in practice and integration in aspiration is an accurate description of what most of us in the integrative movement do most of the time" (p. 44). Our focus in this chapter will be on technique, yet we use the term *integrative* because of its broader acceptance in clinical circles and our belief that clinicians prefer to label themselves as integrative rather than eclectic, a term that some consider to be pejorative.

One form of integrative psychotherapy, about which we have written previously, is pragmatic blending (Halgin, 1985, 1986, 1989; Halgin, Hennessey, Statlender, Feinman, & Brown, 1988; Halgin & Lovejoy, 1991). Pragmatically blended therapy views a psychological problem as emerging from some combination of unconscious, interpersonal, and learned events. Treatment plans are developed from an array of techniques that are considered most responsive to each client's needs with additional attention given to the therapist's unique style, sometimes called the *personal idiom* (Hogan, 1964). The most commonly chosen sources for a pragmatically blended therapy are the psychodynamic, interpersonal, client-centered, and behavioral models of treatment.

An important assumption underlying carefully conceived integrative psychotherapy is the notion that the treatment is planned, rather than the result of a haphazard sampling of techniques selected from a clinical smorgasbord. Numerous authors have laid out strategies for the selection of appropriate therapeutic techniques (e.g., Beutler, 1986; Beutler & Clarkin, 1990; Frances, Clarkin, & Perry, 1984; Lazarus, 1986), with the predominance of attention to client factors as determinants of which technique to employ and when. But what about therapist factors? What factors operate within the thoughts and feelings of the therapist that may affect the choice of therapeutic techniques? In the sections to follow, we will consider some of the conscious and unconscious variables operating in these choice pro-

cesses. Optimally, consideration of these issues by therapists and discussion of these matters between supervisors and supervisees will result in decreased stress for the therapist and diminished confusion for the client in integrative psychotherapy.

Integrative Psychotherapy and the Relationship

Many experts in the field of psychotherapy have pointed to the therapeutic relationship as a central curative factor in psychotherapy (e.g., Frank, 1973, 1982; Linehan, 1988; Waterhouse & Strupp, 1984). Psychotherapy is an event that involves at least two people. Although much that is written about psychotherapy would suggest that psychotherapy is something that is done *to* a client, we need to remind ourselves that the process of psychotherapy is something that we experience *with* the client. Both participants in the therapy relationship are there for personal gain of some sort and each person becomes an important figure in the thoughts and feelings of the other. At a practical level, there is a financial reliance that the therapist has on the client as a source of the therapist's income, but there are presumably many other reasons why most of us continue to work as psychotherapists. Near the top of the hierarchy of values would be our unselfish wish to help others to change, to feel happier, and to make their lives better. But there is a midrange of motivations why many psychotherapists continue to ply this trade; this segment of the hierarchy includes various emotional gains that therapists derive from their professional work, some of which are healthy and others of which are more selfish and neurotic.

It is reasonable and expected that therapists would want to continue providing psychotherapy because they themselves feel good when they observe growth and positive change in those who seek professional help. Not so healthy however are those motivations for conducting psychotherapy that are rooted in the neurotic needs of the therapist, as would be the case when interventions are fueled by voyeuristic drives, needs to control, or wishes to fulfill one's own fantasies vicariously.

There is a great deal written about the therapist's reactions to the client. In the analytic literature, the phenomenon has been called *counter-*

transference, referring to the analyst's unconscious reactions to the patient, especially in response to the patient's own transference (Laplanche & Pontalis, 1973). In recent decades, the term has been broadened substantially. Some authors use the term to connote those aspects of the therapist's responses to the client that are determined by the therapist's own personal history which ultimately may facilitate or hinder therapeutic progress (Pinsof, 1988, p. 310). Other authors use the term in an intentionally overinclusive fashion to refer to the range of the therapist's reactions to the client (Kahn, 1991; Norcross, 1990).

Using this broader understanding of countertransference, it is helpful to consider the fact that responses on the part of the therapist vary along several dimensions. Marshall and Marshall (1988) discuss countertransference as being comprised of three variables: (1) the extent to which the therapist is conscious of reactions to the client; (2) the degree to which the reaction is caused by the client or comes from within the therapist; and (3) the extent to which these reactions are general or specific. It will be useful to keep these dimensions in mind as we discuss what may take place within the therapist, either consciously or unconsciously as particular treatment choices are made.

Therapeutic Shifts, Styles, and Needs: Impact on the Relationship

Psychotherapy is an action-oriented play of sorts, in which the client seeks help in order to make some changes in personal functioning; the psychotherapy session is the stage upon which the script is written and enacted. In integrative psychotherapy, the action may take any of a number of forms ranging from emotional exploration to directive or educative intervention. The integrative psychotherapist faces a countless series of choice points, in which decisions must be made about the extent to which the therapist should promote action or explore mental content, challenge irrational cognitions, discuss relationships, or empathize with the client's distress (Norcross, 1990). Wachtel (1991) points out that many students, when first introduced to multitheoretical approaches, are puzzled by the mechanics of technique shifts and disturbed by a concern that such shifts might prove to be awkward and disruptive.

As therapists work toward helping their clients change, they need to be aware of concomitant changes within themselves that occur within each session and over the course of treatment. In effective psychotherapy, the therapist does not maintain a static attentional and affective state, but responds both consciously and unconsciously to what the client feels, says, and does (Lombardi, 1990). Ideally, therapist actions and reactions are useful and therapeutic, but at times they may be obstructive and countertherapeutic, executed to serve the needs of the therapist rather than the needs of the client (Kahn, 1991). Because integrative psychotherapy often involves shifts in techniques or modalities, particular attention needs to be given to the rationale for such shifts. Integrative therapists should be asking themselves challenging questions about the reasons that underlie intervention choices. In the next section, we will consider several integrative psychotherapy contexts, each with a case example to help give some life to the complexity of the issues involved in moving from one technique or modality to another.

TECHNICAL SHIFTS WITHIN ONE THERAPY: THE POTENTIAL FOR CONFUSING THE CLIENT

In an integrative psychotherapy, a therapist may move from one set of techniques to a dramatically different set, sometimes in a rather brief period of time. For example, the therapist may tap psychodynamically oriented exploratory and interpretive techniques as well as more educative and directive techniques even within a single session. The therapist who is accustomed to such transitions and has become comfortable with such transitions may be oblivious to the confusion that they may engender in the client. The combining of different therapeutic techniques might even alarm a client who infers that he or she must be especially sick because so many different kinds of help are required (Frances, Clarkin, & Perry, 1984).

Case Example: New Techniques for New Problems

A 22-year-old college senior sought professional help in her attempt to resolve longstanding troublesome communication between her and the rest of her family. The therapist conducted a psychotherapy that was primarily exploratory, with the goal of developing an understanding of the developmental history that led up to the client's current difficulties in her relationships with family members and other people with whom she tried to develop intimate relationships. Exploratory and interpretive work was providing the client with an understanding of the roots of her current difficulties, and her insight was freeing her up to make some changes in her relationships. Following three months of work together, a developing relationship with a young man went sour, and the client's academic performance took a nose dive; she became intensely anxious, panicky, and frightened by her own fantasies of hurting herself. The crisislike situation that emerged warranted an abrupt change in therapeutic style that necessitated the inclusion of directive, supportive, and confrontative techniques. Once the turbulent period subsided, the therapist returned to the exploratory work that had been demonstrably effective previously. To minimize potentially jarring effects on the client associated with each transition, the therapist needed to be especially vigilant and take clear steps to inform the client about the timing and rationale for the transitions.

MODALITY SHIFTS: THE POTENTIAL FOR GIVING THE CLIENT THE WRONG MESSAGE

Sometimes it becomes apparent to the therapist that an alternative therapy modality may make more sense. For example, a therapist might recognize that the issues of an individual client might better be treated within a couples therapy modality or vice versa. When making such modality shifts, the therapist needs to be attuned to the tremendous emotional impact such a change can have on the client. For example, if individual therapy is recommended for one member in a couples therapy, will the partner be left feeling rejected and jealous, possibly even wondering about whether the therapist has some seductive fantasies about the partner who has been "selected" for the individual therapy? Therapists should be questioning themselves on these issues as they consider such changes in modality, keeping in mind that such decisions have great therapeutic significance, and therefore involve ethical considerations (Sider, 1984; Sider & Clements, 1982).

Case Example: From Couples to Individual Therapy

A couple in their mid-thirties was referred to a therapist for treatment of a sexual dysfunction. The husband had suffered from premature ejaculation for more than a decade, causing a great deal of disharmony between him and his wife as well as a considerable loss of self-esteem in himself. The couple's problems were compounded by the dramatic contrasts in each personality, the wife being a very strong and critical individual, and the husband seeming passive and weak. In the early sessions, the therapist focused on the sexual issue with the couple and assigned a series of individual and couple exercises. However, as treatment proceeded, the therapist became increasingly disturbed by the wife's recurrent demeaning comments about her husband as well as her intensifying criticism about the therapist's interventions and recommendations. In the fifth session, the therapist recommended that the modality of treatment be changed to individual therapy for the man. The therapist's stated rationale for such a change was her belief that the husband's low self-esteem stood as a barrier to therapeutic progress on the sexual problem; in an individual psychotherapy context she could work more effectively toward addressing this level of impairment. Was there more to the issue than therapeutic need? Perhaps the therapist was looking for an escape from dealing with the difficult wife. Did the recommendation arise from unconscious, possibly even conscious, reactions of the therapist to the woman whose criticism and discontent was too much for the therapist to bear?

DIFFERENTIATING CLIENT NEED FROM THERAPIST NEED

Ideally, all clinical interventions are designed to serve the client's needs. However, in reality, this is not always the case. A disturbed psychotherapist may formulate interventions that serve the therapist's needs rather than the client's. For example, narcissistic therapists may seek out gratification from clients, and neurotically dependent therapists may engender dependency on the part of their clients in an obfuscated attempt to satisfy their own cravings for others. Of course, most cases are not so blatant. However, integrative therapy typically lacks the "script" provided by a particular therapeutic model, such as that provided to psychoanalysts within the analytic tradition. Moving from technique to technique, from model to model, the therapist has greater freedom, but may also be at greater risk of proceeding along intervention lines that are self-serving rather than clinically indicated.

Case Example:
Moving toward a Warm Goodbye

The therapist had worked with a 26-year-old man for two years in a therapy that focused on the client's low self-esteem and chronic substance abuse. Relying on a confrontative style throughout the therapy, the therapist focused on the many ways, including substance abuse, that the client ensured that he would have a life of self-determined inefficacy. Over the course of their work together, the client had become substance-free and had taken steps to get his life on track in terms of getting and keeping a job and returning to complete college. In the minds of both the therapist and the client the therapy had been a "success"—a realization that was understandably pleasing to both parties in this relationship. During the final weeks of their work, the client commented, "I've noticed that lately you have been treating me more like a peer than a patient. It's like you're my friend instead of my shrink." The therapist was a bit startled by the client's comment, leading him to wonder what might be going on within his own feelings about the client. Was the change in the therapist's behavior and affect attributable to a conscious and planned modification of style? Or might the issue be more complex and insidious and have to do with the therapist's own needs. Did the therapist, either unconsciously or even consciously, wish to transform the therapeutic relationship into a friendship? The therapist sought out consultation from a colleague, and came to the conclusion that the change in his behavior was not unlike what many therapists experience as they approach the point of termina-

tion with "successful" clients—a warming up in anticipation of bidding farewell. The therapist came to the realization, however, that alerting clients to stylistic transitions is probably a good idea, in order to avert confusion and anxiety that might otherwise emerge.

THE DILEMMA OF SELF-DISCLOSURE

Many clinicians are attracted to integrative psychotherapy because of the freedoms that a multitheoretical approach affords. Because there are no scripts, there are no explicit rules, other than those dictated by professional and ethical standards of practice. Self-disclosure is one facet of the freedom afforded to integrative therapists that would be considered inappropriate by some of the more analytic models of therapy. In recent years an increasing amount has been written on the topic of therapist self-disclosure (see Mathews, 1988; Hill, Mahalik, & Thompson, 1989; Stricker & Fisher, 1990), and researchers have pointed out the fact that theoretical orientation, with eclecticism in particular, is strongly associated with a disposition toward therapist self-disclosure (Simon, 1988, 1990). When considering the factor of self-disclosure within the therapy relationship, the therapist must attempt to discern the extent to which self-disclosure will serve the needs of the client, and is therefore therapeutically indicated.

Case Example: Using Self-Disclosure in a Misguided Effort to Be Helpful

When a 27-year-old therapist-in-training was assigned one of her first clients, she was immediately struck by the similarity between the client and herself. In the very first session, the 22-year-old college senior described a personal history filled with a great deal of physical abuse by her alcoholic father. Upon hearing the stores of childhood humiliation and beating told by her client, the therapist chose to share her own story with the client. Defining herself as an integrative psychotherapist, she considered it permissible to divulge private issues about herself with the intention of conveying her capacity for empathy and genuineness. She told the client, "I know exactly how you feel. My father did similar things to me." To the therapist's dismay and embarrassment, the client became upset about this revelation. Rather than feeling comforted by the similarity between herself and her therapist, the client became suspicious of the therapist's motives and doubtful about the therapist's ability to remain objective and neutral. Although the therapist tried to smooth over the client's upset, irrevocable damage had been done, and the client refused to return for any further sessions. In supervision, the therapist was able to understand how her intervention was misguided.

TECHNICAL ISSUES

As we noted above, because integrative psychotherapists are choosing from an array of techniques and a variety of modalities, there is considerable potential for confusion. Clients may become confused by the seemingly peculiar juxtaposition of divergent techniques, and therapists may also become confused if they have not planned their interventions in a carefully conceptualized manner. Beyond the issue of confusion on the part of either participant, there is the concern about the underlying rationale determining each intervention and each modality shift.

There is no question that treatment selection and planning should be based on careful and comprehensive assessment of the client's needs. Therapists should be turning to the theoretical models upon which their psychotherapy will be based in order to formulate an appropriate intervention. Using a pragmatically blended therapy for the sake of example, let us consider some of the questions therapists might ask as they formulate a new treatment plan; we will look at questions that emerge from the four most commonly tapped models which form the foundation for pragmatic blending (Halgin, 1989). Later we will consider a fifth set of concerns pertaining to personal issues regarding the therapist's sense of who he or she is, both as a person and as a therapist.

1. *Psychodynamically Informed Questions.* How can I gain access to the client's unconscious issues that might be contributing to the client's problem? How can I help the client develop an understanding of the relationship between his or her developmental history and the problem? How should I go about exploring, uncovering, interpreting, and clarifying those issues that lie below the client's conscious thoughts?

2. *Interpersonally Informed Questions.* How can I use the therapeutic relationship to grasp the client's problematic interpersonal styles? How can I use the therapeutic relationship as a curative context within which the client can observe and alter disturbances in interpersonal relating?

3. *Client-Centered Questions.* How can I make it easier for the client to share personal experiences that may seem too painful or too risky to discuss? How should I go about conveying to the client a sense of caring, genuineness, acceptance, and empathy?

4. *Behaviorally Informed Questions.* What techniques can I prescribe to help the client change maladaptive behaviors? How should I go about helping the client understand the connections between personal distress and faulty learning or thinking?

It is important to point out that the focus of such questioning lies within the therapist rather than the client. Needless to say, a sound treatment approach must be determined by the needs of the client, but the client is only half of the relationship. The therapist, who is the other half, should recurrently ask "How can I . . ." questions within a framework of preconceived inquiry that is designed to assess the various sets of issues determined by each of the two parties in this relationship. This questioning should extend beyond the initial stage of therapy and take place at every stage of treatment. The therapist needs to be constantly vigilant to the client's changing needs, and be prepared to "modify the therapeutic procedure from moment to moment" (Beutler, 1986, p. 107).

PERSONAL ISSUES

Moving to a deeper level of inquiry, let us consider some of the more personal issues, needs, and reactions that affect our thoughts, feelings, and behaviors. In our professional work, we should be considering both the general context within which we define ourselves as therapists and the specific contexts that pertain to each particular therapy we undertake. We need to assess how we see ourselves as people, how we see ourselves as therapists, and how we wish to work with each and every client who asks for help. Usually there is a strong correlation among these factors, such that a "take-charge" individual would probably be inclined to conduct directive psychotherapy, while a more inquisitive problem-solver might lean more toward exploratory techniques.

Just as an individual's personality changes and unfolds over the course of life, so also does a therapist's personal idiom change as the result of life experiences and the accumulation of clinical experience. In the early stages of professional work, many therapists prematurely conclude that they know who they are and what therapeutic approach is best suited for them, and usually have a naïve sense of security, deceptive stability, and simplistic thinking (Loganbill, Hardy, & Delworth, 1982). Although naïveté diminishes with experience, the need to obtain advice and perspective from others in the form of consultations should remain throughout one's career. Next to careful assessment, supervision or consultation is probably the best safeguard against conducting therapy that is fueled by the neurotic or selfish needs that we discussed above.

Presuming that therapists are committed to conducting careful assessments and soliciting ongoing consultation from supervisors or experienced peers, we need to participate in ongoing study of ourselves. As we develop as therapists, we should recurrently confront several sets of questions pertaining to our professional endeavors as therapists. On a general level, it is important for us to ask ourselves why we have opted to be integrative therapists. On a more specific level, we should be assessing our particular responses to each new client, with particular vigilance regarding the ways in which our own personal issues define each intervention.

First, ask yourself why you are an integrative or eclectic psychotherapist. A practical response to questions on this topic would probably sound something like this: each client is different, each with idiosyncratic needs requiring customized interventions derived from an array of methods. Because people are all different, we as therapists must be different with each client. This seems very reasonable, but there are surely other, less obvious, reasons for choosing multitheoretical approaches and techniques. Is the integrative psychotherapist a "peace maker" of sorts, choosing to build bridges between divergent camps rather than alienate one or the other? Is integrationism a good "cover" for the unsure therapist who feels too insecure in his or her knowledge of a single model?

Second, what happens in your thoughts and feelings each time you confront the decision to tap a new technique or move toward a new modality? Many therapists would respond to this question by stating that they do not really think about it; rather, such decisions emerge spontaneously. It probably is true that our work becomes second nature to us, but we need to be vigilant about the possibility that interventions are emerging from our own issues rather than stemming from a treatment plan. We need to be asking ourselves how our personal "stuff" is dictating the therapies we are conducting. Eisenbud (1978) discussed several sets of countertransference factors that can interfere with the work of the therapist. These issues, which occur within the thoughts and experience of the therapist, include such phenomena as situational pressures, unresolved personal issues or neurotic problems, and a certain susceptibility to being influenced by the client's state.

We have all faced situation distractions that accompany us into the treatment room. Perhaps an argument with someone earlier in the day intrudes into the therapist's thoughts during the therapy hour. Is it not possible that the therapist, probably unconsciously, might pursue an intervention style that relates in some way to an antecedent emotional event such as an argument? Perhaps the therapist's intervention will take the form of greater directiveness and control, possibly even expressed with a tone of impatience.

There is also the possibility that the therapeutic work will be rooted in neurotic, longstanding personal issues of the therapist. For example, a therapist who suffers ego-dystonic compulsivity may intervene with a compulsive client in ways that are based on a need for self-cure. Or a therapist suffering from the pain of deprivation experienced in a relationship with an uncaring or abusive parent may neurotically look for ways to be the "good parent" to clients who seem fragile and vulnerable. When such therapeutic styles and interventions are determined primarily by the therapist's needs, the therapy is at risk.

Lastly, therapists may confront the experience of being inappropriately influenced by the behavior or the emotional state of the client in a session. For example, a hostile client may evoke responses within the therapist that mirror the client's hostility. Perhaps the therapist provides a biting interpretation, not so much to help the client develop insight but to "retaliate" against the client. Such behaviors are evidently driven by issues within the therapist rather than the needs of the client, and will certainly prove to be deleterious to the relationship.

Choice of Technique as Influenced by Personal Issues

In trying to understand our countertransferential reasons for incorporating techniques from each model of therapy, it is helpful to look, as systematically as possible, within each model at some of the personal issues that may be tapped. We recognize that in this discussion we are at risk of stereotyping each approach, and we also perceive the fact that our discussion is rooted in a skepticism that implies that treatment choices may be rooted in pathological personal issues of the therapist rather than healthy treatments of choice dictated solely by the client's needs. We resort to such extremism for the purpose of provoking self-study.

Psychodynamic Techniques. Many therapists are attracted to psychodynamic techniques because of the rich tradition and prestige of the psychoanalytic model. Regardless of the vulnerability to criticism of the work of Freud and his followers, therapists may be captivated by the fantasy of achieving the curative miracles they have read about in the psychoanalytic literature of the past century.

The potential for helping a client bring something into conscious awareness from the depths of the unconscious is an exciting undertaking for many therapists. In the process of interpretation, the therapist can in a somewhat magical fashion help the client to understand matters that were previously unintelligible to the individual. What a tremendous source of gratification when clients respond with enthusiastic concurrence and appreciative understanding to an astute interpretation! The therapist may become caught up in the intensity of the client's transference, and treatment strategies may be determined by a hidden wish to enhance the intensity of the client's response.

Interpersonal Techniques. Use of the therapeutic relationship as an analogue of other relationships in the client's life is regarded by many therapists as a very informative and constructive component of psychotherapy. Analysis of the qualities and the behaviors of the transactions between the therapist and the client has its roots in several traditions ranging from some forms of psychodynamic therapy to certain approaches within the humanistic tradition. It seems quite reasonable to rely on analysis of interactions within this relational context to help clients see how they interact with and affect others.

Analysis of the therapeutic relationship is a risky endeavor, however, when the therapist resorts to such work out of a need to satisfy personal needs. Perhaps the therapist has the secret wish that in the discussion of the relationship the client will speak in ways that are gratifying for the therapist. Maybe the therapist is pulling for clients to speak of their admiration for, dependency on, or erotic fantasies about the therapist. Alternatively, the therapist may be excited, in an odd sort of way, by a client's expressed feelings of anger or disappointment with the therapist, rather obscure reflections of the important role the therapist plays in the thoughts and feelings of the client.

Client-Centered Techniques. On the surface it might seem difficult to imagine what neurotic needs might be served by a therapist using client-centered techniques. What could be wrong with conveying genuineness, concern, and empathy? It seems quite admirable that the therapist serve as the accepting and reflective mirror.

But what about the situation in which the kind words of the clinician are maneuvers enabling the therapist to avoid confrontation of the client's maladaptive behavior? When clients are only told things that are pleasant for them to hear, one must question whether the therapist is being motivated by wishes to be the overly nurturant, and therefore well-loved, caregiver. Perhaps the kind, gentle approach that many associate with the client-centered model may serve as a mask for a therapist struggling with personal hostility, either characterologically or in response to a specific client. At times it may be easier for the therapist to "hide" insecurity or incompetence by taking a stance that is unquestioningly supportive and a technical approach that seems comparatively easy.

Behavioral Techniques. The choice of behavioral techniques has great appeal in many instances because of the proven track record of behavior therapy with certain problems. Many integrative approaches incorporate behavioral techniques, and there are dozens of good reasons why and when such choices make sense. But let us consider some of the more problematic reasons why therapists may be attracted to behavioral techniques.

Perhaps a therapist chooses behavioral techniques out of a wish to convey expertise to clients. For example, the precision involved in assigning a series of carefully formulated homework assignments can result in the therapist's being perceived by the client as some kind of a master who possesses a carefully developed formula for success. Sometimes the technology associated with certain behavioral techniques further enhances the image of the therapist as a master of technique, as might be the case when a therapist demonstrates awe-inspiring competence in the use of biofeedback apparatus. Perhaps the behavioral technique serves the therapist's need to be in control; by assuming a directive stance with the client, the therapist may derive enhanced self-esteem resulting from the fact that another person is so trusting, so responsive to directive intervention, and so willing to yield control.

The choice of behavioral techniques may be related to the therapists' issues relating to emotional closeness with the client. Certain behavioral techniques serve to keep the client at an emotional distance, while others serve to enhance a sense of intimacy with the client. At the one extreme are interventions that are quite didactic and educative; for example, the use of behavior rehearsal in assertiveness training can serve to keep the client at a distance as the therapist takes on a role of instructor. At the other extreme, relaxation exercises and hypnotic techniques may engender a sense of intimacy between the therapist and the client as the client

gives over a certain degree of autonomy within the tranquil atmosphere of the therapy session.

Lastly, there is the disturbing possibility that certain behavioral techniques may serve to satisfy sadistic tendencies on the part of the therapist. Therapists who commonly employ aversive techniques need to confront the disturbing question about whether they derive some perverse pleasure from the procedures they employ.

CONCLUDING COMMENTS

In this chapter it has been our intention to raise some provocative and difficult questions for integrative therapists to ask themselves about their overall choice of integrationism, about the particular models upon which they rely, and about the specific techniques they use with each client. By turning to a handful of the more common theoretical models, we have discussed some rather delicate matters that integrative therapists should consider when they develop treatment plans.

With the help of an objective observer, such as a supervisor or consultant, therapists should recurrently assess the extent to which treatment is based on the needs of the client and the degree to which clinical work is determined by personal needs, fantasies, and wishes. Such questioning is never easy, but is so very important for therapists committed to adhering to the highest standards of ethical and professional practice, and providing therapy that is the most effective route to change for each client asking for professional help.

REFERENCES

Beitman, B. D., Goldfried, M. R., & Norcross, J. C. (1989). The movement toward integrating the psychotherapies: An overview. *American Journal of Psychiatry, 146,* 138–147.
Beutler, L. E. (1986). Systematic eclectic psychotherapy. In J. C. Norcross (Ed.), *Handbook of eclectic psychotherapy* (pp. 94–131). New York: Brunner/Mazel.
Beutler, L. E., & Clarkin, J. F. (1990). *Systematic treatment selection: Toward targeted therapeutic interventions.* New York: Brunner/Mazel.
Eisenbud, R. (1978). Countertransference: The therapist's turn on the couch. In G. D. Goldman & D. S. Milman (Eds.), *Psychoanalytic psychotherapy* (pp. 72–90). Reading, MA: Addison-Wesley.
Frances, A., Clarkin, J. F., & Perry, S. (1984). *Differential*

therapeutics in psychiatry: The art and science of treatment selection. New York: Brunner/Mazel.

Frank, J. D. (1973). *Persuasion and healing: A comparative study of psychotherapy* (2nd ed.). Baltimore, MD: Johns Hopkins University Press.

Frank, J. D. (1982). Therapeutic components shared by all psychotherapies. In J. H. Harvey & M. M. Parks (Eds.), *Psychotherapy research and behavior change* (pp. 5–37). Washington, DC: American Psychological Association.

Halgin, R. P. (1985). On learning eclecticism. *International Journal of Eclectic Psychotherapy, 4,* 14–18.

Halgin, R. P. (1986). Pragmatic blending of clinical models in the supervisory relationship. *Clinical Supervisor, 3,* 23–46.

Halgin, R. P. (1989). Pragmatic blending. *Journal of Integrative and Eclectic Psychotherapy, 8,* 320–328.

Halgin, R. P., & Lovejoy, D. W. (1991). An integrative approach to treating the partner of a depressed person. *Psychotherapy, 28,* 251–258.

Halgin, R. P., Hennessey, J. E., Statlender, S., Feinman, J. A., & Brown, R. A. (1988). Treatment of sexual dysfunction in the context of general psychotherapy. In R. A. Brown & J. R. Field (Eds.), *Treatment of sexual problems in individual and couples therapy* (pp. 3–21). New York: PMA-Spectrum.

Hill, C. E., Mahalik, J. R., & Thompson, B. J. (1989). Therapist self-disclosure. *Psychotherapy, 26,* 290–295.

Hogan, R. A. (1964). Issues and approaches in supervision. *Psychotherapy: Theory, Research and Practice, 1,* 139–141.

Kahn, M. (1991). *Between therapist and client: The new relationship.* New York: W. H. Freeman.

Laplanche, J., & Pontalis, J. B. (1973). *The language of psycho-analysis.* New York: Norton.

Lazarus, A. A. (1986). Multimodal therapy. In J. C. Norcross (Ed.), *Handbook of eclectic psychotherapy* (pp. 65–93). New York: Brunner/Mazel.

Lazarus, A. A., Beutler, L. E., & Norcross, J. C. (1992). The future of technical eclecticism. *Psychotherapy, 29,* 11–20.

Linehan, M. M. (1988). Perspectives on the interpersonal relationship in behavior therapy. *Journal of Integrative and Eclectic Psychotherapy, 7,* 278–290.

Loganbill, C., Hardy, E., & Delworth, U. (1982). Supervision: A conceptual model. *Counseling Psychologist, 10,* 3–42.

Lombardi, K. L. (1990). Countertransference: On what constitutes shareable experience. In E. A. Margenau (Ed.), *The encyclopedic handbook of private practice* (pp. 551–559). New York: Gardner Press.

Marshall, R. J., & Marshall, S. V. (1988). *The transference-countertransference matrix.* New York: Columbia University Press.

Mathews, B. (1988). The role of therapist self-disclosure in psychotherapy: A survey of therapists. *American Journal of Psychotherapy, 42,* 521–531.

Norcross, J. C. (1990, April). *Countertransferential confessions of a prescriptive eclectic.* Paper presented at the meeting of the Society for the Exploration of Psychotherapy Integration, Philadelphia, PA.

Pinsof, W. M. (1988). The therapist-client relationship: An integrative systems perspective. *Journal of Integrative and Eclectic Psychotherapy, 7,* 303–313.

Sider, R. C. (1984). The ethics of therapeutic modality choice. *American Journal of Psychiatry, 141,* 390–394.

Sider, R. C., & Clements, C. (1982). Family or individual therapy: The ethics of modality choice. *American Journal of Psychiatry, 139,* 1455–1459.

Simon, J. C. (1988). Criteria for therapist self-disclosure. *American Journal of Psychotherapy, 42,* 404–415.

Simon, J. C. (1990). Criteria for therapist self-disclosure. In G. Stricker & M. Fisher (Eds.), *Self-disclosure in the therapeutic relationship* (pp. 207–225). New York: Plenum Press.

Stricker, G., & Fisher, M. (Eds.). (1990). *Self-disclosure in the therapeutic relationship.* New York: Plenum Press.

Wachtel, P. L. (1991). From eclecticism to synthesis: Toward a more seamless psychotherapeutic integration. *Journal of Psychotherapy Integration, 1,* 43–54.

Waterhouse, G. J., & Strupp, H. H. (1984). The patient-therapist relationship: Research from the psychodynamic perspective. *Clinical Psychology Review, 4,* 77–92.

PART VII

Conclusion

CHAPTER 36

The Therapeutic Interaction in Psychotherapy Integration

Jerold R. Gold

INTRODUCTION

In this chapter, I will examine the ways in which the relationship between therapist and patient has been studied and understood within the context of the progress in psychotherapy integration which has been reported by the contributors to this handbook. In particular, this discussion will be centered upon the commonalities within the discrete approaches to the therapeutic interaction which are overt or implicit. Such convergence in theory and practice concerning this central aspect of psychotherapy may point the way at some time in the future to an integrated psychotherapy or group of therapies. It is the rare student of therapy who would disagree with the notion that the interactive or interpersonal aspect of psychotherapy is critical at the levels of theory, observation, clinical understanding, and intervention. Yet just as we lack currently a unified model of pathology or intervention, we miss a common and open construal of the meaning, process, and utility of the therapeutic relationship.

In some psychotherapies, integrative or otherwise, the conception of the relationship defines and structures the way technique, process, and change are considered, sought after, and evaluated. Other schools of psychotherapy suggest that the therapeutic interaction is more of a dependent variable, and that its evolution and course are determined by interventive and technical issues. Finally, certain therapists (especially those in the humanistic/experiential camp, and others who adhere to the model proposed by Frank, 1961), argue that therapy is relationship and that the two concepts cannot be separated in any significant way. The discussion that follows will examine this debate as well, in terms of the positions taken by writers within the integrative movement, and for its implications for future models of unified psychotherapy.

Lacking a universally accepted framework for discussion of the therapeutic interaction, I now propose and will utilize below three facets of the interaction between patient and therapist which can be examined and compared in a cross-sectional basis. These facets are: the *emotional climate* of the interaction, the *interactional stance*, and the *role of interactional data*.

Jerold R. Gold • Doctoral Program in Clinical Psychology, Long Island University, Brooklyn, New York 11201.

Comprehensive Handbook of Psychotherapy Integration, edited by George Stricker and Jerold R. Gold. Plenum Press, New York, 1993.

THE EMOTIONAL CLIMATE OF
THE THERAPEUTIC INTERACTION

The term *emotional climate* refers to the quality and quantity of affective engagement and involvement between patient and therapist which are thought to be helpful, necessary, or ameliorative. Also important here are the specific types of affective and interpersonal experiences which are deemed to be positive, neutral, or destructive to therapeutic work.

As a group, the integrative therapists represented in this volume seem to be in a broad consensus with each other, and with modern trends in the sectarian schools of psychotherapy which emphasize the need for, and importance of, a warm, respectful, and empathic approach to the patient. The opinions presented in this volume would not be met by much disagreement from many psychoanalysts especially those who would agree with the role of warmth and empathy (Kohut, 1971), the provision of a holding environment (Winnicott, 1971), or the need for a sense of safety, security, and freedom from excessive anxiety in the therapeutic setting (Sandler, 1960; Sullivan, 1953). Cognitive-behavioral therapy, as represented by Beck (1976) and Goldfried and Davison (1976), have emphasized these emotional components as well, as have humanistic therapists since that form of therapy was introduced.

An accepting, safe, and empathic emotional climate is considered to be necessary to allow the patient to reveal his or her intrapsychic and behavior difficulties, and the attachment and closeness which grow out of warmth and empathy are viewed by most writers as serving one of the bases for behavioral experimentation and for cognitive, emotional, and motivational revelation and change.

For the majority of integrative therapists, this emotional climate of empathy and acceptance provides the patient with a new sense of self-worth, confirmation, self-acceptance, and is a significant ingredient in the disconfirmation of old and dysfunctional thoughts, opinions, and feelings about the self and others. This position is exemplified by the chapter by Andrews, who stresses the need for closeness and confirmation of the patient within the therapy before confrontation, challenges, and change can occur. Similarly,

in discussions of integrative therapy with substance abusers and with chronic pain patients, respectively, Cummings and Dworkin and Grzesiak emphasize early bonding and the siding of therapist with patient as a necessary step in the early stages of treatment. Allen's unified systems approach also begins with such efforts at building a safe and sound climate which can serve as a springboard for further work. As a final example, Becker's work with organically impaired patients relies heavily upon monitoring and repairing the damage to the positive bond between patient and therapist which is caused by exploration of the humiliation and shame attendant to neurological dysfunction.

Several chapters, including those by Gold; Hayes and Newman; and Papouchis and Passman, emphasize the role of early attachment experiences in the etiology of psychopathology, and include some stress on the ways pathogenic beliefs and feelings about attachment can be tested and discarded on the basis of a positive and successful experience of relatedness to and with the therapist. This view, which approximates the corrective emotional experience identified by Alexander and French (1946), or the "necessary and sufficient" theory of the therapeutic relationship offered by Rogers (1957), is shared by almost all contributors to one degree or another, though none would suggest that the emotional climate by itself is totally and completely responsible for therapeutic change. Most contributors would argue that empathic engagement is indeed necessary but is not sufficient to produce much meaningful change in and of itself. In the view of Allen; Andrews; Beutler and Hodgson; Cummings; Fodor; Gold and Wachtel; Rieves, Inck, and Safran, among many others, this climate of empathy and safety allows the therapist to be heard when he or she challenges the patient to change an idea, behavior, or self image, and permits and encourages the patient to face a distasteful, fearsome, or painful inner state, interpersonal event, or new behavioral challenge.

INTERACTIONAL STANCE

This facet of the therapeutic interaction is defined in terms of such issues as the therapist's activity level, the roles and responsibilities assigned to both patient and therapist, the place of the specific therapy upon such continua as egalitarian versus authoritarian, directive versus nondirective, and exploratory versus didactic. As a group, there once again exists a surprising level of consensus among the integrative therapists represented in this volume. The large majority defined their role as encompassing both didactic and exploratory dimensions, with freedom of movement between either activity. There exists much agreement about and great emphasis upon the necessity and complementary nature of periods of directive teaching with moments and long expanses of exploration, while the therapist facilitates by nondirective means. Crass authoritarian attitudes and behaviors are nowhere to be found, and the didactic and directive activities of the therapists are typically presented as best set within a context of collaboration and an egalitarian approach to hypothesis testing. As described by Bugenthal and Kleiner, the therapist may best take the role of a consultant who assists through his or her expertise and authority, rather than dictates or controls. The patient most frequently is considered to be the final arbiter of the validity and utility of the therapist's suggestions and interventions. The role definitions provided by many integrative writers for the therapists are thus multidimensional and synthetic of various sectarian positions. The therapist is understood to be a potential model, to be a source of new information about the self and the world, to be someone whose actions stimulate new ideas, feelings, and wishes as well as confirming or disconfirming old experiences and inner states. Moderate to high levels of engagement and activity, at points or throughout the therapy, are prescribed and encouraged. These therapists do not endorse the sanctions against personal influence and guidance shared by classical psychoanalysis or by versions of client-centered and other humanistic therapies. Anonymity, neutrality, and unconditional positive regard are considered to be impossibilities which even if achievable, would not fit or make therapeutic sense in the context of the theories and methods of many, if not most integrative positions.

This consensual stance most resembles the active "collaborative empiricism" described by Beck (1976), and the directed inquiry method favored by Sullivan (1953) in his interpersonal psychotherapy, and therefore it does not come as a surprise that these therapies and their methods are heavily cited as influential, especially by those writers whose work draws in other significant ways from the psychodynamic and humanistic traditions. The relative inactivity and striving for a stance in which the therapist neither teaches nor influences has been understood to be unfortunate and to be among the least helpful aspects of these solitary therapies. As Becker; Gold and Wachtel; Gold and Stricker; Papouchis and Passman, and many others point out, it was these considerations which to a great extent encouraged integration in the first place.

The patient's role in the therapy also is understood in highly similar ways by our various contributors. In an egalitarian, collaborative, and active therapy the patient is considered to be an intelligent, educable, and vigorous participant. Most work in psychotherapy integration stresses or implicitly regards "role induction" (Luborsky, 1984) to be an extremely important activity. Instruction in the roles and behavior associated with patienthood can be critical in helping the patient be clear about what he or she is expected to do, how the therapist will behave and how the therapy will progress, and especially in comprehending the ways in which the patient may help his or her own therapy along. Many integrative therapies have incorporated the cognitive-behavioral and systems methods of homework assignments, in vivo exercises, and environmental manipulation by therapist and patient, thus extending and redefining the role of both parties and their interpersonal stance toward and with each other. In almost all cases the patient is expected to evaluate and to respond to the therapist's interventions and actions on the basis of the patient's successes and failures, emotional, cognitive, imaginative, and systemic experiences, and is taught to expect a respectful and open reaction to such feedback by the therapist. As an example of this emphasis upon activity and responsibility on the part of the patient, the chapters by Bugenthal and Kleiner; Cummings; and Ryle and Low may be cited. Here are three theories and methods which differ greatly in content and form, yet all three explicitly argue that success in treatment is in large part dependent upon the extent to which the patient can take on, or can be moved to accept, an invested, motivated, and responsible role.

THE ROLE OF INTERACTIONAL DATA

Mention of the importance and utility of interactional data in psychotherapy integration is almost ubiquitous. Without exception, a strong and stable therapeutic alliance is deemed critical for ongoing therapeutic activity, and disruptions in the bond, or an inability to form such a bond, will inevitably become the focus of much therapeutic concern and activity in all of the therapies under review.

Certain integrative therapists, most notably Becker; Coonerty; Cummings; Dworkin and Grzesiak; Fitzpatrick; Franklin, Carter, and Grace; and Sollod, do not venture in detail far beyond such notation of the impact of the therapeutic alliance and their views on the use of interactional data must be inferred from their general positions of the processes of therapy. These inferences dovetail considerably with the trends which emerge from reviewing the more developed and specific approaches to interactional data in the other chapters. Two strong and related ways of conceptualizing and working with interactional data seem to be present, and may be labeled the *intrapsychic-tranferential* mode, and the *interpersonal-characterological* mode.

Writers who belong to the intrapsychic-transferential mode typically see the interaction as determined by internalized needs, wishes, conflicts, defenses, and self and object representations. The ongoing, present relationship with the therapist therefore is colored by some degree of regression, distortion and resistance to intimacy, and self-disclosure. Of critical weight in this mode is the assumption of primacy of internal and past experience being recreated and relived, with secondary significance attached to the unique characteristics and behavior of the therapist. This mode is nearly identical to classical and contemporary models of psychoanalysis and is most influential in the work of those integrative therapists who incorporate ideas from a formal intrapsychic psychodynamic model, as do Bugenthal and Kleiner; Fensterheim; Healey; Hellcamp; Papouchis and Passman; Rubin; and Ryle and Low. An intra-

psychic conceptualization of interactional data orients the therapy toward certain interventive decisions and techniques. Interpretation of unconscious distortions, either as a silent guide to the therapist or out loud to the patient, are seen as critical, though interventions from other schools may be used once the transference is formulated. Anxiety and resistance primarily are understood to be intrapsychically generated and as the resultants of past experience, and are worked with accordingly.

The interpersonal-characterological mode of understanding and dealing with interactional phenomena is typical of the efforts at integration which are more indebted to interpersonal theories and psychotherapies, such as Sullivan (1953), and to contemporary systemic and cognitive-behavioral models and methods, than to strictly psychoanalytic constructs. This mode is predominant in the chapters by Allen; Andrews; Beutler and Hodgson; Fodor; Gold; Gold and Wachtel; Hayes and Newman; Rieves, Inck, and Safran; Kirschner and Kirschner; and Westerman and broadens the understanding of the interaction to include the idea that patient and therapist are mutually influencing and that the data of their interaction often is a unique blend of the past and the present. In this mode, the therapeutic interaction is construed as embodying *in vivo* the patient's characteristic ways of engaging other people, and as both expressing and avoiding inner states. Most critically, the ways the patient recreates the past and therefore maintains and reinforces his or her psychopathology by shaping other people to enter into interactions which confirm and reinforce pathogenic ideas, wishes, and feelings, and representations are understood to shape and to be inevitable within the therapeutic interaction. Such patterns of confirmation (Andrews), vicious circles and the creation of accomplices (Gold & Wachtel), or hooking (Rieves, Inck, & Safran) also are known by other names, but are the central construct in all of the chapters which fall within this mode. Technically, this shared understanding of the interaction leads to a consensus about the need for confrontation of such patterns, an examination of the ways both parties colluded in this recreation, and for in session and out of session experiences aimed at breaking the hold of the characterological issues and structures which keep these patterns alive. The interpersonal-characterological approach contains within it implicit or explicit pressures on the therapist to act, within the relationship, in ways which inhibit old patterns from coalescing and which appeal for fresh, novel, and risky new ways of relatedness. In some ways, technique and relationship are more fully blended in this mode than in the alternate intrapsychic mode, which comes closer to the older tradition of talking about relatedness and the need for change, rather than relating in ways meant to produce change.

This mode suggests that anxieties and resistances may be caused by interactional factors or more frequently by variables which are internal to the patient. This view calls on the therapist then to review the interaction and his or her own participation in order to discover any interactional sources of resistance, which, if found, must be met by behavioral and attitudinal changes on the therapist's part. Fensterheim cites an example of a therapy which was stalled by the therapist's fear of the patient's aggression, and which moved to a successful conclusion only after the therapist was desensitized to that experience and was able to comfortably allow the patient to be angry in sessions. Westerman argues that patient and therapist are interdependent actors who cannot help but influence each other in growth promoting or pathogenic ways. Such a conceptualization places much greater and more explicit technical emphasis on the therapist's experience of, and reaction to, the patient than does the intrapsychic mode, wherein such reactions are handled more traditionally as countertransference.

There is no mention in any chapter of rigid strictures or prohibitions against utilizing the subjective experience of the therapist as a source of potential knowledge about the patient. Several writers, including Healy; Rieves, Inck and Safran; and Sollod, explicitly advocate the need for an intensive and extensive inward focus at central points in the therapy. However, within the two modes of approaching the interaction, certain distinctions are notable in the ways these experiences influence further process. Although writers in the intrapsychic-transference mode do not object to judicious self-disclosure, and some (for example, Bugenthal & Kleiner; Healy; and Rubin) explicitly advocate self-disclosure, such action on the part of the therapist is not fully integrated into the technical framework of treatment. That is, the role

of revelation on the part of the therapist cannot be linked to a particular goal *a priori*, and instead such information usually is offered for spontaneous and somewhat idiosyncratic reasons. In the interpersonal-characterological mode, therapist self-examination and interventions drawn from such scrutiny (what Rieves, Inck, & Safran call the therapist's "discipline"), are more fully integrated into the conceptual and technical models of the therapeutic process. When the therapist offers the patient a glimpse of the therapist's experience of the former, this information becomes the starting point for work within the hooking, vicious circles, or characterological patterns of avoidance and confirmation which typify the patient's general life situation. Similarly, while it is doubtful that any integrative therapist would argue against the importance of modeling and vicarious learning within therapy, writers in the interpersonal-characterological mode tend to stress this aspect of the interaction. For example, Fodor suggests that the therapist's experiences in problem-solving and in empowering himself or herself can be told to the patient in order to open up new possibilities of thought and behavior. Gold and Stricker suggest that the therapist can encourage new internal structures through corrective and informative involvement of patient and therapist, whereas Gold and Wachtel point out that answering questions, giving advice, and sharing reactions and ideas may help the patient to end his or her involvement in repetitive and redundant negative relationships with others who refuse to be helpful.

Regression within the therapeutic interaction is acknowledged as a real and frequent phenomenon, but it is one which is not sought after, and often efforts are recommended to counter or undermine extreme regressive and transferential experiences. This opinion seems to be shared by therapists from both interactional modes. Allen points out that a therapist operating within the framework of his unified therapy would seek to inhibit or undo any sign of a transference neurosis, whereas other contributors, such as Andrews; Cummings; and Kirshner and Kirshner, suggest deliberate therapist behavior which will surprise the patient and which will open the patient to the differences between past and present within the interaction. Consensually, integrative therapists appear to avoid extreme reactions within therapy sessions, believing that such upheavals will produce more interference and resistance than is helpful or necessary. Papouchis and Passman, who lean toward the intrapsychic mode, suggest that frequently the transference cannot be acknowledged or worked with openly in work with the elderly but must be "lived" or managed silently by the therapist. In the interpersonal-characterological mode, regression particularly is avoided, as such phenomena are considered to be representative of a very small number of situations in the patient's life, and do not convey more valuable or deeper aspects of the patient's experience. Gold and Wachtel's discussion of the fallacies of the "Wooly Mammoth" aspects of traditional psychodynamic theory is one statement of this position. Interactional data which inform and demonstrate where the patient lives in the here and now, with real figures in his or her life, are valued much more than artificially induced regressive experiences.

In conclusion of this section, I would point out that the two modes which I have described above are not completely contradictory, and in actual practice it is likely that therapists utilize both, while emphasizing one to a degree. The chapter by Gold and Stricker actually includes something of a hybrid model, wherein the intrapsychic and interpersonal are given about equal weight theoretically and practically. Neither mode would dismiss the other completely. It is more a matter of directional emphasis, as discussed by Coonerty, in considering whether the present interaction is a shadow of the past and is caused by distant events, or that the past stays alive because of current interactional experiences.

CONCLUSION AND IMPLICATIONS

Earlier in this chapter, I mentioned that conceptions of the psychotherapeutic relationship can either shape or be shaped by any therapeutic system of process and intervention. Not a single example of the former case can be found in this volume. Without exception, the construal of the interaction follows from the particular ideas about psychopathology and change which mark each chapter's approach to integration. This situation is fairly well equivalent to the state of affairs in the general field of psychotherapy, sectarian or integrative. Few therapies are defined by their

understanding of the therapeutic relationship; instead, technical guidelines and the theory of cure and change inform the therapist with regard to the ideal and sought after relationship. Yet the repeated convergences among integrative therapists in their approach to and use of the interaction mirrors the new similarities between therapists of sectarian schools in both form and in content. Psychotherapy in general seems to be moving toward the greater appreciation of its interpersonal dimension which was first advocated by Sullivan (1953), and which was adapted and expanded by Fromm-Reichman (1950), Singer, (1965), Carson (1969) and Kiesler (1982), among others. Within the integrative psychotherapy community as well as without, the interaction is consensually defined as the arena in which the patient's inner world and character, his or her cognitions, experiences, emotions, and dynamics are displayed and the place in which his or her systemic and interpersonal strengths and weaknesses are experienced and observed *in vivo* by and with the therapist. The therapist's role of participant–observer as first described by Sullivan (1953) is equally valid and applicable today in integrative therapy. In many ways, this is in accordance with Sullivan's (1953) vision of his interpersonal theory, which was perhaps an Ur-integrative therapy in its blending of psychoanalytic ideas with concepts drawn from sociology, social psychology, anthropology, economics, linguistics, and communications theory. This is not an idle or purely academic point. Recently, Alford and Norcross (1991), and Beck (1991) have argued that cognitive therapy be considered an, or perhaps *the* example of a mature integrative psychotherapy. In this *Handbook*, cognitive therapy is powerfully represented as a component of many integrative positions, and yet its ideas and techniques do not possess the same cross-sectional influence as the repeated interpersonal emphases which have been described above in this chapter.

My point is that a start toward a mature and fully expanded theory of the psychotherapeutic interaction might well be found in the convergences in ideas of the contributors to this volume, and in the tenets of interpersonal psychotherapy in general. In turn, such a conceptualization of the therapeutic interaction might in the future give rise to a truly unified or *integrated* form of psychotherapy which would be in fact seamless

(Wachtel, 1991), and which would be impervious to charges of "technical eclecticism" without a consistent and integrated theoretical base (Arkowitz & Messer, 1984). In this hypothetical psychotherapy, interventions would be determined by the state of the therapeutic interaction needed and by which interactional factors, in or outside of the therapy, needed to be addressed in order to move the patient along. A comprehensive theory of any interpersonal relationship, psychotherapeutic or otherwise, must include discussion of psychodynamic, cognitive, emotional, experiential, behavioral, and systemic variables, and must account for the multidirectional nature of causality and influence of those variables (Gold, in press). A theory built from the start which would include all aspects of human experience would surmount and bypass the need for integration at all.

We are far from such an ideal, yet again, the surprising and substantial quantity of agreement within this one collection suggests that some collective level, such as a nascent unity, may exist or at least be forming. In the final chapter, Stricker will review the disparate integrative positions in a broader way and will point out other progress toward an integrative therapy as well. In some ways, the ideas just described are coincident with those of Frank (1961) who brilliantly placed contemporary within the historical and cross-cultural context of healing and interpersonal persuasion. His studies suggested that technique in healing efforts is less important than the ongoing interpersonal union. However, technique serves as an ideological function for the healer, as it separates that person from the untrained and uninitiated. Technique serves a ritualistic function as well, offering comfort and hope and a sense of control through repetitive action. Finally, and perhaps most importantly, technique allows the relationship to continue by justifying ongoing contact between participants.

Frank's description of these processes in psychotherapy frequently has been cited by behavior therapists as indication that only behavior treatment, which has a powerful and specific technology, can go beyond shamanism and persuasion. Yet such studies as Sloane, Staples, Cristol, Yorkston, and Whipple (1975), and Gold (1980) indicated that patients in behavior therapy do not seem to experience it much differently than those in other therapies, and that these patients empha-

sized relationship and interactional factors in their reports of what was most helpful to them. It behooves us then to use these findings in the service of the development of a relationship that unifies the healer with the technician. Obviously some progress has been made, as described herein, but more remains to be done.

REFERENCES

Alexander, F., & French, T. (1946). *Psychoanalytic therapy.* New York: Ronald Press.

Alford, B. A., & Norcross, J. C. (1991). Cognitive therapy as integrative therapy. *Journal of Psychotherapy Integration, 1,* 175–190.

Arkowitz, H., & Messer, S. (Eds.). (1984). *Psychoanalytic therapy and behavioral therapy: Is integration possible?* New York: Plenum Press.

Beck, A. T. (1976). *Cognitive therapy and the emotional disorders.* New York: New American Library.

Beck, A. T. (1991). Cognitive therapy as integrative therapy. (Commentary). *Journal of Psychotherapy Integration, 1,* 191–198.

Carson, R. C. (1969). *Interaction concepts of personality.* Chicago: Aldine.

Frank, J. D. (1961). *Persuasion and healing.* Baltimore: Johns Hopkins University Press.

Fromm-Reichmann, R. (1950). *Principles of intensive psychotherapy.* Chicago: University of Chicago Press.

Gold, J. R. (1980). *A retrospective study of the behavior therapy experience.* Unpublished doctoral dissertation, Adelphi University.

Gold, J. R. (in press). When patients dictate integration. *Journal of Integrative and Eclectic Psychotherapy.*

Goldfried, M., & Davison, G. (1976). *Clinical behavior therapy.* New York: Holt, Rinehart, & Winston.

Kiesler, D. J. (1982). Interpersonal theory for personality and psychotherapy. In J. C. Anchin & D. J. Kiesler (Eds.), *Handbook of interpersonal psychotherapy* (pp. 67–82). New York: Pergamon.

Kohut, H. (1971). *The analysis of the self.* New York: International Universities Press.

Luborsky, L. (1984). *Principles of psychoanalytic psychotherapy.* New York: Basic Books.

Rogers, C. R. (1957). The necessary and sufficient conditions of therapeutic personality change. *Journal of Consulting Psychology, 21,* 95–103.

Sandler, J. (1960). The background of safety. *International Journal of Psychoanalysis, 41,* 352–356.

Singer, E. (1965). *Key concepts in psychotherapy.* New York: Basic Books.

Sloane, R. B., Staples, F. R., Cristol, A. H., Yorkston, N. J., & Whipple, K. (1975). *Psychotherapy vs. behavior therapy.* Cambridge: Harvard University Press.

Sullivan, H. S. (1953). *The interpersonal theory of psychiatry.* New York: W. W. Norton.

Wachtel, P. L. (1991). Towards a more seamless integration. *Journal of Psychotherapy Integration, 1,* 32–41.

Winnicott, D. W. (1971). *Maturational processes and the facilitating environment.* New York: International Universities Press.

CHAPTER 37

The Current Status of Psychotherapy Integration

George Stricker

After reviewing the excellent and varied contributions to this *Handbook*, it is possible to integrate these chapters and to reach some superordinate conclusions. However, let us first begin by drawing distinctions between psychotherapy integration, integrative psychotherapy, and an eclectic approach to psychotherapy. An eclectic approach is one in which the therapist chooses interventions because they work, without any theoretical basis for, or understanding of, or necessary concern with, the reason for using the technique other than the one of efficacy. Psychotherapy integration attends to the relationship between theory and technique. Integrative psychotherapy is presented as a completed, pure-form approach to treatment, whereas psychotherapy integration is a process rather than a school of psychotherapy. Attention is given to the response of the patient as it relates to the goals of the treatment, and techniques are employed in order to pursue those goals, based on some superordinate understanding of the process of treatment. By and large, the

George Stricker • Derner Institute of Advanced Psychological Studies, Adelphi University, Garden City, New York 11530.

Comprehensive Handbook of Psychotherapy Integration, edited by George Stricker and Jerold R. Gold. Plenum Press, New York, 1993.

approaches presented in this *Handbook* are based on some theoretical understanding of the process, but little conviction about the completeness of the system that is presented. There is an understanding of the need for further research and clinical experience to develop the techniques and the theory that are being integrated.

CURRENT DEVELOPMENTS IN PSYCHOTHERAPY INTEGRATION

Gold introduces this *Handbook* with a brief history of psychotherapy integration and places this historical development within the context of the social changes that have occurred over the past decade. We are living at a time when isolationism and nationalism have been replaced by an international perspective, social orthodoxy has given way to a more permissive heterodoxy, revisionist history has placed emphasis on a broader set of contributors, science has become less decontextualized, and disciplinary exclusivity is being replaced by interdisciplinary studies. It is no wonder that the pure-form approaches to psychotherapy of the past are no longer satisfactory to a growing number of practitioners, and the appeal of psychotherapy integration is compelling.

Innovations in theory and technique usually lead, rather than follow, research findings. In psychotherapy integration this also is so, and myriad creative contributions are described by the authors in this *Handbook*, but few are based on, or supported by, research data. Glass, Arnkoff, and Victor, in their companion chapters concerning research on psychotherapy integration and therapeutic change, examine the data that do exist. These data are both disappointingly scant and impressively rich. Much more is needed, but there also are many encouraging leads.

The multiplicity of attempts at integration are substantial, and where data have been collected, the findings are promising. The need for further data is clear, as is the likelihood that ultimately there will be a variety of helpful and appropriate approaches to psychotherapy, perhaps best suited for delivery by different therapists or to different patients, rather than there being a single best approach that will be endorsed by research findings. The data to be collected should be dictated by the theory of the psychotherapy, so that a careful explication of what is to be done, and why, will point to the most critical areas for future research. Further, such explication by each therapist will make clear where common and specific factors lie, and also will point the way toward possibilities for integration across approaches.

Common factors refer to aspects of psychotherapy that are present in most, if not all, approaches to treatment. As the core of psychotherapy, elaborated by the techniques that differentiate the various approaches, common factors either may provide an argument for or against further integration. On the one hand, it is easy to integrate approaches that begin more nearly alike than we had realized. On the other hand, there may be little reason or opportunity to integrate beyond what already is achieved by this common core, and the apparent integration simply may be a translation of old concepts into a common language, reflecting existing similarities but not achieving new integration. The therapeutic underground is aware of this common core and, as a result, we can expect that more experienced therapists will make greater use of the common factors.

Weinberger reviews the theoretical and empirical basis for the establishment of a set of common factors. Although there is no fixed, established list of common factors, consensus suggests that such a list would include a therapeutic alliance, a corrective emotional experience, expectations for change, beneficial therapist qualities, and the provision of a rationale for patient problems. To this list, Weinberger adds values and then summarizes the research support for the efficacy of these common factors. The evidence, although insufficient to establish an integrative common factors model of psychotherapy, does provide support for the importance of these factors in determining therapeutic outcome.

Gold and Wachtel present cyclical psychodynamics, a systematic approach originally introduced by Wachtel, and one that is rooted in interpersonal psychodynamic theory and technique, but that also integrates concepts and techniques of behavioral, cognitive, and systems approaches. The critical contribution is the substitution of mutual influence for linear causation, so that the influence of environmental factors on psychodynamics, as well as vice versa, is considered crucial. This integration at the level of theory then suggests an appropriate integration at the level of technique, the use of interventions that influence behavior and environment in order to augment those factors that have intrapsychic and interpersonal impact.

The patient is seen as acting in ways consistent with intrapsychic dynamics, but selecting accomplices whose response to these behaviors will confirm the anxiety and fears that produced the initial maladaptive response. The description of the resultant vicious circles to the patient is reminiscent of the Procedural Sequence Model of Ryle, although the description is not communicated as early or as explicitly. A break in this vicious circle can lead to a corrective emotional experience and produce important therapeutic change. This break can be expedited by technical interventions drawn from a variety of theoretical positions and encourages a level of therapist activity that goes well beyond that of traditional psychodynamic psychotherapy. Cyclical psychodynamics, with its integration of theory and technique, underlies the approach to entrenched character pathology described by Gold and Stricker.

Fensterheim refers to his integrative method as Behavioral Psychotherapy, although it is an attempt to combine the behavioral and psychodynamic perspectives. It is based on a theory of therapy rather than a theory of personality, with the absence of a theory of personality necessarily leading to a focus on the remediation of pathological behaviors. Choice of interventions is determined by the Law of Parsimony, so that the least inferential method of accounting for a dysfunction usually is assumed until such an assumption is proven to be untenable. Thus, the first level of intervention always is the behavioral, to be followed, in turn, if it proves unsuccessful, by dealing with the obstacle to success and the pursuit of psychodynamic issues. Interestingly, the approach of Gold and Stricker reverses this sequence, beginning with a psychodynamic exploratory phase and introducing behavioral techniques when necessary. Fensterheim's approach, although described as behavioral psychotherapy, goes well beyond the traditional pure-form behavioral approach, not only in terms of the integration with interventions drawn from alternative schools, but by the theoretical recognitions that a behavior may have meaning beyond the superficially apparent, and that a response to the genotypic meaning may be necessary to alter the phenotypic behavioral presentation.

Ryle and Low report on the development of Cognitive-Analytic Therapy (CAT), a theory and approach that was developed by Ryle and is illustrated through a case presented by Low. CAT integrates cognitive psychology and psychotherapy with an object relations approach to psychoanalysis, restated in cognitive terminology. The traps, dilemmas, and snags that comprise many maladaptive patterns of functioning often are based on misconstruals or self-fulfilling prophesies that are subject to reformulation in the treatment. A description of a Procedural Sequence Model (PSM) is developed by the therapist in collaboration with the patient, presented, typically, in the fourth session, and forms the basis for determining appropriate interventions. Just as Andrews describes a sequence of stages, each of which generates different options for intervention, Ryle works with a uniquely derived PSM that provides the direction for intervention. The theory has a developmental dimension that is described carefully and is based on an object relations model.

The therapeutic technique that follows from the developmental theory leads to a short-term therapeutic approach that is presented as far more widely applicable than is most short-term approaches. CAT integrates cognitive-behavioral and psychoanalytic techniques but also draws upon other approaches, such as behavioral or gestalt techniques, if they are applicable for the modification of identified problem procedures. The therapeutic relationship is viewed as a microcosm of the patient's style of relating and is used actively in the treatment, another derivation from a psychoanalytic approach.

Bugental and Kleiner describe existentialism as a philosophical stance that is common to a variety of theoretical approaches, including psychoanalytic, humanistic, and gestalt treatments. The approach they describe is not integrative in the sense of combining prior positions into a new whole, but rather in its overarching relationship to a number of otherwise disparate approaches. The central tenet of this philosophy is that human beings are whole and sentient living organisms, capable of reflexive self-awareness, and beset with the anxiety that is an inherent aspect of the human condition. Existentialism stresses the need to focus on the human experience rather than to engage in reductionistic or objectifying exercises.

The existential perspective can be reflected in a multiplicity of techniques that have in common a primary focus on inner awareness rather than the behavioral consequences of that awareness. The centrality of working with resistance is shared by humanistic and psychoanalytic approaches, both of which see the resistance to be against awareness and change, manifested in maneuvers within the relationship. The relationship, then, becomes an important part of the process, as it is for Ryle as well. Existential-humanistic therapy of the sort described by Bugental and Kleiner is appropriate for a highly select group of patients, but the philosophical stance on which it is based can serve as a backdrop for a broader set of interventions.

The attempt to integrate cognitive, interpersonal, and experiential approaches that Safran has pursued is presented by Reeves, Inck, and Safran. This approach is grounded in cognitive psychotherapy, but it incorporates the affective perspective of the experiential tradition as well as an appreciation of the interpersonal context in which development occurs. The underlying theory postulates the development of interpersonal schema, much as this is seen to occur in object relations theory, leading to the occurrence of interpersonal behaviors that confirm the resultant cognitive frames. This same process has been described in somewhat different language by Gold and Wachtel. The therapeutic attempt to interrupt this pattern is marked by unhooking, an approach that involves the therapist's close attention to feelings aroused in the therapeutic interaction and a resistance by the therapist to being drawn into the client's maladaptive interpersonal pattern. This is similar to the awareness of and resistance to projective identification that is central to many psychodynamic formulations, and often leads to metacommunication in the form of countertransference disclosure, a tactic also familiar to experiential therapists. The experiential changes in the treatment room then can be generalized, with the aid of homework assignments, to interpersonal contexts outside of treatment. This process requires the therapist to be relatively free from maladaptive interpersonal schemata that will distort the therapeutic interaction, and reference is made to Buddhist insight meditation as a model for the maintenance of free-floating attention. This model is described in much greater depth by Rubin, who seeks to integrate Buddhism and psychotherapy. The process by which the therapist unhooks from the pattern established by the client recalls Wachtel's cyclical psychodynamics and the need not to collude with the client's self-perpetuating patterns.

Allen's approach to integration incorporates ideas from a number of orientations and directly addresses the dialectic between self and society. In doing so, he introduces many of the concepts, techniques, and values of family therapy into the individual therapy modality and his approach creates a synthesis between the individual's self-interest and his or her group interest. The continuous, internally generated impetus toward individualism, coupled with a continuous external pressure to maintain the equilibrium of the family (an external pressure that often becomes internalized), leads to a tension that can result in symptomatology and bring a patient to our attention.

Allen believes that the patient's behavior always is rational and comprehensible and his or her motives always are constructive and affirmative, but much exploration may need to be done to discover the rational and affirmative in the appar-

ently irrational and self-destructive. This discovery usually points to the extension of a family situation into role behavior that leads to the construction of a false self. Upon the discovery of the rational and affirmative, the patient can choose alternative paths to reach the affirmative goal. During the process of exploration and discovery, for the therapist to respond with a focus on the issues of individuation may threaten to ignore the systemic consequences of separation from the family. However, for the therapist to respond with a focus on the system may lead to the denial of needs for individuation and the development of an entrenched false self. Allen recognizes that the influence of the family, through introjection, perseveres well beyond the life of the family and may be even more difficult to change without the immediate availability of an external family with whom roles can be appreciated, understood, and renegotiated.

McCullough begins with a modification of a pure-form approach in that traditional psychoanalysis is altered by an emphasis on therapist activity so that it can form the basis of short-term psychotherapy. However, she then goes beyond this model by integrating a number of technical interventions that are drawn from cognitive-behavioral and gestalt orientations. A central role is given to the common factors in psychotherapy, especially as outlined by Weinberger, and each stage of psychotherapy is analyzed by referring to the manner in which it promotes one of the common factors. Further, there is a substantial technical alteration in that the usual stress arousing approach of short-term dynamic therapy is replaced by an emphasis on anxiety reduction, more consistent with self-psychology than with more traditional psychoanalytic approaches.

Beutler and Hodgson describe technical eclecticism, a theoretical approach distinct in its preference for empirical data rather than theoretical formulations. Most of the authors in this *Handbook* begin with theory and incorporate a variety of techniques that fit within and follow from that theory, achieving integration at the level of technique, and perhaps including an integrative approach to their theory as well. In contrast, Beutler and Hodgson begin with technique, assuming therapist factors as a necessary but not sufficient condition for therapeutic success, bypassing any fixed theory of personality or psychopathology, and choosing interventions on the basis of established empirical evidence that considers client, treatment, relationship, and technique variables. The ultimate value of this approach depends on the ultimate adequacy of the data base. The chapters by Glass, Arnkoff, and Victor suggest that there is something to draw upon, but not enough for technical eclecticism to make a comprehensive treatment approach yet likely, if it is to depend on that data base alone.

There is a recognition of the need for the therapist practicing technical eclecticism to obtain training and competence in the use of a wide range of interventions, a heady task indeed. The carefully outlined approach to selecting interventions seems to belie the atheoretical presentation, as it suggests a more well-developed theory of therapy. In any case, technical eclecticism has the potential to be the most broad of any of the approaches described in its use of interventions, assuming both a Renaissance therapist who is master of them all and a data base sufficient to provide adequate direction.

Andrews organizes his integrative efforts around a consistent and novel theoretical position based on his conception of an active self. An identity image is central to each person, and that image is formed and reformed by an active self that guides behavior in a stable manner. The active self seeks out and interprets interpersonal feedback in a manner that is confirmatory of the initial self-schema. This notion is reminiscent of the process described by Gold and Wachtel as cyclical psychodynamics, where a similar interpersonal interdependency is noted and also can lead to a series of self-fulfilling prophesies. Andrews cites research evidence that is consistent with his theoretical formulation.

Having defined a research-based theory of self-development, and having described a series of stages present in the process of on-going self-confirmation, Andrews then can generate a framework for therapeutic intervention. A combination of the stages and of the interventions aimed either at producing awareness or at developing change leads to a matrix of 18 types of interventions. These interventions can be drawn from a plethora of therapeutic approaches thus accomplishing technical integration under the umbrella of a consistent and coherent theoretical approach. Further, that theoretical position itself is integrative, combining concerns of a wide variety of prior theories, including psychodynamic, behavioral, and humanistic formulations.

Westerman integrates a philosophical perspective, hermeneutics, with psychotherapy and then, in the pursuit of developing an approach to psychotherapy, integrates a number of theoretical positions and technical approaches. The hermeneutic circle described by Westerman is not that of the radical subjectivity espoused by some psychoanalysts, but one in which the starting point is the individual's patterns of action within the world. The focus of therapeutic change is not solely the thoughts, the feelings, or the behaviors of the client, but the client's patterns of action. The notion that the therapeutic relationship is a circle involving the client and the therapist is reminiscent of the work of Wachtel and of Safran, and the extension of that circle into the world outside the therapeutic room recalls the formulations of Ryle and of Gold and Stricker. Westerman's perspective leads him to reevaluate behavioral, systematic, and insight-oriented interventions and to suggest ways in which each of them can be conceptualized and incorporated within a hermeneutic approach.

Feminism, as with hermeneutics, more accurately can be considered a philosophy that can be applied to psychotherapy rather than as a complete theory of psychotherapy. Fodor describes this philosophical stance and then shows how it can be integrated with cognitive-behavioral psychotherapy and expanded by the use of techniques to incorporate the affective dimension of gestalt therapy. Although she does not address the integration of feminism and psychoanalysis, Fodor does indicate that this, too, is a possibility. The focus of feminist approaches on the process, the therapist–client relationship, and the possibility of therapist self-disclosure, along with the acceptance of the experience of the client, are reminiscent of Reeves, Inck, and Safran, who also coordinate their theoretical position with cognitive-behavioral and experiential technical interventions.

Although we usually think of integration as occurring across theories of personality or of psychotherapy, or across techniques, it also can occur between the more and the less traditional approaches to healing. Sollod explores the implications and value of spiritual healing techniques for contemporary psychic treatment. Psychotherapy as we know it has a history of less than a century. The need for attention to psychological concerns is as old as humankind. How were these problems addressed before the advent of psychotherapy, and do we need to discard all that had been learned previously in order to give credibility to what we are now discovering? Sollod examines the tradition of spiritual healing, primarily because it may have lessons to be incorporated in contemporary psychotherapy and secondarily because spiritual healing may extend the range of issues with which the therapist can deal.

The common factors in spiritual healing described by Sollod overlap only slightly with the common factors in psychotherapy described by Weinberger, perhaps suggesting a basis for the lack of contemporary mainstream acceptability of spiritual approaches. Nonetheless, many contemporary ideas have historical roots, and it only can help us to be aware of these roots (an idea that echoes psychodynamic approaches to treatment). There seems to be a continuum ranging from some easily accepted spiritual principles of healing, such as the importance of the conscious state of the therapist, to some less readily accepted approaches, such as transpersonal experiences. Each therapist can choose a point of comfort along the continuum, but it seems to be folly to dismiss the entire continuum because of discomfort with one extreme, thereby displaying no regard for the possibility of deriving value from a centuries-old tradition of healing.

In developing further the theme of integration of the psychotherapeutic with the spiritual, Healey describes the integration of one therapeutic orientation, psychoanalysis, with a system of values, Christian religious experience. Although Christianity, at an early stage, was an encompassing approach to psychological and spiritual life, it gradually became dissociated from the psychological, and it was openly condemned for its irrationality by many psychoanalytic writers. Healey finds the bridge between psychoanalysis and religion in relationships, as exemplified both by object relations theory and by the role of community in religious experience. Within this common area, psychology can be used to understand and value the role of religious experience, not to dismiss it reductionistically. In this framework, religion then becomes one among many appropriate and

necessary areas for exploration in psychotherapy. Finally, Healey raises the provocative but supportable question as to whether psychoanalysis itself can be considered to be a religion, for, with the exception of the presence of a transcendent being, it fulfills the definition of a religious system.

Rubin, in a chapter parallel to Healey's, seeks to integrate psychoanalysis with an eastern religion, Buddhism. Unlike Christianity, Buddhism is nontheistic, although it also is a spiritual system. Both psychoanalysis and Buddhism value enlightenment, use similar explanatory processes to reach that goal, and see their version of the self as central to their formulations. However, they diverge in important ways, both theoretical and technical, and the most important point of divergence may be their conception of the nature of the self. Rubin describes how these divergences can be viewed dialectically as stemming from valid but partial viewpoints, thereby underlining the value of integration. This is parallel to psychotherapy integration, in that therapeutic orientations also often combine valid but partial viewpoints. Unlike Healey, who approaches integration by calling for psychoanalysis to appreciate the reality and value of Christian religious experience, Rubin attempts a synergistic blending of psychoanalysis and Buddhism. Interestingly, Rubin emphasizes a theoretical blending and suggests that technical blending may be limited in its utility.

Curtis approaches the task of integration by combining two bodies of knowledge, that of social psychology and of clinical psychology, in order to arrive at an integrated social-clinical theory of psychotherapy. This theory revolves around the goals of the individual, which are actively formulated and pursued, generate affect, and may lead to conflict, both internally and externally. Similar to Andrews, the theory draws upon research and includes an active self, involved in pursuing goals and preserving stability, but the theory focuses on the production of awareness, seeing change occurring as a result of increasing awareness. Subjective constructions of meaning are crucial, and the vital role of the individual in a larger system is a clear heritage from social psychology.

The implications of social-clinical theory for psychotherapeutic technique still are in the process of being developed fully. However, many aspects of psychodynamic and gestalt approaches are clearly involved in the integration. A focus on the therapeutic relationship is recommended, but the therapist appears to be far more active than a traditional psychoanalytic therapist, although this therapeutic activity usually stops short of the directiveness that characterizes a more behaviorally oriented practitioner.

In discussing a therapeutic response to the anxiety disorders, Gold seeks integration at the theoretical level by using attachment experiences as the central etiological agent. This is compatible with psychoanalytic object relations formulations and also is consistent with the interpersonal schemata of cognitive theorists. Much as is the case with Ryle, psychotherapy begins with a very careful assessment phase, in order to establish a differential treatment plan. After the identification of the specific sources of anxiety, graded exposure is conducted, with techniques that include familiar cognitive-behavioral and psychodynamic interventions. This is followed by a stage of treatment that primarily is reconstructive, in a psychodynamic manner, but is supplemented by some cognitive interventions and an experiential framework.

Depression has generated a very large body of literature, and the review by Hayes and Newman makes it clear that it is a complex syndrome with important psychological and social factors involved in its etiology, development, and maintenance. As might be expected, the heterogeneity of the syndrome has led to a multiplicity of therapeutic interventions, each one of which has some evidence for its efficacy, and each one of which focuses on one narrow aspect of the complex syndrome. A comprehensive, integrated formulation is particularly appropriate in such a circumstance. Hayes and Newman, like Gold with regard to the treatment of anxiety, emphasize the importance of a thorough assessment as the foundation for the development of a treatment plan, and, like Ryle, share this formulation with the patient in a direct and explicit manner. This approach is reminiscent of Beutler's emphasis on prescriptive psychotherapy, and is consistent with a view of psychotherapy integration as a process rather than as an orientation. Further, perhaps more than any of the other authors in this *Handbook*, Hayes and Newman attend to the call of Arnkoff, Glass, and Victor for attention to the results of research, and build their techniques using the demonstrated results of research on the treatment of depression.

Gold and Stricker's approach to character pathology is rooted in a psychodynamic framework, but integrates cognitive and behavioral approaches as well. It is consistent with Andrews' approach, displaying an early development of an active self that shapes all experience that follows, and with cyclical psychodynamics, as described by Gold and Wachtel. However, it stands in contrast with Fensterheim, whose theory is of therapy rather than of personality, thereby leading Fensterheim to prefer more parsimonious initial interventions at a behavioral rather than at a dynamic level. Gold and Stricker begin with a theory of personality, which is psychodynamic in origin, and that theory leads to initial exploratory interventions supplemented, when needed, by behavioral and cognitive interventions.

Interestingly, Gold and Stricker describe a three-tier approach, with overt behavioral problems at the most basic tier, and with unconscious schemata at the deepest tier. This tiered conceptualization parallels Fensterheim's view, but Gold and Stricker choose to intervene at the deepest rather than at the most basic level. The focus of Gold and Stricker on character pathology, which is pervasive and resistant to change, may require this approach, whereas more circumscribed symptoms may be more responsive to Fensterheim's approach. The lack of a universal panacea is apparent.

The integration of the treatment of substance abuse, which refers both to alcohol and to drug abuse, requires taking account of medical and 12-step interventions as well as the traditional therapeutic approaches. Cummings's approach integrates the demonstrated success of the 12-step programs with psychodynamic, behavioral, and systems approaches. He outlines a prescriptive assessment schema based on the principle defense employed by the patient and the extent to which the patient is capable of using insight. Addicts are seen as benefitting from insight, hence the value of psychodynamic understanding, but this is at a later stage of the treatment, and must be preceded by a direct confrontation of the problematic behavior, as well as by addressing the medical component of the condition. The foundation role of the therapeutic alliance is recognized, as is the need, skillfully, to confront the problem, to puncture the denial, and to motivate abstinence. Group therapy is the central modality, supplemented by an occasional individual session, and with a substantial use of a 12-step program. Psychotherapy proceeds through some predictable stages, with the therapist assuming an active role guided by an understanding of the dynamics of the addict.

Problems of physical origin pose a particular challenge for therapists. Clearly, a response to the physical symptom is required, and equally clearly, attention to the patient who has the symptom is necessary. Becker discusses the treatment of patients with brain injuries and seeks to integrate, via a cyclic model, the directive approaches that are necessary for rehabilitation with the therapeutic approach, in this case psychodynamic, that is responsive to the personal needs of the patient. In this cyclic model, the directive and cognitive approaches can produce changes that enhance the patient's sense of psychological integrity and well-being, and the self-psychological psychodynamic approach can attenuate the patient's resistance to change and increase the patient's availability to the directive approaches. The attempt to achieve integration in the treatment of the patient necessitates integration in the initial assessment phase. Neuropsychological diagnosis is essential, as is personality diagnosis, and it is crucial to recognize the ways in which organic and psychological dysfunctions create reciprocal problems. For example, cognitive dysfunction will upset the patient's sense of integrity of the self, and an impaired self can exaggerate cognitive problems.

Similar to brain injury, chronic pain is a symptom that has both a physical and a psychological dimension. Thus, the same issues arise concerning the need to combine insight and action techniques, and to combine these with an appreciation of ongoing medical issues. Dworkin and Grzesiak present a stress-diathesis model of chronic pain, and this appreciation of the complex multicausality and consequences of chronic pain leads easily to the need for an integrated approach to the treatment of the patient suffering from that pain. This integrated approach, similar to Becker's approach to brain injury, combines directive, self-regulatory, and cognitive-behavioral techniques that promote change with psychodynamic techniques that promote understanding. Dworkin and Grzesiak also raise the very important issue of patient education. Patients who are not sophisticated about psychotherapy often benefit from an initial explanation of the process of therapy and the roles of the therapist and of the patient. This is particularly important with chronic pain patients, for they present with a physical symptom and often are at a loss as to the relevance of psychotherapy.

In many ways, the treatment of people with serious mental disorders presents problems similar to those encountered in the treatment of people with physical illness. In both cases, there is a need to integrate psychotherapy with techniques that attend directly to the symptoms of the patient, and a need to keep biological issues in mind as psychological approaches to treatment are attempted. Perhaps no area is more in need of integration, and has seen more polarized statements, than is the case with the treatment of people with serious mental disorders. Particularly when the value of medication is considered, proponents not only espouse their preferred approach but disdain integration and even may refer to alternatives as misguided instances of malpractice. In any case, Hellkamp deals with this impasse by describing rehabilitative psychotherapy, an approach that generally integrates rehabilitative techniques with psychotherapy, and further integrates a number of approaches toward psychotherapy. As with the physical illnesses as well as with a number of other integrative approaches, an assessment stage is critical prior to the initiation of psychotherapy, and the establishment of a sound therapeutic alliance is the basis of any successful treatment. Then, directive and educational techniques are integrated with more traditional psychotherapy techniques in order to assist the patient toward both behavior change and increased understanding.

Kirschner and Kirschner describe Comprehensive Family Therapy, their approach to working with couples and families, which necessarily reflects an appreciation of the complex system created by a family unit. Comprehensive Family Therapy integrates this systemic perspective with an understanding of the dynamics of each individual member of the system, based on an object relations approach to psychodynamics, similar to that favored by Ryle. The key aspects of family life are the relationship of the spouses to each other, their ability to rear their children, and the independent functioning of each member of the family. Not only do the first two systems components influence the third, individual component (which, in turn, has an impact on the two systems components), but the systems themselves reflect and influence the individuals who participate in them.

The integration that has been described on a theoretical level then is continued to a technical level. Family systems is not a monolithic approach to psychotherapy, and Kirschner and Kirschner integrate the interventions of a number of prominent family therapists. To this, they add some of the active techniques of the cognitive-behaviorists in order to promote growth. Psychodynamic and humanistic techniques are used to confront the resistance to growth that inevitably occurs. Integration of modalities also takes place, as individual sessions are intermingled with couple and family sessions. A recognition of the possible role of the child as symptom bearer for the family makes Comprehensive Family Therapy an approach that not only is useful for troubled couples and families, but also one that is applicable to dysfunctional children and adolescents.

The treatment of a child necessarily involves a variety of roles because the therapist must respond to the many needs of the child and also must intervene with the important people in the world of the child, as these people are responsible for the care of that child. Coonerty describes an integrative approach to child psychotherapy that is based on a single coherent model, in her case a psychodynamic model based on Wachtel's cyclical psychodynamic approach, and an ability to incorporate a wide variety of techniques drawn from cognitive-behavioral and systemic approaches as well as from psychodynamic play therapy. This integration of techniques within the umbrella of a single theory is a familiar approach to psychotherapy integration and one that is well suited to the multiple roles of the child therapist. The awareness of the reverberations of one intervention through other spheres of functioning is particularly noteworthy and illustrates the value of integrating techniques from outside the usual domain of a pure-form treatment.

Coonerty's discussion of the therapeutic issues and responses that arise in early and middle childhood lead naturally into the issues of, and responses to, adolescence, the subject of Fitz-Patrick's chapter. Here, too, there is the need to work with significant others in the life of the patient and to consider ongoing developmental issues as part of the problem formulation. Fitz-Patrick integrates behavioral and psychodynamic approaches in her work with adolescents, similar to the way in which Fensterheim accomplishes this integration with adults, and then goes beyond that approach by using family therapy in an alternating session format, thereby responding to the unique needs of the adolescent patient.

Papouchis and Passman describe an integrative approach to the treatment of the elderly. Their approach relies on an object relational theoretical orientation to understanding, but is technically integrative in its incorporation of cognitive-behavioral and systemic interventions along with their fundamental object relations approach. Further, there is an appreciation of the significance of physical and environmental factors in the elderly, so that any psychological treatment must be developed in a context defined by these other variables. Papouchis and Passman emphasize the need to recognize the heterogeneity of the elderly, and the need to tailor different therapeutic strategies to different people, but also point to the value of varying strategies during the work with any single patient. These variations in treatment are responsive to an understanding of the person based on a complex, integrated psychodynamic theoretical formulation and lead to a "case-specific" approach to psychotherapy.

It is of interest to note that the specific age groups described, the child, the adolescent, and the elderly, all have a number of issues in common. In each case, some of the therapeutic issues arise from outside the control of the patient and so it is important to appreciate and even to work with significant others in the life of the patient. With adults, some systemic therapists do this as a matter of course, as Kirschner and Kirschner describe, but it is more usual to work solely with the identified patient. An additional similarity across the age span is the need to take developmental issues into account as some apparent symptoms may be normative for the age group and therefore need not be addressed by treatment.

Group therapy is a format that is particularly ripe for integration because of the multiplicity of individual and interpersonal events that can occur with more than one person in the room. Wessler reviews the wide variety of approaches to group therapy and then makes the important point, applicable to individual as well as to group therapy, that integration does not mean that all therapists will converge and do the same thing. If they were to do so, the product would not be psychotherapy integration, a process drawn from many theories, techniques and modalities, but rather would be integrative psychotherapy, another pure-form approach to treatment that brooked no exceptions and allowed no creative integration in the service of a patient's individual needs and circumstances. Wessler then describes Cognitive Appraisal Therapy (CAT, but not the CAT, or Cognitive-Analytic Therapy, of Ryle), his approach to individual psychotherapy as it is adapted to the group therapy modality. This approach contains features of cognitive treatment, interpersonal and object relations approaches, self theory, and an emphasis on the role of affect as a source of information.

Franklin, Carter, and Grace discuss the treatment of the Black American, adopting a multisystems, racial identity model that would be useful in working with any patient who is a member of a racial or cultural subgroup, whether or not identity with that group is a central or an avoided aspect of the self-concept. Although the customs and values vary from group to group, everyone is a member of some racial or cultural subgroup, and so the issues raised in this chapter are of pervasive importance. It is essential to understand the customs and values of the patient as a prerequisite to establishing a therapeutic alliance and to working effectively in psychotherapy. Because no racial group is monolithic and its members differ in their stage of racial identity, it is vital that the therapist be attuned to this factor and prepared to be flexible in therapeutic techniques so that the techniques chosen are most suitable to the individual being treated.

There is a healthy debate concerning the issue as to whether training and supervision in psychotherapy integration should occur early or late in the career of the practitioner. Adherents of the former believe that the concepts and techniques of integration should be introduced at a foundation point, whereas those believing in the latter are concerned about the complexity and ambiguity of the task if it is introduced too early in training. Lecomte, Castonguay, Cyr, and Sabourin review many of the models of training in psychotherapy integration, recognizing the lack of

guidance provided by empirical data, and then present their own model of predoctoral training as it has been implemented at the Université de Montréal. The Montréal experience suggests the importance of a conceptual foundation, as students are prone to identity confusion without a framework for understanding and intervening in psychotherapy. The foundation chosen by Lecomte and his colleagues originated with Rogers but incorporated Kohut and Bandura, thereby having elements of humanistic, psychodynamic, and social-cognitive approaches, and therefore represents integration at the level of theory. The use of the self as the unifying concept is reminiscent of the contributions of Andrews and of Curtis.

There is a parallel process between supervision and therapy, and the supervisor teaching a particular approach to psychotherapy often will model, in the supervisory relationship, the stance of the therapist. For example, the supervision of Kohutian therapy often requires the supervisor to take on the function of a selfobject for the supervisee, with the expectation that the supervisor will then adopt the same function with the patient. If the supervisor is functioning within an integrative framework, the technique of the supervisor becomes enormously more complex, as is the task of the therapist.

Walder's view of training in psychotherapy integration is based on his experiences with the establishment of the Institute for Integrated Training in Psychotherapy, the first postdoctoral training institute designed specifically to provide instruction in psychotherapy integration. Some of his observations are particularly compelling. For example, the candidates at the institute could not integrate what they did not know, so that basic training in pure-form approaches necessarily would seem to precede training in psychotherapy integration, an observation that, contrary to the view of Lecomte, Castonguay, Cyr, and Sabourin, would postpone such training until the latter stages of graduate education at the earliest. Nonetheless, Walder chose a concurrent rather than a sequential curriculum model, preferring to capitalize on the interests and motivation of the candidates, and introducing the models of integration designed by Safran, by Fensterheim, and by Wachtel (each of whom is represented in this *Handbook*) along with the pure-form approaches at the earliest point in training. It is, of course, possible to teach any fully developed model to a capable student, and these were postgraduate candidates, but the encouragement of independent attempts at integration does seem to require some prior knowledge of that which is to be integrated.

Because the integration of psychotherapy requires thorough knowledge of more than one theory, or requires comfort and skill with more than one body of interventions, the demands on the practitioner are greater than those of a pure-form approach. It is not sufficient to be expert in a single approach, but there also must be the knowledge, flexibility, and skill needed to draw upon other approaches as necessary. It is possible that the patient may react to discordances in therapist activity, although all but the very sophisticated patient will assume that whatever the therapist is doing is what should be done, as long as the techniques are not presented in a remarkably disjunctive way. The therapist, however, often is aware of moving from approach to approach, unless therapy is conceptualized and conducted in a seamless way. The responses of the therapist to conducting therapy in an integrative fashion can be conceptualized as countertransference, can influence the choice of approach, and can lead to awkwardness and ineffectiveness. This series of issues is discussed by Halgin and McEntee. They point out that the absence of the strict rules that govern pure-form approaches, although providing room for flexibility and creativity, also provides room for personally determined choices that require the therapist to maintain careful awareness of personal motivation. Considering the complex technical and personal issues, the usual recommendations that a therapist seek regular consultation or supervision, as well as be intensely self-aware, seem even more warranted for therapy practiced in an integrative mode.

CONCLUSIONS

A pure-form approach to psychotherapy is constituted of a series of theory/technique units. It is possible for integration to occur at the level of theory, or at the level of technique, or at both levels. It is unlikely that theory can be integrated without some implications for technique, and interaction at the level of technique often will have implications that lead to the rethinking and possible integration of theory. The data of personal and of patient experience, both within and outside of therapy, also have implications for both the theory and the technique of psychotherapy. Directionality among the tiers of experience, technique, and theory is multiple and circular, as each one can influence the others. Finally, research data should play an increasing role in determining the viability of some of the relationships that are hypothesized to occur within and among the tiers.

If we are to view the patient in the complex manner that is suggested and we are to undertake treatment that incorporates attention to each of the tiers that have been described, the need for a comprehensive initial treatment plan becomes clear. Many of the approaches describe the need for a careful initial assessment, and it seems necessary even for those that do not address this point explicitly. Our theoretical understanding provides the basis for formulating the goals of treatment, the dynamics of the patient, and the relationship between those dynamics and the goals. This leads to a choice of techniques that best will accomplish the passage from the presenting problem to the desired outcome. An integration of theoretical perspectives will allow a more full view of the patient and an integration of techniques will provide more resources in accomplishing therapeutic objectives. Data from our experience with the patient and from the patient's experience in the world will allow for a feedback loop that can modify and correct the treatment plan in the course of the therapy.

A similarly tiered approach, with the tiers now consisting of what the patient does (behavior), what the patient thinks and feels about what is done (cognition and affect), and why the patient does it (motivation and understanding), may be a helpful method of conceptualizing treatment. Here, too, directionality is multiple and circular, each tier reverberates throughout the other tiers, and the optimal point of entrance into the system may vary with the circumstances of the individual case. The attainment of insight and the accomplishment of behavior change are mutually facilitative, there is little point to arguing about which comes first, and most of the approaches to integration that are described attend both to behavior change and to an understanding of the reasons for the behavior.

The approach to understanding that seems most consistent with psychotherapy integration is the variant of psychodynamic theory that embraces either an object relations or a self-psychological view, as these approaches recognize the relationship of the self to the environment. The approach to behavior change that seems most consistent with psychotherapy integration is some variation of cognitive-behavioral work. Further, there is a recognition that both understanding and behavior change can be facilitated by the use of techniques that heighten the affective involvement of the patient in the process of change.

There seems to be value to the notion of an active self involved with the environment, with the self occasionally perceiving the environment in a manner that is discrepant with a consensual view of that environment, thereby creating personal discomfort that is perpetuated by actions consistent with that discrepant view, as these lead to self-fulfilling prophecies. Self-awareness, in a reflexive sense, is vital to any process of change that deals with the active self, and this probably will be necessary for entree at any tier other than the strictly behavioral.

The contrast in some approaches between an inner and an outer locus of change seems resolved by the notion of interdependency, recognizing that the boundary between the inner and the outer is arbitrary and that the two are mutually influenced by each other. Again, the optimal point of entrance, be it with the environment or the self, will vary with the circumstances of the individual case. Another boundary issue that can be dismissed through an appreciation of coexistence and interdependency is that between the conscious and the unconscious. Conscious behaviors have unconscious roots, and unconscious dynamics have conscious manifestations. We may choose to work initially with either, although it is important to recognize the value of attending to the one that is deferred initially.

There is agreement, regardless of the approach chosen, that an integrative approach to psychotherapy requires a great deal more activity than is customary in traditional approaches. The therapist is far more active than in traditional psychodynamic psychotherapy, and the patient is recognized as being far more active than in traditional behavioral psychotherapy.

Some question can be raised as to the locus at which integration should occur. Some believe that integration should take place within the treatment, as a single therapist strives to use a variety of techniques, as appropriate, in order to pursue the goals of treatment. Others favor a prescriptive approach in which the treatment of a single patient is relatively pure form, but integration is espoused within the therapist, so that different patients will evoke different treatment approaches. It is not necessary to choose between the two, as a different set of integrated techniques can be used for different single patients, with this approach most applicable when there is some theoretical understanding that will suggest which combination of techniques to use with which patients, and why.

There are a number of areas where additional work needs to be done in order to develop a more fully rounded approach to psychotherapeutic integration. One of these is the need for a consensually accepted developmental framework. Although some of our authors outlined the developmental process by which the patient arrived at the point where treatment was initiated, this process seemed irrelevant to others. If we incorporate the tier requiring dynamic understanding, it will be necessary to understand the developmental process that produced the current presenting problem.

The role of the therapeutic relationship, too, is an area that is included by some, a focus of others, but ignored by many of the authors. To the extent that the relationship serves as a laboratory in which the patient can enact the problems that produced the need for treatment, attention to that relationship will facilitate the process of treatment. Both the attention to the relationship and the understanding of the developmental antecedents of the presenting problem are central to a psychodynamic approach, and so these features are most likely to be included by those authors who integrate psychodynamic thought, and to be omitted by those authors who are not so inclined. Regardless of the use of specific psychodynamic concepts, the need for developmental and relationship factors to be taken into account in some manner seems compelling.

Finally, the use of research seems minimized by many of the authors. There is little call for confirmation of declared truths through investigatory procedures, and little allowance for the modification of existing approaches by research evidence. The more the authors incorporate the knowledge base of psychology, which usually is reflected in a cognitive or behavioral approach, the more research is likely to be respected and used. With psychotherapy integration, regardless of the use of specific cognitive-behavioral concepts, the need for research findings to be taken into account seems compelling. It is tempting to conclude that, in general, behavioral therapists could learn from psychodynamic therapists to attend more carefully to the developmental antecedents of the presenting problem and to the therapeutic relationship, whereas psychodynamic therapists could learn from behavioral therapists to attend more carefully to the lessons of research.

It also must be noted that this *Handbook* is most deficient in its purposeful failure to incorporate pharmacological approaches. We sought to describe approaches to psychotherapy integration, not more broadly to behavior change or symptom amelioration. Despite that decision, all therapists must recognize that the use of medication often is relevant to a treatment plan, and that the therapeutic implications of the use of medication must be considered in order for the integration to be accomplished in a facilitative way.

There are three additional judgments that will conclude this chapter. The first is that psychotherapy integration is not easy. It requires a range of knowledge, skills, and attitudes beyond what is asked of a therapist functioning within any single approach. The task of the therapist is to overcome a Rashomon-like focus on any single limited and subjective focus, and to expand that focus to make room for the contributions of a number of orientations and approaches.

Not only must more than one approach (at least) be mastered, but the complications resulting from the relationships, implications, reverberations throughout the tiers, and contradictions among the various approaches must also be considered. It is no wonder that integration often is honored more in rhetoric than in performance.

Second, our concern is with psychotherapy integration, not integrative psychotherapy. The active search for an effective approach to intervention, resulting in a plethora of theoretical and technical integrations, seems more likely than the arrival at the single best integrative psychotherapy, which simply would be a more sophisticated pure form approach to treatment. In this line, it must be reiterated that psychotherapy integration is a process rather than an orientation, and therefore is an attitude that marks the approach of the therapist to the therapeutic situation. Parenthetically, the Society for the Exploration of Psychotherapy Integration (SEPI) captures this distinction in its carefully chose name, and the development and rapid growth of SEPI is testimony to the vitality of the interest in this phenomenon.

This leads naturally to the final point, that there is unlikely to be a single best solution to the problem of psychotherapy integration. Instead, there may be a need for a match of therapeutic approaches to patient problems, not in a prescriptive fashion, as all people cannot do all things, but in a triage fashion, with appropriate referrals being made to practitioners who are expert in the approach most suitable for the patient's presenting issues. In that way, the art and science of psychotherapy can be advanced and the mental health needs of the patient can be served in the most efficient and effective manner possible.

Index

Printed in the United Kingdom
by Lightning Source UK Ltd.
117916UK00005B/47